The LEARN® Program for Weight Control

Special Medication Edition

for Use with MERIDIA®

(sibutramine hydrochloride monohydrate) C-IV Capsules

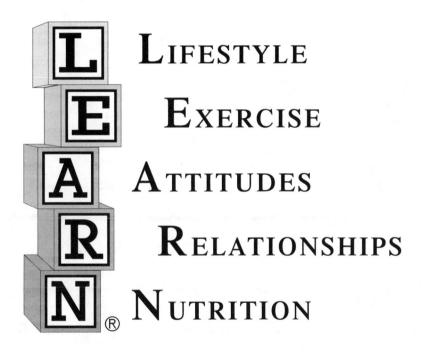

LIFESTYLE

EXERCISE

ATTITUDES

RELATIONSHIPS

NUTRITION

Kelly D. Brownell, Ph.D.
Yale University

Thomas A. Wadden, Ph.D.
University of Pennsylvania School of Medicine

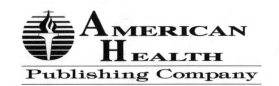

AMERICAN **H**EALTH Publishing Company

Permissions Department
American Health Publishing Company
P.O. Box 35328, Department 10
Dallas, Texas 75235–0328
Facsimile: 817–545–2211

Library of Congress
ISBN 1–878513–16–8

Address orders to:

The LEARN® Education Center	In Dallas (817) 545–4500
P.O. Box 35328, Department 70	Toll Free (800) 736–7323
Dallas, Texas 75235–0328	Facsimile (817) 545–2211
World Wide Web address	www.LearnEducation.com
E-mail address	Learn@LearnEducation.com

ACKNOWLEDGMENTS

We are grateful to several trusted colleagues and friends for providing comments and suggestions for this manual. Their help was invaluable. They are:

Dr. Steven N. Blair, Director of Epidemiology, The Cooper Institute for Aerobics Research, Dallas, Texas.

Dr. John P. Foreyt, Professor of Medicine and Director, Behavioral Medicine Research Center, Baylor College of Medicine, Houston, Texas.

Dr. G. Alan Marlatt, Professor of Psychology, University of Washington, Seattle, Washington.

Dr. Sachiko T. St. Jeor, Associate Professor and Director, Nutrition Education and Research Program, Department of Family and Community Medicine, University of Nevada School of Medicine, Reno, Nevada.

Permission to reprint cartoons was granted by the Cowles Syndicate, Inc., the Universal Press Syndicate, Chronicle Features, King Features, North American Syndicate, Newspaper Enterprise Association, Tribune Media Services, *The Washington Post*, United Features Syndicate, Inc., and James Estes.

Finally, we thank our students, colleagues, and especially our clients for providing the challenges and stimulation that encouraged us to undertake this writing.

LEARN® is a registered trademark of American Health Publishing Company.

MERIDIA® is a registered trademark of Knoll Pharmaceutical Company.

Table of Contents

Introduction and Orientation 1
   The Promise of Combining
   Medication and Lifestyle Change 1
   Our Welcome 1
   Medication and Lifestyle Modification: A Winning Combination 1
   MERIDIA and the New Era in Medications for Weight Control 3
   A Description of The LEARN Program 3
   The Schedule of LEARN Lessons 4
   A Revolution in Thinking about Weight Loss 5
   Your Goals and Expectations 5
   Weight Loss Readiness 6
   The Weight Loss Readiness Test Categories 7
   A Word of Caution 8
   Optimizing Your Success 9
   Your Quality of Life 10
   Helpful Resources 11

Lesson 1 17
   Understanding Your Weight Loss Medication 17
   Starting Medication 17
   Diet vs. Lifestyle Change 19
   Record Keeping 19
   The Food Diary 20
   Using the Calorie Guide 21
   The Weight Change Record 22
   Rating Your Diet 24
   A Note About Exercise and Relationships 24
   Your Self-Assessment 24
   Setting Personal Goals 24

Lesson 2 33
   Reviewing Your Diary 33
   Taking Your Medication 33
   Following a Balanced Diet 35
   The Food Guide Pyramid 36
   Selecting an Eating Plan: Calorie Counting vs. Exchange Plan 38
   On Being a Good Group Member 39
   Setting Personal Goals 39

Lesson 3 43
   Taking MERIDIA 43
   An Expanded Food Diary 43
   Small Changes in Your Diet 44
   The Mysterious Calorie 44

Not All People Are Created Equal. 45

Determining Your Target Calorie Level 46

The Role of Exercise in Weight Control 47

A New View of Exercise 47

The Benefits of Exercise 48

Setting Personal Goals. 49

Lesson 4 53

Analyzing Your Expanded Food Diary 53

Medication Diary. 54

How Often Should You Weigh Yourself? 54

On the Move 55

Is Exercise Safe for You?. 55

Barriers to Exercise 57

The 15-Minute Prescription 59

You Can Win a Presidential Sports Award 59

A Walking Partnership 60

Building Skills and Confidence 61

Setting Personal Goals. 61

Lesson 5 65

Quality of Life 65

Factors Affecting Your Weight Loss. 67

Compulsive Eating and Binge Eating. 68

Perfecting Your Walking Program 70

Benefits of Increasing Physical Activity 71

Setting Personal Goals. 72

Lesson 6 75

The ABC's of Behavior 75

Taking Control of Your Eating 76

Bracing Yourself Against a Toxic Environment 79

Checking on Your Physical Activity. 80

Servings from the Five Food Groups 81

Introducing a New Monitoring Form 81

Setting Personal Goals. 83

Lesson 7 87

Why Social Support Can Be So Important 87

Solo and Social Changing 88

Slowing Your Eating Rate 89

An Impressive Reason to Be Active 90

Continuing Walking and Lifestyle Activity 91

A Pulse Test for Positive Feedback 92

Setting Personal Goals. 94

Lesson 8 97

Reasons for Overweight 97

Weight Loss Medications and Causes of Overweight. 99

Why Losing Weight Is Difficult 100

Choosing a Support Person. 101

Communicating with Your Partner 101

Making Physical Activity Count 103

Setting Personal Goals 105

Lesson 9 107

A Two-Month Review 107

The Role of Fat in Your Diet 108

Planning Healthy Meals 113

Cravings vs. Hunger 114

Shaping the Right Attitudes 115

Setting Personal Goals 117

Lesson 10 121

Physical Activity and Good News 121

Great News about Activity 122

A New Activity Formula for Americans 123

The Mighty Calorie 125

The Calorie Values of Physical Activity 126

The Importance of Food 126

Nutrients Without Energy 128

Food and Weight Fantasies 130

Setting Personal Goals 130

Lesson 11 133

Thinking Your Way to Success 133

Attribution: Thinking about Your Medication 135

Shopping for Food 136

Revisiting the Food Guide Pyramid 138

Milk, Yogurt, and Cheese in Your Diet 138

Setting Personal Goals 140

Lesson 12 143

Internal Attitude Traps 143

Dichotomous (Light Bulb) Thinking 144

Storing Foods (out of Sight, out of Mouth) 146

The Importance of Protein 147

What Is Protein? 147

The Meat, Poultry, Fish, Eggs, and Nut Group 148

Setting Personal Goals 151

Lesson 13 153

Medication and Your Rate of Weight Loss 153

Meet Cindy 154

Impossible Dream Thinking 155

Serving and Dispensing Food 157

Carbohydrates and Your Diet 159

Vegetables in Your Diet 162

Reevaluating Your Quality of Life 163
Setting Personal Goals 164

Lesson 14 167
Selecting and Starting a Programmed Activity 167
Something for Your Partner to Read 172
Ways to Increase Fruit in Your Diet 174
Setting Personal Goals 177

Lesson 15 179
Follow-Up on Programmed Activity 179
More on Activity 179
Breads, Cereals, Rice, and Pasta in Your Diet 182
Breakfast Cereal: The Good, the Bad, the Sugar Coated 184
Setting Personal Goals 186

Lesson 16 189
Taking Stock of Your Progress 189
Your Body and Your Self-Esteem 194
More about Dietary Fat 197
High-Risk Situations—Triggers for Eating 198
A Note about Parties, Holidays, and Special Events 199
Continuing Your Medication 199
Transition from Weekly to Monthly Lessons 200
Setting Personal Goals 200

Lesson 17 203
For You and Your Family to Read 203
Dealing with Pressures to Eat 205
Another Attitude Trap: Imperatives 207
More about Water Soluble Vitamins 209
Reading Food Labels 211
A New Weight Change Record 213
Setting Personal Goals 213

Lesson 18 217
Quality of Life Assessment 217
Eating and Activity Habits 217
The Role of Medication 222
More Facts about Vitamins 223
Setting Personal Goals 225

Lesson 19 229
Let's Consider Jogging and Cycling 229
Facts, Fantasies, and Fiber 231
Warning: Alcohol and Calories 233
Stress and Eating 234
Setting Personal Goals 236

Lesson 20 239
    Eating Away from Home 239
    Are Aerobics for You? 244
    Pleasurable Partner Activities 245
    More about Fat Soluble Vitamins 245
    Setting Personal Goals 247

Lesson 21 251
    Bringing it All Together: The Behavior Chain 251
    Using the Stairs 257
    Poultry: Better than Red Meat? 258
    Fast Food 259
    A Review of Your Quality of Life 260
    Setting Personal Goals 261

Lesson 22 265
    Preventing Lapse, Relapse, and Collapse 265
    Identifying Urges and High-Risk Situations 267
    Making a List, Checking it Twice 270
    Hard Work at the Office 270
    Setting Personal Goals 271

Lesson 23 275
    Coping with Lapse and Preventing Relapse 275
    Becoming a Forest Ranger 277
    Life on Chutes and Ladders 278
    Cholesterol 280
    Setting Personal Goals 280

Lesson 24 285
    The Master Monitoring Form 285
    Using the Master List of Techniques (Appendix A) 286
    Holidays, Parties, and Special Events 287
    The National Walking Movement 288
    More on Minerals 290
    A Note about Breakfast 293
    Setting Personal Goals 294

Commencement Lesson 297
    Interpreting Your Progress 297
    Remember Reasonable Weight? 299
    Making Your Habits Permanent 300
    Examining Your Master Monitoring Form 300
    Doing a Master Self-Assessment 301
    A Special Guide for Weight Maintenance 301
    Where to Go from Here 301
    Looking at Your Quality of Life 303
    Our Salute to You! 304
    Ending Where We Began 305

A Final Weight Change Record 305
Saying Farewell. 305
Appendix A. 309
Lifestyle Techniques 309
Exercise Techniques 309
Attitude Techniques 309
Relationship Techniques 310
Nutrition Techniques. 310
Appendix B 311
Appendix C 317
Appendix D 323
Guidelines for Being a Good Group Member 323
Importance of the Group 323
Guidelines and Responsibilities 324
In Summary. 327
Appendix E. 329
Appendix F. 335
Ordering Information 347
The LEARN Education Center. 347
The LEARN Institute for LifeStyle Management. 347
The American Association of LifeStyle Counselors 348
Other Materials 348
About the Authors *349*

Introduction and Orientation

The Promise of Combining Medication and Lifestyle Change

We hope you are as excited as we are about the innovative program you are about to begin. It wraps into a single package the best the field has to offer on lifestyle change with information on optimizing the potential of medication.

Breakthroughs in science have provided you this opportunity to take a medication that helps with long-term weight management. The medication, however, is only part of the picture. The lifestyle changes you make will be the key to permanent results.

You might wonder whether you can make changes when you may have tried before. Sure you can—you are motivated, and you now have the help of medication. Most of all, you are starting a state-of-the-art program, and you now have us on your team.

Our Welcome

We have put together a program that we hope will make you feel welcome, will be easy to follow, and will work. There will be times you will laugh and other times you will struggle, but with the right information and right effort, you'll be surprised by what you can accomplish.

Medication and Lifestyle Modification: A Winning Combination

We believe that MERIDIA and The LEARN Program are helpful as separate actors, but when put together, an exciting picture emerges. It is our belief that when medication and a lifestyle change program are combined, a person has the greatest chances for success.

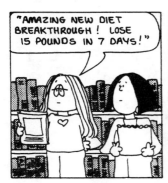  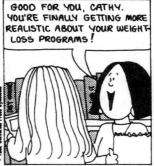 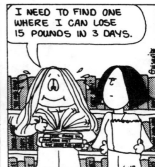

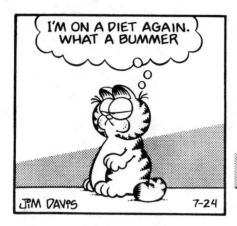
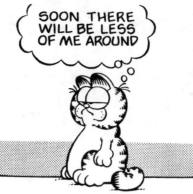
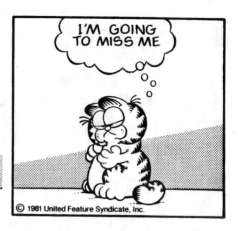

The beauty of a combined program is clear from the results of a classic study by researchers at the University of Pennsylvania. People in one group were given a weight loss medication (not MERIDIA) and attended 26 weekly meetings in which they discussed ways of adopting a healthier diet and a more active lifestyle. Those in a second group were given the identical medication but received no lifestyle counseling. Those in the first group lost 34 pounds compared with only 13 pounds for those using medication alone.

Medication and lifestyle modification go hand-in-hand. For instance, you will probably feel less hungry when you take MERIDIA, which can decrease snacking between meals. The medication can help you lose weight, but you must also control your appetite with lifestyle changes such as carefully selecting the foods you buy, planning what to eat when you go out to dinner, and not giving up when you make small mistakes. The LEARN Program helps you develop strategies like these.

To make lifestyle changes, do you need to see a professional weight loss counselor? Not necessarily. Can you do this on your own with the help of LEARN? Very likely. Consider a recent study of ours. People in one group were prescribed a weight loss medication for one year and were asked to attend 32 lifestyle modification classes (of 75 minutes each) at which they discussed topics covered in The LEARN Program. They were also seen briefly on ten occasions by a doctor who checked their health. People in a second group were prescribed the same medication and were given a copy of The LEARN Program, but they did not attend group treatment sessions. Instead, they discussed topics from The LEARN Program during ten brief visits with their doctor. At the end of the year, patients in both groups had lost about 30 pounds. Those who used The LEARN Program on their own did just as well as those who attended all of those group meetings. These results contributed to the development of this edition of The LEARN Program by combining the use of weight loss medications with lifestyle change.

We would like to emphasize that this book is not intended to give medical advice. We discuss side effects and the schedule you use to take your medication, but do so to help support the medical input you receive from your doctor. Your doctor is the best source of information on the medication and on individual issues in general.

MERIDIA and the New Era in Medications for Weight Control

MERIDIA has been approved by the Food and Drug Administration for the management of weight problems, including "weight loss and maintenance of weight loss," in conjunction with a reduced-calorie diet. Many experts in the field now believe that weight problems are chronic and require long-term help, much the same as high blood pressure and diabetes.

MERIDIA can help you lose weight, but may be most helpful in keeping it off. Two separate year-long studies showed that people who received MERIDIA achieved their maximum weight loss in about the first six months. They remained on medication for an additional six months and maintained statistically significant weight loss. This excellent maintenance contrasts sharply with the usual results of most diet programs, in which people start gaining weight almost as soon as they finish.

This program combines the tested techniques of The LEARN Program, now more than 20 years in the making and in its seventh edition, with the benefits you can receive from MERIDIA. This combination, together with your motivation and energy, can be a real winner.

A Description of The LEARN Program

We named this program LEARN for two reasons. The first is that learning implies an educational process in which the learner must master crucial informa-

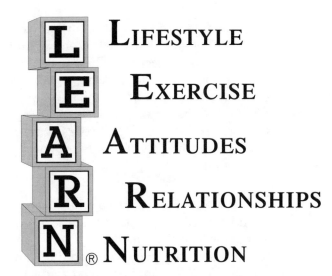

LIFESTYLE

EXERCISE

ATTITUDES

RELATIONSHIPS

N® **N**UTRITION

tion and apply it in everyday life. The second reason is that the word LEARN is an acronym created from the first letter of the five essential components of the program: **L**ifestyle, **E**xercise, **A**ttitudes, **R**elationships, and **N**utrition.

This special version of The LEARN Program contains 24 lessons designed to provide you a one-year program. If you follow the typical program, you will read a lesson each week for the first four months and then a lesson each month for the last eight months. The five components of the program—Lifestyle, Exercise, Attitudes, Relationships, and Nutrition—will be covered throughout the 24 lessons.

Each lesson has a Self-Assessment Questionnaire and an assignment for setting personal goals. The Self-Assessment Questionnaire is for *you* to decide whether you have acquired the important information in each lesson. It will highlight the key points and will alert you to areas that need more detailed work. The assignments on setting personal goals ask you to experiment with different approaches, so you can learn what works best for you and remind yourself about the progress you are making.

You will become a student of your habits. You will learn when, how, and why your habits occur and how to change them. You will practice your new techniques so they will become part of your lifestyle. This is what separates the approach of The LEARN Program from most programs—the focus is on permanent results.

We should mention two other aspects of the program. First, there are no assigned or forbidden foods. We resist the idea of dictating what you can and cannot eat. You will not be asked to rid your life of apple pie or faint with envy when your friends dip into the Haagen-Dazs. Likewise, you will not be running to the fruit stand for papaya and mangoes so you can abide by a senseless series of magical foods. The program is structured around your lifestyle, not vice-versa.

The second factor is that you can individualize the program to your unique circumstances. The focus is on learning new habits, whatever the necessary habits are for you. You can weave the principles and techniques of the program into the fabric of *your* life.

The Schedule of LEARN Lessons

As we mentioned, The LEARN Program is designed to cover an entire year. Lessons 1–16 are written as weekly lessons. The aim is for you to read one lesson each week and to work on the material in that lesson before proceeding to the next. The first 16 lessons, therefore, cover a four-month period. During this time we will introduce you to dozens of ideas for changing your eating, physical activity, and attitudes. You will discover the ones that work best for you. In the later stages of the program you will refine, fine-tune, and practice these changes so they become permanent.

After the initial four months, we provide monthly lessons to cover weeks 20 through 52 of the program. The focus at this point becomes even stronger on practicing the new behaviors you have learned so they become automatic and routine. Our commitment is to work with you as long as it takes, knowing that lifestyle change does not occur overnight. We'll be together for a year or more, so let's work together to make the best team possible!

The LEARN Program Schedule
A 12-month Program

Lessons 1–16 (one lesson each week)

Lessons 17–24 (one lesson each month)

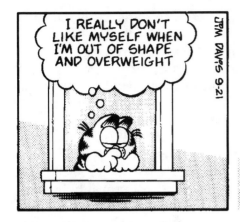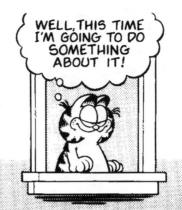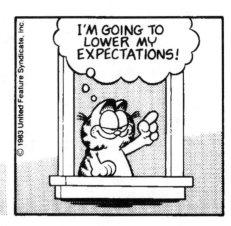

A Revolution in Thinking about Weight Loss

Most of us have had years of worrying about "ideal weight." Height-weight tables are everywhere, and in many programs, people are given a goal weight based on the ideals from the tables. The message is that you must lose to a magic level to benefit from weight loss. Far from being "ideal," these weight tables are a source of enormous frustration given their unrealistic view that "one size fits all." Say goodbye to this thinking.

A large collection of scientific evidence now converges on an important conclusion—that even modest weight losses can have important health benefits. High blood pressure, diabetes, elevated cholesterol, sleep disturbances, and a variety of other medical problems are often improved, if not controlled, by modest weight loss. This changes everything.

Two prominent scientific groups recently recommended that people initially try to lose as little as 5 percent to 10 percent of their starting weight. A woman, for example, who weighs 200 pounds would set an initial goal of losing 10 to 20 pounds. Her top priority would be to maintain this initial loss. Once this was

certain, she could decide whether to lose more weight. She might still lose more, but if not, would feel good in knowing that the modest loss she did accomplish was worthwhile.

The new weight loss goals are designed to help people achieve a healthier weight, and to push aside the notion of ideal weight. Virtually everyone can achieve a healthier weight, at which they feel better, have more energy, and reduce their risk of health complications.

Your Goals and Expectations

This program can help you achieve a "healthier" weight. People who follow the program lose an average of about 10 percent of their starting weight during the first six months. Some lose more, others less. By the way, you are more likely to achieve your best results by reading this manual faithfully and completing the assignments in each lesson. A recent study showed that the more assignments people completed, the larger their weight losses.

You will be most satisfied with your results if you set clear and realistic goals that you have a good chance of attaining. We will speak often in this program about realistic goals, appropriate expectations, and what we have written about extensively, "reasonable weight."

Take a minute now and think about what a 10 percent weight loss would be for you. This is a good starting goal. Whether or not you lose more, the 10 percent loss will be an important achievement.

A 10 percent weight loss for me will be ___21___ pounds

Weight Loss Readiness

Losing weight requires time and effort. MERIDIA can help you lose weight, but the key results will come from your own efforts. It is important to ask yourself if you are ready.

Think ahead to the next few months. Does it look like "all's calm on the horizon" or "a storm's brewing?" Concentrating on weight control can be difficult when you're experiencing major upsets at home or work, when a parent or loved one is seriously ill, or when you have serious financial problems. If you know that such events will be time limited—meaning they will end in the near future—then you will probably be more successful if you wait until these stressors pass. Your goal, until that time, is to prevent weight gain rather than trying to lose weight.

Weight loss readiness also involves whether you feel ready to lose weight. Do you feel motivated and optimistic? Do you believe that you have the skills required to develop healthy eating and activity habits? We hope that you do and encourage you to talk with your doctor or family members if you do not feel

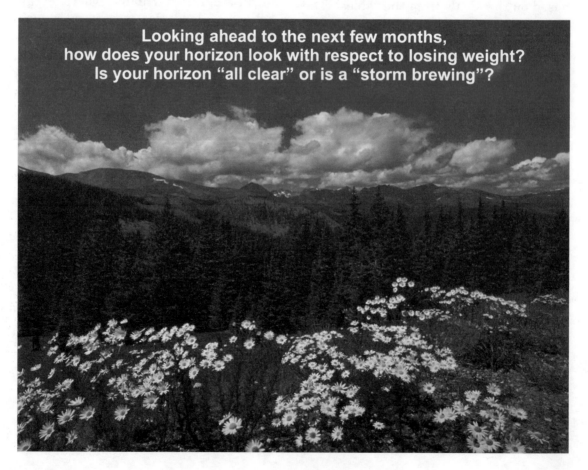

Looking ahead to the next few months, how does your horizon look with respect to losing weight? Is your horizon "all clear" or is a "storm brewing"?

motivated right now. It may be better to wait until your motivation increases, rather than to start on an empty tank.

You can check your readiness by taking The weight loss Readiness Test at the end of this lesson (see page 13). The test has 23 items divided into six sections, with a scoring key at the end of each section. The sections deal with goals and attitudes, hunger and eating cues, control over eating, binge eating and purging, emotional eating, and exercise patterns and attitudes.

It is important that you understand what this test is and what it is not. The test was developed to pinpoint the areas you should consider when assessing your weight loss readiness. The categories and the specific questions were derived from clinical experience and from research on predictors of weight loss. The test is still in its early stages of development, so only limited information on its scientific utility is available.

The test should not be used, therefore, to make specific decisions on starting a program. This is why we do not use the test to provide a single summary score for readiness. It can be used to help you think through the readiness concept and to decide how the concept applies to you. You are in the best position to make a judgment on readiness.

The Weight Loss Readiness Test Categories

The questions in The Weight Loss Readiness Test are grouped into six categories. The discussion that follows covers the rationale for each of the six sections.

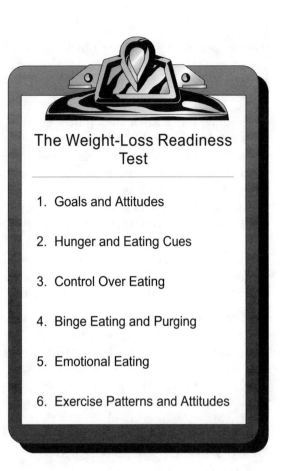

The Weight-Loss Readiness Test

1. Goals and Attitudes

2. Hunger and Eating Cues

3. Control Over Eating

4. Binge Eating and Purging

5. Emotional Eating

6. Exercise Patterns and Attitudes

Section 1: Goals and Attitudes

The questions in this section are designed to help you evaluate how motivated you are, how long you anticipate the motivation will last (commitment), and whether you can envision a weight loss program being woven into your lifestyle. In addition, it deals with setting realistic goals. This is relevant because many people have unrealistic expectations about how quickly they will lose weight and how easy the process will be. When the fantasies fail to become reality, you may feel discouraged and may be more likely to relapse.

Section 2: Hunger and Eating Cues

It is common lore that overweight people eat not in response to physical hunger, but instead out of habit, in response to some psychological need, or simply because food is available. This may or may not be true. It is also possible that overweight people experience physical hunger more often, perhaps because they are driven by internal pressures.

Science has shown that many people, regardless of weight, are responsive to external cues to eat. Seeing a dessert cart after a meal, driving past a bakery, or realizing that it is a regular snack time can make many people want to eat. This section of the test is designed to help you recognize how responsive you are to cues to eat.

Section 3: Control Over Eating

People vary in how much control they feel they have over eating. Some people exert strict control, while others can be thrown off course by seemingly trivial events. The questions in this section deal with whether external pressures to eat threaten your control.

Section 4: Binge Eating and Purging

Binge eating is a common problem in overweight persons. Research on this topic is relatively new, but what we know suggests that weight loss may be especially difficult when binge eating. Purging, which involves the use of vomiting, laxatives, or diuretics to rid the body of weight, is less common, but is a serious matter. Individuals who indicate frequent binge eating and purging should be evaluated by an eating disorders specialist to determine whether additional help is necessary.

Section 5: Emotional Eating

Emotional upheaval can weaken dietary restraint which, in turn, sets the stage for overeating. This can occur when people are depressed, anxious, angry, or lonely. In some cases, feeling good or relieved about some aspect of life can lead to overeating. This section of the test is designed to help you identify whether eating occurs in response to emotional changes.

Section 6: Exercise Patterns and Attitudes

As discussed elsewhere in this book, exercise is one of the key components to a comprehensive weight loss program. People who exercise are most likely to keep off lost weight. This section contains questions about readiness to exercise. Your prediction on the likelihood of regular exercise should be discussed because of its central role in weight control.

A Word of Caution

We want to underscore that the readiness test should not be used as the only basis for deciding whether to begin a program. You should use it to ask yourself questions about readiness, not to make a final decision. As much information as possible should be gathered so that you can think through issues, such as motivation, commitment, and life circumstances. Then you decide whether the time is right based on your feelings, attitudes, and behaviors.

Please note also that overall readiness may be a less helpful notion than thinking of readiness in different areas. For instance, most people enter a weight loss program expecting to change their diet, so the majority would be in a high state of nutrition readiness. People vary more widely in their readiness to be physically active.

Low scores in one area may be a signal to take action to improve readiness in that specific area. A low physical-activity score might be a tip-off to think about obstacles to exercise, either physical or emotional, and then to devise ways to remove the obstacles. We will discuss such obstacles in an upcoming lesson. Remember that readiness can change, if you take the right steps.

Having you assess your readiness is an important process. Even people who are not highly motivated may do an honest self-assessment and then find ways to motivate themselves. Low readiness is not necessarily permanent. It is a snapshot in time to show whether the conditions are right at this moment. Because you may not be ready at this point does not mean that you will not be ready later.

Optimizing Your Success

You may have already started taking MERIDIA and passed The weight loss Readiness Test with flying colors. You are more than eager to lose weight. Let's review a few final points that will help ensure that you get your best possible results.

Friends and Family

It can be very helpful to talk with family members and close friends about your weight control plans. Take a minute to explain the program and to answer any questions they may have. Loved ones may worry that you are taking a weight loss medication. You can reassure them with information in this book and information you receive from your physician or pharmacist.

You may also want to tell friends and family members how they can support your weight control efforts. As we discuss in future lessons, little things such as inviting you to go on a walk, or not offering you snack foods, can make a big difference. Express your appreciation when loved ones support you.

Ultimately, you know your family and friends best. If you think that talking about your weight control efforts is going to cause problems, we trust your judgment. Such discussions are a help rather

My Additional Resources

Family

Friends

Doctor

Other Support

than a hindrance in most cases, but as with all we discuss, you will know best what is effective for you.

Your Doctor

Your doctor has prescribed MERIDIA for you and obviously wants to support your weight loss efforts. In addition to monitoring your health your doctor can help in the following ways:

❶ Ask your doctor to specify the approximate schedule of visits for the first six months so you will know what support to expect. We anticipate that your doctor will want to see you after your first month on MERIDIA, to review your weight loss, and to ask whether you have any side-effects. You should call your doctor before this time if you become ill, whether or not you think it is related to the medication. After the one-month visit, your doctor may see you less frequently—once every other month or even less.

The two of you together should map out the schedule of visits.

❷ At each visit, plan to tell your doctor about the lifestyle changes you are working on in The LEARN Program and identify the lessons that you plan to complete before the next visit. You may not have a lot of time to review your accomplishments, but the discussion can be informative for both of you.

❸ Ask if you can stop by the doctor's office for a non-medical visit, just to get weighed. Many people find that such visits, as brief as one minute, keep them motivated. A smile from the office manager or your favorite nurse may give you an added boost.

Other Support

Some people enjoy the support of a weight loss group, while others like to "fly solo." If you know from experience that you enjoy attending group meetings, because of the social support or valuable information provided, feel free to do so. If such meetings aren't for you, don't attend them. As we mentioned, people who took weight loss medication and read The LEARN Manual on their own (with the support of their doctor) lost just as much weight as those who took medication and attended weekly lifestyle modification classes.

We encourage you to seek additional support—preferably from a professional—if you feel that you are having a particularly difficult time with your mood, your eating, or some personal issues. If such events are significantly disrupting your work or your enjoyment of life, talk with your doctor about places you can get help. Dealing with these problems directly will give you more energy for weight control.

Enlist the help and support of others

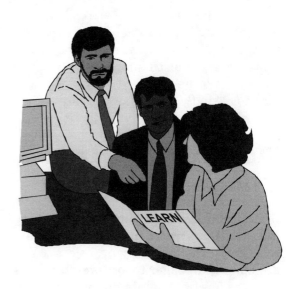

Your Quality of Life

People begin a weight loss program because of the benefits they hope will occur with weighing less. Looking better, feeling better, having more energy, and having more self-confidence are examples of what we call "quality-of-life" issues. These and other factors shape how you feel every day.

As you progress through this program, you will have a natural tendency to focus on the scale. This can be a problem when the scale shows no change, even when you might be making positive strides. Keeping your eye on the many changes that might occur in this program can be helpful. This helps you appreciate the positive effects of your hard work, shows just how many areas of your life can be affected by better eating and physical activity, and gives you more than one means of evaluating your progress.

Quality of Life Self-Assessment

Please use the following scale to rate how satisfied you feel now about different aspects of your daily life. Choose any number from this list (1 to 9) and indicate your choice on the questions below

1 = Extremely Dissatisfied   6 = Somewhat Satisfied

2 = Very Dissatisfied   7 = Moderately Satisfied

3 = Moderately Dissatisfied   8 = Very Satisfied

4 = Somewhat Dissatisfied   9 = Extremely Satisfied

5 = Neutral

1. _3_ Mood (feelings of sadness, worry, happiness, etc.)
2. _6_ Self-esteem
3. _7_ Confidence, self-assurance and comfort in social situations
4. _4_ Energy and feeling healthy
5. _7_ Health problems (diabetes, high blood pressure, etc.)
6. _7_ General appearance
7. _6_ Social life
8. _6_ Leisure and recreational activities
9. _6_ Physical mobility and physical activity
10. _6_ Eating habits
11. _6_ Body image
12. _7_ Overall quality of life

Please complete the Quality of Life Self-Assessment provided above to get a feeling about various aspects of daily life. We will ask you to complete this assessment several times later in the program, to see if the scores have changed.

Helpful Resources

Additional materials have been developed which may be helpful to you while working through this program. *The LEARN Program Cassettes* contain four cassette tapes where one of us (Dr. Brownell) discusses the essential elements of The LEARN Program, lesson by lesson. These tapes were developed to help individuals acquire and apply the skills necessary for long-term weight control. *The LEARN Program Monitoring Forms* were developed at the request of many people who had completed The LEARN Program. Although we provide you with daily monitoring forms throughout this manual that you may copy, some individuals find it more convenient to have a pocket-sized form that contains a week's supply of food monitoring.

Looking ahead, we want to alert you to *The Weight Maintenance and Stabilization Guide*, an in-depth companion and follow-up to The LEARN Program. After losing weight, a looming issue is how to make the changes permanent over time. There is a great deal of information on this in The LEARN Program, but more help is available for the long-term process of losing more weight, maintaining the loss, and stabilizing how you feel, how you think, and how you act in order to make your changes permanent.

The Weight Control Digest was developed as a newsletter for both professionals and nonprofessionals to keep abreast of the latest developments in the field as well as keep up-to-date on the latest methods and techniques that help individuals maintain their weight. A complimentary copy of *The Weight Control Digest*, along with information on other materials, can be obtained by calling or writing to the address shown below.

The LEARN Education Center

P.O. Box 35328, Department 70

Dallas, Texas 75235–0328

Telephone   817–545–4500

Toll Free: 800–736–7323

Fax: 817–545–2211

E-mail: Learn@LearnEducation.com

Internet: www.LearnEducation.com

Another helpful resource is the Point of Change^{SM} weight-management program offered by Knoll Pharmaceutical, makers of MERIDIA. You may enroll at no cost. After completing a simple questionnaire, you will receive regular mailings with state-of-the-art information tailored to your individual needs. Receiving this information while you are following The LEARN Program can be quite helpful. You may enroll by calling 1–888–566–5502 or by visiting the www.healthyweight.com web site.

Congratulations on your decision to take control of your weight and health. You can be proud for making an important decision.

If you have seen your doctor, filled your prescription for MERIDIA, and completed this lesson, you are ready to begin. You can read Lesson 1 at any point.

We wish you every success and look forward to working with you. So, without further delay, let's move on!

Good Luck!

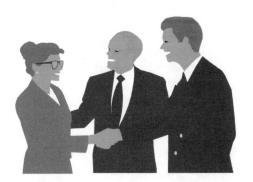

The Weight Loss Readiness Test

Answer the questions below to see how well your attitudes equip you for a weight loss program. For each question, circle the answer that best describes your attitude, then write the number of your answer on the line before each question number. As you complete each of the six sections, add the numbers of your answers and compare them with the scoring guide at the end of each section.

Section 1: Goals and Attitudes

_5_ 1. Compared to previous attempts, how motivated are you to lose weight at this time?

    1 Not at all motivated

    2 Slightly motivated

    3 Somewhat motivated

    4 Quite motivated

    5 Extremely motivated

_4_ 2. How certain are you that you will stay committed to a weight loss program for the time it will take to reach your goal?

    1 Not at all certain

    2 Slightly certain

    3 Somewhat certain

    4 Quite certain

    5 Extremely certain

_4_ 3. Consider all outside factors at this time in your life (the stress you're feeling at work, your family obligations, etc.). To what extent can you tolerate the effort required to stick to a program?

    1 Cannot tolerate

    2 Can tolerate

    3 Uncertain

    4 Can tolerate well

    5 Can tolerate easily

_4_ 4. Think honestly about how much weight you hope to lose and how quickly you hope to lose it. Figuring a weight loss of one to two pounds per week, how realistic is your expectation?

    1 Very unrealistic

    2 Somewhat unrealistic

    3 Moderately unrealistic

    4 Somewhat realistic

    5 Very realistic

_4_ 5. While losing weight, do you fantasize about eating a lot of your favorite foods?

    1 Always

    2 Frequently

    3 Occasionally

    4 Rarely

    5 Never

_4_ 6. While losing weight, do you feel deprived, angry and/or upset?

    1 Always

    2 Frequently

    3 Occasionally

    4 Rarely

    5 Never

_25_ **Section 1—TOTAL Score**

If you scored:

6 to 16: This may not be a good time for you to start a weight loss program. Inadequate motivation and commitment, together with unrealistic goals could block your progress. Think about those things that contribute to this, and consider changing them before undertaking a program.

17 to 23: You may be close to being ready to begin a program but should think about ways to boost your readiness before you begin.

24 to 30: The path is clear with respect to goals and attitudes.

Section 2: Hunger and Eating Cues

_2_ 7. When food comes up in conversation or in something you read, do you want to eat even if you are not hungry?

    1 Never

    2 Rarely

    3 Occasionally

    4 Frequently

    5 Always

_4_ 8. How often do you eat because of **physical hunger**?

    1 Always

    2 Frequently

    3 Occasionally

    4 Rarely

    5 Never

_4_ 9. Do you have trouble controlling your eating when your favorite foods are around the house?

    1   Never

    2   Rarely

    3   Occasionally

    4   Frequently

    5   Always

_10_ **Section 2—TOTAL Score**

If you scored:

3 to 6: You might occasionally eat more than you would like, but it does not appear to be a result of high responsiveness to external cues. Controlling the attitudes that make you eat may be especially helpful.

7 to 9: You may have a moderate tendency to eat just because food is available. Weight loss may be easier for you if you try to resist external cues, and eat only when you are physically hungry.

10 to 15: Some or most of your eating may be in response to thinking about food or exposing yourself to temptations to eat. Think of ways to minimize your exposure to temptations, so that you eat only in response to physical hunger.

Section 3: Control Over Eating

If the following situations occurred while you were on a weight loss program, would you be likely to eat **more** or **less** immediately afterward and for the rest of the day?

_3_ 10. Although you planned on skipping lunch, a friend talks you into going out for a meal.

    1   Would eat much less

    2   Would eat somewhat less

    3   Would make no difference

    4   Would eat somewhat more

    5   Would eat much more

_3_ 11. You "break" your diet by eating a fattening, "forbidden" food.

    1   Would eat much less

    2   Would eat somewhat less

    3   Would make no difference

    4   Would eat somewhat more

    5   Would eat much more

_3_ 12. You have been following your diet faithfully and decide to test yourself by eating something you consider a treat.

    1   Would eat much less

    2   Would eat somewhat less

    3   Would make no difference

    4   Would eat somewhat more

    5   Would eat much more

_9_ **Section 3—TOTAL Score**

If you scored:

3 to 7: You recover rapidly from mistakes. However, if you frequently alternate between eating out of control and dieting very strictly, you may have a serious eating problem and should get professional help.

8 to 11: You do not seem to let unplanned eating disrupt your program. This is a flexible, balanced approach.

12 to 15: You may be prone to overeat after an event breaks your control or throws you off the track. Your reaction to these eating events can be improved.

Section 4: Binge Eating and Purging

_2_ 13. Aside from holiday feasts, have you ever eaten a large amount of food rapidly and felt afterward that this eating incident was excessive and out of control?

    2   Yes

    0   No

_1_ 14. If you answered yes to question 13 above, how often have you engaged in this behavior during the last year?

    1   Less than once a month

    2   About once a month

    3   A few times a month

    4   About once a week

    5   About three times a week

    6   Daily

_0_ 15. Have you ever purged (used laxatives, diuretics, or induced vomiting) to control your weight?

    5   Yes

    0   No

_6_ 16. If you answered yes to question 15 above, how often have you engaged in this behavior during the last year?

    1 Less than once a month

    2 About once a month

    3 A few times a month

    4 About once a week

    5 About three times a week

    6 Daily

_3_ **Section 4—TOTAL Score**

If you scored:

0 to 1: It appears that binge eating and purging is not a problem for you.

2 to 11: Pay attention to these eating patterns. Should they arise more frequently, get professional help.

12 to 19: You show signs of having a potentially serious eating problem. See a counselor experienced in evaluating eating disorders right away.

Section 5: Emotional Eating

_4_ 17. Do you eat more than you would like to when you have negative feelings, such as anxiety, depression, anger, or loneliness?

    1 Never

    2 Rarely

    3 Occasionally

    4 Frequently

    5 Always

_2_ 18. Do you have trouble controlling your eating when you have positive feelings—do you celebrate feeling good by eating?

    1 Never

    2 Rarely

    3 Occasionally

    4 Frequently

    5 Always

_3_ 19. When you have unpleasant interactions with others in your life, or after a difficult day at work, do you eat more than you would like?

    1 Never

    2 Rarely

    3 Occasionally

    4 Frequently

    5 Always

_9_ **Section 5—TOTAL Score**

If you scored:

3 to 8: You do not appear to let your emotions affect your eating.

9 to 11: You sometimes eat in response to emotional highs and lows. Monitor this behavior to learn when and why it occurs, and be prepared to find alternative activities.

12 to 15: Emotional ups and downs can stimulate your eating. Try to deal with the feelings that trigger the eating, and find other ways to express them.

Section 6: Exercise Patterns and Attitudes

_4_ 20. How often do you exercise?

    1 Never

    2 Rarely

    3 Occasionally

    4 Frequently

    5 Always

_5_ 21. How confident are you that you can exercise regularly?

    1 Not at all confident

    2 Slightly confident

    3 Somewhat confident

    4 Quite confident

    5 Extremely confident

_4_ 22. When you think about exercise, do you develop a positive or negative picture in your mind?

    1 Completely negative

    2 Somewhat negative

    3 Neutral

    4 Somewhat positive

    5 Completely positive

_5_ 23. How certain are you that you can work regular exercise into your daily schedule?

    1 Not at all certain

    2 Slightly certain

    3 Somewhat certain

    4 Quite certain

    5 Extremely certain

_18_ **Section 6—TOTAL Score**

If you scored:

4 to 10: You are probably not exercising as regularly as you should. Determine whether your attitudes about exercise are blocking your way, then change what you must and put on those walking shoes.

11 to 16: You need to feel more positive about exercise so you can do it more often. Think of ways to be more active that are fun and fit into your lifestyle.

17 to 20: It looks like the path is clear for you to be active. Now think of ways to get motivated.

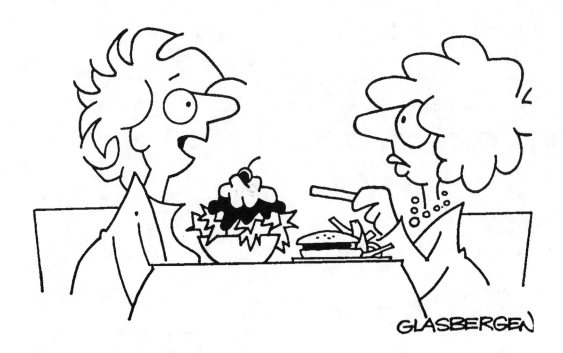

"*I'm easing into my diet gradually. It's a hot-fudge salad!*"

Lesson 1

Today you begin The LEARN Program. It contains the best of what science and clinical practice have to offer. In writing this manual, our intention is for us to form a partnership. Together we can make it work.

When you lose weight on this program, only one person deserves credit. We would be happy to claim credit, but we deserve no more than Rand McNally does when you use their atlas to drive from one city to the next. The atlas supplies the possible routes, and may even suggest the best, but you choose the route and you determine whether you reach your destination. Most important, you do the driving. With that in mind, let's go!

Understanding Your Weight Loss Medication

Your doctor has prescribed MERIDIA to help you lose weight and maintain that weight loss. This medication reduces your appetite by acting on chemicals in the brain such as norepinephrine and serotonin. People who take MERIDIA report that they feel full more quickly and, thus, eat less. The result—steady weight loss and maintenance of weight loss.

We want to emphasize a point from the Introduction and Orientation Lesson before addressing several new issues about medication. MERIDIA will be most effective if you combine its appetite-reducing properties with your own efforts at lifestyle change. The medication will help you eat less, but there is so much more you can do on your own. The LEARN Program will show you how in the lessons to come.

Starting Medication

MERIDIA is typically taken in the morning and only needs to be taken once a day. That is an advantage MERIDIA has over other weight loss medications, some of which have to be taken two or three times a day.

MERIDIA needs to be taken once daily. Your doctor will advise you about the dose. We will suggest ways to help you take your medication as part of your routine.

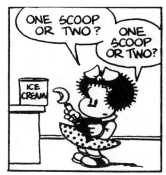 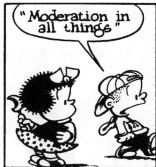 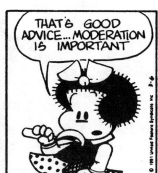 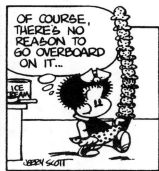

Plan to take your medication at the same time and in the same place each day to make it a habit. Decide now where you will keep your capsules and when you will take them. Many people keep their medication on the kitchen table so they remember to take it at breakfast. Others keep the medication next to their tooth brush. They take their capsule first thing in the morning. Record your plan below:

Place: _____

Time: _____

Keep a record of your medication schedule for at least the first month until you have this new habit firmly in place. The daily Food Diary, that we will discuss later, contains a medication box at the top. Check it each day when you take your capsule.

Missed Medication

What should you do if you forget to take your medication? Speak with your physician to see how much later in the day he or she would advise you to take the capsule.

Do not be surprised if it takes some effort to remember to take your medication every day, seven days a week. Even a little behavior, as simple as this one, requires attention.

Side Effects

Your doctor may have told you that you could experience side effects. She or he is in the best position to describe these. Some side effects will go away with time, but be certain to contact your physician if you have concerns or questions about what you are experiencing.

Sometimes people stop taking their medication before first speaking to their doctor. This can be unfortunate because the doctor can often decrease the side effects by lowering the dose or by explaining that the symptoms are not connected to the medication. Speak with your doctor if you have concerns about your health that would lead you to discontinue your medication.

You will find that you have the best appetite control if you take your medication regularly. This is why we encourage you to develop a medication schedule and stick to it.

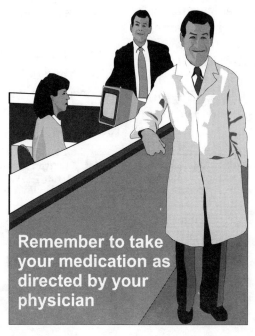

Remember to take your medication as directed by your physician

Positive Effects

Some people worry when they have minor side effects. Others interpret side effects as evidence that the medication is working—working to increase their feelings of fullness (known as satiety) and to facilitate weight loss. During the first couple of days and weeks, see if you can identify any positive effects that the medication gives you. Evaluate whether you are less preoccupied with food, have fewer cravings, or eat less between meals. Determine if the size of your dinner meal or lunch changes. If you are like most people, you will notice a change in some aspect of your appetite.

Diet vs. Lifestyle Change

The LEARN Program is not a diet. It is a system for lifestyle change. This is more than just a matter of words—it is a fundamental difference in philosophy that affects nearly every aspect of the LEARN approach.

The word *diet* conjures up a number of images. It implies deprivation and suffering, but most of all, it is something that you go on or off. Whether someone is "on a diet" or "off a diet" is part of modern language. This is a problem, of course, because changing habits is not something that happens while a person is *on* a diet and then stops later when the diet ends. This implies a temporary solution, a quick patch job that only requires minor effort over the short term.

We are seeking a permanent solution. Instead of a quick but temporary fix, we want a reorientation of lifestyle. This involves establishing new habits and working hard to make these part of day-to-day life. Most people who struggle with weight have a chronic problem. Chronic

problems require attention over the long-term.

Think for a moment of this difference between going on a diet and changing your lifestyle. The lifestyle approach, which emphasizes gradual, sustainable, and permanent changes in eating, exercise, thinking, and feeling, is the hallmark of this program.

Record Keeping

Its Purpose and Importance

The first and perhaps most important lifestyle behavior you will learn is to keep records. You will be keeping records of your eating, exercise, and weight. You will have more records than an accountant! Don't worry, there is a good reason for this.

This lesson introduces two records. The first is the Food Diary, which is a daily record of the food you eat. The second is the Weight Change Record, which is a weekly graph of your weight. Both will increase your awareness of eating and its effects on your weight.

Awareness is a key step in changing habits. You may already know a great deal about your habits and your weight patterns, particularly if you have kept records for an earlier program. You will be surprised by how much more there is to learn. The awareness you gain from record keeping has several benefits. These will become clear within a few weeks.

> ▶ **You learn about calories.** There are calories lurking where you least suspect. Do you think yogurt is a good diet food? One cup of fruit yogurt can have more calories than an ice cream cone. Ten innocent potato chips contain 110 calories, more than five cups of plain

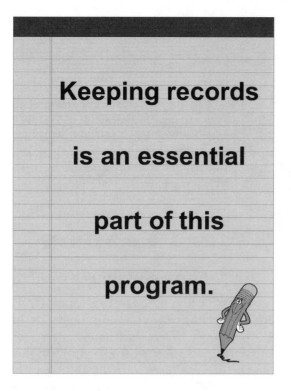

Keeping records is an essential part of this program.

feelings (anger, anxiety, etc.), and others find they eat when doing something else (watching TV). Knowing your patterns is a big help in changing habits.

▶ **The records help you *bank* calories.** Your body is like a bank account in which you make calorie deposits and withdrawals. If you eat less, you have some calories to bank for a special occasion. If you have a party to attend on the week-end, you can cut back during the week and can afford to indulge with some special dessert. Calorie records give you the information to make such a decision.

▶ **The weight change record prevents despair**. There may be one or more weeks when you fail to lose weight, or even worse, gain weight! There are many reasons for this, as we will discuss later. Such a discouraging bout with the scale can make life difficult. This despair can be prevented by reviewing your change in weight over many weeks. A slight gain is easier to tolerate when you are reminded by your records that you have been losing weight in a steady manner.

popcorn. Becoming a calorie expert insures you won't be derailed by calorie surprises.

▶ **You are aware of what you eat.** You might be thinking, "Of course I know what I eat." However, one does not always recall the exact number of Doritos consumed at happy hour or the ounces of milk poured into the bowl of Wheaties. These are forgotten calories, some-times because we like to forget them!

▶ **You increase control over eat-ing.** Knowing exactly where you stand with the day's calorie count permits you to judge whether you can afford certain foods. You may have the calories banked to have that snack you are considering. Knowing where you stand makes the choice easier.

▶ **Eating patterns become clear.** You may discover that most of your eating is done between dinner and bedtime. Another person might eat throughout the day. Some peo-ple eat when they have certain

The Food Diary

The Food Diary is your holy book dur-ing this program. You will use it to rec-ord amounts and calories of the foods you eat. You may resist this part of the pro-gram. It will be hard initially to record everything you eat and to estimate calo-ries. When it becomes easy, you may find it repetitive. It is important to conquer this resistance and keep the records. Re-search has shown this to be one of the most, if not the most important part of habit change.

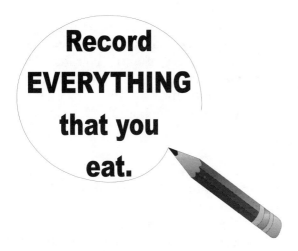

Record EVERYTHING that you eat.

A blank Food Diary is provided on page 27, along with a sample that has a typical person's eating filled in on page 26. Make photocopies of the blank Food Diary and use it for your own. Here are the instructions for completing the Diary:

- ▶ **Record everything, forget nothing.** Every morsel of food goes in the Diary. If you eat pretzels, count how many. Every ounce of food or beverage must be entered. Don't forget when you taste foods you are preparing.

- ▶ **Record the food, the amount, the calories.** Record the type of food you eat, how it is prepared (baked, fried, etc.), how much, and the number of calories.

- ▶ **Record immediately after eating.** Do not wait until you are ready for bed, until the next morning, or even later! It is hard to remember how many peanuts you ate at the cocktail party or how much juice you had for breakfast. As soon as you finish eating, whip out the Food Diary and make your entries. If you are with others and are embarrassed, excuse yourself and find a private place, like a phone booth. If Clark Kent can do it, so can you!

- ▶ **Carry the Food Diary always.** There is food everywhere waiting to leap into your mouth. Keep your Food Diary with you (except when swimming or in the shower) so you won't be caught unaware. Some people use a pocket notebook during the day and then transfer the information to their Food Diary later.

- ▶ **Take and record your medication each day.** This is an important aspect of your program. A section to record whether you took your medication is added to the Food Diary. For some people, this is a helpful reminder. Checking off your medication is a cue that you have taken a positive step, just like changing the food you eat.

Using the Calorie Guide

You will need a calorie guide to estimate the calories in foods. The Calorie Guide for The LEARN Program appears at the end of this manual (Appendix F). Previous versions of this manual recommended that people purchase calorie guides at a bookstore, but we were convinced by our clients to develop an official guide. As you know, many calorie books are available, and they do not always agree. Feel free to use another guide if you wish, but first check it for accuracy against the guide given here.

You will have to do some arithmetic to calculate calories. The guide may list one pat of margarine at 36 calories. If you have two pats on a roll, the contribution from margarine will be 72 (36 x 2) calories. If you have only half the pat, mark down 18 calories.

Your judgment is important when estimating calories because a calorie guide provides only estimates and may not apply to the food you are actually eating. For instance, a calorie guide may show

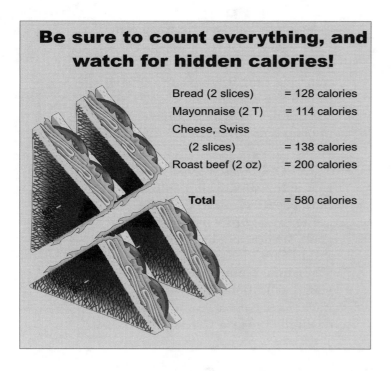
that a roast beef sandwich has 347 calories. This refers to a regular sandwich with about two ounces of meat with no mustard, mayonnaise, or whatever else you use. If you get a deli sandwich with two inches (rather than two ounces) of roast beef, the calories could be three or four times what the guide lists.

The challenge is to estimate the portion sizes and composition of the foods you eat. This can be difficult, especially when you eat out. At home, the job can be simplified by using a food scale. Many people feel they do not need a scale, especially the veterans of weight loss programs who have been keeping calorie records for years. We did a study on this with some colleagues by having individuals in our program estimate the quantities and calories in common foods and beverages, such as milk, green beans, meat, and soda. Some estimated high and some low, but the average error was 60 percent! Food scales are widely available and are not expensive.

Finding the hidden calories in foods is also important. Examples are butter on vegetables, whipped cream on desserts, dressings on salad, and sugar used as a sweetener. Be painfully honest since these are sources of extra pounds. Did you know that one extra pat of margarine per day, which has only 36 calories, can add up to four pounds of weight in one year?

As you progress through the program, you will be able to estimate food portions, the composition of foods, and calories more easily and accurately. The Food Diaries will be easier to keep and the exact calories will become less important.

The Weight Change Record

The Weight Change Record is a weekly graph of changes in your weight. Once each week, record the date and your weight change from the previous week. A sample is given on page 23.

Keeping the Weight Change Record has several advantages. First, it is a reminder of how you are faring with the program. Second, it shows the relationship between your eating and your weight. You can make a rough estimate of how many calories you need to lose weight by taking the average daily calorie values from several weeks of your Food Diary and checking weight changes from your Weight Change Record. Third, the graph puts your weight change in perspective. If you gain a pound during your eighth week, you can take heart from the steady loss in earlier weeks.

You will notice that the Weight Change Record is a graph of change, not of weight per se. This is done so people can place the graph in a public spot, like on the refrigerator door, if they wish. Your weight does not appear on the graph, just your progress. Many people

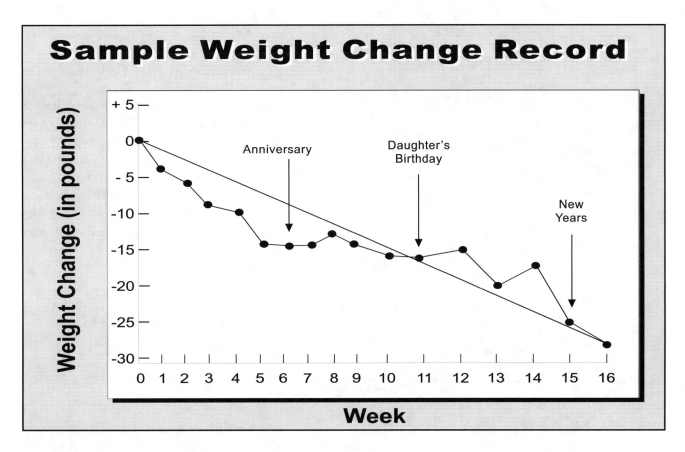

Sample Weight Change Record

Weight Change (in pounds) vs Week

Anniversary

Daughter's Birthday

New Years

like to have the graph posted in a place where they see it frequently, so it can act as a source of encouragement. The sample here shows how this could happen.

On the sample graph provided here, you will see a straight line. This represents what weight would look like if a person lost exactly the same amount of weight each week. Of course, life does not occur in a straight line. The realistic line on the graph shows some weeks where weight stays stable and even weeks when weight increases.

A terrific help in setting reasonable goals is to think ahead to how much weight you are likely to lose by landmark dates. Let's use the sample graph above as an example. A person's anniversary might be at week 6 of the program, a daughter's birthday at week 11, and New Years at week 15. Since a good weight loss is one to two pounds a week, this individual might lose about 9 pounds by

the anniversary, 16 pounds by the daughter's birthday, and 22 pounds by New Years. When the person reaches these dates, he or she can see if what they accomplish is in line with what they expect. People usually expect too much!

Take a few minutes to pencil in some landmark dates for your own graph, using holidays, birthdays, or other special dates. When those dates roll around, compare your weight loss to the graph. A weight loss that might feel disappointing looks good when compared to a reasonable standard.

You should know right now that there may be weeks when your graph looks more like the realistic line than the straight line. What matters in a given week is where you are compared to where you started, not what you weighed the week before. Gaining a pound is a small setback in the scheme of your total program, but your reaction to the pound

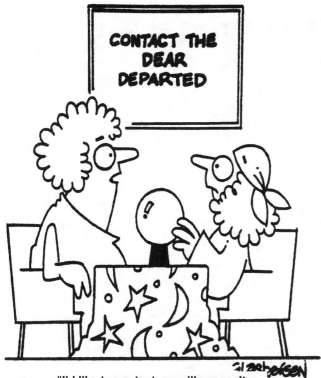

"I'd like to contact my willpower. It died last night at Angelo's Pizza Palace!"

can be devastating. Therefore, think of this sample graph often, and remember that you are a real person and that the realistic line may best reflect your experience.

Rating Your Diet

Nutrition is one key to successful weight control. What you eat affects how you feel, whether you are healthy, and how you look. A great deal of information on nutrition awaits you in this program. To start the process, let's evaluate your diet.

We have provided on page 29 the Rate Your Diet Quiz developed by the Center for Science in the Public Interest and published in the *Nutrition Action Healthletter*. Take a few minutes to complete the quiz and to score your answers. You have probably changed your diet since beginning the program. Complete

the quiz as you would have before starting the program, so you will see how you would score ordinarily. Then, toward the end of this program, you can take the quiz again to see how your eating habits have changed.

Better diets will receive higher scores on this quiz. You will see which choices for each question contribute to or subtract from the total score. Taking the quiz can be educational because it may help provide new ideas for healthy food choices.

A Note About Exercise and Relationships

The emphasis this week is on your medication, lifestyle (record keeping), and nutrition. We will cover exercise and relationships in detail later. They will receive much attention as we progress through The LEARN Program.

Your Self-Assessment

After each lesson there will be a Self-Assessment Questionnaire. This will be a simple true-false quiz to help you decide whether you have learned the important points of the lesson. If you answer all the questions correctly, you can boast about being a weight loss whiz! When you answer a question incorrectly, check the material in the lesson.

Setting Personal Goals

Each lesson of this program will end with a section on setting personal goals. This section will include specific issues for your attention, based on the material in that lesson. In some ways, it is an assignment to practice the new activities you read about. In addition, it will offer you a time to reflect on what you want to accomplish before moving on to the next lesson. Sometimes the goal will be broad, like being more aware of temptations to eat, but others will be more specific, such as being physically active for a certain number of minutes each day.

Setting goals is important. It gives you something to strive for, a standard against which to judge your progress. It is essential to remember several things as you establish personal goals. The first is to set goals that are reasonable. The tendency is to set goals too high. This makes good progress seem trivial. We will discuss this issue of setting realistic goals in great detail as the program moves ahead.

The second key issue in goal setting is to reward yourself, even with a few kind words. Too often people dismiss important changes they make and focus instead on how far they have to go. People are notoriously reluctant to reward themselves, perhaps because it seems like bragging. But you can be your biggest booster. Most people would not dream of praising themselves for something they would routinely praise in a friend. Getting in the habit of praising yourself is a good habit indeed.

There are two primary program goals for this week. The first is to take your medication each day at the same time, in the same place. The second is to learn about your eating and weight habits from the Food Diary and the Weight Change Record. Specific calorie levels will be described in Lesson 2. Your assignment for this week is to make copies of the Food Diary provided here and to fill in one for each day of the week, and to begin your Weight Change Record. We

have provided you with a blank form on page 28.

Completing these forms is critical, for three reasons. First, it is a good test of your motivation. Difficulty in keeping the records may reflect inadequate motivation. If this is the case, you might start the program later when motivation is higher. Second, the information will teach you about your habits. Third, the information will be valuable to a group leader or professional who may be working with you.

Self-Assessment Questionnaire

Lesson 1
(Circle either T for true or F for false)

T F 1. It is best to call your doctor if you have any questions about the side effects of your medication.

T F 2. A good way to be certain to take a medication on schedule is to take it at the same time and place every day.

T F 3. People who take weight loss medications don't need to worry about the foods they choose to eat. The medication does all the work.

T F 4. Very few people can accurately estimate the quantity and calories of food.

T F 5. Record keeping may be the most important aspect of a weight loss program.

(Answers in Appendix C)

Food Diary—Lesson 1 *(sample)*

Today's Date_____

☑ **Medication Taken Today**

Description	Calories
Breakfast	
Orange juice, ½ cup	60
Cheerios, 1 cup	89
Skim milk, 1 cup	86
White toast, dry, 1 slice	64
Total calories from this meal	299
Lunch	
Apple, 1 medium	81
Vegetable soup, 2 cups	144
Chicken salad sandwich, 2 oz, with 2T mayonnaise	332
Ritz crackers, 5	70
Diet Pepsi, 12 oz	1
Total calories from this meal	628
Dinner	
Sirloin steak, lean, 3.5 oz	208
Green beans, 1 cup	26
Cauliflower, 2 cups	60
Wheat bread, 1 slice	61
Apple pie, 1 slice (1/6 of pie)—water to drink	231
Total calories from this meal	586
Snacks	
Yogurt, low-fat, 8 oz	144
Total calories from snacks	144
Total calories for the day	1,657

Food Diary—Lesson 1

Today's Date_____

☐ Medication Taken Today   Description   Calories

Breakfast	
Total calories from this meal	
Lunch	
Total calories from this meal	
Dinner	
Total calories from this meal	
Snacks	
Total calories from snacks	
Total calories for the day	

My Weight Change Record

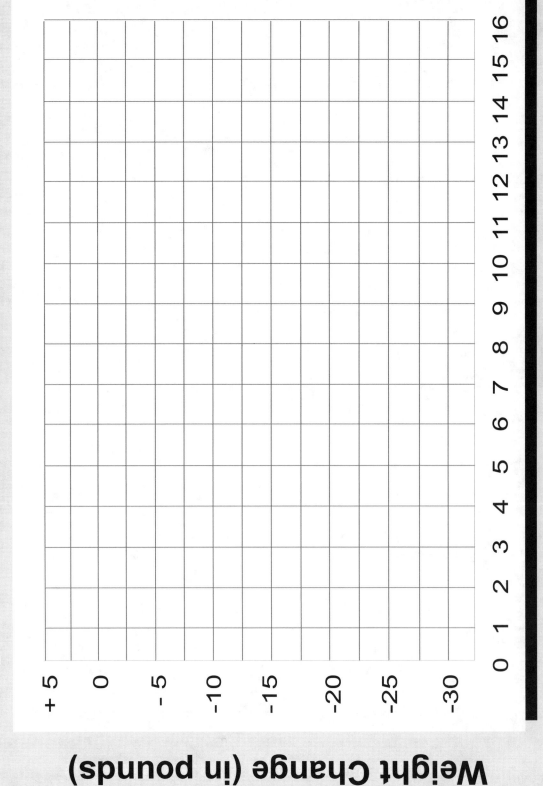

Weight Change (in pounds)

Week

Rate Your Diet Quiz

The following questions will give you a rough sketch of your typical eating habits. The (+) or (-) number for each answer instantly pats you on the back for good eating habits or alerts you to problems you didn't even know you had. The quiz focuses on fat, saturated fat, cholesterol, sodium, sugar, fiber, and fruits and vegetables. It doesn't attempt to cover everything in your diet. Also, it doesn't try to measure precisely how much of the key nutrients you eat.

Next to each answer is a number with a + or - sign in front of it. Circle the number that corresponds to the answer you choose and write that score (e.g., +1) in the space provided in front of each question. That's your score for the question. If two or more answers apply, circle each one. Then average them to get your score for the question.

How to average. In answering question 19, for example, if your sandwich-eating is equally divided among tuna salad (-2), roast beef (+1), and turkey breast (+3), add the three scores (which gives you +2) and then divide by three. That gives you a score of +⅔ for the question. Round it to +1.

Pay attention to serving sizes, which are given when needed. For example, a serving of vegetables is ½ cup. If you usually eat one cup of vegetables at a time, count it as two servings. If you're ready, let's start.

Fruits, Vegetables, Grains, and Beans

____ 1. How many servings of fruit or 100% fruit juice do you eat per day? (*OMIT fruit snacks like Fruit Roll-Ups and fruit-on-the-bottom yogurt. One serving = one piece or ½ cup of fruit or 6 oz of fruit juice.*)

    -3   None
    -2   Less than 1 serving
    0   1 serving
    +1   2 serving
    +2   3 serving
    +3   4 or more servings

____ 2. How many servings of non-fried vegetables do you eat per day? (*One serving = ½ cup. Include potatoes.*)

    -3   None
    -2   Less than 1 serving
    0   1 serving
    +1   2 serving
    +2   3 serving
    +3   4 or more servings

____ 3. How many servings of vitamin-rich vegetables do you eat per week? (*One serving = ½ cup. Only count broccoli, Brussels sprouts, carrots, collards, kale, red pepper, spinach, sweet potatoes, or winter squash.*)

    -3   None
    +1   1 to 3 servings
    +2   4 to 6 servings
    +3   7 or more servings

____ 4. How many servings of leafy green vegetables do you eat per week? (*One serving = ½ cup cooked or 1 cup raw. Only count collards, kale, mustard greens, romaine lettuce, spinach, or Swiss chard.*)

    -3   None
    -2   Less than 1 serving
    +1   1 to 2 servings
    +2   3 to 4 servings
    +3   5 or more servings

____ 5. How many times per week does your lunch or dinner contain grains, vegetables, or beans, but little or no meat, poultry, fish, eggs, or cheese?

    -1   None
    +1   1 to 2 times
    +2   3 to 4 times
    +3   5 or more times

____ 6. How many times per week do you eat beans, split peas, or lentils? (*Omit green beans.*)

    -3   None
    -1   Less than 1 time
    0   1 times
    +1   2 times
    +2   3 times
    +3   4 or more times

____ 7. How many servings of grains do you eat per day? (*One serving = 1 slice of bread, 1 oz of crackers, 1 large pancake, 1 cup pasta or cold cereal, or ½ cup granola, cooked cereal, rice, or bulgur. Omit heavily sweetened cold cereals.*)

    -3   None
    0   1 to 2 servings
    +1   3 to 4 servings
    +2   5 to 7 servings
    +3   8 or more servings

____ 8. What type of bread, rolls, etc., do you eat?

    +3   100% whole wheat as the only flour
    +2   Whole-wheat flour as 1st or 2nd flour
    +1   Rye, pumpernickel, or oatmeal
    0   White, French, or Italian

____ 9. What kind of breakfast do you eat?

    +3   Whole-grain (like oatmeal or Wheaties)
    0   Low-fiber (like Cream of Wheat or Corn Flakes)
    -1   Sugary low-fiber (like Frosted Flakes or low-fat granola)
    -2   Regular granola

Rate Your Diet Quiz (continued)

Meat, Poultry, and Seafood

____ 10. How many times per week do you eat high-fat red meats *(hamburgers, pork chops, ribs, hot dogs, pot roast, sausage, bologna, steaks other than round steak, etc.)*?
  +3   None
  +2   Less than 1 time
  -1   1 time
  -2   2 times
  -3   3 times
  -4   4 times

____ 11. How many times per week do you eat lean red meats *(hot dogs or luncheon meats with no more than 2 grams of fat per serving, round steak, or pork tenderloin)*?
  +3   None
  +1   Less than 1 time
   0   1 time
  -1   2 to 3 times
  -2   4 to 5 times
  -3   6 or more times

____ 12. After cooking, how large is the serving of red meat you eat? *(To convert from raw to cooked, reduce by 25 percent. For example, 4 oz of raw meat shrinks to 3 oz after cooking. There are 16 oz in a pound.)*
  -3   6 oz or more
  -2   4 to 5 oz
   0   3 oz or less
  +3   Don't eat red meat

____ 13. If you eat red meat, do you trim the visible fat when you cook or eat it?
  +1   Yes
  -3   No

____ 14. What kind of ground meat or poultry do you eat?
  -4   Regular ground beef
  -3   Ground beef that's 11 to 25% fat
  -2   Ground chicken or 10% fat ground beef
  -1   Ground turkey
  +3   Ground turkey breast
  +3   Don't eat ground meat or poultry

____ 15. What chicken parts do you eat?
  +3   Breast
  +1   Drumstick
  -1   Thigh
  -2   Wing
  +3   Don't eat poultry

____ 16. If you eat poultry, do you remove the skin before eating?
  +2   Yes
  -3   No

____ 17. If you eat seafood, how many times per week? *(Omit deep-fried foods, tuna packed in oil, and mayonnaise-laden tuna salad—low-fat mayo is okay.)*
   0   Less than 1 time
  +1   1 time
  +2   2 times
  +3   3 or more times

Mixed Foods

____ 18. What is your most typical breakfast? *(Subtract an extra 3 points if you also eat sausage.)*
  -4   Biscuit sandwich or croissant sandwich
  -3   Croissant, Danish, or doughnut
  -3   Eggs
  -1   Pancakes, French toast, or waffles
  +3   Cereal, toast, or bagel (no cream cheese)
  +3   Low-fat yogurt or low-fat cottage cheese
   0   Don't eat breakfast

____ 19. What sandwich fillings do you eat?
  -3   Regular luncheon meat, cheese, or egg salad
  -2   Tuna or chicken salad or ham
   0   Peanut butter
  +1   Roast beef
  +1   Low-fat luncheon meat
  +3   Tuna or chicken salad made with fat-free mayo
  +3   Turkey breast or humus

____ 20. What do you order on your pizza? *(Subtract 1 point if you order extra cheese, cheese-filled crust, or more than one meat topping.)*
  +3   No cheese with at least one vegetable topping
  -1   Cheese with at least one vegetable topping
  -2   Cheese
  -3   Cheese with one meat topping
  +3   Don't eat pizza

____ 21. What do you put on your pasta? *(Add one point if you also add sautéed vegetables.)*
  +3   Tomato sauce or red clam sauce
  -1   Meat sauce or meat balls
  -3   Pesto or another oily sauce
  -4   Alfredo or another creamy sauce

____ 22. How many times per week do you eat deep-fried foods (*fish, chicken, French fries, potato chips, etc.*)?

+3 None
0 1 time
-1 2 times
-2 3 times
-3 4 or more times

____ 23. At a salad bar, what do you choose?

+3 Nothing, lemon, or vinegar
+2 Fat-free dressing
+1 Low- or reduced-calorie dressing
-1 Oil and vinegar
-2 Regular dressing
-2 Cole slaw, pasta salad, or potato salad
-3 Cheese or eggs

____ 24. How many times per week do you eat canned or dried soups or frozen dinners? (*Omit lower-sodium, low-fat ones.*)

+3 None
0 1 time
-1 2 times
-2 3 to 4 times
-3 5 or more times

____ 25. How many servings of low-fat calcium-rich foods do you eat per day? (*One serving = ⅔ cup low-fat or nonfat milk or yogurt, 1 oz low-fat cheese, 1½ oz sardines, 3½ oz canned salmon with bones, 1 oz tofu made with calcium sulfate, 1 cup collards or kale, or 200 mg of a calcium supplement.*)

-3 None
-1 Less than 1 serving
+1 1 serving
+2 2 servings
+3 3 or more servings

____ 26. How many times per week do you eat cheese? (*Include pizza, cheeseburgers, lasagna, tacos or nachos with cheese, etc. Omit foods made with low-fat cheese.*)

+3 None
+1 1 time
-1 2 times
-2 3 times
-3 4 or more times

____ 27. How many egg yolks do you eat per week? (*Add 1 yolk for every slice of quiche you eat.*)

+3 None
+1 1 yolk
0 2 yolks
-1 3 yolks
-2 4 yolks
-3 5 or more yolks

Fats & Oils

____ 28. What do you put on your bread, toast, bagel, or English muffin?

-4 Stick butter or cream cheese
-3 Stick margarine or whipped butter
-2 Regular tub margarine
-1 Light tub margarine or whipped light butter
0 Jam, fat-free margarine, or fat-free cream cheese
+3 Nothing

____ 29. What do you spread on your sandwiches?

-2 Mayonnaise
-1 Light mayonnaise
+1 Catsup, mustard, or fat-free mayonnaise
+2 Nothing

____ 30. With what do you make tuna salad, pasta salad, chicken salad, etc.?

-2 Mayonnaise
-1 Light mayonnaise
0 Fat-free mayonnaise
+2 Nothing

____ 31. What do you use to sauté vegetables or other food? (*Vegetable oil includes safflower, corn, sunflower, and soybean.*)

-3 Butter or lard
-2 Margarine
-1 Vegetable oil or light margarine
+1 Olive or canola oil
+2 Broth
+3 Cooking spray

Beverages

____ 32. What do you drink on a typical day?

+3 Water or club soda
0 Caffeine-free coffee or tea
-1 Diet soda
-1 Coffee or tea (up to 4 a day)
-2 Regular soda (up to 2 a day)
-3 Regular soda (3 or more a day)
-3 Coffee or tea (5 or more a day)

____ 33. What kind of "fruit" beverage do you drink?

+3   Orange, grapefruit, prune, or pineapple juice

+1   Apple, grape, or pear juice

0   Cranberry juice blend or cocktail

-3   Fruit "drink," "ade," or "punch"

____ 34. What kind of milk do you drink?

-3   Whole

-1   2% fat

+2   1% low-fat

+3   skim

____ 35. What do you eat as a snack?

+3   Fruits of vegetables

+2   Low-fat yogurt

+1   Low-fat crackers

-2   Cookies or fried chips

-2   Nuts or granola bar

-3   Candy bar or pastry

____ 36. Which of the following "salty" snacks do you eat?

-3   Potato chips, corn chips, or popcorn

-2   Tortilla chips

-1   Salted pretzels or light microwave popcorn

+2   Unsalted pretzels

+3   Baked tortilla or potato chips or homemade air-popped popcorn

+3   Don't eat salty snacks

____ 37. What kind of cookies do you eat?

+2   Fat-free cookies

+1   Graham crackers or reduced-fat cookies

-1   Oatmeal cookies

-2   Sandwich cookies (like Oreos)

-3   Chocolate coated, chocolate chip, or peanut butter cookies

+3   Don't eat cookies

____ 38. What kind of cake or pastry do you eat?

-4   Cheesecake

-3   Pie or doughnuts

-2   Cake with frosting

-1   Cake without frosting

0   Muffins

+1   Angle food, fat-free cake, or fat-free pastry

+3   Don't eat cakes or pastries

____ 39. What kind of frozen dessert do you eat? *(Subtract 1 point for each of the following toppings: hot fudge, nuts, or chocolate candy bars or pieces.)*

-4   Gourmet ice cream

-3   Regular ice cream

-1   Frozen yogurt or light ice cream

-1   Sorbet, sherbet, or ices

+1   Nonfat frozen yogurt or fat-free ice cream

+3   Don't eat frozen desserts

_____   **Total Score**

Add up your score for each question and write it in the "total score" line above. **If your score is:**

1 to 29   Don't be discouraged. Eating healthy is tough, but you can learn to eat healthier.

30 to 59   Congratulations. Your are doing just fine. Pin your Quiz to the nearest wall.

60 or above   Excellent. You're a nutrition superstar. Give yourself a big pat on the back.

Source: Adapted with permission from *Nutrition Action Healthletter*, May 1996, V23/N4. (*Nutrition Action Healthletter*, 1875 Connecticut Ave., N.W., Suite 300, Washington DC 20009-5728. $24 for 10 issues.)

Lesson 2

Welcome back after your first lesson! We hope you did well and are on your way to permanent weight loss.

Reviewing Your Diary

Your Food Diary contains information about two important things you did last week—took your medication and recorded the foods you ate. We will examine medication first.

Taking Your Medication

We hope you devised a plan for taking your medication every day at the same time, in the same place. Review your diary to see how you did. If you can couple your medication with other morning activities, whether eating breakfast, brushing your teeth, having that first cup of coffee or watching your favorite news show, you'll be sure to take it each day. Taking medication will become part of your morning routine (just like hitting the snooze alarm!).

Remember that pharmacies sell medication boxes with separate compart-ments for each day's capsule. These boxes can be loaded in advance so when you are puzzled about whether you took your medication some morning, you can look at the compartment, see if the capsule is still there, and be assured that you have or have not had your medication for the day. These boxes are especially handy if you are taking more than one medication or just your weight control medication and a multivitamin.

Symptoms

You may have experienced a few symptoms in adjusting to the medica-tion. Side effects generally decline in intensity over the first few weeks. If your mouth feels dry, not an uncommon symp-tom, drink plenty of water or other non-caloric beverages. This will help, as can sugar-free mints.

If you have any significant symptoms that disrupt your concentration or daily functioning, call your doctor. Your doc-tor may be able to reduce your symptoms by decreasing the amount of medication you take or by determining that you ac-tually have a separate illness, such as a cold or the flu, which needs attention.

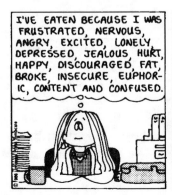
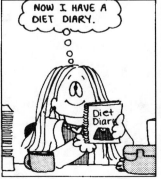
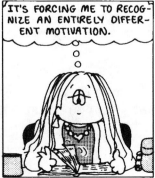
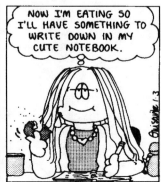

Positive Effects

We hope that you experienced some positive effects of the medication. Did you notice a change in your hunger level in the afternoon or evening? Did you eat less at mealtime? Many people report that they are less preoccupied with food and have fewer cravings when they take medication. These changes should make it easier for you to eat a healthy diet and to lose weight.

Searching for Patterns

One purpose of completing the Food Diary is to examine your eating patterns. Much of our eating is automatic and occurs with little thought or appreciation. We miss much of the pleasure in food and eat more than we need. Think of munching from a large bag of potato chips. Would you remember how many you ate? Would you taste each bite of each chip? Would you have just the right amount to satisfy yourself?

What are the times you eat during the day?

How much are you eating—do you enjoy every bite?

What are your food choices—do you eat a variety of foods?

Where do you eat—are you doing other things while you eat?

A nice example of automatic eating is from a client of ours named Ginny. She loved ice cream and would have a bowl every night. With instruction, she began counting her bites and noting the pleasure in each. She averaged 16 bites. She found that the first four bites were delicious, then there were about ten where she paid little attention (automatic eating). The final few bites were good again because she was nearly finished. With her increased awareness, Ginny decided that the middle ten bites were needless calories.

Examine your Food Diaries for the past week and look for patterns. The patterns you find will be the foundation for later parts of the program. This is where we work together with you. We will give you guidelines for tailoring techniques to your specific eating and exercise patterns. Here are some ideas for patterns.

➤ **Time.** Look for times of the day when you are likely to eat. A typical pattern shows little eating at breakfast and lunch, but much eating and snacking at dinner and after. Do you crave a snack just before bed? Do you always have something in mid-afternoon? Are your meals irregular? Do you skip meals?

➤ **Amount.** Look over the quantities and calories of the food you eat. One key is to enjoy the food you eat so there are no wasted calories. Are there foods you could eat less of or avoid completely? Do you eat specific amounts each time, without thinking about how much you need and want?

➤ **Foods.** Pay close attention to the foods you eat. Are there patterns to the foods you choose? Which foods contribute most to your calories? Can you think of substitutes for high-calorie foods?

▶ **Places.** Are there certain places where you eat? Do you frequently eat in places other than your kitchen or dining room? Some likely candidates are the den, the office, and the car.

Following a Balanced Diet

Recording what you eat and the times, places, and activities associated with eating will make you more conscious of your food choices. Some people can use this information to craft a healthy meal plan, but many like to learn more about the components of a nutritious, well-balanced diet.

There is no end to advice on nutrition. When we visit bookstores or listen to the radio, we are amazed at the half-baked schemes concocted by "experts." One day it is apricot pits for cancer or papaya juice for arthritis. The next day it is mega-doses of vitamins for stress and prune pulp for bad breath.

It is inviting to believe some of these nutty plans because they provide hope for difficult problems. But think back over the years. There was the Scarsdale Diet, The Rotation Diet, The Beverly Hills Diet, The Carbohydrate Addicts Diet, among many, many others. Each promised breakthroughs, grand solutions, and results that seemed guaranteed. Do you know anyone who lost weight and kept it off on one of those programs? Where are the programs now? How much would you bet that the miracle book that comes along next week, next month, or next year will be different than the rest—that it will deliver on what it promises and offer a final solution?

When it comes to nutrition, there is no magic, just common sense and rational eating. The key word to remember is balanced. This means eating a variety of foods from the different food groups. This may sound like what you learned in the sixth grade, but the message is just as important today.

The body needs a balance of nutrients. It does not function well with too little or too much of any nutrient. If your body needs a certain amount of vitamin E each day, you will be worse off with one-half that amount or with 100 times more. This is similar to making your favorite cake. Each ingredient is important. One ingredient may give the cake a very good taste, but too much will ruin it.

Some clients in our clinic ask why nutrition is so important. The answer is simple. What we eat helps determine

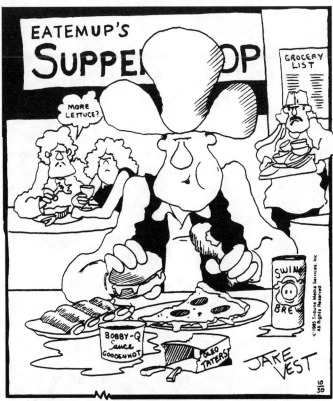

'A balanced meal has something from each of The Five Major Food Groups -- hamburgers, fried chicken, pizza, ribs and French fries.'

35

how healthy we are, which in turn influences how we cope with life both physically and psychologically. You could lose weight by eating nothing but grapefruit, but your body would suffer greatly from deficiencies in the nutrients grapefruit does not provide. How much you eat (calories) is only part of the answer. How well you eat must also be considered.

You will notice that we say not a word about forbidden foods. We do not believe in prohibition for people losing weight. Such an approach is doomed to fail. If you like cheesecake, but feel it is illegal, you will eventually eat it and feel guilty. This will weaken your restraint even more. If you have the expectation that the first bite will send you into a frenzy and you will eat all the cheesecake in sight, you are setting yourself up to fall apart when you might otherwise have a little and be satisfied. It is fine to eat cheesecake, as long as it occurs within the guidelines for sensible nutrition.

The Food Guide Pyramid

The pyramid is a graphic illustration of the research-based food plan developed jointly by the U.S. Department of Agriculture (USDA) and the Department of Health and Human Services (HHS). The following represent the dietary guidelines developed for Americans by the USDA and the HHS:

- ► **Eat a variety of foods.** Eating a variety of foods will help you to get the energy, protein, vitamins, minerals, and fiber you need for good health.
- ► **Maintain a healthy weight.** Many studies show that maintaining a healthy weight can reduce your chances of having high blood pressure, heart disease, certain

cancers, a stroke, and the most common kind of diabetes.

- ► **Choose a diet low in fat, saturated fat, and cholesterol.** Diets that are low in fat, saturated fat, and cholesterol may reduce your risk of heart attack and certain types of cancer. Fat contains more than twice the calories of an equal amount of carbohydrates or protein, so a diet low in fat can help you maintain a healthy weight.
- ► **Choose a diet with plenty of vegetables, fruits, and grain products.** These foods provide the essential vitamins, minerals, fiber, and complex carbohydrates. Since these foods are naturally low in dietary fat, they can help to lower your intake of fat.
- ► **Use sugars only in moderation.** A diet that includes high amounts of sugar has too many calories and may not provide the nutrients your body needs to be healthy. Too much sugar can also contribute to tooth decay.
- ► **Use salt in moderation.** A diet that is low in sodium can help reduce your risk of high blood pressure.
- ► **If you drink alcoholic beverages, do so in moderation.** Alcoholic beverages add calories, but provide little nutrition. Alcohol can also contribute to many other health problems and may lead to addiction.

You can see from these dietary guidelines that the key message is moderation. As we progress through the program these guidelines will become more and more familiar to you. Review each of the guidelines again and check to see how many you are now following. At this point in the program we want you to be familiar with the guidelines so that you can be thinking of how they apply to you and your eating habits.

A Graphic Illustration

The design of the Food Guide Pyramid divides foods into five separate groups as shown below. The pyramid also includes a category for fats, oils, and sweets. Each group in the pyramid includes suggested daily servings which are listed beside the groups. Small circles are used throughout the pyramid to identify food groups that contain high-fat foods, and triangles are used to identify foods that have added sugars.

At the top of the pyramid is the section containing foods that should be eaten sparingly. It should not be surprising that this smallest section consists of fats, oils, and sweets. As the food groups progress toward the bottom of the pyramid they become a larger part of your diet. For instance, the bread and cereal group is the largest section. Foods from this group should make up the largest portion of your daily diet.

Many things we eat are a mixture of foods from the five groups. Pizza, for example, has bread (dough), vegetables (tomatoes, peppers, etc.), cheese, and meat in some cases. A chicken pot pie has pastry, vegetables, meat, etc. You will become an expert at identifying the components of combination dishes.

In this lesson, we want you to become familiar with the five food groups in the pyramid. This graphic will become more familiar to you as you continue through the program. In the lessons that follow, we will describe in more detail each tier of the pyramid. At this point in the pro-

The Food Guide Pyramid

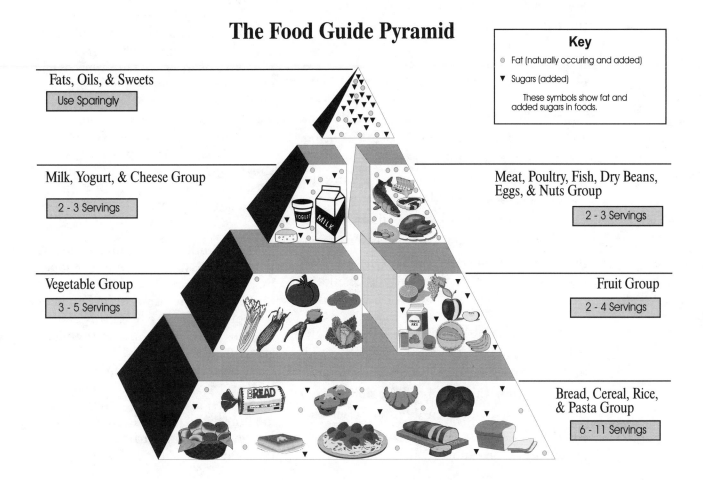

Key

○ Fat (naturally occuring and added)

▼ Sugars (added)

These symbols show fat and added sugars in foods.

Fats, Oils, & Sweets
Use Sparingly

Milk, Yogurt, & Cheese Group
2 - 3 Servings

Meat, Poultry, Fish, Dry Beans, Eggs, & Nuts Group
2 - 3 Servings

Vegetable Group
3 - 5 Servings

Fruit Group
2 - 4 Servings

Bread, Cereal, Rice, & Pasta Group
6 - 11 Servings

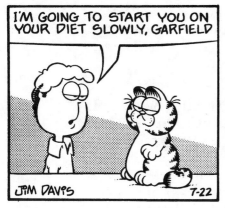
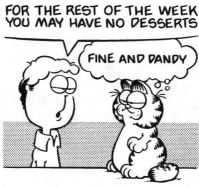
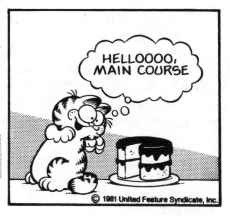

gram do not be concerned with the number of servings you should be eating from the various food groups or how much food it takes to make one serving. We will discuss this and other information about each of the five food groups in later lessons. For now, be aware of the five different food groups and try to include each group in your diet. In your Food Diary this week, note whether you are eating foods from all five food groups.

The Food Guide Pyramid is a useful way to see that you get balanced nutrition, but it is possible to follow the guide and still take in too many calories to lose weight. Eating the recommended number of servings will generally help the average person maintain his or her weight, but since you want to reduce, the number of servings will have to be reduced. As you find the level of calories you need to lose weight, you will be able to adjust the number of servings from the pyramid.

In thinking about good nutrition while losing weight, both the Food Guide Pyramid and a means of counting calories are important. Within the number of calories you budget for yourself each day, try to choose the right balance of servings across the food groups in the pyramid.

Selecting an Eating Plan: Calorie Counting vs. Exchange Plan

There are several available plans for eating nutritiously. One prevailing plan is to count calories while eating a specified number of servings in the five food groups. This approach is one many individuals are familiar with because counting calories is the way most people learn to judge how they are doing with a weight loss plan. This is the approach used in this program. We introduce it in this lesson and then expand on it in the lessons that follow.

An excellent alternative eating plan is the Exchange Plan developed by the American Dietetic Association (ADA) and the American Diabetes Association. The exchange plan places foods into six categories: starch/bread, meat and meat substitutes, vegetables, fruit, milk, and fat. Within each category, amounts of foods are provided so that in the amount listed, all foods have approximately the same carbohydrate, protein, fat, and calories. A food in a given category, therefore, can be exchanged with any other food in the same category. Copies of the exchange list guide are available for $1.50 each plus $4.95 shipping & handling. If you would like to receive a complete guide for the exchange plan, you can call 800-745-0775 or write to:

The American Dietetic Association
P.O. Box 97215
Chicago, IL 60678-7215

Both the calorie counting and exchange plans represent sound nutrition. If you are in a program run by a health professional, he or she may have a preference, so both plans are provided here. Otherwise, choose the plan you feel best meets your needs, and then follow it throughout the program. If you choose the exchange plan over the calorie counting approach, you can obtain a copy from the American Dietetic Association as outlined above.

Try this week to eat the recommended number of servings from the Food Guide Pyramid. You can experiment with the number of servings required for you to lose weight. In the next lesson we will discuss the number of calories you might try to eat each day.

On Being a Good Group Member

Many people who use this program do so on their own. Others are part of a group program. If you are part of a group and are with others who struggle with problems like yours, there are several important matters to consider.

Being in a group can be a wonderful experience. Support, encouragement, and good ideas can flow from one member of the group to another. This is why groups can be so beneficial. To make a group a positive experience, each member must realize that working in a cooperative way, with a team spirit, will allow the group to reach its potential. Each member has the opportunity and responsibility to follow certain guidelines. Some effort will be required, but the payoff will make it worthwhile.

Detailed guidelines for being a good group member are presented in Appendix D. If you are participating in a group program, we urge you to read these over, and to take the advice seriously. Being a contributing and constructive member of the group will support the other group members, who in turn will support you. This can go a long way toward motivating you when times are tough and providing you with fresh ideas for specific problems.

Setting Personal Goals

The program goals for this week are to continue taking your medication each day, seeing to it that you have established a routine, and to continue keeping the Food Diary to increase your awareness of eating. There will be food diaries (later we'll call them Monitoring Forms) for each remaining lesson in the program. You may make photocopies from this book, or you can order blank diaries (to carry you through the entire program) from The LEARN Education Center, either by telephone (1–800–736–7323) or through the Internet (www.LearnEducation.com).

Think also of the goals you would like to accomplish this week. A good food goal would be to eat a diet consistent with the Food Guide Pyramid. Try to make the goal as specific and reasonable as possible, and remember that you deserve to feel good about yourself if you meet these goals.

Self-Assessment Questionnaire

Lesson 2

T F 6. Automatic eating is common in overweight people and distracts them from the taste of food.

T F 7. The Food Diary helps uncover patterns in your eating habits.

T F 8. The five food groups are Milk and Yogurt Products, Vegetables, Fruits, Meats and Proteins, and Breads and Cereals.

T F 9. Ice cream and several other high-sugar desserts are not allowed in this program.

(Answers in Appendix C)

Food Diary—Lesson 2 *(sample)*

Today's Date_____

☑ **Medication Taken Today**   **Description/Amount**   **Calories**

Breakfast		
	Coffee, 6 oz	0
	Poached egg, 1 med	79
	Bagel, ½ med	92
	Orange juice, 1 cup	111
Lunch		
	Roast beef sandwich, 2 oz, with 2T mayonnaise	442
	Water, 1 glass	0
	Raspberry yogurt, 8 oz	90
Dinner		
	Chicken breast-grilled, 3.5 oz	198
	Green beans, 1 cup	44
	Carrots, 1 cup, cooked	70
	Wheat bread, 1 slice, dry	86
Snacks		
	Celery, 4 stalks	24
	Apple, 1 med	81
Total calories for the day		1,373

Food Groups from the Food Guide Pyramid

Milk, yogurt, and cheese	☑ ☑ ☐
Meat, poultry, etc.	☑ ☑ ☑
Fruits	☑ ☑ ☐ ☐
Vegetables	☑ ☑ ☑ ☑ ☑
Breads, cereals, etc.	☑ ☑ ☑ ☑ ☐ ☐ ☐ ☐ ☐ ☐

Food Diary—Lesson 2

Today's Date_____

☐ **Medication Taken Today**   **Description/Amount**   Calories

Breakfast		
Lunch		
Dinner		
Snacks		
Total calories for the day		

Food Groups from the Food Guide Pyramid

Milk, yogurt, and cheese   ☐ ☐ ☐

Meat, poultry, etc.   ☐ ☐ ☐

Fruits   ☐ ☐ ☐ ☐

Vegetables   ☐ ☐ ☐ ☐ ☐

Breads, cereals, etc.   ☐ ☐ ☐ ☐ ☐ ☐ ☐ ☐ ☐

Lesson 3

You have now taken MERIDIA for two weeks and probably have lost some weight. Congratulations! We hope you are pleased with your progress, both with your weight and your behavior change.

Taking MERIDIA

Any symptoms you had the first few days you took MERIDIA may have declined. If, however, you are still troubled by side effects, you may want to call your doctor's office. Your doctor may decide to reduce your dose of medication. Many people lose weight satisfactorily on a lower dose and are able to reduce their symptoms. Alternatively, your doctor may determine that your symptoms are not related to the medication.

If you have trouble falling asleep at night, ask your doctor about taking your medication earlier in the day, perhaps first thing when you wake up. Taking your medication earlier may allow you to fall asleep earlier. And as we mentioned, drink lots of noncaloric fluids—particularly water—if your mouth feels dry. Sugar-free mints can also help.

Medication Schedule

Taking your medication every day is one of the most important things that you can do to ensure your success—both now and in the future. Failing to take it regularly is likely to slow your weight loss.

So, how have you done with developing a medication schedule? Take out your Food Diaries from last week. How many days did you take your medication? All seven? Congratulations, if you did. If you missed one or more days, what happened? Did you wake up late and have to rush out the door? Whatever

the circumstances, make a plan now to prevent this from happening again.

Remember, try to link taking your medication with other things you do. Make MERIDIA a part of your morning routine, right along with washing your face, brushing your teeth, or having breakfast. If you are having trouble developing a routine, use Post-it® notes on the bathroom mirror, the breakfast table, or even your steering wheel. If you work outside of the home, be sure to keep a couple of extra capsules of MERIDIA at the office. Taking your medication daily will provide the best control of your appetite and weight!

An Expanded Food Diary

Since you have your Food Diary out, take a few minutes to review your eating habits from this past week. After two

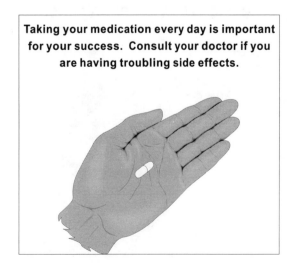

Taking your medication every day is important for your success. Consult your doctor if you are having troubling side effects.

weeks of recording, you should have a better idea of how many meals you typically eat each day, the types of food you enjoy, when you are hungriest, and the places in and outside the home where you are most likely to eat. Your job is to become a detective who analyzes your eating habits and tries to correct the troublesome ones. Sometimes this requires only small changes such as taking a piece of fruit or a small bag of pretzels to work so you will be prepared for the three o'clock munchies. In other cases, you may have to take more time to plan your meals and to make sure you get to the supermarket at least once a week.

This week you will find several categories added to your new Expanded Food Diary. These categories are Time, Feelings, and Activity. In addition to the food and calories, you will be able to record the times you eat, how you feel, and whether you do something else while eating.

These are important factors in the eating habits of many overweight people. Therefore, use the Expanded Food Diary as you did the Food Diary for Lessons 1 and 2. In the next lesson, we will discuss the interpretations of the new diary. A blank diary is provided in this lesson, and a sample from one of our clients is given to show you how the diary might be completed. Make copies of the blank diary to use between now and the next lesson.

Small Changes in Your Diet

You may be feeling a bit overwhelmed by all the information you read last week about different methods of following a balanced diet. You learned about the Food Guide Pyramid and the number of servings that you should eat from each of the food groups. Don't be alarmed if your present meal plan would not win an award (or even Honorable Mention) from the nutrition experts.

It takes time to change eating habits. For example, if you eat no fruit most days, start by adding just one serving a day, and make it an easy one. You can probably add a small banana to your morning cereal or have four ounces of orange juice for an afternoon snack. Each week, try to make one small change you can live with. These small changes will yield big results over the long-term.

Like Sherlock Holmes, your job is to become a detective who analyzes your eating habits.

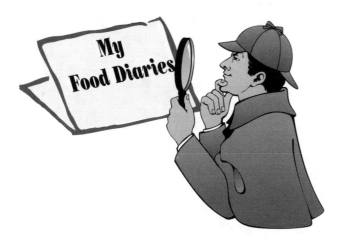

The Mysterious Calorie

The lesson last week discussed your option of counting calories versus food exchanges. Regardless of which option you choose, you need to know more about calories.

The word "calorie" is on the lips of millions of Americans. Food products boast about being "low calorie" and diet soft drinks sell because they have "no calories." Just what is this thing we call a calorie?

A Calorie Is

The calorie is a measure of energy available to the body, much like a gallon is a measure of volume, the inch a measure of length, and the pound a measure of weight. When you eat something, the number of calories it contains is the number of energy units it provides to the body. The calorie is also a measure of energy your body uses, so it is a measure of both intake and expenditure. That is why we talk about the number of calories burned during exercise.

How do we measure the calories in foods? This is done by burning food in a special instrument called a bomb calorimeter. The food is first dried to remove water and then is placed in a special container which rests in water. When the food is burned, heat is transferred to the water. The amount the water is heated is the measure of calories. One calorie is the energy needed to raise the temperature of one gram of water one degree centigrade. Foods contain proteins, carbohydrates (sugars and starches), and fats, each of which provides calories. The water, vitamins, and minerals in food provide no calories.

Most foods are measured in kilocalories, which is 1000 times the energy in a calorie. In common usage, as in diet books and calorie guides, the word calorie actually refers to kilocalorie.

This may sound technical, but you need only know the calorie values of foods. A piece of apple pie has 400 calories, and a fresh apple has 100. The pie gives you four times the energy (calories) as the apple. This would be fine if you were starving, but when your basic energy requirements are met, the body stores the excess as fat. The pie contributes four times as many calories to your fat stockpile.

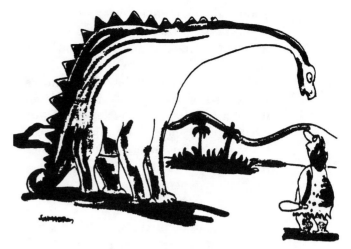

"How many calories are you?"

Not All People Are Created Equal

People differ greatly in how their bodies use calories. We all know people who eat like crazy and gain very little. These fortunate folks are well served in a society where food is abundant and thin is in. In a famine, however, they would be the first to go because their bodies are not efficient at converting ingested calories to precious energy stores (fat).

The unfortunate ones among us are those who are food efficient. Their bodies make very good use of calories, so they are prone to gain weight. This is adaptive if food is scarce, but promotes weight gain when food supplies are adequate. To lose weight, such a person must cut intake to very low levels.

This is one reason why some heavy people have a more difficult time losing weight than others. Let's consider two individuals (Sheri and Bonnie) who fight different battles. Both weigh 180 pounds. Sheri eats 2500 calories each day to maintain that weight and will lose about one pound each week by cutting to 2000 calories. Bonnie, on the other hand, maintains the 180 pounds on only 1800 calories each day, and must reduce to 1300 calories to lose the one pound each week. Is it surprising, then, that Bonnie will have a more difficult time losing weight than Sheri? Because of these individual differences, it would not be fruitful to prescribe the same calorie goal to these two people.

In a related matter, we often hear that 3500 calories equals a pound (it takes 3500 extra calories to gain one pound). If we decrease intake by 3500, one less pound will adorn our bodies. The typical arithmetic is as follows. If you eat 500 fewer calories each day than your ordinary intake, you will create a 3500 calorie deficit in a week and will lose one pound. These numbers are helpful to show how calories can be translated into pounds, but again, the numbers are rough averages. People are highly variable in the number of calories necessary to lose a pound, so these numbers may or may not apply to you. The key question is, therefore, "How do you choose a calorie goal for you?"

Determining Your Target Calorie Level

It is time to identify your target calorie level. As we explore your body's calorie requirements, you will soon learn (if you do not know already) whether you are more like Sheri or Bonnie, the two people mentioned above.

The guidelines are simple. We want to find the calorie level at which you can lose one to two pounds each week. Faster loss can be a clue that you are making drastic changes that can be difficult to maintain. You can probably make a good

guess about what this level might be. Start there, and experiment to see whether you need to increase or decrease the calories.

If you are uncertain about the calorie level, consider using 1200 calories per day for women and 1500 for men. These are commonly used figures which represent calorie levels at which most people will lose weight. As you know, however, this is just an average, which means that some people will need fewer calories and some can afford more. In the space provided below, write in the calorie level you will use as the first step in identifying your long-term target.

Over the next few lessons, you will have time to experiment with this beginning calorie level and to arrive at your target number. This number is important and will be entered into your Monitoring Form for each week in future lessons. You will make note of your target number in each lesson and will have a record of whether you attained the goal each day of the program. The space for the precise calorie level in the Monitoring Form is left blank, so you can fill in your personal number.

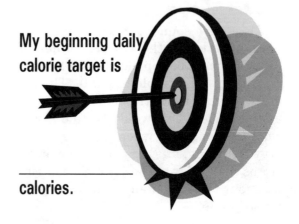

Your Calorie Target

My beginning daily calorie target is

_____

calories.

It is not advisable to drop your calorie level below 1000 calories per day. It is extremely difficult to pack the necessary nutrients into fewer calories than this, so by eating fewer than 1000 calories, you may be losing weight at the expense of good nutrition. Diets of less than 1000 calories per day should be supervised by a physician.

Diets that fall below this level are labeled very-low-calorie diets (VLCDs). Again, these are to be used only under medical supervision, preferably in a program where a registered dietitian is available to provide expert nutritional input. The body goes through complicated changes when on such diets. There is the potential for danger if a person is not screened and monitored adequately and if the food or supplement to be eaten does not contain the right mix of nutrients.

The Role of Exercise in Weight Control

We have talked a lot about the benefits of MERIDIA for controlling your appetite, as well as different methods of eating a balanced diet. These two approaches will reduce your calorie intake, thus leading to weight loss. Now it is time to talk about the other side of the weight loss equation—increasing the number of calories you expend by increasing your physical activity. Are you ready?

It is hard to overstate the importance of increasing physical activity. Theoretically, you can eat less, exercise more, or do both to alter your energy balance and hence your weight. We feel strongly that doing both is the best approach. This comes from experience with hundreds of clients and from research showing that people who exercise are most likely to achieve long-term weight loss.

The Importance of Being Active

Don't get nervous! Increasing your activity does not have to involve calisthenics, weight lifting, or marathon running. Many overweight people avoid exercise because it hurts, it takes time, they are embarrassed, and they are not skilled at athletic activities. There are solutions to these problems. We will discuss these in upcoming lessons. For now, we want you to be aware of the importance and benefits of being active.

A New View of Exercise

Most of us labor under the old idea that exercise has to be taxing to be bene-

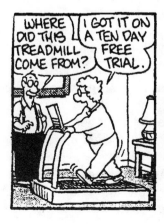
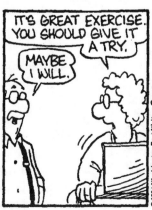
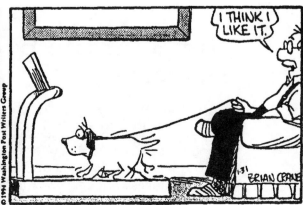

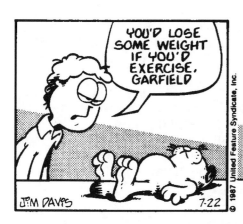

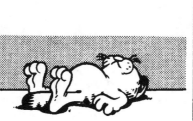

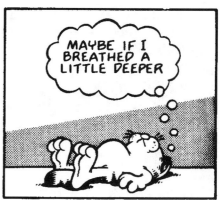

ficial. In fact, this is what most experts preached for years and years. Much to the delight of people struggling with their weight, the view of exercise has changed entirely in the last several years. What we know now, and what has been emphasized by prestigious groups like the American College of Sports Medicine and the Centers for Disease Control and Prevention, is that low levels of activity can be beneficial for health. We also know that low levels can be helpful for weight loss.

This turns everything upside down. It means that making small increases in physical activity counts as exercise. It means that even with modest changes, you may improve your health. It also means that we can set aside the biggest barrier to exercise—the thought that high levels are the only acceptable amounts. We hope you don't tire of us saying that any amount of exercise is beneficial, because it will come up a number of times in the program.

The Benefits of Exercise

There are seven reasons why physical activity is central to weight loss. Most people know only the first—that it burns calories.

▶ **Burns calories.** Exercise does burn calories, but this may be its least important benefit. Be careful to avoid feeling that a modest amount of exercise entitles you to more calories at the table. You will probably eat more calories than the exercise expended.

▶ **Counteracts the ills of overweight.** Exercise can help change the physical and psychological problems associated with being overweight. It can lower blood pressure and cholesterol and improve carbohydrate metabolism.

▶ **Helps control appetite.** Studies with both animals and humans suggest that exercise can help control appetite. It certainly does not stimulate appetite when people exercise in moderate amounts. If you exercise and feel increased hunger, your mind is at work rather than your body.

▶ **Preserves the body's muscle.** Your body loses both muscle and fat when you lose weight. The aim is to maximize fat loss. Combining exercise with diet does this more effectively than using diet alone.

▶ **Increases metabolic rate.** Eating less and losing weight slow down your metabolism. This is bad news because your body then uses less energy (calories) for basic functioning at a time when you want to burn more calories. Exercise speeds up metabolism, although the degree and duration of this increase is subject to debate. Exercising and eating less may help offset this drop in metabolic rate.

▶ **Improves confidence and psychological factors.** Exercise makes people feel good. Each time you are active is a symbol that you are making positive changes. This improves confidence and gives you a boost that can carry over to your eating plan. In addition, many people exercise to relieve stress. If you are one of the people who eats to relieve stress, exercise may accomplish the same thing but will burn rather than add calories.

▶ **Correlates with long-term success.** Exercise is the factor which best predicts who will lose weight and keep it off. If people are followed a year or more after a weight loss program, those who are exercising tend to be the ones who keep weight off. Furthermore, those individuals who are prescribed a structured exercise program during weight loss typically do better than those who just diet.

As you can see, the evidence in favor of exercise is clear and powerful. In the next lesson we will begin with specific suggestions for increasing activity. Walking will be the first step, so if you are walking now, keep up the good work! If not, don't hesitate to begin—but don't overdo it.

Dr. Steven Blair of The Cooper Institute for Aerobics Research in Dallas has written an excellent book for those individuals who find it difficult to find time to exercise. *Living With Exercise* is a step-by-step guide designed to help people incorporate increased physical activity into their daily lifestyle. For more information on this guide, contact The LEARN Education Center (1-800-736-7323).

Setting Personal Goals

You have several goals this week—some old, some new. Continue to take your medication every morning and keep a record. Troubleshoot instances when you forgot to take your medication last week, so you can prevent them in the future. Make copies of the new Expanded Food Diary and complete it each day, recording the types and amounts of food you eat, as well as times, places, and activities associated with eating. Most women should set a goal of eating approximately 1200 calories a day and men 1500 calories a day. Continue to search for patterns in your eating habits.

Finally, think about your attitudes toward physical activity, as you prepare to increase yours this week. Can you see exercise in a more positive light after reading the lesson? Increased activity brings many rewards, only one of which is long-term weight control. And, even small increases can help.

Self-Assessment Questionnaire

Lesson 3

T F 10. Exercise isn't of much use for weight loss because it burns relatively few calories.

T F 11. Exercise can help prevent the loss of muscle tissue during weight loss.

T F 12. The calorie is the measure of the amount of fat in food.

T F 13. The calorie level necessary to lose weight is the same for all people.

(Answers in Appendix C)

Expanded Food Diary—Lesson 3 *(sample)*   Today's Date_____

Description	Time	Feelings	Activity	Calories
Breakfast				
Coffee, 6 oz	7:30	Tired	Reading paper	0
Poached egg, 1 med				79
Bagel, ½ med				92
Orange juice, 1 cup				111
Total this meal				282
Lunch				
Roast beef sandwich, 2 oz, with 2T mayonnaise	12:30	Hurried	Working at desk	442
Water, 1 glass				0
Raspberry yogurt, 8 oz				90
Total this meal				532
Dinner				
Chicken breast-grilled, 3.5 oz	7:30	Relaxed	Watching TV	193
Green beans, 1 cup				44
Carrots, 1 cup, cooked				70
Wheat bread, 1 slice, dry				61
Skim milk, 1 cup				86
Total this meal				454
Snacks				
Celery, 4 stalks	10:00	Tense	Working at desk	24
Apple, 1 med	3:00	Frustrated	On break	81
Total snacks				105
Total calories for the day				1,373

Medication Taken Today   ☑ Yes   ❏ No

Food Groups from the Food Guide Pyramid:

Milk, yogurt, and cheese	☑ ☑ ❏
Meat, poultry, etc.	☑ ☑ ☑
Fruits	☑ ☑ ❏ ❏
Vegetables	☑ ☑ ☑ ☑ ☑
Breads, cereals, etc.	☑ ☑ ☑ ☑ ❏ ❏ ❏ ❏ ❏

Expanded Food Diary—Lesson 3   Today's Date_____

Description	Time	Feelings	Activity	Calories
Breakfast				
Total this meal				
Lunch				
Total this meal				
Dinner				
Total this meal				
Snacks				
Total snacks				
Total calories for the day				

Medication Taken Today   ❑ Yes   ❑ No

Food Groups from the Food Guide Pyramid:

Milk, yogurt, and cheese	❑ ❑ ❑
Meat, poultry, etc.	❑ ❑ ❑
Fruits	❑ ❑ ❑ ❑
Vegetables	❑ ❑ ❑ ❑ ❑
Breads, cereals, etc.	❑ ❑ ❑ ❑ ❑ ❑ ❑ ❑ ❑

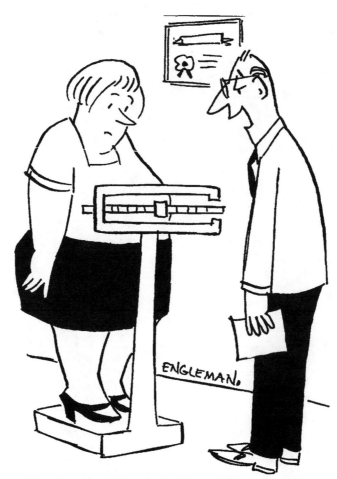

"To give my patients the incentive to diet, I've
decided to charge by the pound."

Lesson 4

We are ready to move on to new and exciting things. Our emphasis in this lesson will be on Lifestyle and Exercise, with information also on the other parts of The LEARN Program. You will begin to see how the areas of the LEARN model complement each other. For example, we will begin a structured walking program (Exercise) and will discuss the virtues of walking with a partner (Relationships). Our interpretation of the Expanded Food Diary (Lifestyle) will teach you to be aware of when you are eating from hunger or habit. We hope you can see how the different aspects of the program are woven together.

Analyzing Your Expanded Food Diary

Now that you have experience with the Expanded Food Diary, let's discuss what the information means. We are looking for several things. The first involves eating patterns that tell us whether your eating follows a reliable course from day-to-day. The second are triggers—the circumstances which provoke overeating.

The Search for Patterns

The Expanded Food Diary included spaces for the time of eating, feelings, and other activities. Did you find any patterns?

► **Time.** Did your eating cluster in certain parts of the day? Your eating times may vary depending on the day of the week. Some people keep a strict schedule on weekdays and then have less control on weekends. If you find times when control is difficult, think about scheduling alternative activities (like exercise).

► **Feelings.** Did you eat when you were bored, depressed, anxious, angry, or lonely? Other feelings may also be involved, like resentment, hostility, jealousy, or even joy. Seeing a pattern is a sure sign that you can learn more adaptive ways to cope with difficult feelings.

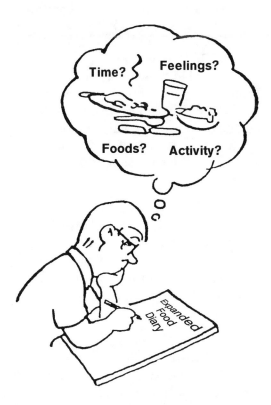

Searching for Patterns

► **Activity**. What do you do while eating? Watching television is the main culprit, but reading a newspaper, listening to a radio, or browsing through magazines can also be a problem. Doing two things at once insures that neither gets full attention. Eating already gets less attention than it deserves. Later we will discuss how eating can be separated from other activities.

► **Foods.** What types of foods do you eat? Do you crave carbohydrates at certain times? Do you eat foods because they are available or do you seek out the foods you love? Are some foods very difficult to eat in moderation?

Medication Diary

Just as you have reviewed your Food Diary, take a few minutes to examine your medication patterns. We hope you took MERIDIA every morning last week and recorded this information on your Expanded Food Diary. Congratulations if you did. If you forgot your medication on one or more days, can you identify the circumstances that led you to do so? These are the situations that need your attention.

Why is it so important to take MERIDIA regularly? Because you eat less at meals and throughout the day. This is the kind of appetite control that you can use every day.

It is common for people to adjust to the medication and for the side effects to fade with time. If this is not the case and you are troubled by symptoms, call your doctor. He or she can advise you on what steps to take.

How Often Should You Weigh Yourself?

We encouraged you at the outset of the program to weigh yourself weekly and to record the results on your Weight Change Record (on page 28). Many people wonder how frequently they should weigh themselves. One popular self-help group, Overeaters Anonymous, does not weigh its members at all. The theory is that more frequent weighing gives "too much power to the scale." Other programs recommend that members weigh regularly to get feedback on their progress. Some people weigh themselves many times each day. The average for people who enter weight loss programs is about once per day.

Feedback from the scale can be a nice incentive for some individuals. It reminds them of the progress they have made and spurs their efforts. Others despair when the scale shows no change,

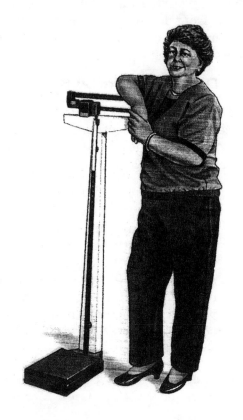

and they look with horror at how much weight they have to lose to reach their goal. Since the scale represents various things to different people, it can be either friend or foe. Please remember that it can be a *powerful* friend or foe, so think seriously about how often you and the scale should communicate.

This is where *your* judgment must prevail. Weigh yourself as often as you see fit. We recommend no less than once each week and no more than once each day. If you are a frequent weigher you may get discouraged by weight gains beyond your control. Fluid shifts alone can lead to gains or losses of several pounds. However, if you feel the scale can be a motivating factor, try weighing more often.

One problem with paying too much attention to the scale is that it can lead to undeserved euphoria or disappointment. An example would be a person who does not do well on their eating plan, but shows a weight loss anyway, perhaps due to water loss from a menstrual cycle. The person may think she can stray from the plan and still lose weight. The opposite side of the coin is the person who does well on the program and gains weight anyway. Again, this can happen for several reasons, including fluid shifts. The danger lies in the person assuming that his or her efforts are going for nothing.

The scale should be a general guide about progress, not a day-to-day index of whether your program is working. This is why the Food Diaries (Monitoring Forms) at the end of each lesson ask you to record your calorie intake, your behavior changes, and your exercise. If these change, you *will* lose weight. Paying attention to these will make you less vulnerable to the vagaries of the scale.

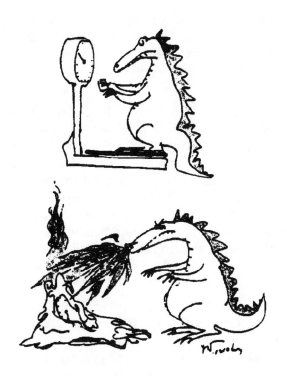

On the Move

Much has been said about the glories of exercise. Some joggers boast of a runner's high, and others feel that sweating and panting are the path to heaven. Some overweight people react to this hysteria by giving up on exercise. However, the LEARN concept of physical activity is not your usual exercise program. The object is to make it fun and to increase the number of activities you consider *exercise*. The first example is walking. Other activities will follow later in the program.

Is Exercise Safe for You?

Today we begin a walking program. If you are doing more vigorous activity, keep it up if you feel comfortable and have medical clearance. If you are not exercising regularly, the walking program may be for you. Walking has many virtues. It is healthy and helps you lose weight. It is easy and poses little physical risk (depending on where you walk!). But before we begin, we must ask if it is safe for you to exercise.

Moderate activity, including the walking discussed here, is safe for most people. There are, however, some people with physical problems who should not begin an exercise program without being checked carefully by a physician. This should extend beyond a simple checkup, and the physician should be alerted that the person is being checked to determine whether regular exercise is advisable.

The Physical Activity Readiness Questionnaire (PAR-Q) on page 58 provides a simple questionnaire you can complete to see if it is safe for you to increase your physical activity. Read and answer each question carefully. If any factor applies to you, see your physician before doing any exercise. This is serious and goes beyond the usual warning to *see your doctor* that is found in every diet book. If you are uncertain about what the terms mean or about whether you qualify, play it safe, and consult a physician. The list is adapted from the Canadian questionnaire by Dr. Steven Blair of The Cooper Institute for Aerobics Research.

Starting Your Walking Program

Walking has many advantages. Here are a few:

▶ **Almost anybody can do it.** Compared to many activities like swimming, basketball, or horseback riding, walking is an activity available to most people.

▶ **Do it at your pace**. You can walk fast or walk slow, and you can do it whenever you want—not just when the health club is open.

▶ **Walking is easy.** You need not strain with exertion when you walk. Even low levels are helpful.

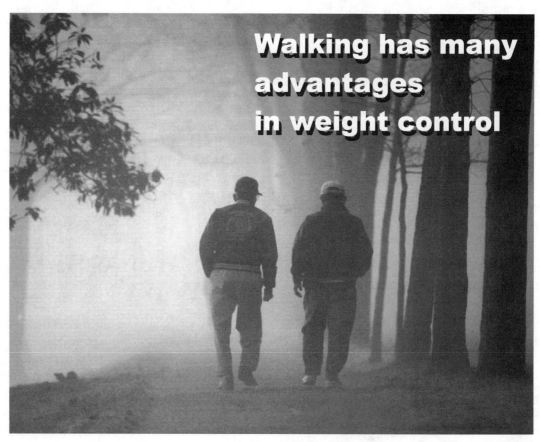

Walking has many advantages in weight control

- **Walking is enjoyable.** Think of all you can see while walking. You can enjoy the sights, listen to a portable tape player, or walk with friends.
- **It is cheap.** You do not need a health club membership or expensive equipment.
- **It can be a social event.** You may like company while you walk. It is a nice time to be with someone you enjoy.

This may surprise you, but walking burns almost the same number of calories as running the same distance. How far you go is more important than how fast you go. It needn't knock you out for it to help.

Clothes, Shoes, and Weather

Before you begin, consider clothes, shoes, and weather. Wear clothes that make you feel comfortable. There is nothing special about expensive jogging suits. Walking will help just as much if you are adorned with an old sweatshirt and jeans.

Shoes are important and may be worth the money for a good pair. Go to a sporting goods store and try on several brands. Pick one that feels good. Good shoes can help your feet, keep you from tiring, and reduce the chance of orthopedic injury.

Weather can be tricky. Avoiding exercise when it is too hot or too cold is wise. If the temperature is above 90 degrees or is below zero, it is best to get your exercise inside. This still leaves most days of the year available. Most people manage to do their walking in nearly any weather.

Wear layers of clothing in cold weather. When it gets quite cold you might wear a cotton T-shirt, several sweatshirts, and a windbreaker. The cotton will absorb the perspiration. You may feel cold for the first few minutes, but you will warm up rapidly. If you get too hot, you can remove one of the layers. Wear a hat because much of the body's heat loss occurs through the head (especially if you are a hot head!). Mittens will keep hands warmer than gloves.

Being careful in hot weather is also important. Walking in the morning or evening may help avoid the hottest parts of the day. Wear as few clothes as possible, and never wear rubber suits or other clothes designed to make you sweat. Whatever weight you lose in sweating will be regained, and trapping the body's heat in hot weather can be dangerous. Drink plenty of water. It is safe to drink water before, during, and after exercise.

Mall Walking

Shopping malls are a good place to walk in inclement weather, or even when the weather is nice. In many parts of the country, *mall walkers* go to malls early in the morning and walk alone or in groups. This is a terrific idea.

The walkers who go with friends or who make new friends find the social contacts helpful in adhering to a regular schedule. Also, walking by the stores each morning leaves you poised for action the minute new "SALE" signs are posted!

Barriers to Exercise

Many overweight people are reluctant to exercise because they are embarrassed. This occurs for several reasons. The extra weight can make exercise physically difficult. People who have been overweight all their lives may have little experience with vigorous exercise, and the experiences they do have may be unpleasant (being picked last for teams,

The Physical Activity Readiness Questionnaire (PAR-Q)

The PAR-Q is designed to help you help yourself. Many health benefits are associated with regular exercise, and the completion of the PAR-Q is a sensible first-step to take if you are planning to increase the amount of physical activity in your life.

For most people, physical activity should not pose any problem or hazard. The PAR-Q has been designed to identify the small number of adults for whom physical activity might be inappropriate or those who should have medical advice concerning the type of activity most suitable for them.

Common sense is your best guide in answering these few questions. Please read them carefully, and circle the YES or NO for each question as it applies to you.

1.   YES   NO   Has your doctor ever said you have heart trouble?

2.   YES   NO   Do you frequently have pains in your heart and chest?

3.   YES   NO   Do you often feel faint or have spells of severe dizziness?

4.   YES   NO   Has a doctor ever said your blood pressure was too high?

5.   YES   NO   Has your doctor ever told you that you have a bone or joint problem, such as arthritis, that has been aggravated by exercise, or might be made worse with exercise?

6.   YES   NO   Is there a good physical reason, not mentioned here, why you should not follow any activity program, even if you wanted to?

7.   YES   NO   Are you over age 65 and not accustomed to vigorous exercise?

If you answered YES to one or more questions:

If you have not recently done so, consult with your personal physician by telephone or in person BEFORE increasing your physical activity and/or taking a fitness test. Tell him or her what questions you answered YES.

After a medical evaluation, seek advice from your physician as to your suitability for:

Unrestricted physical activity, probably on a gradually increasing basis, or

Restricted and supervised activity to meet your specific needs, at least on an initial basis. Check in your community for special programs or services.

If you answered NO to all questions:

If you answered the questions on the PAR-Q accurately, you have reasonable assurance to your present suitability for:

A graduated exercise program. A gradual increase in proper exercise promotes good fitness development while minimizing or eliminating discomfort.

An exercise test. Simple tests of fitness may be undertaken if you so desire.

Postpone exercise or exercise testing:

If you have a temporary minor illness, such as a common cold.

Adapted with permission from Blair SN. (1991). *Living With Exercise*. Dallas, TX: American Health Publishing Company.

---

teasing, etc.). Most important, however, is the fear of what others will think when a heavy person jogs by or cruises past on a bike.

Put aside these feelings right now! You have nothing to be ashamed of. Your weight loss program is more important than being shy or embarrassed. Losing weight is a long process as it is and will be even longer if you wait to trim down before starting to exercise. Don't worry about what others think. In fact, most normal-weight people give heavy people much credit for making positive changes.

The 15-Minute Prescription

After all this information on walking, it is time to begin. Begin gradually and work your way up. There is no danger in starting with less than you can tolerate, but starting with more can be painful and discouraging.

Begin walking for 15 minutes each day. If you have difficulty doing this all in one bout, try three five-minute walks. When you can do this with ease, increase by five minutes each day to the point you feel some exertion. If the 15-minute walk is too difficult, subtract time until you feel comfortable. *The goal is to walk 30 minutes to one hour each day.* Try to gradually increase your walking to this level, so as not to make it difficult or unpleasant.

You know best when your schedule can accommodate your walking. Here are six suggestions:

❶ Get up 30 minutes early to walk
❷ Walk at lunch
❸ Walk during work breaks
❹ Walk after work
❺ Walk after dinner
❻ Walk before bedtime

Do your level best to walk every day. Making it part of your routine is important, like brushing your teeth, making your bed, or taking a shower. This is the only way it will be integrated into your lifestyle. However, do not despair if you miss a day now and then. The long-term picture is more important than if you miss a day occasionally. We will discuss your attitudes about exercise later in the program.

Experiment with walking different places, at different times, and with different people (or try it alone). Find the

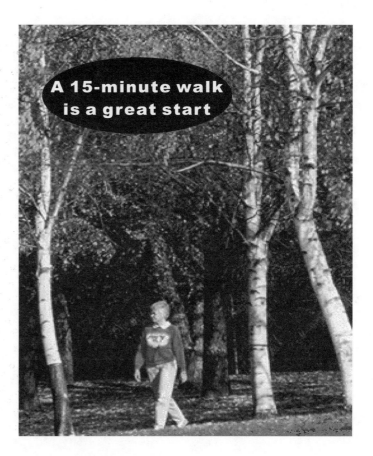

A 15-minute walk is a great start

way you like it best. In Lesson 5, we will present specific ideas about making walking fun.

You Can Win a Presidential Sports Award

A program sponsored by the President's Council on Physical Fitness and Sports now makes awards available to adults for participation in a number of activities. The award, called the *Presidential Sports Award*, can be earned by participation in one or more of 43 qualifying sports. Examples of these sports are backpacking, bicycling, bowling, fitness walking, golf, jogging, racquetball, rowing, running, sailing, swimming, tennis, and general types of exercise that you might do at a spa, aerobics class, a gym, or even at home. Chances are whatever activities you like and can do are on the list.

These awards are for regular people doing regular exercise—you do not have to be an Olympic athlete. You simply write to the address below and receive a sheet called the Personal Fitness Log. The sheet explains which activities are included and what you must do to be granted the award. You fill out the sheet as you exercise, send it in, and receive a handsome Personalized Certificate of Achievement with your name and qualifying sport, suitable for framing. You can also receive a nice lapel pin, and can win as many awards in as many sports as you would like. To receive the information on the award, just send a stamped, self-addressed envelope to:

> Presidential Sports Award
> President's Council on Physical
>   Fitness and Sports
> 200 Independence SW, Suite 738H
> Washington, DC 20201
> Telephone (202) 690-9000

To show how these awards are truly achievable, we will list the criteria for earning awards in the "Fitness Walking" and "Tennis" categories. For Fitness Walking, a person must do the following within a four-month period:

❶ Walk a minimum of 125 miles,

❷ Each walk must be continuous, without pauses for rest, and the pace must be at least four m.p.h. (15 minutes per mile), and

❸ No more than two and one-half miles in any one day may be credited to the total.

For tennis, one must:

❶ Play tennis a minimum of 50 hours,

❷ No more than one and one-half hours in any one day may be credited to the total, and

❸ The total must include at least 25 sets of singles and/or doubles.

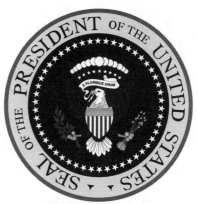

**The Presidential
Sports Award**

These examples show that you can win the awards, even if you are struggling with your weight. Some effort will be required, but then effort is just what we want, right? This program can be very motivating. You may or may not be up to the required amount of exercise now, but you probably will be before long. So, write now! You may win the award before you know it.

A Walking Partnership

This is a good time to introduce the "R" (Relationships) part of the LEARN approach. Since we are focusing on walking, we can discuss its social aspects. Some people like to walk with others while some like to go solo. You are the best judge of what is right for you.

Walking with another person can be a powerful way to make walking more enjoyable. The company is a nice distraction because you can talk about politics, speculate about the stock market, bet on ball games, or best of all, gossip! A partner can also help by establishing a regular time for walking. There may be days when you would stay home, but knowing that a partner is waiting is just the stimulus you need to get out and get going.

Having a partner is not for everyone. Walking can be a nice time to enjoy yourself, to reflect, and to think about important matters. Don't feel pressured to have a partner, because going it alone may be best for you. Think about the advantages of walking with a partner or walking alone. You might try it both ways to see which you like.

Building Skills and Confidence

Albert Bandura, a highly respected psychologist at Stanford University, developed a concept known as self-efficacy. The concept states that an individual's chance of accomplishing some goal depends on having the skills to make the change and the confidence that the change can occur. The concept applies beautifully to weight control.

Skills are what this program is all about. You will be exposed to many approaches. You'll take each for a test drive and will find the ones that work best for you. The skills will deal with what you eat, whether you are active, and perhaps most importantly, the thoughts, feelings, and attitudes you have about many important factors. Thinking helpful thoughts, and looking at the world in a constructive way involves skills that you can cultivate.

Confidence is the second part of the picture. If you are confident that you can handle high-risk situations, that you can bounce back when you falter, and that you can keep your motivation high, you'll have the strength to hang in there when things get tough. You'll approach situations with a new sense of control. We will be speaking many times about confidence.

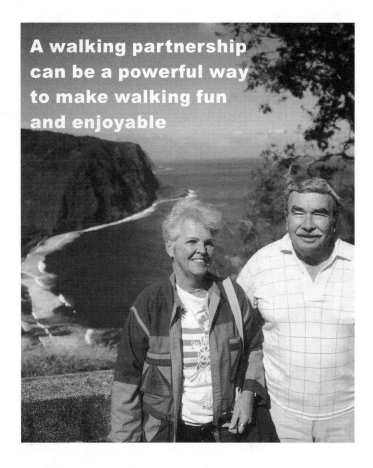

A walking partnership can be a powerful way to make walking fun and enjoyable

Sometimes these discussions of confidence will sound like a pep talk, but pep talks can be pretty helpful. One of the most important things you can do is to hold your own internal pep talks. What you say when you do well, when you do not do well, or when you are pondering how best to proceed will be central to your success. You may be surprised by how often we will discuss the talks you have with yourself.

Setting Personal Goals

The main goal for this week is to begin your walking program. Walk as many days as possible by using the guidelines provided in this lesson. Be sure to take it easy if you have not been exercising regularly. Continue to use the Expanded Food Diary. It will help you identify patterns and triggers. Remember what you learned the previous week and see if you can develop even more insight into situations which place you at high risk for overeating. Last, continue to take MERIDIA every morning and record when you do so.

Self-Assessment Questionnaire

Lesson 4

T F   14. Walking one mile burns almost as many calories as running the mile.

T F   15. Expensive exercise suits are worth the money because the special materials help the body.

T F   16. Everyone should walk with a partner because the company increases pleasure.

T F   17. You can identify your triggers and high-risk situations for overeating by keeping a food diary and examining it carefully.

T F   18. You should weigh yourself every morning.

(Answers in Appendix C)

Food Diary—Lesson 4

Today's Date_____

Description	Time	Feelings	Activity	Calories
Breakfast				
Total this meal				
Lunch				
Total this meal				
Dinner				
Total this meal				
Snacks				
Total snacks				
Total calories for the day				

Medication Taken Today   ❏ Yes   ❏ No

Food Groups from the Food Guide Pyramid:

Milk, yogurt, and cheese	❏ ❏ ❏
Meat, poultry, etc.	❏ ❏ ❏
Fruits	❏ ❏ ❏ ❏
Vegetables	❏ ❏ ❏ ❏ ❏
Breads, cereals, etc.	❏ ❏ ❏ ❏ ❏ ❏ ❏ ❏ ❏

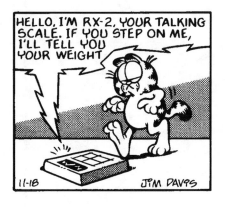 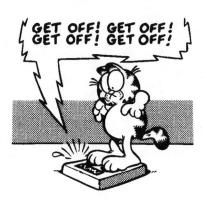 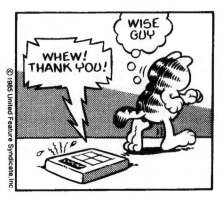

Lesson 5

Congratulations! You have now completed the first month of The LEARN Program. We hope you are pleased with your progress. Take a few moments to review —and enjoy—your many accomplishments this past month. You may be surprised to see all that you have done.

Quality of Life

One way of assessing the changes you have made in the first month is to complete the Quality of Life Self-Assessment on the next page. Rate how satisfied you are with each of the 12 areas listed, including your mood, eating habits, and body image. Complete these items based on how you feel today.

Now compare your responses to those before you began the program. You will have to turn back to the Introduction and Orientation on page 11 to see how you felt back then. Look at each item, then and now. We suspect that your satisfaction has increased in at least one area, if not several. Many people report increased satisfaction the first month with their mood, energy level, general appearance, eating habits, and physical mobility and activity. What is remarkable is that these changes occur relatively quickly and with only a modest weight loss. That is an excellent return on your weight loss investment!

Satisfaction may come more slowly in other areas, such as with your social life or leisure and recreational activities. If you have specific desires in these areas, such as wanting to meet new people or taking up tennis or golf, make a plan for how you can start achieving these goals. Do not make the mistake of thinking you have to be at some magical goal weight in order to socialize more or take up a new hobby.

Your Health

You may have noticed changes in your health over the past month. You may feel more alert and energetic or may be sleeping better. People frequently report such changes with only small weight losses. You might be scheduled to meet with your doctor at about this time in the program. Tell your doctor about any symptoms you still have.

Your doctor can also assess other changes in your physical health. For example, if your blood pressure, cholesterol, or blood sugar were high before you started this program, they may be slightly lower by now. These reductions are a result of your weight loss and your improved eating and activity habits. Your overall health should continue to improve over the next few months as you

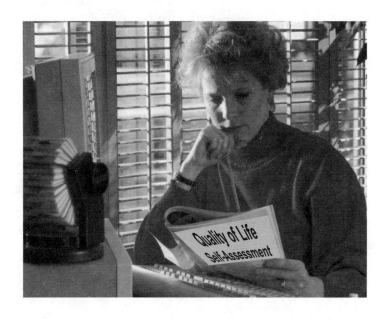

Quality of Life Self-Assessment

Please use the following scale to rate how satisfied you feel now about different aspects of your daily life. Choose any number from this list (1 to 9) and indicate your choice on the questions below

1 = Extremely Dissatisfied

2 = Very Dissatisfied

3 = Moderately Dissatisfied

4 = Somewhat Dissatisfied

5 = Neutral

6 = Somewhat Satisfied

7 = Moderately Satisfied

8 = Very Satisfied

9 = Extremely Satisfied

1. ___ Mood (feelings of sadness, worry, happiness, etc.)
2. ___ Self-esteem
3. ___ Confidence, self-assurance and comfort in social situations
4. ___ Energy and feeling healthy
5. ___ Health problems (diabetes, high blood pressure, etc.)
6. ___ General appearance
7. ___ Social life
8. ___ Leisure and recreational activities
9. ___ Physical mobility and physical activity
10. ___ Eating habits
11. ___ Body image
12. ___ Overall quality of life

progress through the program. What a wonderful accomplishment—to improve your health and well being!

Weight Loss

We believe that improvements in quality of life and physical health are the real measures of success. However, it's hard not to focus on weight loss. People frequently want to know how they are doing as compared with others. During the first month of this program, most women lose approximately four to six pounds and most men approximately six to eight pounds. Don't worry if you have lost slightly more or less; people vary just like cars and gas mileage.

If you have lost fewer than four pounds, you and your doctor will want to review your progress. If this is the first time in years that you have been able to lose weight, you will probably want to remain on the medication. If, however, you feel that the medication is not helping (to feel fuller at meals) you should notify your doctor so she or he can reevaluate your situation. Your doctor may wish to change your dose of MERIDIA. Doctors do not understand why, but some people are more responsive to MERIDIA than are others. The same is true of pain remedies. One brand may cure your headaches but do nothing for your best friend. We'll discuss below some possible reasons for small weight losses the first month but want you to know that the

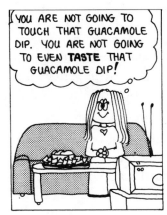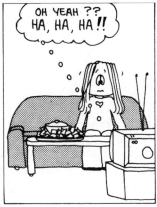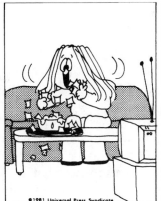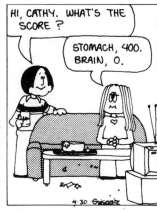

medication does appear to be more effective with some people than others. This is true of all medications.

You may have had the opposite experience the first month and lost far more weight than you had expected. Women who have lost more than 8 pounds and men more than 12 pounds should talk to their doctors. Women should make sure that they eat at least 1200 calories a day and men 1500 calories. Increasing your calorie intake above these levels may be necessary if your weight loss does not slow in the next few weeks. Rapid weight loss can increase the risk of developing gallstones and other health complications.

Factors Affecting Your Weight Loss

Two principal factors have probably affected your rate of weight loss this past month. They include:

❶ How faithfully you have taken MERIDIA

❷ Your daily calorie intake

Let's review these briefly.

Medication Adherence

Taking MERIDIA every morning will help ensure that you achieve your opti-

mal weight loss. The medication will help you feel fuller at meals and may reduce unwanted eating between meals. Check your medication log by reviewing your Food Diary for the past week. If you took your medication six or seven days, that is terrific. You have developed an effective routine. If you took it fewer than six days, try to determine how you can adjust your schedule to make medication a part of your morning routine. You may want to ask a family member or friend to remind you.

Calorie Intake

A smaller-than-anticipated weight loss can also result from not decreasing your calorie intake sufficiently. As we discussed in Lesson 2, if you eat 500 fewer calories a day than your body burns, you will lose a pound a week. If, instead, you eat only 250 fewer calories a day, you will lose only about a half-pound a week.

If you lost less than four pounds the first month, plan to pay extra attention to your Food Diary this week. Try to incorporate these tips:

▶ Record your foods and beverages immediately after consuming them. This will ensure that you remember everything.

▶ Measure portion sizes to ensure that you are eating the amounts that you think you are. Most people underestimate their daily calorie intake by 20–40 percent, so be careful.

- ▶ When reading food labels, be sure to determine how many servings the item contains. For example, a 20-ounce soda contains two and one-half servings (one serving equals eight ounces). Each serving has 100 calories or a total of 250 calories for the whole bottle. That is a big difference from thinking that the bottle contains one serving and only 100 calories.

- ▶ Keep a running total of your calories throughout the day. That way, you will know if you have enough calories for a second serving at dinner or for a bedtime snack.

- ▶ Set a calorie goal for the week, not just each day. That way if you exceed your goal on Thursday, you can eat a bit less on Friday, Saturday, and Sunday—and still make your goal for the week. The closer you come to your calorie goal each week, the better your weight loss will be.

Compulsive Eating and Binge Eating

Doctors increasingly recognize that a small but significant minority of overweight individuals struggle with epi-sodes of compulsive eating or binge eating. Overeaters Anonymous popularized the most widely used term for this problem—compulsive overeating. Researchers have called this binge eating.

The official definition of binge eating has two features. The first is eating what others would consider a large amount of food and the second is feeling out of control. When this happens with sufficient frequency (two times a week or more) and over a sufficient period of time (six months) a person can qualify for a diagnosis called Binge Eating Disorder. We hasten to add that some people have binges many more times than this, and some people have fewer or less frequent binges but still have a troubling problem.

In the early stages of research on binge eating, some experts felt that individuals who ate compulsively needed treatment for this type of eating disorder in addition to whatever help they needed for weight. More recently, research has shown that individuals who participate in a program like The LEARN Program stop binge eating as well as people who get a program focused specifically on the binge eating, but in addition, lose more weight. Therefore, if you have a problem with binge eating, you may find that this program helps with both the control over eating and with weight loss.

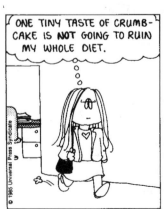

ONE TINY TASTE OF CRUMB-CAKE IS **NOT** GOING TO RUIN MY WHOLE DIET.

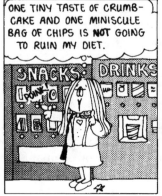

ONE TINY TASTE OF CRUMB-CAKE AND ONE MINISCULE BAG OF CHIPS IS **NOT** GOING TO RUIN MY DIET.

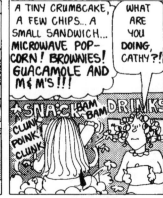

A TINY CRUMBCAKE, A FEW CHIPS... A SMALL SANDWICH... MICROWAVE POP-CORN! BROWNIES! GUACAMOLE AND M&M'S!!!

WHAT ARE YOU DOING, CATHY?!

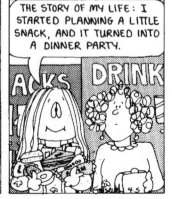

THE STORY OF MY LIFE: I STARTED PLANNING A LITTLE SNACK, AND IT TURNED INTO A DINNER PARTY.

The Neighborhood

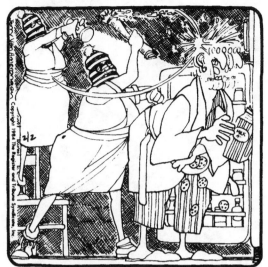

Since joining Diet Watchers Anonymous, Noel Cramer continues to be surprised at just how comprehensive the group's services are.

There will be some people who need additional help. If by this time in the program you are having problems with eating compulsively, you might examine whether additional resources would be helpful. We can suggest three approaches.

The first approach is to use a book entitled *Overcoming Binge Eating* written by Dr. Christopher Fairburn, a leading authority from Oxford University in England. The book is an excellent guide that has been tested thoroughly and brings the best of science to the reader in a useable and friendly format. The book is published by Guilford Press in New York and can be ordered by calling 1–800–736–7323. This is the best such guide of its type in the world today.

The second, but more expensive alternative, is to seek counseling. If you choose this course, try to see someone with special experience in treating eating disorders. Several organizations can provide the names of professionals in your area who have experience with eating disorders, although there is no guar-

---

Support Organizations for Eating Disorders
(Potential Help for Compulsive Eating/Binge Eating)

United States

National Eating Disorders Organization
445 E. Granville Road
Worthington, OH 43085-3195
614-436-1112

American Anorexia/Bulimia Association
418 E. 76th Street
New York, NY 10021
212-734-1114

National Association of Anorexia Nervosa and Related Diseases
P.O. Box 7
Highland Park, IL 60035
708-831-3438

Anorexia Nervosa and Related Eating Disorders
P.O. Box 5102
Eugene, OR 97405
503-344-1144

Canada

National Eating Disorder Information Centre
200 Elizabeth Street
College Way
Toronto, Ontario M5G 2C4
416-340-4156

Bulimia, Anorexia Association
3640 Wells Street
Windsor, Ontario N9C 1T9
519-253-7545

United Kingdom

Eating Disorders Association
Sackville Place
44 Magdalen Street
Norwich
Norfolk NR3 1J3
01603-621414

---

antee that such professionals are truly skilled. These organizations are listed in the table above. The two approaches that have been proven effective for binge eating are cognitive behavior therapy and interpersonal psychotherapy, so you might ask if the professional you contact offers one of these.

A final approach is to consider help from Overeaters Anonymous (OA). While OA has not been evaluated, it does offer strong support and a focus on compulsive eating. For some people, the

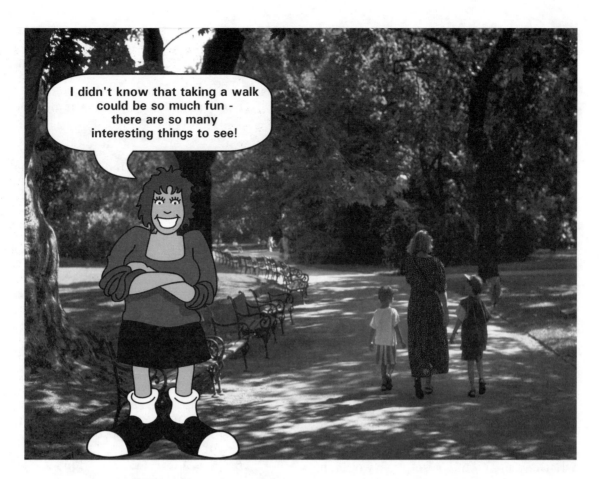

support, the around-the-clock help available from a sponsor, and the group meetings can be quite helpful.

Perfecting Your Walking Program

How are you doing with your walking program? Do you feel good about this positive activity? It may still be too early to know how you will like it, but if your initial reactions are positive, then you are on the right track.

Maximizing the Pleasure of Walking

Walking can be lots of fun if you consider a few facts. The more fun you have, the more you will walk. Making the exercise a permanent habit is one key to success in this program.

▶ **Pay attention.** There are many interesting things to see wherever you walk. Look at the style of the houses or buildings you pass, or what your neighbors plant in their yards. What sort of cars go by and what type of people do you see? This is a good way to take advantage of what has always been available.

▶ **Bring entertainment.** Some walkers like to carry portable radios and cassette players. It is fine to listen to the news or music. Decide whether you want to enjoy the outside world or drown it out.

▶ **Don't overdo it.** A sure way to undermine an exercise program is to do too much too soon. You will be sore, frustrated, and discouraged. Beware of the tendency to increase your exercise too fast, even though you may be enjoying it.

> **Take a gradual approach.** *Gradual* is a key word in this program. Start exercise at the level you need, not what some book or videotape tells you. Work your way up from there, but do it sensibly. This is the principle of *shaping* discussed later in the program.

Increasing Your Walking

In Lesson 4, we recommended that your walking program begin with 15 minutes each day. If you can do this comfortably, increase the time. Again, your judgment must prevail. Do no more than you can handle, but try to make it a routine part of your day.

We recommend that you add five minutes of walking each day until you reach our goal of one hour of walking each day. As you add time, stop when you feel tired or uncomfortable. For example, you may feel fine when increasing from 15 to 20 minutes, but may feel fatigue or discomfort when going to 25 minutes.

Back up to the 20-minute comfort level and stay there until you are ready to move ahead. Some people will stay at one level for many weeks before moving ahead while others can progress more rapidly. Tailoring these guidelines to your needs is important.

Benefits of Increasing Physical Activity

We want you to have a clear understanding of what exercise is and what it *can* and *cannot* do for you. The more realistic your expectations and the more positive your outlook, the more likely you are to enjoy physical activity, both now and in the future.

As we view it, exercise involves any activity in which you move your body and expend calories. Moving your arms in circles is a type of exercise, as is rolling down a car window (if you can still find a car without electric windows). Similarly, walking up the stairs in your home or apartment counts as exercise and so does driving to a health club to work out on a Stair Master. We prefer the first method of climbing stairs; it is more practical and not as sweaty!

Any duration of physical activity counts, whether 15 seconds, 15 minutes, or 15 hours. You burn calories when you get up to change the TV channel, take a walk during your lunch break, or ride all day in the Tour de France (the famous French bike race). Over the course of a day, brief bouts of activity can add up to a lot of exercise. Just ask anyone who has waited tables. You do not to have to exercise for a certain amount of time to improve your well-being or health—any type and amount of activity counts.

Improved Health, Fitness, and Fun

You now know what exercise is. What are its benefits? We believe that the principal benefits are improved physical and emotional well-being. Exercise improves blood pressure, cholesterol, blood sugar and overall health. This was shown in a recent study in which overweight individuals who exercised regularly had a lower risk of heart disease and premature death than did people who were thin but inactive.

Perhaps the best reason to exercise is that it makes you feel good about yourself. Even a quick two-minute walk can help clear your mind and give you a lift. Over time, longer bouts of activity can make you feel more self-confident and more attuned to your body. Many of our clients tell us that simple activities such as stretching, dancing, and walking help

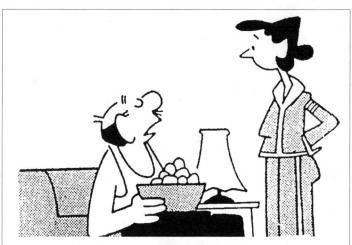

"Stop nagging me about exercise. For your information, opening a bag of chips involves more than 25 different muscles!"

them rediscover their bodies and enjoy movement for the sake of movement.

Exercise and Weight Loss

You probably noticed that we have not emphasized the weight-reducing benefits of exercise. This is for two reasons. First, it takes a lot of exercise to lose one pound of fat. For most people, it requires walking at least 25 to 30 miles or spending five to six hours a week in an intensive aerobics class. That is a lot of activity. Most people cannot exercise enough each week to lose more than about a third of a pound of fat. Second, judging the benefits of exercise on the basis of weight loss is bound to disappoint you some weeks. Your bathroom scale probably cannot reliably detect a weight loss of a half-pound or less. Sooner or later you will get on the scale and hear yourself exclaiming, "It's not fair. I exercised five days this week and didn't lose anything! What's the point?"

The way out of this trap is to separate activity from weight loss. Increase your physical activity for the sake of the pleasure and improved health that it will bring. These are important payoffs in themselves. And, there is a long-term reward. People who exercise regularly are far more likely to maintain their weight loss than are those who are not physically active. Exercise can facilitate long-term weight control by improving mood, food choices, and self-control—in addition to burning calories. During weight maintenance, most of our clients tell us that they exercise because they love it. Keeping off lost weight is only one of many benefits.

We hope you will keep these points in mind over the next few weeks as you increase your physical activity. Enjoy your walking program.

Setting Personal Goals

Your goals this week include scheduling a visit with your doctor if you have not already seem him or her during the first month. This will give you a chance to ask questions and to review your progress. You may want to make a list of topics to discuss with your doctor. Continue to take MERIDIA each morning and to complete your Food Diary. Keep up the search for patterns in your eating habits by identifying times, places, or activities that prompt your eating. Finally, focus on ways to maximize your pleasure while walking this week. Enjoy the scenery or an audio tape while walking. Try to become more aware of muscles and movements that you may not have noticed for years. Find something rewarding in your activity other than the promise of weight loss. That will increase your enjoyment—both today and a year from today.

Self-Assessment Questionnaire

Lesson 5

T F   19. Weight loss is the best measure of success in The LEARN Program.

T F   20. Most people have difficulty estimating the amounts of food they eat and the calories they consume.

T F   21. Exercise produces large weight losses on a short-term basis.

T F   22. Binge eating is characterized by eating large amounts of food with an accompanying sense of loss of control.

T F   23. Exercise must be strenuous in order to be beneficial.

(Answers in Appendix C)

Food Diary—Lesson 5

Today's Date _____

Description	Time	Feelings	Activity	Calories
Breakfast				
Total this meal				
Lunch				
Total this meal				
Dinner				
Total this meal				
Snacks				
Total snacks				
Total calories for the day				

Medication Taken Today   ❏ Yes   ❏ No

Food Groups from the Food Guide Pyramid:

    Milk, yogurt, and cheese   ❏ ❏ ❏

    Meat, poultry, etc.   ❏ ❏ ❏

    Fruits   ❏ ❏ ❏ ❏

    Vegetables   ❏ ❏ ❏ ❏ ❏

    Breads, cereals, etc.   ❏ ❏ ❏ ❏ ❏ ❏ ❏ ❏ ❏

Lesson 6

We have made significant progress in dealing with issues of medication and lifestyle change. In this lesson, we will deal with a new approach to change—the ABC's of behavior. We will also cover ways to seize control over your eating and strategies to deal with something you may not have considered—our toxic food environment. Finally, we will introduce you to a new Monitoring Form that will help you track your personal goals.

The ABC's of Behavior

As we progress through the program, you will learn ways to change your behavior. We will use the ABC approach. The letters stand for Antecedents, Behavior, and Consequences.

Antecedents

Antecedents are the events, feelings, and situations which occur *before* eating. These usually occur together in a series of steps called the Behavior Chain, which will be discussed in Lesson 21.

Behavior

Behavior refers to eating itself and to the related events and feelings. The relevant factors are the speed of eating, rate of chewing, taste of food, and the events that take place *during* eating.

Consequences

Consequences are the events, feelings, and attitudes that follow eating. These factors happen *after* eating and can determine whether the eating will occur again.

You can see each aspect of the ABC approach in the case of Steve. He was home on the weekend watching a football game. Steve was excited by the game because he bet $20 with his neighbor. He went to the kitchen to get his favorite TV snack, cheese curls. He ate the cheese curls rapidly and did not taste each one. He ate until he was very full and then felt guilty about eating so much.

The antecedents were being at home, watching the football game, being excited, and having the cheese curls available. The behavior was eating rapidly until very full. Steve did not taste all the cheese curls. The consequences were an unpleasant, full feeling in his stomach and guilt about overeating.

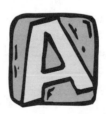

Antecedents occur BEFORE

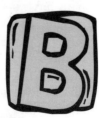

Behavior occurs DURING

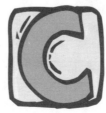

Consequences occur AFTER

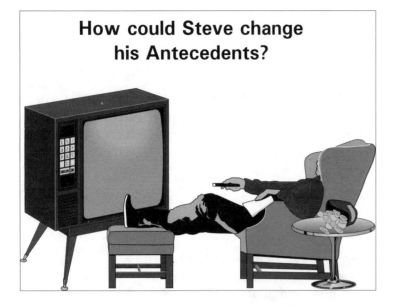

How could Steve change his Antecedents?

This analysis gives us many ideas about reducing Steve's chances for overeating. Steve could alter the antecedents by doing something other than watching the game, which is a high-risk situation, or by not having the cheese curls in the house. The behavior could be changed by eating slowly and savoring every bite. The consequences could change if he had different attitudes and could prevent the guilt and self-doubt that might stimulate more eating.

We will use the ABC approach in upcoming lessons. You can prepare yourself by thinking about the antecedents, behaviors, and consequences related to your eating. One way to do this is to review your Food Diaries from the past weeks and to raise your level of analysis a notch or two. You have been thinking about events that trigger eating (the antecedents), but think of the eating itself and the consequences. If you think ahead to situations that may be risky for you, you can predict in advance what the A, B, and C parts are likely to be. This puts you in a good position to cope with even the greatest challenges.

Let's use the example of Sandy. Her greatest risk is after work when she is driving home. She is happy her day is over, she is tired, and she is used to stopping at the convenience store or McDonald's for something to help her unwind. When she gets home she feels guilty and loses more of her control, and then bingo, she has a bad night. Because she has done this so many times, the pattern may seem impossible to control.

What can Sandy do? She can look at the antecedents, the behavior, and consequences, and can change this sequence of events in a number of ways. She could have something healthy to eat (like an apple) just before she leaves work. Sandy could take a few minutes to relax before leaving work, drive a different way home, or react differently by not falling apart when she arrives home. And these are only a *few* ways to use the ABC approach. See if you can apply it to events that happen in your life.

Taking Control of Your Eating

The Food Diaries have helped you discover patterns in your eating, and this section will give you some concrete advice on how to disrupt those patterns. These are classic strategies that have been used successfully by countless people. Let's see if they might work for you.

Many people have situations, times, or activities that stimulate eating. These events become *paired* with eating so that the event can make you feel hungry. Here are a few examples. You may read the paper every day at breakfast. You may watch television every evening and have a snack. You may always eat when you sit in a certain chair. If eating is paired repeatedly with these events, the events can make you feel like eating. If you sit in your chair, watch TV, or read the morning paper, you will feel like eating, irrespective of physical hunger.

It is important to separate eating from other activities. This will remove the ability of these activities to stimulate eating, freeing you to respond to actual hunger. There are several ways to make this happen. We will present four such techniques below.

Do Nothing Else While Eating

You may be one of those individuals who does other things while eating. It could be working on a hobby, talking on the phone, writing letters, watching TV, reading a magazine, and so forth. This has two disadvantages. The first is mentioned above; eating can become paired with other activities. Second, the activity distracts you from eating, so you get all the calories but only part of the pleasure.

Calories Should Be Tasted, Not Wasted

Many a food diary shows people who eat half a bag of popcorn, 45 Fritos, 22 pretzels, or three-quarters of a pound of mixed nuts. Many of the calories are wasted, not tasted. The following rule will actually help you enjoy food more.

Do nothing else while eating. This means reading the paper at another time, eating before or after you watch TV, waiting to read the book, etc. Eating should be a pure experience. Don't contaminate it with extraneous activities. If this seems awkward, it is a sure sign that you are hooked on the association of eating with other activities. The more this technique bothers you, the more you need it.

Follow an Eating Schedule

You may have uncovered *time* patterns from your Food Diaries. If you eat many times each day, and if you always feel like eating at those times, a schedule will help. This does not necessarily mean three meals a day at conventional

Do nothing else while eating, and taste every bite. Remember—calories should be tasted, not wasted!

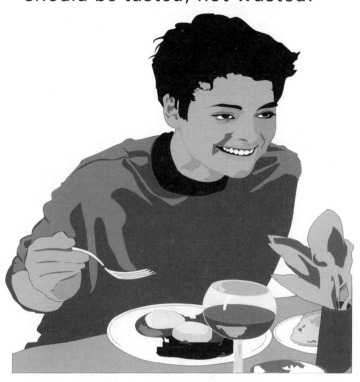

times. It does mean finding a schedule that is convenient for you.

Plan a schedule for your eating. If you eat breakfast at 7:00 a.m., put it in. If you have a mid-evening snack, add it (if necessary). Keep the number of times you eat under control. This may involve eating three conventional meals, but remember to choose a plan you can tolerate.

Following a schedule will help you eat less and think more. You might have a snack planned at 9:00 p.m. If you feel like eating at 8:15, you can wait out the urge, and then see if you are still hungry at 9:00. You may get by with no snack at all! Above is an example of an eating schedule made by Judy, one of our clients.

Time	Meal
7:00 am – 7:20 am	*Breakfast*
10:30 am – 10:45 am	*Morning snack*
12:30 pm – 1:15 pm	*Lunch*
6:30 pm – 7:00 pm	*Dinner*
9:00 pm – 9:20 pm	*Evening snack*

Sample

The space on the next page contains blanks for you to plan your eating schedule. List the times and meals you can live with, and do your best to stick with the schedule. There will, of course, be times when you violate your schedule, but do your best. When you feel like eating at times other than your schedule permits, think carefully about whether you are hungry or are responding to associations of eating and other factors.

Eat in One Place

Some people can eat *anywhere*. They eat standing up, sitting down, at the kitchen counter, in an easy chair, lying in bed, or driving the car. They eat in the den, living room, bedroom, basement, and bathroom. One of our former clients even tied Oreo cookies in a bag and hung them with a rope out the window into the shrubs. She could eat with her head hanging out the window! Places can also be associated with eating, so it is important to limit the places you eat.

Here is a hypothetical example we use with our clients. Let's say that for the next ten years you came to our clinic every day to eat a delicious meal while seated in a yellow chair. At the same time, we would have a chair in your home where no eating would occur. After the ten years and 3650 meals, your response to the two chairs would be quite different. You would feel hungry in the yellow chair even after eating. This would not happen in the chair at home.

Select one place in your home where you will eat. Do *all* your eating there, but do *nothing else*. Do not use the place to play chess, pay the bills, plot a way to beat the stock market, or win the lottery.

Do Not Clean Your Plate

It is time to turn the tables on your plate. Until now, you may have been a slave to the rule issued by every mother, "Clean Your Plate!" It is nice to avoid wasting food, but think for a minute of the folly in cleaning your plate.

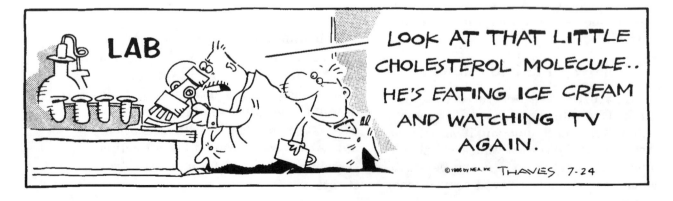

LAB

LOOK AT THAT LITTLE CHOLESTEROL MOLECULE.. HE'S EATING ICE CREAM AND WATCHING TV AGAIN.

© 1986 by NEA, Inc   THAVES 7-24

When you eat everything on the plate, you are at the mercy of the person doing the serving. Unless the person has mystical powers and knows your body's energy requirements, you will be served too much or too little. Given our cultural tendency to overdo it, you will usually be served more than enough. If you clean your plate, you are responding to the *sight* of food, and eating stops only when no more food is in sight. When you serve yourself, remember that you do so *before* you have eaten, so you might be inclined to serve large amounts.

You can exert control by breaking the habit of cleaning your plate. Try to leave some food on your plate each time you eat. Leave only small portions if you like (two peas or one bite of mashed potatoes), but leave a bit of everything. You can ask for second servings, but only if you are really hungry. This puts *you* in control of what you eat, not the chef.

Bracing Yourself Against a Toxic Environment

People with weight problems face a difficult, even toxic environment. The temptations to eat are constant, powerful, and compelling. If you pause for a moment to think, you might be surprised by how we accept this without the slightest protest.

Think of the number of fast food restaurants you find within a 15-minute drive of your home. In addition to the national chains like McDonald's, Burger King, Wendy's, and Kentucky Fried Chicken, there are local and regional restaurants. Most now have drive-thru windows, which make it easier and faster to get loads of calories and fat. Most now serve breakfast, and some are open 24 hours. Nearly every service sta-

My Eating Schedule	
Time	**Meal**

tion has been closed and remodeled to contain a mini-market and almost every mall has a food court. There are vending machines everywhere and fast food chains like McDonald's are showing up in airports, airplanes, and even hospital lobbies!

Let's take another example. Many of the fast food restaurants offer package meals called value meals. More unhealthy food for less money—some value, eh? They also offer, at a seemingly good price, the opportunity to get extra large drinks and fries, when you "supersize it." This is so much a part of our landscape that the word "supersize" has become a verb in our vocabulary.

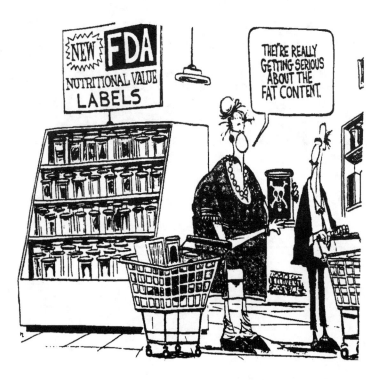

The value meals and the supersize portions are a powerful and effective means the companies have of marketing their foods.

Food advertising is also a problem. Madison Avenue's brightest minds set to work to convince us that we should eat foods that can often be very high in calories, fat, and sugar. The average American child sees 10,000 food commercials each year, 95 percent of which are for fast foods, sugared cereals, candy, and soft drinks.

It is not stretching the language to say that we are exposed to a toxic food environment. We are exposed to and are encouraged to consume things that can cause deadly diseases such as heart disease and cancer. We rail against the tobacco companies for exposing us to temptations to smoke (especially when the inducements are aimed at children), but we remain remarkably quiet when the same thing happens with unhealthy food. We expect that over time a more militant attitude will begin to occur with the public.

What does this mean for you? It means that you must find creative ways to resist the environmental pressures to buy unhealthy foods. Part of this lies in developing an attitude, in some cases an angry one. When you see the drive-thru sign, remember that it is designed to make it easier for you to spend your money on products that can harm you. When you see the junk food stores in the food court, remember that they are in business to feed their high-fat food to as many people as possible. When you fill your car with gas, remember that there is an industry that sells chips, pastries, ice cream, and soft drinks that wants you to succumb. Get mad, and resist!

The other way to deal with this pressure is be aware of it and avoid exposure as much as possible. When you can, avoid going around these places. If at the mall, stay away from the food court. Use a credit card to pay for gas at the pump rather than go inside where the food is. Try not to drive by the fast food places when you are hungry. Most of all, keep alert to these inducements to eat and see that you—not a multi-billion dollar food industry—are in charge of your eating and your health.

Checking on Your Physical Activity

Now that we are part way through the program, let's stop for a moment and assess how you are doing with being more physically active. Let's first give you some perspective on what others are usually doing at this stage.

There will be the jocks who grew up doing sports and can readily adopt a program of exercise. They might be discouraged being in poor shape, but they can see themselves being quite active as their condition improves. Others may have been active in the past, but feel this is forever gone, given how little exercise they do now. Still others have never been active and are having a hard time getting mobilized. Being in the last group, if you are, is perfectly natural. After all, weight gets in the way of physical activity for both physical and emotional reasons, and becoming active requires a major shift in thinking for many people.

We have spoken a great deal about having reasonable weight goals, and having reasonable goals for physical activity is also important. The object is not to have you do some magic amount of exercise, but to increase your level of activity from where you started. If you have been successful thus far, you deserve to be pleased. And remember, being more active is important beyond its effect on your weight—it is good for your health in its own right. So, get as much activity as you can, and have fun at it. You'll benefit in many ways.

Servings from the Five Food Groups

The five food groups of the food guide pyramid were introduced in Lesson 2. We can now be more specific about the number of servings to have every day. First, we need to know what constitutes a serving. A serving from each group can be defined as the amount shown on the next page.

It is important to select the correct number of servings from each group to insure the right mix of nutrients. Look again at the graphic illustration of the Food Guide Pyramid (see next page). As we continue through the program, the pyramid will become a familiar friend. The average numbers of servings per day recommended for adults are listed in the graph. Use this as a guide to structure your diet. Do your best to eat the recommended number of servings every day. We will focus on each of the groups in later lessons, and we will provide you with lists of servings from each group.

Introducing a New Monitoring Form

This lesson ushers in a new Monitoring Form. An example of a completed form appears at the end of this lesson. The new form has three sections. The section on the top is to record food intake, time, and calories, just as you have done with the Food Diary. There are no longer separate sections for breakfast, lunch, dinner, and snacks. List foods in the order you eat them. This will be a part of the Monitoring Form for the remainder of the program—that's how important it is.

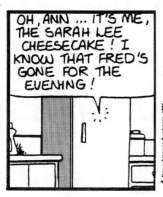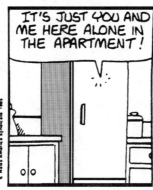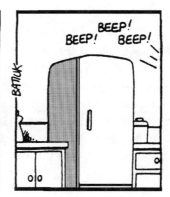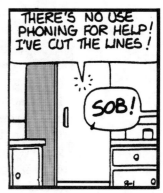

The Food Guide Pyramid

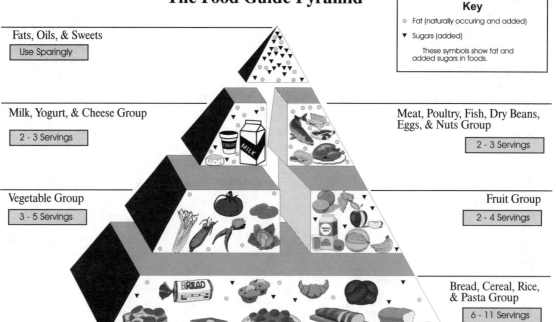

Fats, Oils, & Sweets
Use Sparingly

Key
○ Fat (naturally occuring and added)
▼ Sugars (added)
These symbols show fat and added sugars in foods.

Milk, Yogurt, & Cheese Group
2 - 3 Servings

Meat, Poultry, Fish, Dry Beans, Eggs, & Nuts Group
2 - 3 Servings

Vegetable Group
3 - 5 Servings

Fruit Group
2 - 4 Servings

Bread, Cereal, Rice, & Pasta Group
6 - 11 Servings

The Food Guide Pyramid

(Amounts listed are for one serving)

Milk, Yogurt, and Cheese

☞ 1 cup of milk or yogurt

☞ 1½ ounces of natural cheese

☞ 2 ounces of process cheese

Meat, Poultry, Fish, Dry Beans, Eggs, and Nuts

☞ 2–3 ounces of cooked lean meat, poultry, or fish (a 3-ounce piece of meat is about the size of an average hamburger, or the amount of meat on a medium chicken breast half)

☞ Count ½ cup of cooked dry beans, 1 egg, or 2 tablespoons of peanut butter as 1 ounce of meat (about ⅓ serving)

Vegetables

☞ 1 cup of raw leafy vegetables

☞ ½ cup of other vegetables, cooked or chopped, raw

☞ ¾ cup of vegetable juice

Fruits

☞ A medium apple, banana, or orange

☞ ½ cup of chopped, cooked, or canned fruit

☞ ¾ cup of fruit juice

Bread, Cereal, Rice, and Pasta

☞ 1 slice of bread

☞ 1 ounce of ready-to-eat cereal

The middle portion of the new form is for recording the behavior changes prescribed for each lesson. For this week, the prescribed activities are:

❶ Note the ABC's of eating

❷ Do nothing else while eating

❸ Follow an eating schedule

❹ Eat in one place

❺ Eat servings from the five food groups

❻ Eat less than _____ calories

You simply mark down whether you follow the recommended behavior always, sometimes, or never. Different behaviors will be listed for each lesson.

Some of the techniques you will be trying will be listed under the Always, Sometimes, or Never part of the Monitoring Form, even though the behaviors do not fit neatly in these categories. For example, in Lesson 11 you will be encouraged to shop from a list to avoid impulse buying. However, most people do not shop for food each day, so it is difficult to note on the Monitoring Form each day whether you shopped from a list always, sometimes, or never. In cases like this, put NA (for Not Applicable), if Always, Sometimes, or Never do not apply.

The third section, on the bottom, is to keep a record of your physical activity and your medication use, and to keep track of the number of servings you eat daily from the five food groups. In the lessons that follow, we will discuss the five food groups of The Food Guide Pyramid in more detail. There are also spaces for the type of exercise you do and the number of minutes you do it. This section will also be part of the form from now on. List everything here, like using stairs more than usual, working in the yard, walking, and playing sports.

Setting Personal Goals

Let's review once again why we have this section on "Setting Personal Goals" in each lesson.

➤ The process of setting goals helps you take stock of the changes that are most important to make.

➤ Thinking about specific changes gives you a standard against which to compare your progress.

➤ Setting behavior-change goals shows that there is more to focus on than just the scale. What the scale shows is the end-product of many changes you make. Emphasizing the behaviors rather than the scale is a good way to keep motivated when the scale doesn't move as fast as you'd like.

➤ Setting concrete goals allows you to test whether your expectations are reasonable.

➤ Most important of all, you deserve to feel good about changes you make. Without goals, many people make positive changes but dismiss them as unimportant. We want you to take advantage of every opportunity to feel good about your progress. Feeling good makes everything go better.

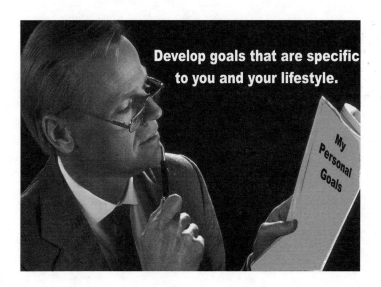

Develop goals that are specific to you and your lifestyle.

My Personal Goals

In each lesson, we discuss goals you might set based on the material in the lesson. We also urge you to develop goals that are specific to you that may or may not be based on that lesson. For example, we will not mention in every lesson things like thinking positively or eating a balanced diet. You might feel, however that these are goals you would like to set for yourself.

Based on the material from this lesson, and from earlier lessons, we recommend you consider the following goals:

▶ Continue to record your food intake and monitor your behaviors on the Monitoring Form

▶ Analyze your behavior using the ABC approach

▶ Continue your program of walking or other physical activity

▶ Take your medication each day

Think of any additional goals you feel might be important for you, being sure they are specific, concrete, and attainable. As you meet the goals, think about what we would say if we were with you — things like, "Nice going!," "Good job!," and "Congratulations, we know you worked hard to do that." But, since we can't be there, you'll have to do this yourself. Be your own strongest supporter!

Self-Assessment Questionnaire

Lesson 6

T F 24. The ABC approach stands for Alternatives, Behavior, and Consciousness.

T F 25. It can be helpful to develop a militant attitude about the "toxic food environment" we face.

T F 26. By Lesson 6 in this program, nearly everyone has developed a plan of regular, vigorous physical activity.

T F 27. It is helpful to set specific, concrete, and attainable goals at each step of the program.

T F 28. If you eat an equal number of servings from the five food groups of the Food Guide Pyramid, you will have a balanced diet.

T F 29. Eating on a schedule is not advisable because it is too regimented.

(Answers in Appendix C)

Monitoring Form—Lesson 6 *(sample)*

Today's Date:

Time	Food and Amount	Calories
7:15	Apple juice, ½ cup (4 oz)	58
	Special K cereal, 1⅓ cups (1 oz)	111
	Skim milk, 4 oz	43
12:30 pm	Club sandwich	590
	Orange, 1 med	65
	Coffee, black (4 oz)	0
6:30 pm	Broiled chicken breast, w/o skin (3 oz)	148
	Broccoli, steamed (1 cup)	46
	Butter, 1t	36
	French bread, 1 slice	81
	Ice tea	0
9:10 pm	Celery, 3 stalks	18
	Skim milk, 8 oz	86
	Total Daily Calories	1,282

Personal Goals This Week	*Always*	*Sometimes*	*Never*
1. Note the ABCs of eating		✓	
2. Do nothing else while eating	✓		
3. Follow an eating schedule		✓	
4. Eat in one place		✓	
5. Eat servings from the five food groups		✓	
6. Eat less than ____ calories each day	✓		

Medication Taken Today ☑ Yes ❑ No	*Physical Activity*	*Minutes*
Milk, yogurt, and cheese ☑ ☑ ❑		
Meat, poultry, etc. ☑ ☑ ❑		
Fruits ☑ ☑ ❑ ❑		
Vegetables ☑ ☑ ☑ ❑ ❑		
Breads, cereals, etc. ☑ ☑ ☑ ☑ ❑ ❑ ❑ ❑ ❑ ❑		

Monitoring Form—Lesson 6

Today's Date:

Time	Food and Amount	Calories
	Total Daily Calories	

	Personal Goals This Week	*Always*	*Sometimes*	*Never*
1.	Note the ABCs of eating			
2.	Do nothing else while eating			
3.	Follow an eating schedule			
4.	Eat in one place			
5.	Eat servings from the five food groups			
6.	Less than _____ calories each day			

Medication Taken Today ❑ Yes ❑ No	*Physical Activity*	*Minutes*
Milk, yogurt, and cheese ❑ ❑ ❑		
Meat, poultry, etc. ❑ ❑ ❑		
Fruits ❑ ❑ ❑ ❑		
Vegetables ❑ ❑ ❑ ❑ ❑		
Breads, cereals, etc. ❑ ❑ ❑ ❑ ❑ ❑ ❑ ❑ ❑		

Lesson 7

In this lesson, we will bring to you in all its glory the "R" part of LEARN—Relationships. We will introduce this section on social support by discussing how important support can be and then will discuss ways you can get support from family and friends. We will also cover the "L" (Lifestyle) part of LEARN by discussing the benefits of eating more slowly. Finally, we expand the "E" (Exercise) part of LEARN by discussing ways to increase your lifestyle activity.

Why Social Support Can Be So Important

Many scientists have studied the impact of social networks on health and well-being. In early days, researchers evaluated whether people had friends and interacted frequently with family members. They then studied whether these events were related to health. The problem with this approach is that a person might have a lot of social contacts, but the contacts might not be positive (say in the case of a distressed marriage). More recently, experts have agreed that the quality of a person's relationships is the key. People who have relationships they can count on for emotional support (e.g., love, caring, concern, etc.) and tangible support (e.g., baby-sitting, financial assistance, and other practical issues), live longer, are healthier, and are happier than people who do not have these relationships.

If support can be so helpful, we have to ask ourselves two questions:

❶ Why is it so helpful?
❷ What we can do to get more support or to take advantage of the support we have?

As for the first issue, support may be helpful for many reasons. Just feeling cared for may help by inspiring us to lead a health-ier lifestyle, to do things that make us happier, and perhaps even influence things like our immune system. Whatever the reason, it is clear from many studies that support can be beneficial.

The question then becomes how to get support. Before talking about this, let us first say that support is something that benefits some people more than others. Some people are perfectly content doing things on their own and they do not want or need others involved in their business. This is perfectly fine—in fact we will speak about different personality types and how some people are

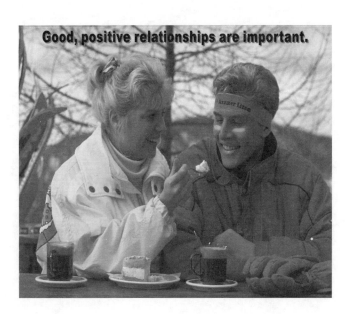

Good, positive relationships are important.

more social types and others more solo types. For those who feel they would benefit from support, even if it occurs at a modest level from only one person, there is a lot to discuss.

Solo and Social Changing

Individuals come in many packages with many personalities. Some like to make changes on their own and do not want other people involved. Others like the aid and support they might get from family and friends. We call the first group *solo* changers and the other group *social* changers.

Solo changers like to travel the weight loss path alone. They often do not tell others when they go on a program. They do not enjoy questions about their weight or their eating. No other person knows their weight. Social changers, on the other hand, like company. They talk with others about their program and are pleased when others notice their progress. They might join a program with a friend or enlist someone in the family to exercise.

Being a social changer is fine. Being a solo changer is fine. What is important is to determine which type best fits you and to structure your program accordingly. There is much material in this manual about enlisting the aid of family and friends. This is likely to help the social person but not a solo type. Solo changers can be upset when others attempt to assist them, even when the assistance is offered for the right reasons.

Think about whether you are a social or solo person. If you are social, the "Relationships" part of The LEARN Program may be helpful, starting with the information on partners in the next section.

Think of support from others as a resource to be cultivated. If you are a solo person, decide exactly when and how you would like others to be involved. Support from others is a resource only if you find it helpful. There are many other resources at your disposal.

Would a Partner Help?

Program partnerships can be very powerful. They occur when a person enlists the aid of another. Sometimes the partner is also on a g program, but fine partnerships can occur when the partner is thin. How can you tell if a partnership is for you?

First, there are different types of partnerships. The most logical one is with a spouse. A husband or wife can be a real aid, but not in all cases. Many of our clients have formed successful partnerships with coworkers, good friends, neighbors, or relatives.

You may already have a partner in mind. In Lesson 8, you can complete the Support Partner Quiz to determine whether this person would be a good choice. In this lesson, you can decide

Are you a Solo or Social changer?

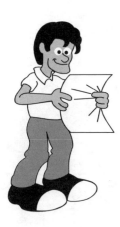
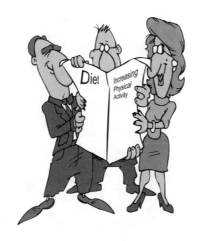

whether your personality is best suited for a partnership or a solo program.

A program partnership is much like a friendship. It is based on give and take. All the support does not flow from the partner to you. You must reciprocate. There will be good times and bad. Some energy is required to keep the partnership intact, as with any relationship.

Do you think you would profit from a partnership? While you decide, let us explain what scientific studies have shown. There have been about 20 studies on partnership programs, including several that we have conducted with our colleagues. In some studies, working with a partner greatly increased weight loss. In others, there was no advantage to the partnership approach. We interpret these inconsistent findings to show that losing weight with a partner is helpful for some, but not for all.

Several examples may illustrate how others can help or hurt. Marjorie enlisted the aid of her husband in her program. He was supportive and showed his concern by walking with her and by not eating treats when she was around. This encouragement helped Marjorie.

Sharon's case was different. Her husband made fun of her and was bitter about her weight problem. He ate in front of her and was nearly always discouraging in his comments. It would have been difficult for Sharon to engage her husband in a partnership. Only you know whether this approach will work for you.

Think about having a weight loss partner. Remember, this person does not have to be overweight. It is important that you feel comfortable with this person and that he or she is able to motivate you. Next, think about your own style and personality. Do you like to do things with others or alone? Can you confide in others or do you keep things to yourself? Could you discuss weight control troubles with another person or would you rather not share them? Finally, what is your *gut* feeling? Do you think the partnership approach would work for you?

You will have time to ponder these important matters, because guidelines for starting a partnership will appear in the next lesson. Think about your own style and decide if a partnership would help. Sort through your friendships and form a pool of possible partners. The partnership may work for you. Do not feel guilty if you are a solo person. Many people do best this way.

Slowing Your Eating Rate

Could you qualify for the Olympic speed eating trials? Many people, both heavy and thin, eat so fast that their taste buds see only a blur as the food speeds by. This minimizes the enjoyment of food. More importantly, eating rapidly can fool your body's defense against eating too much.

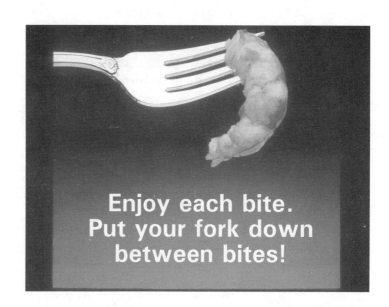

Enjoy each bite.
Put your fork down
between bites!

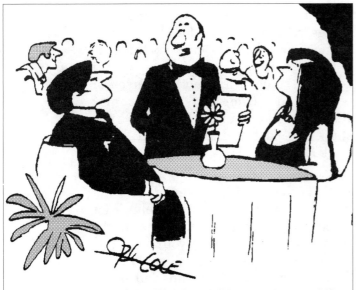

"I'm sorry, but part of the 'Diet Special' is a two-hour wait!"

Your body has an internal satiety (fullness) mechanism. When you have eaten enough, the mechanism sends out signals saying "Enough is enough!" We think this takes about 20 minutes, although this is a very complex process involving the stomach, hormones in the small intestine, brain chemicals, and other factors. If you eat rapidly, you will consume too much food before the mechanism kicks in. You will outpace your body's internal controls.

Slowing down eating can be like halting a runaway freight train. You have had many meals in your life, so the habit of eating fast can be practiced thousands of times. Be patient and practice the following techniques until the old patterns are replaced by new ones.

Techniques to Slow Your Eating

There are two main ways to slow your eating. Both can help put the brakes on eating and can increase the enjoyment of food.

Put your fork down between bites. When you take a bite of food, put your fork down, chew the food com-pletely, swallow, and then pick up the fork for another bite. Do the same with a spoon, and if you are eating finger foods like a sandwich, put the food down between bites.

Pause during the meal. Take a break during your meal. Start with a brief pause, of perhaps 30 seconds. Gradually increase the time to one, then two, and finally three minutes. This pause gives you time to reflect on what you have eaten, so you can make a conscious decision to proceed with more. This may also help you eat less. One study with animals found that interrupting the meal led to fewer total calories, even though the animals could eat all they wanted after the break.

An Impressive Reason to Be Active

Previously, we mentioned that people who are regularly active tend to lose weight better over the long-term. Scientists have used nearly every known psychological and medical test to predict who will lose weight and keep it off. The most consistent finding is that exercise is associated with weight maintenance.

An impressive example of the research on this topic is a study by Kayman, Bruvold, and Stern published in the *American Journal of Clinical Nutrition*. They studied people in a large Health Maintenance Organization who had taken part in a weight loss program. Many months after the program, the individuals were contacted to see what distinguished those who had maintained their weight losses from those who regained.

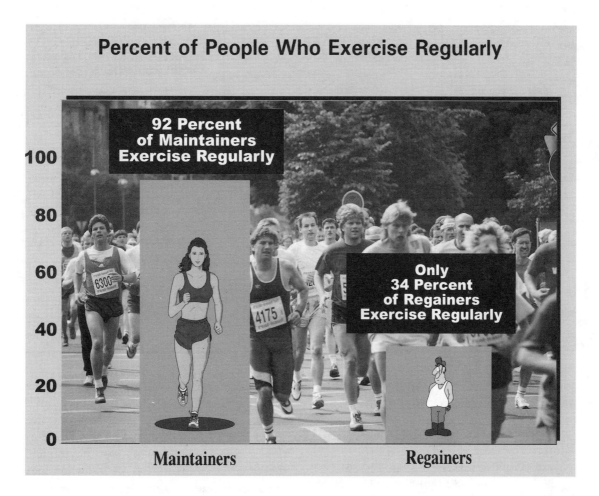

Percent of People Who Exercise Regularly

92 Percent of Maintainers Exercise Regularly

Only 34 Percent of Regainers Exercise Regularly

100 · 80 · 60 · 40 · 20 · 0

Maintainers   **Regainers**

As the graph above shows, exercise was a key factor. Of those who maintained their weight loss, 92 percent were getting regular physical activity. Only 34 percent of the regainers were exercising.

The effect of physical activity on weight maintenance could occur in many ways. There may be physical effects on metabolism or other factors, but almost certainly the psychological advantages of activity are operating. When we are active, even in a modest way, we are doing something positive—we are making a statement to ourselves that we are committed to lifestyle change. This goes a long way in making a person feel good and in boosting confidence for weight control. So, if you are in this for the long run, regular physical activity is one of the best companions you can have.

Continuing Walking and Lifestyle Activity

Let's review your progress with walking and lifestyle activity. This is a good time to look back at the section on the "Benefits of Exercise" from Lesson 5. As you may recall, being active brings many physical and emotional benefits. Two of the most important benefits, at this stage of your program, are that exercise may help control appetite and may bolster self-confidence.

Remember that exercise is one predictor of who will keep weight off over the long-run. On average, people who exercise are more likely to maintain their weight loss long after a program ends. There are exceptions, however. Some people exercise and do not lose weight, and others lose weight without exercising. Where you fit in this

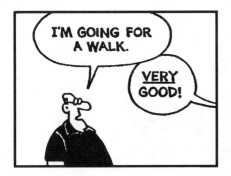
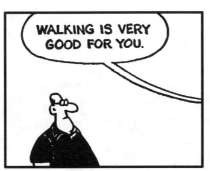
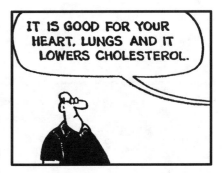
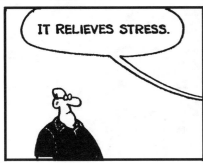
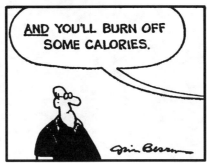
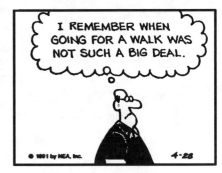

scheme may not be evident for many months, but increasing your activity now may pay nice dividends later.

How much are you walking, and do you enjoy it? Lesson 5 contained ideas for making walking pleasurable, so please review that material if you feel the ideas would help. You should be walking between 15 and 60 minutes each day. It is best to walk as much as possible without feeling discomfort. If you tire from walking, take several short walks rather than one long one. Having two brisk 30-minute walks or four 15-minute walks can help you as much as an hour walk in a single bout.

What types of lifestyle activities have you been doing? Have you found opportunities to use stairs, to park some distance from your destination, or to do some extra walking? These lifestyle activities are nice because they remind us that we are doing something positive.

One reason we use the term *lifestyle* activity is the hope of developing permanent habits. Each trip up the stairs may not make you lose a pound, but summed over many days,

months, or years, the effect can be powerful. New habits can be difficult to acquire, so it is important to practice, and then practice some more. Some of our clients say they now search out stairs wherever they go and feel that an opportunity is missed when they must use an elevator or escalator.

A Pulse Test for Positive Feedback

The Pulse Test is a simple means of feedback on your progress with exercise. The directions on the following page explain how to take your pulse and how to estimate your heart rate. Doing this every few weeks can reveal one important physical change due to exercise—a lower heart rate.

Your pulse, or heart rate, is the number of times your heart beats per minute to supply the body with blood. A high pulse means that your heart must beat many times to do its job. A low pulse means the heart is in better condition and can do its job with less effort (fewer beats).

An example can illustrate the benefits of lowering your heart rate. Consider a woman whose resting heart rate is 75 beats per minute. If she lowers her heart rate to 70 beats per minute, her heart has five fewer beats to make each minute. This is 300 fewer beats per hour and 7200 fewer per day! By taking your pulse periodically, you can estimate the positive changes you make.

Before we move on to the actual Pulse Test, a few facts are important to mention. First, this is not a sophisticated exercise fitness evaluation that a cardiologist or exercise specialist would do. The numbers you estimate for your heart rate cannot be used to judge your overall fitness or your cardiovascular condition.

Second, some people improve their fitness in leaps and bounds but show no change in heart rate. This is particularly true of people who exercise regularly and/or have low heart rates. Betablocker drugs, which are prescribed for hypertension, lower heart rate so only small changes may be possible with exercise. Do not get discouraged if you walk like a real trooper and your pulse stays the same. You will be able to feel your improvement in many other ways. For most people, however, the Pulse Test will detect changes in heart rate as their condition improves.

Steps for Taking Your Pulse

❶ Select either wrist.

❷ Wrap fingers of other hand around back of the wrist.

❸ Press the index and middle fingers on the upturned wrist until you feel the regular pulsing of the blood through the vessel.

❹ Count the number of beats (pulses) in exactly 15 seconds.

❺ Multiply the number by four to calculate your beats per minute.

Take Your Pulse

My Resting Heart Rate is _____ beats per minute.

My Exercise Heart Rate is _____ beats per minute.

_____(distance walked).

_____(time to walk that distance).

There are two times to take your pulse. The first is when you are at rest. Be still for at least five minutes, then take your pulse. The second time is during exercise. Do this during your walking program. Walk for at least three to four minutes at a comfortable pace. Stop walking, and take your pulse immediately. How rapidly your heart rate recovers to its resting level is one index of fitness. Write down the distance you walked, how long it took, and record your pulse rate.

Take your resting and exercise pulse rates as soon as possible, and write them in the spaces provided above. You can refer back to these figures as your condition improves. For the exercise figures, you should find improvements in the time it takes to walk a given distance, in heart rate, or in both. Take your pulse and write it down every two weeks. This will show your improvement over time.

Setting Personal Goals

This is a great time to think about the issue of social support. Think how support may have helped you in the past and how it may be helpful in your attempts to control your weight now. If you have not focused on support in past attempts at weight loss, this might be a good time to try something new. We have not yet discussed the specific ways to get and maintain support, so you may not be able to set a concrete goal at this point, but you can think about support and begin asking yourself who might be supportive and how they might be able to help you.

One specific goal you can set is to eat more slowly. This helps most people and is worth making a habit. In addition, think of the personal goals you'd like to set at this point, and try your best to reach those goals. Continue walking and find ways to increase your lifestyle activity. We hope you will continue to include taking your medication each day and keeping your Monitoring Form.

T F   *30.* Research has shown that social support can be intrusive and does not help with lifestyle changes such as weight loss.

T F   *31.* Eating rapidly helps you enjoy food more because the taste buds get more stimulation.

T F   *32.* Pausing during a meal increases food intake because the body digests food and sends out signals to eat more.

T F   *33.* Your resting pulse will increase as you lose weight and get in better condition.

T F   *34.* Exercise is not a good predictor of who will keep weight off over the long-run, but the health benefits are reason enough to do it.

(Answers in Appendix C)

Monitoring Form—Lesson 7
Today's Date:

Time	Food and Amount	Calories
	Total Daily Calories	

Personal Goals This Week	*Always*	*Sometimes*	*Never*
1. Fork down between bites			
2. Pause during meal			
3. Increase lifestyle activity			
4. Take medication every day			
5. Eat from the five food groups			
6. Less than ___ calories each day			

Medication Taken Today ❑ Yes ❑ No	*Physical Activity*	*Minutes*
Milk, yogurt, and cheese ❑ ❑ ❑		
Meat, poultry, etc. ❑ ❑ ❑		
Fruits ❑ ❑ ❑ ❑		
Vegetables ❑ ❑ ❑ ❑ ❑		
Breads, cereals, etc. ❑ ❑ ❑ ❑ ❑ ❑ ❑ ❑ ❑		

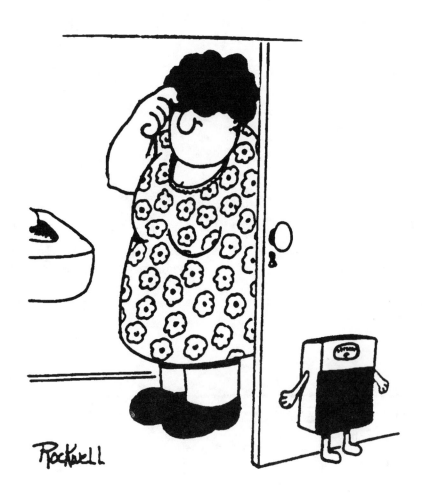

Lesson 8

In the last lesson, we spoke about the importance of social support. We noted that not everyone would want or need support, but for those who do, having others available to help can make a big difference. We urged you to consider who might be helpful and promised that we would discuss ways to pick a support person and then obtain and maintain a supportive relationship. We will do just this, right after covering the reasons people become overweight and the implications this has for you.

Reasons for Overweight

Why people are overweight is still somewhat of a mystery, even though scientists from many countries have been working on the problem for years. Exciting discoveries occur frequently, yet there is still a long road to travel before we can unravel the complex causes and consequences of weight problems. In the meantime, it is helpful to examine the popular reasons people use to explain overweight.

We cover this information here because the reasons we use to explain weight problems create attitudes that can help or hinder efforts to lose weight. A person who feels their weight is determined by genetics may be discouraged from attempting to lose weight. The information that follows may counter some misconceptions.

▶ **Glands.** Having an underactive thyroid used to be a popular reason to explain weight problems. The truth is, most overweight people have no gland problems, or if they do, the problems are not serious enough to account for much of their excess weight. If you suspect gland problems, do not hesitate to see your doctor, but remember that fewer than 5 percent of overweight persons have these difficulties.

▶ **Metabolism.** The issue of metabolism will be covered later in our discussion of exercise. Metabolic rate, which is the energy (calories) your body uses for living, varies widely among people. This influences the way they gain or lose weight. Some women will lose weight rapidly on 1600 calories per day while there are rare individuals who lose slowly on 800 per day. These people are cursed by a thrifty metabolism that conserves energy and promotes weight gain. Determining your exact metabolic needs is

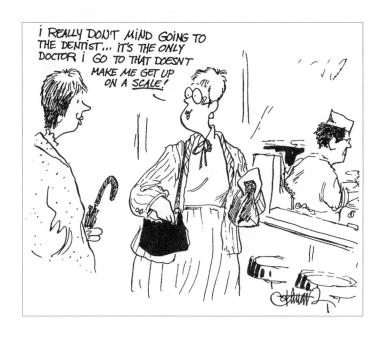

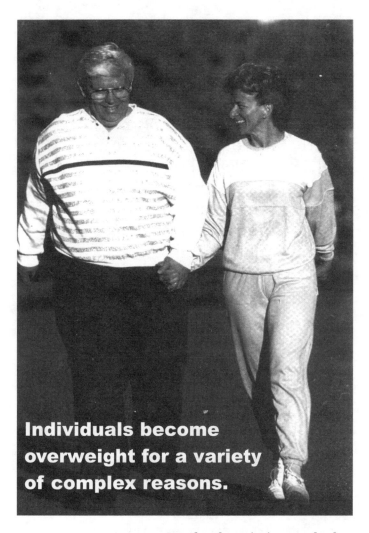

Individuals become overweight for a variety of complex reasons.

meat you buy at the supermarket comes from an animal bred to have a certain percentage of body fat. But what do we know about humans?

The past 15 years have brought an explosion of research on the genetics of body weight regulation. Among the ways to study genetics is to examine identical twins. Studies have compared body weights of twins who are reared together to weights in twins reared apart. If genes are important, we would expect the weights within twin pairs to be similar regardless of whether they were reared together. If the twins reared apart are more dissimilar than twins reared together, the environment would seem to exert an important influence. The studies show that the similarity in body weights within twin pairs is nearly the same whether twins are reared apart or reared together. This indicates that genes are important.

This does not mean that weight is completely controlled by genetics, because how we eat and exercise will determine whether our genetic predisposition to be heavy or thin is expressed. One virtue of this research is that it relieves some of the blame people place on themselves for being overweight. One danger is that people overstate the importance of genetics and come to feel they are destined to be heavy and there is nothing to be done.

more costly than it is worth, because you approach weight loss in the same way regardless of metabolism. If you have a thrifty metabolism, exercise is especially important.

► **Genetics**. Overweight runs in families. A child with no overweight parents has less than a 10 percent chance of being overweight. If one parent is overweight, the chances increase to 40 percent. With two overweight parents, the odds are 70 percent. This could, of course, reflect the tendency of families to pass along their eating and exercise habits to children.

We have known for years that animals can be bred to be fat. The

► **Fat Cells.** The body accumulates and stores fat in fat cells, also called adipose tissue. Some people have too many fat cells (hyperplastic obesity) while others have the normal number but their fat cells are too large (hypertrophic obesity). Still others have both types. People who were overweight in childhood or are very heavy tend to have an excessive number of fat cells as well as enlarged cells. Early researchers in this area speculated that people with too many fat cells would have difficulty losing weight. This has not been tested sufficiently to know whether it is true.

▶ **Family Upbringing.** Some families foster overeating for emotional or even cultural reasons. Some people may eat for psychological reasons related to family upbringing. A program aimed at behavior change is the right approach for these people because it helps to separate emotions from eating and helps to identify other sources of gratification.

▶ **Psychological Factors.** Many overweight people have trouble controlling their eating in response to stress, depression, loneliness, anger, and other emotions. Does this mean that being overweight is a symptom of deep psychological distress? If so, the remedy would be to root out the underlying psychological problems in hopes that the symptom (overeating) would disappear.

This theory rings true intuitively for many people, but does not have much support among experts. Many normal weight persons have psychological problems but cope without overeating. In people who undergo intensive psychotherapy, weight problems generally remain after the psychological difficulties have been resolved. If you feel that psychological problems are at the root of your weight problem, deal with either the weight (through this program) or the psychological problems (with therapy). Do not labor under the notion that the psychological problems must be

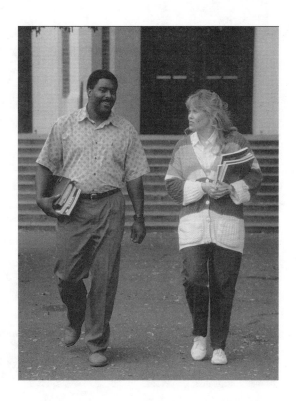

remedied before you can lose weight.

When all is said and done, and all the reasons for overweight are debated, the fact remains that people gain weight because they consume more calories than their bodies use. Becoming overweight is usually a gradual process and may result from small errors in what we eat. One business executive gained five pounds each year for 20 years. He did not notice the five pounds each year, but he was unhappy with the total of 100 pounds. This could have occurred from nothing more than two to three drinks per week. The solution to such a problem is gradual change in eating habits so that long-term weight loss can occur.

Weight Loss Medications and Causes of Overweight

Since you have been prescribed medication for weight loss, it is natural to ask

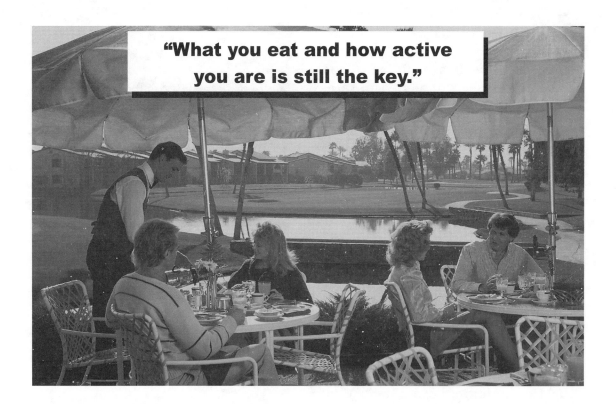

"What you eat and how active you are is still the key."

whether the drugs are designed to correct some biological cause of your weight problem. As we mentioned, MERIDIA acts on chemicals in your brain such as serotonin and norepinephrine. If the drug is helping you lose weight, does this mean you had problems with these chemicals?

The answer is only maybe. Knowing why any one person is overweight is difficult. Some cases may occur because of low levels of these or other chemicals, but the fact the drug helps does not prove this to be true. The medication helps with appetite, and whether biology, emotions, or a combination governs appetite, the drug helps because it affects behavior. Behavior—what you eat and how active you are—is still the key, so let's view the drug as a way to help you manage your behavior. It is an aid to your change, but don't forget that you are making the changes yourself.

Why Losing Weight Is Difficult

Let's face it—losing weight is hard work. Most overweight people really want to lose weight, but find it difficult. There are many reasons. We will discuss several here. It is important for you to appreciate the complexities of weight loss so you don't get demoralized when you encounter tough times.

Eating is a complex activity. When you face temptation from food, say a piece of cake after dinner, many factors combine to determine whether you will eat it. There is physiology at work because hunger might be stimulated. Your family upbringing can enter the picture because you may have learned that foods (especially desserts) are associated with love. Culture plays a part, particularly if you are dining with someone else and you feel obliged to eat everything, including dessert. Psychology might take part if you are feeling depressed or lonely and want food for gratification.

No one reason can be pinpointed. To keep your attitudes on the right track, remind yourself that getting the actual eating and exercise habits under control is the best course to weight loss. Instead of feeling guilty about what you eat or resentful about what you cannot eat, you can learn about food and calories and enjoy yourself!

Choosing a Support Person

People who feel they would benefit from the support of another person have a number of choices for doing so. The most extensive involvement is to have a weight loss partnership. In this case, you and another person would both be losing weight and would work with each other as support partners. This can work wonderfully in some cases, but again, it is not for everyone.

You can obtain less intensive but equally important support from others, including a spouse, parent, child, friend, coworker, or anyone who encourages you. The person could be involved in a big way, say by asking you each day about your goals and accomplishments, or in a smaller way, by just being there when you ask for help. Who you choose and what you ask them to do is, of course, best decided by you.

We will discuss how to decide whether a given individual would be a good support person. A quiz for this follows. Then we will discuss how to work with such a person and whether it should be in a full-blown partnership or some other type of helping relationship.

A Quiz for Choosing a Support Partner

We promised in the last lesson to give you a quiz for evaluating whether a person would make a good partner to go through the program with you. Your job was to think of possible partners, and then to use the quiz to make a final decision.

To take this quiz (see the Support Partner Quiz on the next page), think of the person you would have as a partner, and answer the questions honestly. First, answer each question either true or false. Beside each of your answers is a number. Write this number in the space provided immediately before each question number. Add the numbers of your responses, then use the scoring guide at the bottom of the quiz.

These guidelines should help in choosing a partner. Once you have done so, discuss the possibility with the person you have in mind. The next lesson will bring specific suggestions on how to proceed.

Let us stress again that you need not have a partner. The decision is left to you. If you do decide on the partner approach, these questions could help in selecting a supportive partner. If you are uncertain about proceeding with a partner, even after taking the quiz, experiment with it. Use what you learn about partnerships to see if you profit from the aid of another person. If not, consider yourself a solo changer and move ahead.

Communicating with Your Partner

The Support Partner Quiz can help you decide whether one or more people

Support Partner Quiz

_____ 1.   It is easy to talk to my partner about weight.

        True—5   False—1

_____ 2.   My partner has always been thin and does not understand my   weight problem.

        True—1   False—3

_____ 3.   My partner offers me food when he or she knows I am trying to   lose weight.

        True—1   False—5

_____ 4.   My partner never says critical things about my weight.

        True—3   False—1

_____ 5.   My partner is always there when I need a friend.

        True—4   False—1

_____ 6.   When I lose weight and look better, my partner will be jealous.

        True—1   False—3

_____ 7.   My partner will be genuinely interested in helping me with my weight.

        True—6   False—1

_____ 8.   I could talk to my partner even if I was doing poorly.

        True—5   False—1

If you scored between 30 and 34, you may have found the perfect partner. A score in this range indicates that you and this person are comfortable with one another and can work together.

If you scored between 25 and 29, your friend is potentially a good partner, but there are a few areas of concern. Try asking the partner to take the quiz and predict how you answered the questions. This may help you make a decision.

If you scored between 17 and 24, there are potential areas of conflict, and a program partnership with this person could encounter stormy going. Think of another partner.

If you scored between 8 and 16, definitely look to someone else as a partner. A program partnership in this case would be a high-risk undertaking.

might be good support partners. Now you are ready to discuss your program with this person and start the ball rolling. There is a lot you can do to get the most out of this effort.

In later lessons we will discuss methods for dealing with family and friends. This is different from a partnership where someone can be very involved with your program. With the family, there are more ways that support can be provided and sabotage can be prevented. If you feel your family is a problem or can be a useful resource now, it may be helpful to read Lesson 18. In the meantime, let's discuss partnerships.

Here are specific ideas for starting a program partnership. Communicating is the first and most important step. If you and your partner can communicate effectively, you are on the way to a successful partnership. Here are some ideas for making this happen.

It is essential that you and your partner talk together. Sit down and have a friendly talk with the person you have chosen as a partner. Discuss the topics below in an open and honest way.

▶ **Are you both ready for a partnership?** Is your partner ready to listen to requests for help and make the required effort? Is he or she ready to help you during good times and bad? Are you ready to help your partner in return? Some degree of commitment is necessary from both of you.

▶ **Tell your partner how to help.** A common and crucial mistake is to expect your partner to read your mind. If it is your spouse, you may think he or she should know what you want and need. Most people are not good mind readers, so leave nothing to chance. Tell your partner what he or she can do. Do you want to be praised when you do well or scolded when you do poorly? Should the person avoid eating in your presence? Can your partner help by exercising with you?

▶ **Make specific requests.** The more specific your requests, the easier it will be for your partner to comply. If your request is vague and general, like "Be nice," your partner is at a disadvantage. A more specific request is better, such as "Please tell me you love me when I lose weight." Instead of saying, "Don't eat in front of me," say "It helps me when you eat your evening bowl of ice cream in the other room." Replace a general statement like, "Exercise ewith me" with "Please take a half-hour walk with me each morning."

▶ **State your requests positively**. It is better to ask for something positive than to criticize something negative. Clever changes of words can help. If your partner nags, you can say "It really helps me when you say nice things." If your partner offers you food, you can say "I appreciate the times when you don't offer me food. It is easier to control my eating then." Human nature responds well to the chance to do something positive, so try this approach with your partner.

▶ **Reward your partner.** For your partner to help you, you must help your partner. One-way relationships don't last long. If you are going through this program together, you can work out weight control related ways of helping. If your partner is not on a program, be forward, and ask what you can do in return. Remember, being a partner can be challenging, so you need to acknowledge your partner's help.

Use these techniques to start the ball rolling with your partner. Upcoming lessons will give you more ideas for working with your partner. It is important to lay this groundwork first.

Making Physical Activity Count

It is time to distinguish between *lifestyle* and *programmed* activity. Lifestyle

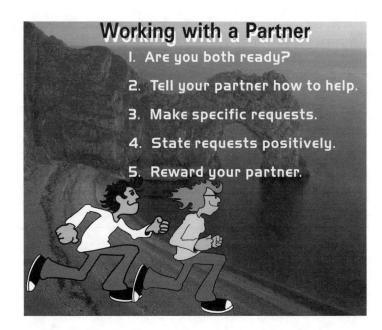

Working with a Partner
1. Are you both ready?
2. Tell your partner how to help.
3. Make specific requests.
4. State requests positively.
5. Reward your partner.

activity is simple and can be done in your day-to-day routine. An example would be using stairs rather than an elevator when you go to work. Programmed activity is a traditional exercise regimen of jogging, biking, aerobics, racquetball, and so forth. We will discuss programmed activities beginning with Lesson 10. For now, let us consider lifestyle activities.

Lifestyle Activity

You can imagine the virtues of lifestyle activity. It is easy, takes little time, does not hurt, does not require special clothes or equipment, and can become habit with little effort. It makes you feel better both psychologically and physically.

The idea here is to sneak in activity whenever possible. The suggestions that follow may help you get started with another part of the assignment for this lesson—*Increase Your Lifestyle Activity*.

Use Stairs

Stairs can be a good friend because they are so readily available. Climbing stairs burns more calories per minute than rigorous activities like jogging and cycling. If you work on the fifth floor of a

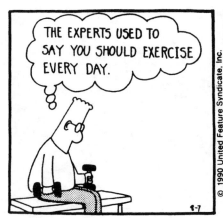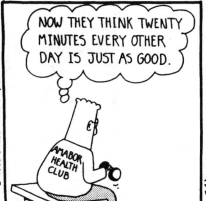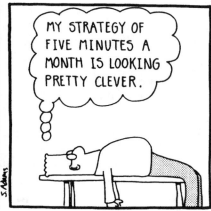

building, take the elevator to the fourth floor and walk the remaining flight. As your condition improves, get off on lower floors. One of our favorite examples is a client who lived in a two-story house with bathrooms on each floor. She decided to use the bathroom on the floor where she wasn't located, which gave her several extra trips per day up and down the stairs.

Park Further Away

When you drive to the mall, don't circle around like a vulture in search of a spot by the door. Park where only the people with new cars pull in—away from the crowd.

Walk More

If you take the bus downtown, get off one or two stops early and walk the extra distance. If someone gives you a ride to the store, have them drop you off a few blocks away. At home, take things up the stairs in several trips instead of letting them accumulate for one trip.

Make it Count

Count everything you do as exercise. When you do housework, turn on a timer and keep moving. Use the vacuum an extra day each week. Time yourself as you wash the car, rake the leaves, or mow the lawn. You will be surprised how fast the minutes go by, and you will accomplish another task as well.

The beauty of these small bouts of activity is that each one provides an opportunity for you to feel virtuous—to be reinforced for doing something positive. And this is not just a trick—you really are doing something positive. Anything you do to be more active is beneficial, and you should acknowledge it as such. You deserve a pat on the back whenever you make an effort to do something good, and you're the closest one around to do it. Our hope is that you will count yourself among the ranks of people who consider themselves exercisers. This can build on itself to the point where you are feeling much better about your body and your physical condition. It doesn't take much to notice improvement.

These are just examples of the general *principle* of increasing lifestyle activity. Think of more methods to fit your own routine. The section that follows, on the calorie values of exercise, may give you more ideas. Be sure to record your lifestyle activities on your Monitoring Form. You deserve credit for doing these activities, so they should show up in your records.

Tracking Your Progress with Activity

When you are making positive changes, it is important to *feel* like you are making progress and to reinforce yourself accordingly. To do this, it can help to have a way of assessing how you are doing. The activity section on the monitoring forms at the end of each lesson is an excellent place to begin, but some people like to do more.

Some people like to keep a graph or a log of when they are active. Either could include the number of minutes being active, how fast you do some activity (like walking a certain distance), or how far the activity takes you (distance). Another helpful index of progress can be to use a pedometer. These are available in sporting goods stores and have been refined in the last several years to be much more accurate than earlier models. Some devices measure how far you walk and others give the number of steps you take. The ones with the number of steps are nice because you can see evidence of even small increases in activity.

We have worked with individuals who set up reward systems for themselves by making a contract. The contract states that certain rewards (e.g., a movie, a new CD, clothing, etc.) will be rewards for attaining a certain level of activity. These are fine, but whether or not you have a reward system, it is important to track your activity so you have a sense of how much you are improving. This helps you feel virtuous when you deserve it.

Setting Personal Goals

The main focus of this lesson was on social support. Think seriously about whether your effort would be aided by involving another person. You might be shy, reluctant to discuss your program, or embarrassed about your weight. It may be worth looking past these barriers and taking action to get more support. It can go a long way in times of need.

For your personal goals, see about establishing a support partnership and begin working with the person or persons you have chosen. In addition, make specific goals for other changes you would like to make and record whether you are meeting these goals. These might be goals that have become standard for you, such as completing your Monitoring Form or being physically active.

Self-Assessment Questionnaire

Lesson 8

T F 35. Discovering the psychological roots of your weight problem is the most important factor in weight reduction.

T F 36. All overweight people have an excessive number of fat cells.

T F 37. There is no such thing as a slow or underactive metabolism.

T F 38. You should tell your program partner in specific terms how he or she can help.

T F 39. It is important to reinforce your partner for helping you.

(Answers in Appendix C)

Monitoring Form—Lesson 8

Today's Date:

Time	Food and Amount	Calories
	Total Daily Calories	

Personal Goals This Week	*Always*	*Sometimes*	*Never*
1. Work with a partner			
2. Complete my Monitoring Form			
3. Increase lifestyle activity			
4. Take medication every day			
5. Eat from the five food groups			
6. Less than _____ calories each day			

Medication Taken Today ❑ Yes ❑ No	*Physical Activity*	*Minutes*
Milk, yogurt, and cheese ❑ ❑ ❑		
Meat, poultry, etc. ❑ ❑ ❑		
Fruits ❑ ❑ ❑ ❑		
Vegetables ❑ ❑ ❑ ❑ ❑		
Breads, cereals, etc. ❑ ❑ ❑ ❑ ❑ ❑ ❑ ❑ ❑		

Lesson 9

It is time to dive into nutrition in more detail. We will cover a topic of great interest and importance—the role of fat in your diet. There is much to say about fat, and there is good news ahead on how to deal with fat in a positive way. We will also discuss planning healthy meals, cravings, and attitudes.

A Two-Month Review

This lesson marks another milestone in our program. For eight weeks now, you have taken MERIDIA, changed your eating and activity habits, and made other efforts to improve your health and fitness. Congratulations on your progress! Let's briefly review your efforts in these areas.

Medication Schedule

We hope you have continued to take MERIDIA every morning to achieve optimal control over your appetite. Review your medication records for the past two weeks to see how you have done. If you missed any days, determine what happened so you can prevent such episodes in the future.

Eating and Activity Habits

We did not review your eating and activity habits in detail in the last few lessons, but we hope you are still focused on them. Keeping your Monitoring Forms and increasing your physical activity are two of your keys to long-term success. Your Monitoring Forms will tell you if you are eating the appropriate number of calories which, as we discussed before, is roughly 1200 a day for women and 1500 a day for men. Check your records to determine your intake for the last two weeks. In addition, continue to use your records to identify patterns in your eating.

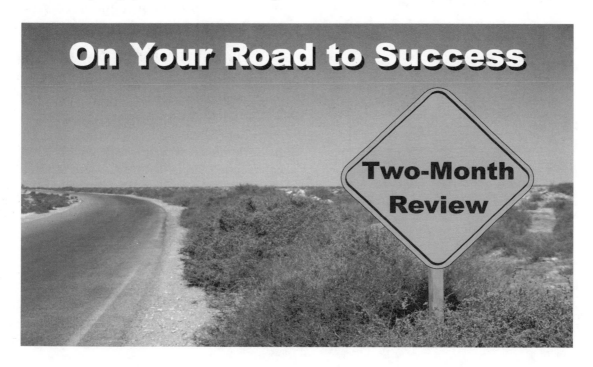

On Your Road to Success

Two-Month Review

Some people dislike keeping the Monitoring Forms. They say that it takes too much time, is too bulky to carry through the day, or prevents them from enjoying their meals. If this is true for you, then stop using our Forms and develop one of your own. You may want to use a 3" x 5" spiral pad or index cards. Similarly, you may want to develop your own system of recording in which you only keep records on weekends or at times when you usually eat more. There are dozens of ways in which you can track the foods you eat. Find one that works for you if you don't like ours.

We hope that you are enjoying your walking program or whatever other activity you are pursuing. Remember, the object is to make sure you enjoy your program by choosing an activity you like, setting modest goals, and focusing on additional ways of making activity pleasurable, such as walking with a friend or listening to audiotapes. Take a few minutes to review your activity during the past two weeks.

Weight Loss

After eight weeks of the program, most people have lost about 4 to 6 per-

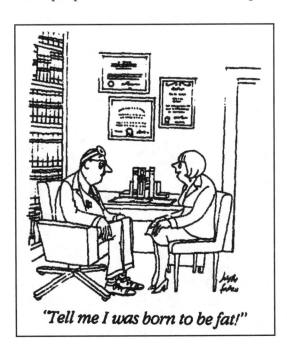

"Tell me I was born to be fat!"

cent of their starting weight. So, if you weighed 200 pounds before the program, we suspect you have lost about 8 to 12 pounds. If you have lost substantially less than this (less than 3 percent of your starting weight) or much more (more than 10 percent of starting weight), you may want to talk to your doctor. While rapid weight loss is exciting it can increase the risk of gallstones and other complications.

More likely, your health has continued to improve with weight loss. If you have high blood pressure or blood sugar, these conditions have probably improved even more since the first month of the program.

The Role of Fat in Your Diet

Fat is what it's all about, right? You want to eat less fat and get rid of body fat. How are dietary fat and body fat different, and what role should fat play in your diet? You might think that fat is just what we see on meats and that it goes right to our store of body fat. The picture is more complex and is very interesting.

The Importance of Fat

Fat plays an important role in everyone's diet and has received a lot of attention lately due to its associations with heart disease and cancer. Dietary fat provides *essential* fatty acids that carry fat soluble vitamins (A,D,E, and K) throughout the body and a *semi-essential* fatty acid that helps to prevent growth deficiencies and build the membranes of cell walls. Fat in your body protects vital organs and prevents excessive heat loss. Fat is also a valuable source of energy, particularly for endurance activities; carbohydrate is used for quick energy. Fat also provides flavoring to many of the foods that we eat.

Our bodies can manufacture many of the essential fatty acids we need from carbohydrate or protein, however, there are some that it cannot make—these must be included in the food that we eat. The fat we eat is a combination of fatty acids and glycerol. All fats in foods are mixtures of three types of fatty acids: saturated, monounsaturated, and polyunsaturated. The fatty acids consist of carbon atoms that are attached to oxygen and hydrogen atoms. Each carbon atom has four possible binding sites. When the hydrogen/oxygen atoms are attached to all four binding sites, the fatty acid is *saturated* (i.e., the carbon atom is saturated with the maximum number of hydrogen/oxygen atoms). When the hydrogen/oxygen atoms are attached to less than all four binding sites, the fatty acid is said to be *unsaturated*. You can visually identify saturated fats because they are usually solid at room temperature and come primarily from meat and dairy products, although they are also found in some vegetable fats, such as coconut, palm and palm kernel oils.

When two nearby carbon atoms are each missing one molecule from one of their four binding sites, a double bond can be formed between the two atoms. When this happens the fat is considered to be *monounsaturated*. Monounsaturated fats are found mainly in olive, peanut, and canola oils. If more than one double bond is formed, the fat is said to be *polyunsaturated*. Polyunsaturated fats are generally liquid or soft at room temperature and are found mainly in safflower, sunflower, corn, soybean, and cottonseed oils and some fish.

This distinction between saturated and unsaturated fats is important for health reasons. Again, the saturated fats are easy to distinguish because they are usually solid at room temperature and come primarily from animal sources (butter, lard, meat). High consumption

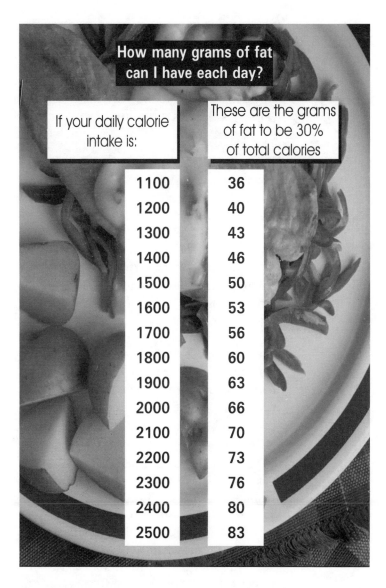

How many grams of fat can I have each day?

If your daily calorie intake is:	These are the grams of fat to be 30% of total calories
1100	36
1200	40
1300	43
1400	46
1500	50
1600	53
1700	56
1800	60
1900	63
2000	66
2100	70
2200	73
2300	76
2400	80
2500	83

of these fats has been associated with heart disease and is likely related to increased risk for colon and breast cancers.

On the other hand, polyunsaturated fats are usually liquid or soft at room temperature and are from vegetable sources (vegetable oils, margarine). These are healthier than the saturated fats. This is why so many people have switched from butter to margarine, reduced their intake of high-fat meats like beef and pork, and cook more with vegetable oils. The best unsaturated oils are corn, soy, sunflower, and safflower (the most highly unsaturated oil). A noteworthy point is that all fats contain the same number of calories.

Calculating My Daily Fat Intake (*Example*)		
Total Daily Caloric Intake (calories)		1500
Target Percentage of Total Calories	x	30%
Daily Calories from Fat		450
Number of Calories in One Gram of Fat	÷	9
Daily Grams of Fat		50

Calculating My Daily Fat Intake		
Total Daily Caloric Intake (calories)		_____
Target Percentage of Total Calories	x	30%
Daily Calories from Fat		_____
Number of Calories in One Gram of Fat	÷	9
Daily Grams of Fat		_____

How Much Fat Should I Eat?

There are three basic facts to remember for your diet. The first is that fat provides a lot of energy, which is bad news for a person trying to lose weight. Fat contains twice the calories (nine per gram) of either protein or carbohydrate. You will get more calories from the fat on a single steak than from an equal amount of pure sugar.

Second, the amount of fat you eat is associated with risk for several serious diseases. The average American gets close to 40 percent of total calories from fat. It is recommended that this be reduced to no more than 30 percent. Saturated fat should be limited to less that 10 percent of calories, or about one-third of total fat intake. Reducing your fat intake should help with weight and with general health.

Third, we mentioned earlier that fat calories are more easily converted to body fat than are calories from other sources. Therefore, keeping fat intake under control can go a long way toward helping you reduce your weight.

To calculate the amount of fat you should eat each day, begin with your total daily calorie goal. Multiply this number by 30 percent to determine your daily calories from fat. Since each gram of fat contains nine calories, divide your daily calories from fat by nine to determine your daily grams of fat. See the example in Calculating My Daily Fat Intake. Use the blank chart at the top of this page to calculate your daily fat gram goal.

Sources of Fat

We generally don't realize how much fat we eat. About 60 percent of the fat we eat cannot be seen (hidden fat) because it is contained in other food products, such as meat, cheese, nuts, breads, etc. In determining the amount of fat in your diet, it is important to account for both visible and hidden fat.

The chart on the next page provides you with a sampling of foods from the five food groups of the Food Guide Pyramid. This chart includes the number of servings of each food and the amount of fat for each. Use this chart along with the calorie guide in Appendix F to help you reduce your dietary fat.

Dietary Fat Adds Up

The fat in some foods adds up quickly. As mentioned earlier, fat contains more than twice the calories of protein or carbohydrate. One gram of fat has nine calories, whereas one gram of carbohydrate or protein has only four calories. One teaspoon (one pat) of butter or margarine has four grams of fat; that's 36 calories of fat for every teaspoon. It is important to watch out for those extras that

Food Group Choices

Foods	Servings	Grams of Fat
Fats, Oils, and Sweets		
Butter, margarine, 1t	–	4
Mayonnaise, 1T	–	11
Salad dressing, 1T	–	7
Reduced calorie salad dressing, 1T	–	A
Sour cream, 2T	–	6
Cream cheese, 1 oz	–	10
Sugar, jam, jelly, 1t	–	0
Cola, 12 fl. oz	–	0
Fruit drink, 12 fl oz	–	0
Chocolate bar, 1 oz	–	9
Sherbet, ½ cup	–	2
Fruit sorbet, ½ cup	–	0
Gelatin dessert, ½ cup	–	0
Milk, Yogurt, and Cheese Group		
Skim milk, 1 cup	1	Trace
nonfat yogurt, plain, 8 oz	1	Trace
Low-fat milk, 2 percent, 1 cup	1	5
Whole milk, 1 cup	1	8
Chocolate milk, 2 percent, 1 cup	1	4
Low-fat yogurt, plain, 8 oz	1	4
Low-fat yogurt, fruit, 8 oz	1	3
Natural cheddar cheese, 1 ½ oz	1	14
Process cheese, 2 oz	1	18
Mozzarella, part skim, 1 ½ oz	1	10
Cottage cheese, 4 percent fat, ½ cup	¼	5
Ice cream, ½ cup	⅓	7
Ice milk, ½ cup	⅓	3
Frozen yogurt, ½ cup	½	2
Meat, Poultry, Fish, Dry Beans, Eggs, and Nuts Group		
Lean meat, poultry, fish, cooked,	3 oz	6
Ground beef, lean, cooked	3 oz[B]	16
Chicken, with skin, fried	3 oz[B]	13
Bologna, 2 slices	1 oz[B]	16
Egg, 1,	1 oz[B]	5

Foods	Servings	Grams of Fat
Dry beans and peas, cooked, ½ cup	1 oz[B]	Trace
Peanut butter, 2T	1 oz[B]	16
Nuts, ⅓ cup	1 oz[B]	22
Vegetable Group		
Vegetables, cooked, ½ cup	1	Trace
Vegetables, leafy, raw, 1 cup	1	Trace
Vegetables, non leafy, raw, chopped, ½ cup	1	Trace
Potatoes, scalloped, ½ cup	1	4
Potato salad, ½ cup	1	8
French fries, 10	1	8
Fruit Group		
Whole fruit: medium apple, orange, banana	1	Trace
Fruit, raw or canned, ½ cup	1	Trace
Fruit juice, unsweetened, ¾ cup	1	Trace
Avocado, ¼ whole	1	9
Bread, Cereal, Rice, and Pasta Group		
Bread, 1 slice	1	1
Hamburger roll, bagel, English muffin, 1	2	2
Tortilla, 1	1	3
Rice, pasta, cooked, ½ cup	1	Trace
Plain crackers, small, 3–4	1	3
Breakfast cereal, 1 oz	1	A
Pancakes, 4" diameter, 2	2	3
Croissant, 1 large (2 oz)	2	12
Doughnut, 1 medium (2 oz)	2	11
Danish, 1 medium (2 oz)	2	13
Cake, frosted, 1/16 average	1	13
Cookies, 2 medium	2	19
Pie, fruit, 2-crust, 1/6 8" pie	2	19

A Check product label.

B Serving sizes vary with the type of food and the meal.

Source: Adapted from Home and Garden Bulletin Number 252, U.S. Department of Agriculture, 1992.

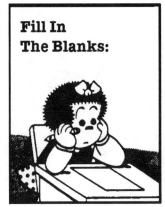
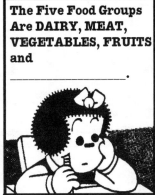
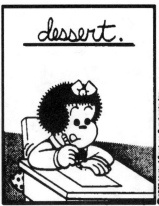
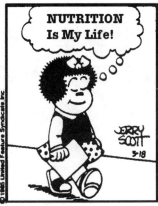

contain high amounts of fat. For example, a bologna-and-cheese sandwich made with two slices (two oz) of bologna, two slices (1½ oz) of cheese, and two teaspoons of mayonnaise, counts up to about 36 grams of fat, approximately nine teaspoons. A similar sandwich, however, made with lean beef, lettuce, tomato, and low-fat mayonnaise, and served with a cup of nonfat milk instead of cheese, has only about six grams of fat.

Reducing the Fat in Your Diet

There are many tips available for lowering the amount of dietary fat we eat every day. The first step is to determine a target intake of fat as we did in the calculation on page 110. Next, you should become aware of the fat content of the foods that you eat. In addition to reading food labels, there are many good books available that can help you. Here are some additional tips that will help you decrease the level of fat in your diet.

From the Milk, Yogurt, and Cheese Group

Use skim or low-fat milk (two grams of fat per serving) instead of whole milk (16 grams of fat per serving) for drinking as well as cooking. Also, use nonfat or low-fat fruit yogurt (two grams of fat per serving) over whole-milk yogurt (seven grams of fat per serving). Frozen yogurt or ice milk (two to three grams of fat per one-half cup) is a nice substitute for ice cream (seven grams).

From the Meat, Poultry, and Fish Group

Eat modest portions of meat, poultry, and fish. Three cooked ounces is the recommended portion size. Choose lean cuts of meat, such as sirloin tip and round steak, and choose lean and extra lean ground beef, center cut ham, loin chops, and tenderloin. Limit your use of processed meats which tend to be high in fat. When in doubt, read the food label. If the fat content is not listed on the food product, be extra cautious. If cholesterol is a problem, limit your use of organ meats (liver, kidneys, brains, etc.) and limit the number of egg yolks to three or less per week. Legumes (dried beans and peas) are good alternative sources of protein and have little or no fat. Use them in mixed dishes instead of meat, or combine them with a small portion of meat or poultry.

From the Vegetable and Fruit Groups

Fruits and vegetables provide a good supply of fiber, vitamins, and minerals—all with low fat and no cholesterol. Use them generously at mealtime and for snacks. For both cooked and fresh vegetables (including salads) try seasonings and substitute flavorings, such as herbs, spices, or a splash of lemon instead of butter or salad dressings. Remember, there are four grams of fat in each teaspoon of butter, margarine, or mayonnaise. Cutting out the salad

The Food Guide Pyramid

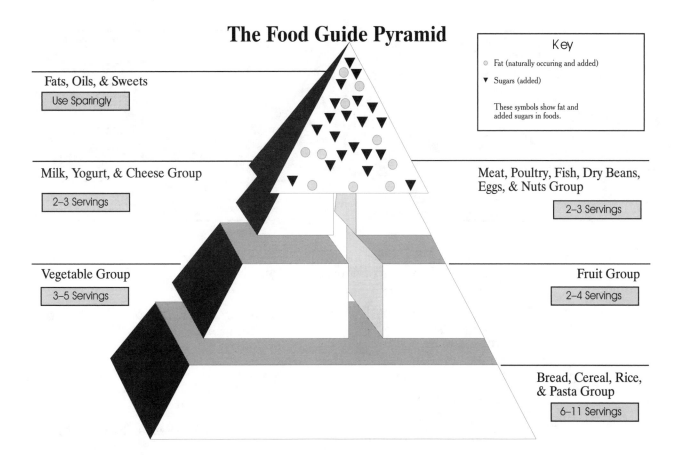

Key
- ○ Fat (naturally occuring and added)
- ▼ Sugars (added)

These symbols show fat and added sugars in foods.

Fats, Oils, & Sweets
Use Sparingly

Milk, Yogurt, & Cheese Group
2–3 Servings

Meat, Poultry, Fish, Dry Beans, Eggs, & Nuts Group
2–3 Servings

Vegetable Group
3–5 Servings

Fruit Group
2–4 Servings

Bread, Cereal, Rice, & Pasta Group
6–11 Servings

---

dressing can save up to nine grams of fat for each tablespoon.

From the Bread, Cereal, and Rice Group

Use rice, pasta, and other grain products as the mainstay of a low-fat eating plan. Small portions of meat, fish, and poultry go a long way when combined with grain products. Eating whole grain products will help you maximize your intake of fiber and other nutrients. Choose a dinner roll (two grams of fat) rather than a croissant (12 grams of fat).

Cooking Tips

Trim away all visible fat from meat before cooking. Remove skin and fat from chicken and turkey before cooking. Use nonstick pans and sprays for cooking. In sauces, salads, and soups, substitute low-fat or nonfat plain yogurt for sour cream or mayonnaise. Broil or bake meats instead of frying.

Snacks and Desserts

Eat plenty of fresh fruit and vegetables every day. Pop popcorn in a microwave or air popper. To add flavor, spray the popcorn lightly with hot vegetable oil or vegetable spray and add seasoning salts. Sorbet, flavored ice, and frozen fruit bars are a nice snack. Danish, doughnuts, cookies, and frosted cakes are high in fat and should be eaten sparingly. Also, potato chips and other crunchy snacks are high in dietary fat. Be sure to read the food label for the fat content of these foods.

Planning Healthy Meals

Many excellent resources are available for planning healthy meals. These include cookbooks and guides for buying, preparing, and serving healthy foods.

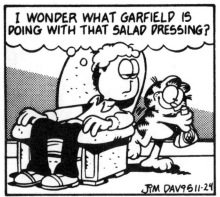 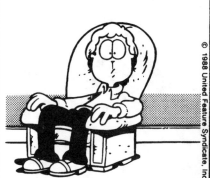 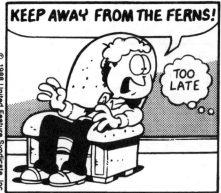

These are handy aids because losing weight conjures up impressions of deprivation and boring food. A trip to the bookstore can help prevent this boredom. The following books are filled with ideas and recipes that can help you eat delicious foods while reducing calories, fat, sodium, cholesterol, and increasing fiber. Get those taste buds ready!

American Heart Association Quick and Easy Cookbook. New York: McKay, 1997.

Better Homes and Gardens Eat & Stay Slim. Des Moines, Iowa: Meredith, 1997.

Better Homes and Gardens Eating Well With the Food Guide Pyramid. Des Moines, Iowa: Meredith, 1996.

Better Homes and Gardens Family Favorites Made Lighter. Des Moines, Iowa: Meredith, 1992.

Better Homes and Gardens Healthy Family Cookbook. Des Moines, Iowa: Meredith, 1996.

Better Homes and Gardens Healthy Meals Fast. Des Moines, Iowa: Meredith, 1996.

Better Homes and Gardens Low-Fat Meals. Des Moines, Iowa: Meredith, 1996.

Betty Crocker's New Choices Cookbook. New York: Prentice-Hall, 1993.

Cooking Light Five Star Recipes. Birmingham, AL: Oxmoor House, 1996. 1-800-633-4910 to order.

Eat Right Lose Weight: 7 Simple Steps. Birmingham, AL: Oxmoor House, Inc., 1997. 1-800-633-4910 to order.

Low-Fat Ways To Lose Weight. Birmingham, AL: Oxmoor House, 1996. 1-800-633-4910 to order.

Low-Fat Ways To Cook Vegetarian. Birmingham, AL: Oxmoor House, 1996. 1-800-633-4910 to order.

Light Chinese Dishes. New York: HP Books, 1995.

Secrets of Low-Fat Cooking. New York: Eating Well Books, 1997.

Southern Living Soup & Stew Recipes. Birmingham, AL: Oxmoor House, 1996. 1-800-633-4910 to order.

Southern Living Best Recipes Made Lighter. Birmingham, AL: Oxmoor House, 1997. 1-800-633-4910 to order.

30-Minute Vegetarian Recipes. Des Moines, Iowa: Meredith, 1995.

Cravings vs. Hunger

Here is the place where your mind and body deceive each other, and where the "A" (Attitudes) part of The LEARN Program comes to the fore. When you eat, are you responding to physical hunger or to psychological cravings? Take the Cravings and Hunger Quiz here to find out. Which is the mind and which is the body?

Situations 1, 3, and 5 usually indicate psychological cravings. Situations 2 and 4 signal physical hunger. Situation 6 could be either. Distinguishing cravings from hunger is important. Once you can distinguish the cravings, we will work on special anti-craving techniques.

You can identify cravings by paying careful attention to when you want to eat. Does something stimulate the urge beside actual hunger? Does someone offer you food? Does something make you think about food? Do you have bad feelings that food would help satisfy? You can make note of these cravings on your Monitoring Form. This will remind you of the situations in which food will be hard to resist. Information on conquering the cravings is in the next lesson.

Shaping the Right Attitudes

Conquering the Cravings

In the discussion above, we learned to separate food cravings from physical hunger. Once you can spot the cravings, there are two ways to deal with them: distraction and confrontation.

The *distraction* approach involves ignoring the cravings. When you know a craving is about to engulf you, do something else. Think about something wonderful, plan a dream vacation, or do anything to take your attention away from the urge to eat. The craving will usually pass.

The distraction method works best for people who have a good imagination or can change activities or thoughts at an instant's notice. You only have to do these things for a few moments, because cravings generally pass within minutes or even seconds. If you are bombarded by

---

Cravings and Hunger Quiz

Answer each question below by circling either T for true or F for false.

T F 1. Even after a large meal, I still want dessert.

T F 2. I often have a gnawing feeling in my stomach.

T F 3. When someone mentions a food I love, I feel like eating.

T F 4. I feel lightheaded after not eating for hours.

T F 5. When I drive by a fast-food restaurant, I want to eat.

T F 6. There is a time every day when I feel hungry.

---

cravings throughout the day, confronting the cravings may be most effective.

The *confrontation* approach pits you against the craving. Let's say you want to raid the refrigerator for ice cream. You could pretend the urge is another person trying to convince you to eat the ice cream. Argue with this person and say why you will not give in to the urge. Another approach is to visualize the ice cream container beckoning to you and tempting you with promises of fulfillment. Imagine how silly it is to let the ice cream get the best of you.

A typical confrontation scene might be as follows. You get the urge to stop for a snack while driving home from work. You recognize the craving and decide to get the best of it. You say, "You nasty craving! You want me to stop for Peanut Butter Cups when I'm not really hungry. I'll show you who's boss. I am in charge of my own life and my weight."

Think of these two approaches now and decide which will work for you. If you are in doubt, experiment with both. Try to arrive at a strategy as soon as possible, be it distraction or confrontation. This will prepare you in advance for the

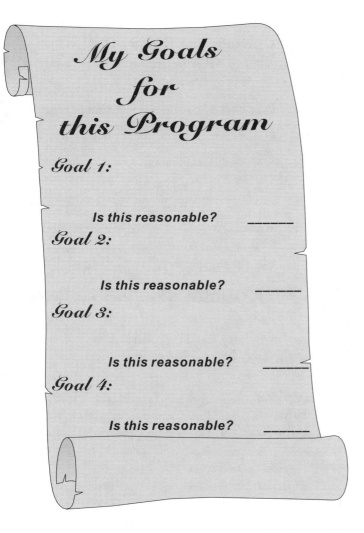

My Goals for this Program

Goal 1:

Is this reasonable? _____

Goal 2:

Is this reasonable? _____

Goal 3:

Is this reasonable? _____

Goal 4:

Is this reasonable? _____

❶ How much weight do you expect to lose each week?

❷ How soon do you expect to be thin?

❸ Will your life be different when you lose weight?

❹ Do you expect losing weight to be easy and quick?

These are just examples of some tricky areas. You are a sensible person and can formulate reasonable goals. Do you think your hidden or unconscious goals are not realistic? If so, remind yourself time and time again that setting unrealistic goals is a setup for trouble.

In the space to the left, list your four major goals for this program, and decide whether they are realistic. The goals may be specific weight-loss accomplishments (to lose one pound each week, or to lose 25 pounds in total) or other changes (clothes will fit better, look better for daughter's wedding).

The Principle of Shaping

Shaping refers to making gradual, step-by-step changes in your behavior. Two examples can highlight how this works. If your weakness is donuts and you begin every day with three of your favorite kind, dropping them completely may be difficult. You could start by cutting down to two donuts, then one, and finally to none. Our approach to exercise is another example of shaping. We began with comfortable levels of walking with the goal of increasing in a gradual way to a final level.

You can see how the shaping principle applies to goal setting. Setting realistic goals means starting from a point you can master and then working up gradually to the level you desire. This will come through many times in the lessons that follow.

inevitable cravings you will face. Do your best not to give in.

Goal Setting

One common attitude problem is having unrealistic goals. Some individuals do not recognize they are setting unattainable goals, but they do so nonetheless. Examples of this are starting a program in May for swimsuit season when you have 50 pounds to lose. Having fantasies of being thin and having life improve immediately is another example. These things may happen, but not right away.

Think about your goals for the program. Think of specific answers to these four questions:

Quality of Life Self-Assessment

Please use the following scale to rate how satisfied you feel now about different aspects of your daily life. Choose any number from this list (1 to 9) and indicate your choice on the questions below.

1 = Extremely Dissatisfied   6 = Somewhat Satisfied

2 = Very Dissatisfied   7 = Moderately Satisfied

3 = Moderately Dissatisfied   8 = Very Satisfied

4 = Somewhat Dissatisfied   9 = Extremely Satisfied

5 = Neutral

---

1. ___ Mood (feelings of sadness, worry, happiness, etc.)
2. ___ Self-esteem
3. ___ Confidence, self-assurance and comfort in social situations
4. ___ Energy and feeling healthy
5. ___ Health problems (diabetes, high blood pressure, etc.)
6. ___ General appearance
7. ___ Social life
8. ___ Leisure and recreational activities
9. ___ Physical mobility and physical activity
10. ___ Eating habits
11. ___ Body image
12. ___ Overall quality of life

Quality of Life Assessment

It is time again to complete the Quality of Life Self-Assessment. We ask you to do this about once a month to track changes in important areas of your life. Following a healthier diet, being more physically active, and losing weight can have multiple benefits. The problem is that we are so focused on the scale that we overlook some of the most important benefits of all. Having more energy and more self-confidence are just examples. One reason we do this self-assessment periodically is to keep you going even when the scale seems stuck. If the assessment shows change, things are going well and you have cause to feel good. Compare your score today with the scores from the Quality of Life Self-Assessments you filled out in the Introduction and Orientation (page 11) and in Lesson 5 (page 66). Remember, the scale is only one index of your success.

Setting Personal Goals

For your personal goals, consider being aware of fat in foods, and if you feel you would benefit from reducing fat, be active in doing so while still eating a tasty diet. Cutting back the fat can be a great way to reduce calories, and since fat intake is related to risk of heart disease and probably some cancers, your body will thank you for more than the weight loss.

Think also of our principle of shaping. Some people do well with making abrupt, massive changes, but it is usually easier to break down long-term goals into short-term goals you are pretty sure you can reach.

And, as always, think of the personal goals that are important for you to reach. Only you can decide what these will be. This is the way to tailor the program to your needs.

Self-Assessment Questionnaire

Lesson 9

T F 40. Since too much dietary fat has been linked to heart disease and other health-related risks, it's best to eliminate all fat from your diet.

T F 41. The recommended daily intake of dietary fat is 30 percent or less of total calories.

T F 42. One gram of fat contains more than twice the calories of one gram of carbohydrate or protein.

T F 43. Saturated fat is usually solid at room temperature and is found only in animal foods, such as meats and dairy products made from whole milk or cream.

T F 44. Since all fruits and vegetables have only small amounts of fats, it is not as important to count the amount of fat in these foods as it is to count the dietary fat from meat and dairy products.

T F 45. To conquer food cravings, distraction will be helpful for some people and confirmation will be helpful for other.

T F 46. Shaping refers to encouraging others to help you lose weight.

(Answers in Appendix C)

Monitoring Form—Lesson 9

Today's Date:

Time	Food and Amount	Calories
Total Daily Calories		

Personal Goals This Week	*Always*	*Sometimes*	*Never*
1. Take medication every day			
2. Keep fat intake to 30 percent or less of total calories			
3. Separate psychological cravings from physical hunger			
4. Set realistic goals			
5. Less than _____ grams of fat each day			
6. Less than _____ calories each day			

Medication Taken Today ❏ Yes ❏ No	*Physical Activity*	*Minutes*
Milk, yogurt, and cheese ❏ ❏ ❏		
Meat, poultry, etc. ❏ ❏ ❏		
Fruits ❏ ❏ ❏ ❏		
Vegetables ❏ ❏ ❏ ❏ ❏		
Breads, cereals, etc. ❏ ❏ ❏ ❏ ❏ ❏ ❏ ❏ ❏		

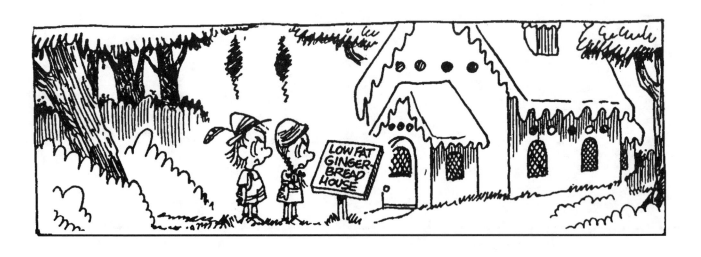

Lesson 10

We are now far enough into The LEARN Program to reflect on what you have learned, the behaviors you have practiced, and the new outlook on diet and lifestyle changes we have been discussing. Have some of the techniques become habits? Is this a program you can live with? These are the key questions we must consider for the long-term outlook.

In this lesson we will talk more about some exciting news about physical activity (we introduced this discussion in Lesson 5). You might be delighted to learn that there is scientific evidence to show that you do not have to knock yourself out to benefit from being physically active. You will also learn the calorie values of different types of physical activity in this lesson. We'll talk about the importance of food and the different types of nutrients that are essential for good health. Finally, we will discuss your forbidden fantasies—at least those dealing with food!

Physical Activity and Good News

We have focused on lifestyle activity, particularly walking. This is where most overweight individuals should start. By now, however, you may feel more comfortable with being physically active and may be ready for more. It is time to introduce the topic of regular, programmed exercise. In Lesson 14 we will talk about this more and help you select appropriate activities.

We expect that about half the people who read this manual will be ready for more rigorous activity. The others can continue walking and lose more weight before taking on programmed activity. If you are in the latter, read this section for its information, and remember to refer back to it when you are ready to increase your activity. In the meantime, continue to increase your walking by adding time or by increasing the speed with which you walk.

As we mentioned earlier, programmed activities include jogging, walking, aerobics, racquetball, swimming, cycling, or any regular activity. Selecting the right activity is something of an art and will be discussed later in Lesson 14. For now, we want to address the issue of how much exercise is necessary.

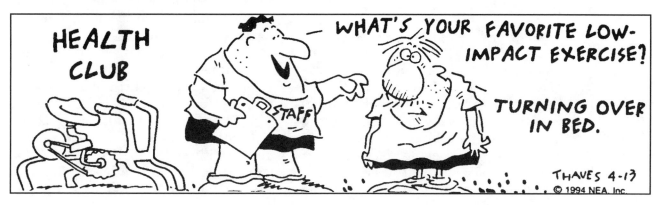

HEALTH CLUB — WHAT'S YOUR FAVORITE LOW-IMPACT EXERCISE?

TURNING OVER IN BED.

THAVES 4-13
© 1994 NEA, Inc.

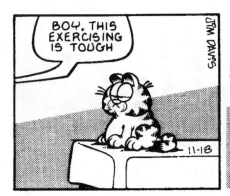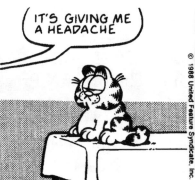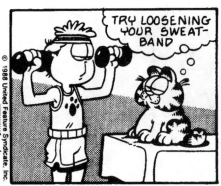

Great News about Activity

For many people, exercise is a major factor in their long-term prospects for weight control. It is true that many people lose weight without exercise, but for others, exercise makes an enormous difference. Do you remember the graph in Lesson 7 on page 91 that showed the difference between the maintainers and the regainers?

Exercise helps people lose weight for both physical and psychological reasons. It burns calories and may boost your metabolic rate. Perhaps as important are the ways exercise makes us feel good. Each time we exercise, we are sending a signal to ourselves that we are making positive changes. The exercise may reduce stress and may give us more energy for life's other activities (like planning our weekly diet). Some people find exercise especially helpful by scheduling it at times they are most likely to eat.

One bit of very good news about exercise comes from work by Dr. Steven Blair and his colleagues at The Cooper Institute for Aerobics Research in Dallas, Texas. These researchers studied physical fitness and health in 10,224 men and 3,120 women. Each person in the study had undergone a detailed medical exam that included a maximal stress test on a treadmill. The people were grouped into categories of physical fitness based upon their performance on the treadmill test. They were then followed for an average of eight years.

Dr. Blair and his colleagues placed these people into five categories of fitness, ranging from the very unfit (Fitness Level 1) to the very fit (Fitness Level 5). The graphs shown on the next page give the risk ratio (which represents the death rate) for both men and women depending on their level of fitness. The risk for the most fit people is given a value of one, and then risks for the other categories are given in reference to that number. For instance, in the figure showing risk rates for men, the men in Fitness Level 5 (the most fit) have a risk factor of one. The risk increases to 1.17 (a 17 percent increase) for men in Fitness Level 4 and to 1.46 (a 46 percent increase) for men in Fitness Level 3.

There are several striking aspects to this study. First, it is yet another piece to the puzzle showing that people who exercise and are physically active live longer. For our purposes, however, the important news is that even modest levels of fitness are associated with greatly reduced risk. Look at the figure showing numbers for the men. Men in the lowest level of fitness (Fitness Level 1) have a risk ratio of 3.44 compared to a ratio of 1.37 in Fitness Level 2. There is a substantial decline in risk by moving from the least fit group to the next group.

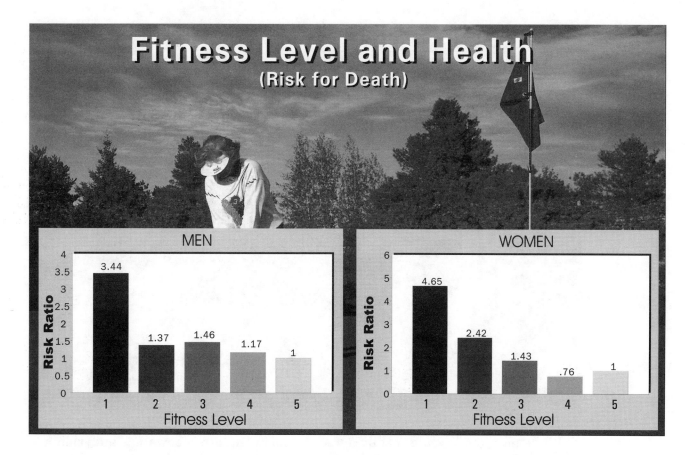

Fitness Level and Health
(Risk for Death)

MEN

Risk Ratio

3.44 | 1.37 | 1.46 | 1.17 | 1

Fitness Level: 1 2 3 4 5

WOMEN

Risk Ratio

4.65 | 2.42 | 1.43 | .76 | 1

Fitness Level: 1 2 3 4 5

There are certainly gains made by increasing fitness further, but the big drop occurs as people go from being completely sedentary to moderately active. The figure for women shows much the same pattern.

The moral to this story is that you do not have to kill yourself to keep from dying. Even small amounts of exercise are likely to have a big impact on health and will certainly be helpful for weight loss. In the Blair study, one only had to do regular walking at a moderate pace to be fit enough to be in Level 2, which had about half the risk of the group who were least fit. How much exercise should you do? You should do as much as you can and still have fun. Don't worry so much about how much or what type, just try to do it regularly.

Remember, any type of activity should be considered exercise. If you take an extra flight of stairs, rake the leaves, walk an extra block, or chase the rabbits out of your vegetable garden, you have exercised and should say so in your own mind. You deserve to feel good about these activities and can feel confident that you are making progress.

A New Activity Formula for Americans

The work of Dr. Blair and other experts in the field has provided a growing body of evidence that regular, moderate-intensity physical activity can result in substantial health benefits. One of the primary benefits is protection against coronary heart disease. Other health benefits may include protection against several other chronic diseases, such as adult onset diabetes, hypertension, certain cancers, osteoporosis, and depression.

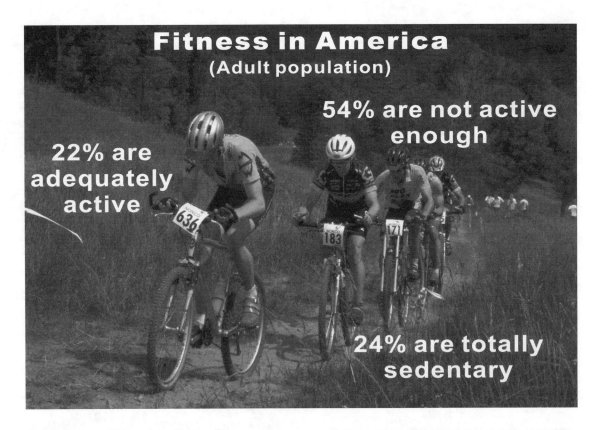

Fitness in America
(Adult population)

22% are adequately active

54% are not active enough

24% are totally sedentary

While most of us would readily agree that regular physical activity is beneficial, most of us are not physically active on a regular basis. Only about 22 percent of adults in this country engage in leisure time physical activity. About 24 percent of adults are completely sedentary, and the remaining 54 percent are inadequately active. They too would benefit from more regular physical activity. With all of this scientific evidence, why are we a nation of inactivity? Two reasons come to mind.

We live in a high-tech society. The more technologically advanced we become, the more inactive we become. Cars, garage-door openers, portable telephones, television, remote controls for most electrical devices, and many other labor-saving gadgets have changed the way we work, take care of our homes, and use our leisure time. Technology entices us to be inactive. Further, our environment presents many obstacles and barriers to physical activity. Walking to the corner store is difficult if there are

not adequate sidewalks, and riding a bicycle or walking to work is difficult because of the way suburbs have moved many people further from their work.

The second reason people may be inactive is that they have a misconception about exercise. Many people have thought that the exercise prescription for cardiovascular training (we will discuss this later) is THE prescription for exercise. It is NOT! This led to the belief that if a person could not follow the prescription, then why exercise at all? The following new guidelines may help to dispel this old myth.

New Guidelines for Exercise

In July of 1993, the American College of Sports Medicine and the U.S. Centers for Disease Control and Prevention, in cooperation with the President's Council on Physical Fitness and Sports, released new exercise guidelines and recommendations for Americans. The new guidelines recommend 30 minutes or more of moderate intensity physical activity over the course of most days of the week (at least five days).

This is great news. Six five-minute walks count as 30 minutes of activity. Activities that can also contribute to the 30-minute total include walking up stairs, gardening, cleaning house, raking leaves, and walking part or all of the way to and from work. The recommended 30 minutes of physical activity may also come from planned exercise or recreation, such as jogging, riding a bicycle, playing golf or tennis, or swimming. A brisk two-mile walk is another way to achieve 30 minutes of physical activity.

As you can see, there are many reasons to increase your physical activity. The best advice is to build physical activity into your daily routine—make it become part of your lifestyle just like eating, working, and sleeping. The physical and psychological aspects of a more active lifestyle can be quite rewarding.

The Mighty Calorie

In Lesson 3 we explained what a calorie is. We eat at least a half-million calories each year. You might wonder, therefore, what difference a few calories can make. They can make a big difference.

As we mentioned earlier, 3500 calories will translate into a pound of body weight. If you consume 7000 calories more than your body uses, you will gain two pounds. These are rough estimates, and people vary greatly in the precise number of calories needed to gain or lose weight. What is clear is that calories do count. Let's examine the effects of add-

ing an innocent 10 calories per day to your total.

If you add ten calories per day to what you ordinarily eat, you will gain an extra pound in a year. Added over a decade or two, this is 10–20 pounds; and all from 10 crummy calories per day! If the difference each day were 100 calories, this would be 10 pounds per year and 100 pounds for 10 years! Let's look at the 10 calorie difference for the moment. The chart below shows you how little you have to eat to get 10 extra calories.

Think how easy it is to have an extra teaspoon of ketchup, one bite of an orange, or less than one ounce of Pepsi. This shows the need for careful calculation of calories in your Monitoring Form and a vigilant attitude about foods.

You can also take a positive outlook on this calorie equation. Cutting out 10 calories each day will save you a pound each year. You certainly won't miss the 10 calories, but you can easily do without the pound.

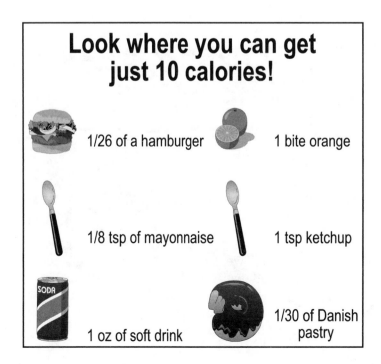

Look where you can get just 10 calories!

1/26 of a hamburger

1 bite orange

1/8 tsp of mayonnaise

1 tsp ketchup

1 oz of soft drink

1/30 of Danish pastry

The Calorie Values of Physical Activity

How many calories do you burn when you wash the dishes? Is it more than when you rake leaves? Is it easier to burn calories by swimming, jogging, or cycling? Your questions will be answered in the table on the next page.

Several important points are highlighted by the calorie chart. First, any activity uses energy (calories), so any increase in activity can help. Sitting uses approximately 15 calories per 10 minutes, while standing uses 17, and walking briskly uses 60. Even something as simple as standing rather than sitting can use a few extra calories. Second, heavier people burn more calories than other people while doing the same activity, because more energy is required to move the extra weight. Third, several routine activities like using stairs and walking are useful methods of burning calories.

Several facts must be considered when viewing these calorie figures. One is that calorie expenditures vary enormously for many activities, depending on their intensity. Two people shoveling snow may differ greatly in how quickly they shovel, how much snow is lifted with each shovel, and how much they move around while shoveling. Similar differences can occur with skiing, tennis, yard work, and so forth. Therefore, the figures in the tables are only averages.

The second fact is that the table shows the calories burned for 10 minutes of continuous activity. If you do an activity for five minutes, divide the value in the table by two. If you are active for 30 minutes, multiply the value by three.

The word *continuous* is important to understanding the table. The table shows that a 125 pound person burns 56 calories for 10 minutes of bowling. This is 10 minutes of nonstop bowling and does not include time to keep score, chat with friends, polish your ball, or visit the snack bar. The 10 minutes for skiing would not include time waiting in the lift line, marveling at the scenery, or falling down! So, to calculate the calories you burn for a given activity, add the time you are truly active, and then use the table on the next page as a guide.

The Importance of Food

In simple terms, food is energy; it is the fuel our body uses to enable us to carry on our daily activities. Like most energy sources, quality is as important as quantity, and having the right mixture of nutrients at the right time is also important. Some nutrients have energy (calories) and others do not, but both are critical to our bodies. The nutrient needs of our bodies are comparable to the different needs of our automobiles. Gaso-

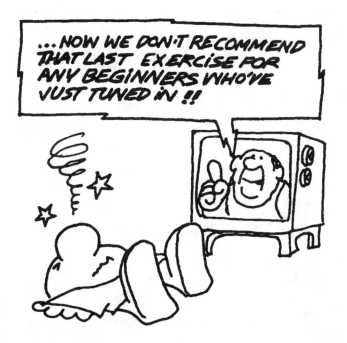

Calorie Values for 10 Minutes of Activity

Activity	Body Weight 125 Pounds	175 Pounds	250 Pounds	Activity	Body Weight 125 Pounds	175 Pounds	250 Pounds
Personal Necessities				*Light Work*			
Sleeping	10	14	20	Assembly line	20	28	40
Sitting (watching TV)	10	14	18	Auto repair	35	48	69
Sitting (talking)	15	21	30	Carpentry	32	44	64
Dressing or washing	26	37	53	Bricklaying	28	40	57
Standing	12	16	24	Framing chores	32	44	64
Locomotion				House painting	29	40	58
Walking downstairs	56	78	111	*Heavy Work*			
Walking upstairs	146	202	288	Pick & shovel work	56	78	110
Walking at 2 mph	29	40	58	Chopping wood	60	84	121
Walking at 4 mph	52	72	102	Dragging logs	158	220	315
Running at 5.5 mph	90	125	178	Drilling coal	79	111	159
Running at 7 mph	118	164	232	*Recreation*			
Running at 12 mph	164	228	326	Badminton	43	65	94
Cycling at 5.5 mph	42	58	83	Baseball	39	54	78
Cycling at 13 mph	89	124	178	Basketball	58	82	117
Housework				Bowling (nonstop)	56	78	111
Making beds	32	46	65	Canoeing (4 mph)	90	128	182
Washing floors	38	53	75	Dancing (moderate)	35	48	69
Washing windows	35	48	69	Dancing (vigorous)	48	66	94
Dusting	22	31	44	Football	69	96	137
Preparing a meal	32	46	65	Golfing	33	48	68
Shoveling snow	65	89	130	Horseback riding	56	78	112
Light gardening	30	42	59	Ping-Pong	32	45	64
Weeding garden	49	68	98	Racquetball	75	104	144
Mowing grass (power)	34	47	67	Skiing (alpine)	80	112	160
Mowing grass (manual)	38	52	74	Skiing (cross country)	98	138	194
Sedentary Occupation				Skiing (water)	60	88	130
Sitting (writing)	15	21	30	Squash	75	104	144
Light office work	25	34	50	Swimming (backstroke)	32	45	64
Standing, light activity	20	28	40	Swimming (crawl)	40	56	80
Typing (electric)	19	27	39	Tennis	56	80	115
				Volleyball	43	65	94

line and diesel fuel provide fuel or energy. Oil, water, transmission fluid, and other lubricants are also critical to a car's operation, but they do not provide energy.

There are over 45 different nutrients that our bodies need every day. They are essential for our health and must be provided in the food we eat. There are six classes of these nutrients, and they can be divided into two categories:

❶ Nutrients with energy (calories)

❷ Nutrients without energy

Nutrients with energy include carbohydrates, proteins, and fats. In Lesson 9 we discussed the role of fat in your diet;

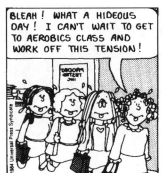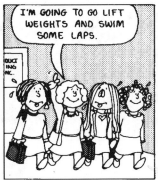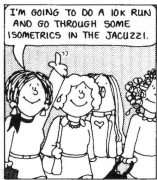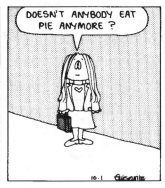

proteins and carbohydrates will be covered in later lessons. The nutrients without energy include minerals, vitamins, and water.

Nutrients Without Energy

There are three classes of nutrients that are essential to our bodies, are contained in the food that we eat, and provide no energy or calories. These nutrients include minerals, vitamins, and water.

Minerals

Our bodies contain over 60 different minerals, of which about 22 are essential. The amount or quantity needed of the different minerals varies greatly. The 22 essential minerals are classified by their presence in the body as either *Macronutrients* (those having a greater presence) and *Micronutrients* (those of lesser quantity). It is important to remember that this classification is based upon presence in the body and not on importance. For example, a deficiency in cobalt, which comprises only two parts per trillion of body weight, can have more damaging effects than a deficiency in calcium, which accounts for two percent of body weight.

Minerals serve many functions. They help to aid in the growth of body tissue, transmit nerve impulses, regulate muscle contraction, maintain water balance in the body, form parts of essential body compounds, maintain the acid-base balance in the cells, and facilitate many biological reactions. Minerals are found together in the foods we eat and interact with each other as well as with other nutrients in the body. Because of this interaction and combination, certain foods are considered better sources than others.

Vitamins

Vitamins are also essential nutrients that are needed to sustain life. They are required for the regulation of the body's metabolism and for the transformation of energy (protein, carbohydrates, and fat) in the body. Some vitamins help to form important enzymes, and others act as catalysts to speed certain chemical reactions. There are two types of vitamins:

❶ Fat soluble
❷ Water soluble

Fat Soluble Vitamins

The four fat soluble vitamins are A, D, E, and K. These vitamins are found in dietary fat and are stored in the body's fat tissue if consumed in excess amounts. Since these vitamins are stored, toxic doses can be an important issue. You should be cautious of people who promote large quantities of these vitamins. No more than the Recommended Daily Allowance (RDA) is suggested.

Vitamin A is essential for the growth of skin, bones, and teeth. It is also important in vision. The RDA for vitamin A is 5000 International Units. Vitamin D is essential for bone and tooth development. In addition, it helps the body utilize calcium and phosphorus. The RDA for vitamin D is 400 International Units. Vitamin E is essential for the functioning of red blood cells and helps the body utilize the essential fatty acids. The RDA for Vitamin E is 30 International Units. Vitamin K is used by the liver to produce prothrombin, a factor in blood plasma that combines with calcium to help in blood clotting. An RDA has not been established for vitamin K.

Water Soluble Vitamins

Water soluble vitamins consist of seven primary vitamins: Vitamin C and the B complex vitamins that include vitamin B_1 (thiamine), vitamin B_2 (riboflavin), vitamin B_3 (niacin), vitamin B_6 (pyridoxine), folacin, and vitamin B_{12} (cobalamin). Unlike the fat soluble vitamins, these are absorbed in the body's water, and excess amounts are usually excreted.

The Six Classes of Nutrients

Nutrients with Energy (Calories)

1. **Carbohydrates**—starches, sugar, and fiber.
2. **Protein**—includes 22 amino acids.
3. **Fats**—saturated, monounsaturated, and polyunsaturated fatty acids.

Nutrients Without Energy

4. **Minerals—22 in total**

7 Macronutrients	15 Micronutrients	
calcium	arsenic	manganese
chlorine	boron	molybdenum
magnesium	cobalt	nickel
phosphorus	copper	selenium
potassium	chromium	silicon
sodium	fluorine	vanadium
sulfur	iodine	zinc
	iron	

5. **Vitamins**

Fat Soluble	*Water Soluble*
Vitamin A-RDA 5000 IU	Vitamin C-RDA 60 mg
Vitamin D-RDA 400 IU	Vitamin B₁ (thiamine)-RDA 1.5 mg
Vitamin E-RDA 30 IU	Vitamin B₂ (riboflavin)-RDA 1.7 mg
Vitamin K	Vitamin B₃ (niacin)-RDA 19 mg
	Vitamin B₆ (pyridoxine)-RDA 2.0 mg
	Vitamin B₁₂ (cobalamin)-RDA 6 micrograms
	Folicin-RDA 400 micrograms

6. **Water**

Vitamin C is used by the body for teeth, bones, cells, and blood vessels; it is essential for good health. The RDA for vitamin C is 60 mg. Vitamin B_1 is essential for the heart and nervous system and plays an important role in carbohydrate metabolism. A deficiency of this vitamin can result in beriberi and certain nervous disorders. The RDA for vitamin B_1 is 1.5 mg. Vitamin B_2 is also important in carbohydrate metabolism and body tissue repair. It is necessary for the skin and helps prevent light sensitivity in the eyes. A deficiency of this vitamin in the diet can lead to stunted growth and loss of hair. The RDA for vitamin B_2 is 1.7 mg. Vitamin B_3 (more commonly known as niacin) is important for metabolism and absorption of carbohy-

drates in the body and plays an important role in converting food to usable energy. The RDA for vitamin B_3 is 19 mg. Vitamin B_6 aids in the metabolism of protein, carbohydrate, and fat. The RDA for vitamin B_6 is 2.0 mg. Vitamin B_{12} is essential for normal growth and neurological function. This vitamin also helps prevent anemia. The RDA for vitamin B_{12} is 6 micrograms. Folacin is also important and helps the body metabolize food and is useful in preventing certain anemias. The RDA for folacin is 400 micrograms.

As a general rule, nutrition experts believe that people in the U.S. receive an adequate supply of minerals and vitamins if they eat a balanced diet. Following the dietary guidelines of the Food Guide Pyramid will help insure a balanced diet. Therefore, most people do not need or benefit from mineral or vitamin supplements, much less the megadoses promoted by some people, including seemingly credible nutrition stores.

Water

Many people overlook the importance of water in their diets, not realizing that water is an essential nutrient. Considering that water makes up about 60 percent of our body and that water is needed by every cell in our body, water is indeed an important nutrient. Most people in the U.S. do not consume enough water. It should be consumed generously. As a rule of thumb, about four cups of water should be consumed for every 1000 calories eaten. For most adults, this is equivalent to about10cups (2½ quarts) of water each day.

Food and Weight Fantasies

Many individuals have fantasies of foods. It is common, for example, to fantasize about having a celebration or letting go meal when the program ends. Some people even think about specific foods or the ability to eat large quantities again. There are also common weight fantasies. These usually are visions of a sleek body and huge weight losses.

Food or weight fantasies are a sign of unrealistic expectations. Weight loss is not easy, and pounds do not fly off as we'd like. Food fantasies reveal an expectation that the rigors of going through a program will end some magic day and that old eating habits will return.

We must keep up what we learn. You can eat your favorite foods now and will be able to eat them later. You will not, however, be able to return to uncontrolled eating. Identify what you want to eat, and eat a small quantity in a controlled manner. Most of all, enjoy it. By not overeating you will not feel guilty, and by eating a small portion you will not deprive yourself and feel resentful.

Setting Personal Goals

We covered a lot of ground in this lesson. For the next week, carefully monitor your physical activity and think of additional activities you enjoy doing. Review your Monitoring Forms from last week and look for places to cut10 calories from your diet. Remember, over time,10 calories do add up.

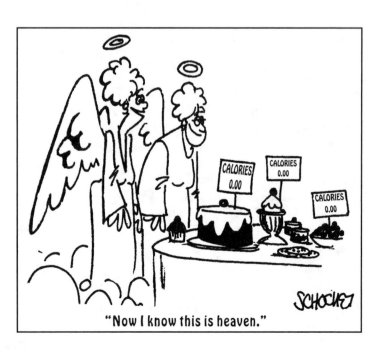

"Now I know this is heaven."

Self-Assessment Questionnaire

Lesson 10

T F   47. Most people get enough exercise to realize the many health benefits of an active lifestyle.

T F   48. Exercise must be done in specific amounts for it to aid you with weight loss.

T F   49. Thirty minutes of moderate-intensity physical activity is now recommended for Americans.

T F   50. Climbing stairs requires more energy per minute than many traditional exercises like swimming and jogging.

T F   51. All nutrients that we eat contain calories.

(Answers in Appendix C)

Monitoring Form—Lesson 10

Today's Date:

Time	Food and Amount	Calories
	Total Daily Calories	

Personal Goals This Week	Always	Sometimes	Never
1. Take medication every day			
2. Keep fat intake to 30 percent or less of total calories			
3. Look for ways to cut 10 calories			
4. Increase lifestyle activity			
5. Less than _____ grams of fat each day			
6. Less than _____ calories each day			

Medication Taken Today ❑ Yes ❑ No	*Physical Activity*	*Minutes*
Milk, yogurt, and cheese ❑ ❑ ❑		
Meat, poultry, etc. ❑ ❑ ❑		
Fruits ❑ ❑ ❑ ❑		
Vegetables ❑ ❑ ❑ ❑ ❑		
Breads, cereals, etc. ❑ ❑ ❑ ❑ ❑ ❑ ❑ ❑ ❑		

Lesson 11

This lesson will focus in part on what you think about your eating. This issue is central to your ability to persist over the weeks, months, and years it takes for successful weight control. How you think will determine whether you get discouraged and feel like giving up, or instead feel positive, upbeat, and energized. We will also discuss the notion of shopping for food and shopping with a partner. In the nutrition area we discuss the Milk Group from the Food Guide Pyramid. So, if you're ready, let's forge ahead.

Thinking Your Way to Success

We cannot overstate how important your thoughts are. Your thoughts will determine how you feel about yourself, which in turn effects your mood, your interactions with others, and your interpretation of your progress in the program.

People in weight loss programs have some common ways of thinking. Examples are expecting too much, being upset with anything less than perfection, and letting small mistakes build to catastrophe. We have seen these take root in hundreds of people. They get in the way, can sour a person's outlook, and can be difficult to change. It is our job to help you pull these out by the root and plant more constructive thoughts in their

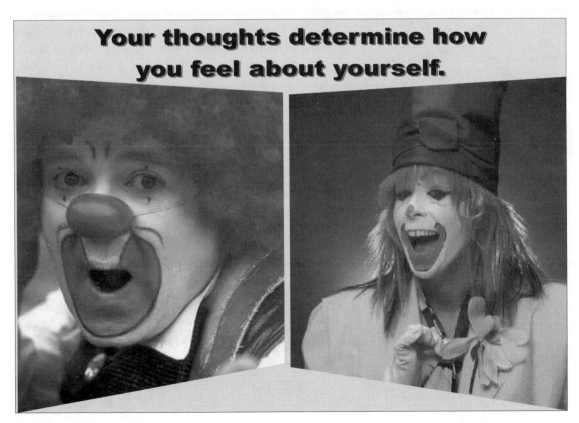

Your thoughts determine how you feel about yourself.

Measuring Up to Your Own Goals

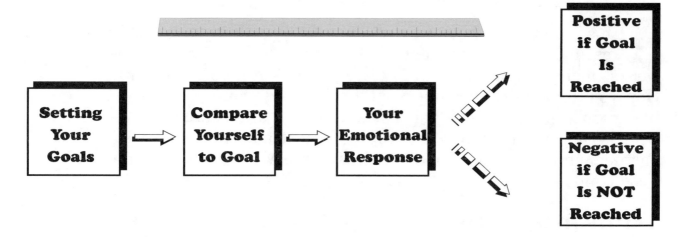

place. This may sound puzzling to do, but stay with us and we'll explain.

Your Thinking Process

We discussed goal setting in Lesson 9 and concluded that setting unrealistic goals can halt your progress. It is time to explore this matter further. We set goals for everything we do. Although we do not articulate a goal for every activity, hidden within our mind are expectations of how well we should perform. If you mow the lawn, write a letter, buy clothes, or simply talk to a friend, you expect a certain level of performance. If you scalped the lawn, wrote an unintelligible letter, bought gaudy clothes, or said insensitive things to your friend, you would be upset because you expected more—you did not satisfy your internal standard.

You can see how difficult life would be if your goals were absurdly out-of-reach. If you expected *Better Homes and Gardens* to lust after your lawn, for the National Archives to enshrine your letter, for the President's wife to wear your clothes to the Inaugural Ball, or for your friend to memorialize your words in a book of quotes, you would be crushed by what is otherwise an acceptable performance. Unfortunately, it is just such out-of-reach goals that people losing weight

tend to set for themselves about their eating, exercise, and weight loss. When the goals are not met, the negative emotional response can send your progress into a tailspin.

This occurs in a three-part process. Setting the goals comes first and is often unconscious. You then compare actual performance to that goal. Finally, there is a positive emotional reaction if the goal is achieved and a negative one if it is not. The model above shows this three-step process.

At the top of the next page are a few examples of how this process pertains to weight loss goals. These are common examples, so while you are reading, think if these or similar situations occur with you.

This emotional response is what worries us. Many people have enough trouble controlling their eating and exercise without the extra burden of negative feelings and thoughts. You can change the emotional response by altering the two steps that precede it, namely the goal setting and the comparison you make to the goals.

Setting Goal	Comparing Performance	Emotional Response
Will never cheat on a program.	Cheating on program does occur.	Guilt and resignation.
Will be good at sports.	Others do better and look better.	Embarrassment.
Will lose weight each week.	Some weeks weight stays stable or goes up.	Discouragement and self-blame.

When you have negative feelings, examine them and trace them to the goals you set. If you feel guilty because you sneak a Snickers, think about your goal, which is probably something like, "I should never cheat on this program." You can examine the comparison to this goal by understanding that you or anyone else could never be satisfied with this as a standard. This will change the emotional response.

Below are the same situations with different goals, comparisons, and emotional responses. Use these examples to analyze your own goals, comparisons, and responses. This can lift the weight of negative feelings from your shoulders.

Attribution: Thinking about Your Medication

One key issue in using medication for weight control is what scientists call at-

tribution. Whether you attribute success to your own efforts or to the medication is an important matter.

Research has shown that people are more likely to maintain changes they make if they attribute the changes to their own efforts rather than to some external factors. Here's a simple example.

A person who wants to lose weight for their own reasons and begins a program by their own choice should do better in the long run than someone who was pushed by a family member and began a program due to the pressure.

This attribution process relates directly to using medication for weight loss. When some people lose weight using medication, they feel the medication is helping, but know that their own hard work is a big part of their success. These people are likely to be confident about keeping control when facing challenges such as going to a buffet dinner. They

Setting Goal	Comparing Performance	Emotional Response
Will follow the program as much as possible.	Meet goal on most occasions.	Satisfaction and desire to do better.
Will increase level of exercise.	Increase is steady and substantial.	Pride in doing something positive.
Will lose weight most weeks.	Lose weight 10 out of 12 weeks.	Feel good about hard work.

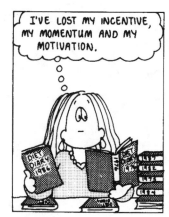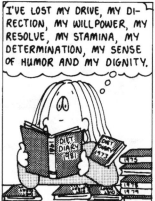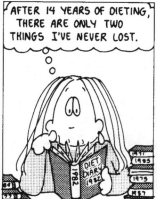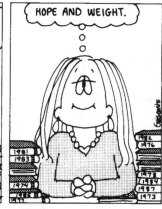

know they can choose foods wisely. Other people give all the credit to the drug and believe they are incapable of controlling their eating without it. Guess which group will do better in the long run?

You may have a hard time accepting that it is you who makes the changes, but it is true. Believing it is true is one key to maintenance, so you must do your best to convince yourself of this. It can be done—it just takes repetition. So, whenever you do something positive, give yourself credit and acknowledge you have made a worthwhile effort. These changes will become easier with time, sometimes to the point of being automatic. This can give you a special confidence that can be a great ally as time goes on.

Shopping for Food

Let's look back on the ABC approach introduced in Lesson 6. The "A" refers to the antecedents that set the stage for eating. One important antecedent is shopping for food. If you buy good foods, you will eat good foods. This may sound obvious, but too few people plan their shopping accordingly.

Having problem foods available in the house, office, car, briefcase, purse, or pocket can be asking for trouble, even if you vow to "eat only a little." If something threatens your restraint, say fatigue or boredom, you can pay a dear price for a decision to buy the food made hours or days earlier. On the other hand, if your refrigerator resembles a salad bar because of wise shopping, weakened restraint can inflict only minor damage. There are several clever methods you can use while shopping to make prudent food choices.

▶ **Shop on a full stomach**. It is easy to buy impulsively when you are hungry because everything looks appetizing. An innocent trip to the store to buy a few essentials can become an eating excursion. The supermarket to a hungry person is like water to someone stranded in the Sahara. The stores are made to tempt you. Your restraint is high when you first walk in, but little good it does when you are in the produce section! As you move through the store, you get worked up just as you pass the cookie aisle. Desire reaches its peak as you travel down Dessert Lane (the frozen food and ice cream section). Shop only after you have eaten. You will be surprised how much grief this can prevent.

▶ **Shop from a list**. Prepare a shopping list before you leave the house, and shop only from the list. Decide what to buy *before* you are tempted by the foods in the store. Make the list when you are not hungry.

▶ **Buy foods that require preparation**. With this age of prepackaged foods, microwave ovens, and fast food restaurants, you can eat at an instant's notice. Eating requires little thought and can be done impulsively. Buying foods that require preparation can halt this process.

Let's use an example of a common food. If you have a hankering for fried chicken, you could visit the Colonel and procure 1000 calories in an extra crispy three-piece dinner. Little time would separate craving and consumption. If you chose the preparation route, you would buy a whole chicken, cut it, prepare it, then fry it. You could think about how much you wanted the chicken and might eat less (if you eat it at all). In addition, preparing the chicken yourself would give you the option of baking it, which would bring far fewer calories than deep frying.

A Shopping Partnership

Partners can often help with your food shopping. There are several ways to do this, as discussed below. If your partner is also on a program, you can swap shopping duties. If not, the partner can help you shop in exchange for favors from you. This was the case with Tom and Sheila. On Saturdays, Tom did yard work while Sheila (the one on a weight loss program) did the food shopping. Sheila had trouble with impulse buying because food beckoned her like the sea nymph sirens beckoned Odysseus. They switched tasks, so Tom did the shopping and Sheila did the yard work. This even added some lifestyle activity to Sheila's routine. Here are a few examples of putting the partnership to work.

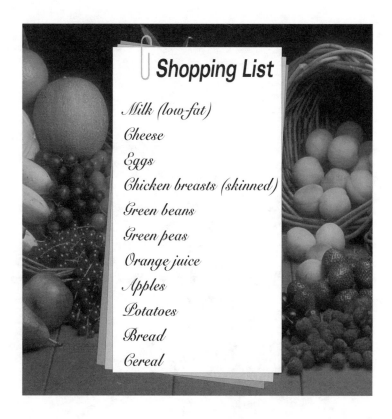

▶ **Shop with a partner**. Shopping can become a social event if your partner journeys with you to the supermarket. You can resist the goodies if you know someone has their eye on your cart. Your partner could help you design your shopping list and could carry it in the store.

▶ **Switch tasks with your partner.** This is what Tom and Sheila did in the example earlier. Your partner may be willing to do the shopping in exchange for help with another job.

▶ **Swap shopping duties with your partner**. If your partner is on a program, trade shopping lists. You do your partner's shopping and your partner can do yours. Unless your partner stuffs your bag with treats, you will come away with the foods you need.

The Food Guide Pyramid

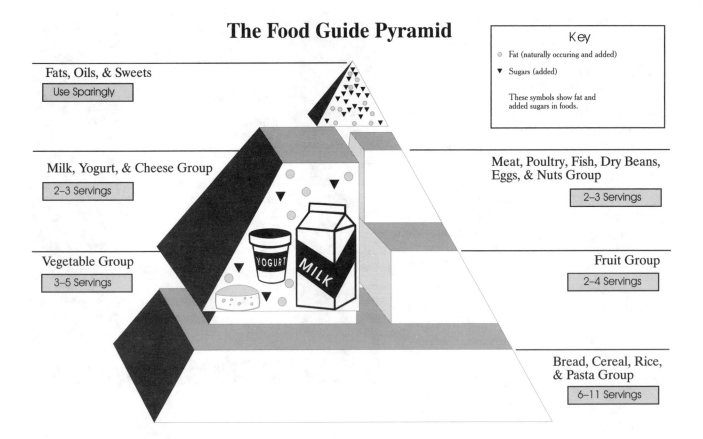

Key

- ● Fat (naturally occuring and added)
- ▼ Sugars (added)

These symbols show fat and added sugars in foods.

Fats, Oils, & Sweets
Use Sparingly

Milk, Yogurt, & Cheese Group
2–3 Servings

Meat, Poultry, Fish, Dry Beans, Eggs, & Nuts Group
2–3 Servings

Vegetable Group
3–5 Servings

Fruit Group
2–4 Servings

Bread, Cereal, Rice, & Pasta Group
6–11 Servings

Revisiting the Food Guide Pyramid

Over the next few weeks, we will be working on the "N" part of LEARN—Nutrition. We cannot emphasize enough the importance of a balanced, healthy diet. Diet is a key ingredient to weight management and overall good health.

The Food Guide Pyramid is an excellent way to help individuals develop sound nutrition skills. In Lesson 9 we discussed the top tier of the pyramid—fats, oils, and sweets. In this lesson we move down the pyramid to the second tier and discuss the Milk, Yogurt, and Cheese Group. We want you to pay close attention this week to the foods you eat from this food group. Try to eat the recommended number of servings each day. This may take a little planning at

first, but we're confident you can master the task.

Milk, Yogurt, and Cheese in Your Diet

The second tier of the Food Guide Pyramid represents foods that come essentially from animal sources—milk, yogurt, and cheese; and meat, poultry, fish, dry beans, eggs, and nuts. The focus in this lesson will be on the Milk, Yogurt, and Cheese Group.

Food items in this group include milk, yogurt, and cheese. These foods are good sources of protein and carbohydrate, but can provide large amounts of unwanted dietary fat (see the food list on page 139). In addition, foods from the Milk Group are good sources of vitamin A, vitamin D, and calcium. Vitamins A and D are es-

Milk, Yogurt, and Cheese

Each of the following counts as one serving.

Description	Calories	Protein (g)	Carbo. (g)	Fat (g)
Milk, skim—1 cup (8 oz)	86	8.4	11.9	Trace
Milk, 1%—1 cup (8 oz)	104	8.5	12.2	2.4
Milk, 2%—1 cup (8 oz)	125	8.5	12.2	4.7
Milk, whole—1 cup (8 oz)	150	8.0	11.0	8.0
Yogurt, nonfat—1 cup (8 oz)	90	10.0	13.0	Trace
Yogurt, light—1 cup (8 oz)	100	9.0	17.0	Trace
Yogurt, low-fat—1 cup (8 oz)	144	11.9	16.0	3.5
Yogurt, skim—1 cup (8 oz)	127	13.0	17.4	Trace
Yogurt, whole—1 cup (8 oz)	139	7.9	10.6	7.4
Yogurt, frozen 1 cup (8 oz)	210	6.2	33.2	6.2
Ice cream, 10% fat—1½ cup (12 oz)	404	7.2	48.0	21.5
Ice cream, 16% fat—1½ cup (12 oz)	524	6.2	48.0	35.6
Ice milk, vanilla—1½ cup (12 oz)	276	7.8	43.5	8.4
Ice milk, soft serve—1½ cup (12 oz)	335	12.0	57.6	6.9
Cheese, American processed—2 oz	212	12.6	1.0	17.8
Cheese, cheddar—1½ oz	171	10.6	.6	14.1
Cheese, colby—1½ oz	168	10.0	1.0	13.7
Cheese, cottage, creamed—2 cups (16 oz)	434	52.4	11.2	19.0
Cheese, cream—1½ oz	149	3.2	1.2	14.9
Cheese, mozzarella—1½ oz	120	8.3	.9	7.2
Cheese, mozzarella part skim—1½ oz	108	10.4	1.2	6.8
Cheese, ricotta whole milk—½ cup (4 oz)	216	14.0	3.8	16.1
Cheese, ricotta part skim— ½ cup (4 oz)	171	14.1	6.4	9.8

Note: This table should be used as a guide for the foods listed. Since food values vary by brand name it is important to read the food labels for these foods.

sential for the growth and development of skin, bones, and teeth. Calcium is an essential mineral for good health. Approximately 2 percent of the body is calcium, most of which is teeth and bones. Food items from the Milk Group are the best source of calcium and generally supply the greatest amount of calcium in our diet. One cup of milk (8 fl oz), for example provides 500 IUs of vitamin A (i.e., 10 percent of the 5000 RDA) and 100 IUs of vitamin D (i.e., 25 percent of the 400 RDA). The same cup of milk also provides about 313 mg of calcium (i.e., 40 percent of the 800 mg RDA).

Cheese items have proportionally more calories from protein than carbohydrate. Milk and yogurt, on the other hand, provide more carbohydrates per serving than protein.

How Many Servings?

The Food Guide Pyramid suggests two to three servings per day from the Milk Group. For most people, two servings from this group is sufficient; however, for teenagers, young adults, and women who are pregnant or breast feeding, three servings per day is recommended. It is important to know what makes up a serving size. Many people may know that servings from this group are important, yet most do not know how many servings are optimal.

How Much Is a Serving?

The guide here lists single serving portions for many common food items from this group. The following items count as a single serving:

- ▶ 2 oz processed cheese
- ▶ 1 cup (8 oz) milk
- ▶ 1 cup (8 oz) yogurt
- ▶ 1½ oz natural cheese
- ▶ 1½ cups (12 oz) ice cream
- ▶ 2 cups (16 oz) cottage cheese

Eating food items from the Milk Group should be balanced during the day. In other words, it is best not to eat all of the required servings at the same time. An example of balance would be to have a cup of milk at breakfast (with cereal or in a glass), cheese or yogurt for lunch, and a serving of milk, yogurt, cheese, or ice cream for dinner.

Watch out for Fat

Most products from the Milk Group come from animal sources. As such, these food items also contain cholesterol and fat. The fat content as well as the number of calories in each serving can vary greatly. For instance, one serving of skim milk (8 fl oz) has 86 total calories, compared to one serving of ice cream (12 oz) which can have as many as 524 calories. Moreover, the one serving of skim milk has only a trace (less than 1 percent) of fat. Compare this to the ice cream with 35.6 grams of fat—that is 61 percent of total calories from fat!

Setting Personal Goals

In addition to whatever goals you design on your own, give some thought to a goal dealing with your thinking and your attitudes. Thoughts are ever so important because they determine how we feel and how we act. Being able to identify thoughts that help or hinder you, and having confidence that you can change your thoughts, can be a powerful asset.

A good goal for this week would be to write down the thoughts you feel get in your way and are obstacles to your success. Then, write down more positive thoughts and find at least five times a day you can review these positive thoughts in your mind. More repetition will lead to more permanent, positive thoughts. Your nutrition goal for the week might be to include the recommended number of servings each day from the Milk Group. And, of course, set goals in other areas that you feel are important (an activity goal, a nutrition goal, etc.).

Self-Assessment Questionnaire

Lesson 11

T F 52. Thoughts and attitudes generally occur out of our control and are automatic when we are confronted by certain situations.

T F 53. When taking medication for weight loss, it is important to appreciate how essential the drug is to your success.

T F 54. It is wise to shop for food when you are hungry to test the new restraint you have learned.

T F 55. Buying foods that require preparation can increase your awareness of eating and help you eat less.

T F 56. The recommended number of daily servings from the Milk, Yogurt, and Cheese Group is two to three.

(Answers in Appendix C)

Monitoring Form—Lesson 11

Today's Date:

Time	Food and Amount	Calories
	Total Daily Calories	

Personal Goals This Week	*Always*	*Sometimes*	*Never*
1. Shop on a full stomach			
2. Shop from a list			
3. Eat foods that require preparation			
4. Write down positive thoughts			
5. Daily servings from the Milk Group			
6. Less than ___ calories each day			

Medication Taken Today ❑ Yes ❑ No	*Physical Activity*	*Minutes*
Milk, yogurt, and cheese ❑ ❑ ❑		
Meat, poultry, etc. ❑ ❑ ❑		
Fruits ❑ ❑ ❑ ❑		
Vegetables ❑ ❑ ❑ ❑ ❑		
Breads, cereals, etc. ❑ ❑ ❑ ❑ ❑ ❑ ❑ ❑ ❑		

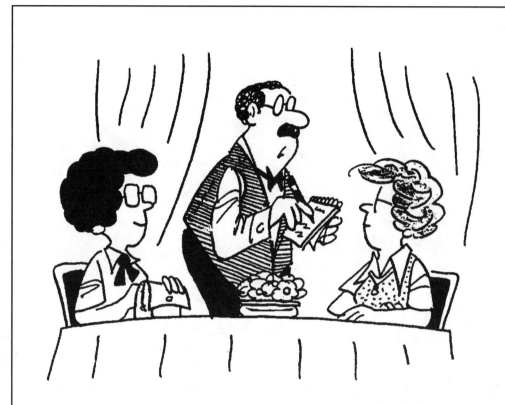

"That's 15 percent of your lunch in protein, 50 percent in carbohydrate, 25 percent in unsaturated fat, and 10 percent in saturated fat—with a drink on the side."

Lesson 12

In the last lesson we spoke about the importance of thoughts and the role they can play in your success. You may want to refer back to the diagrams and tables in that lesson to recall just how thoughts are placed in the sequence linking how we think to how we feel and finally to our eating and activity. In this lesson, we will speak about a specific area of attitude change, something we call internal attitude traps. Here we begin to show you how to challenge thoughts that hold you back and replace them with positive ways of thinking. We will also talk about storing food to help you keep temptation under control and discuss the importance of protein in your diet.

Internal Attitude Traps

We all talk to ourselves, albeit silently. We discussed this earlier regarding goal setting and emotions. How you view your lifestyle changes can help or hinder you greatly. There are several common traps you may encounter. If you are prepared with counter thoughts and attitudes, your job will be easier.

Countering the Traps

You might visualize the part of yourself that pressures you to eat. You can be more than a match for this part, but only if you are conscientious and face the problem directly. What follows are some common traps, called *fat thoughts*. We will give you material for possible counter measures.

> **Internal Trap Number 1**
> **"The diet is the key."**

Fat Thought: The diet and this program are the only reasons I lose weight. When the program is over, I will have real trouble keeping the weight off.

Counter: I am losing weight because of my own efforts. Just because the program ends does not mean my new habits will vanish. The program helps me along, but I get the credit.

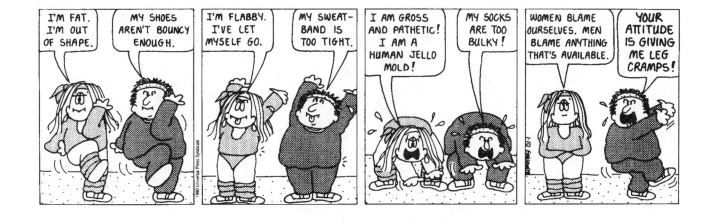

143

Fat Thought: I have been on my program for weeks, and I still have lots of weight to lose. I can't wait till this program ends so I can get back to normal.

Counter: Stop this right now! Who said this would be easy? It took a long time to gain the weight, and it will take a long time to lose it. I would like to lose fast and easy, but facts are facts. I don't want to let down now and waste the effort. I can stick with it.

Fat Thought: I have heard this nutrition stuff before, and we covered behavior modification in the last program I was in. It didn't help me then and will not help me now.

Counter: I have never been taught these things in such a concentrated way,

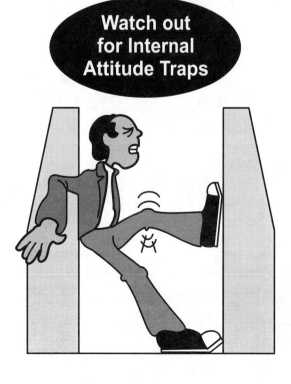

Watch out for Internal Attitude Traps

and my motivation to learn may be different now. I know deep down this is the only way to get permanent results, so putting down the approach just means I have trouble doing the work. Only I can do it, so I must forge ahead.

Try to recognize these and other internal traps. The fat thoughts you have lived with for years will do their best to control your attitudes and eating. Now you can blast them with a counterattack.

Dichotomous (Light Bulb) Thinking

This is the classic attitude problem that plagues many people on weight-loss programs. It involves viewing the world and losing weight as either right or wrong, perfect or terrible, good or bad, friend or foe, legal or illegal. We see this in nearly every client we work with.

Here are some examples. You might have six straight days in which you meet your calorie level and then splurge the seventh day by eating cake and boosting your calorie total to 2000. The common response would be "I really blew it now. I am off my program."

Notice the phrase "off my program." This is the dichotomous view that you are either perfect or terrible, that you are either on or off a program. This is where the term *Light Bulb Thinking* was born, because a light bulb is either on or off.

The danger is the despair that you feel about making inevitable mistakes. Having 2000 calories is insignificant in your total calories for a week, month, or year. However, your *reaction* to those calories can be devastating. If you feel guilty and depressed, the likely response to soothe the feelings is eating.

Another example is the tendency for people to classify foods as good or bad, dietetic or fattening, and legal or illegal. The specific foods that are good or bad vary from person to person. For you, ice cream might be the illegal food, but for another person it might be corn chips, beer, donuts, potato chips, or fast food. Dichotomous thinking occurs when you slip and feel you have blown the program. A slight transgression can send you into a tailspin.

It is essential that you be aware of your dichotomous thoughts. Have you made internal rules about foods that you can and cannot eat, a calorie level you *must* maintain, things you must do to stay "on the program," or what constitutes proper dietary behavior? Notice how you feel when you violate the rules. Negative feelings usually indicate dichotomous thinking.

You can contend with dichotomous thinking by talking back to yourself. You realize how illogical it is to feel terrible about one slip or to make rules where eating some food throws you off your program.

Please realize that attitudes are habits just like any other. Simply reading this material and knowing that attitudes

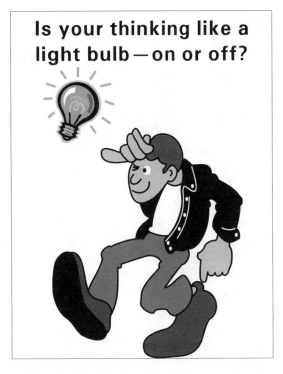

Is your thinking like a light bulb — on or off?

might be hindering your progress is not enough. It will help to practice the new thinking and then to practice again. Try not to be a passive recipient of our advice. Be active and search for these thoughts, and be poised to counter them when they occur.

In the spaces below, write down your most common dichotomous thoughts and write a counter statement for each. You can then be prepared in advance when the fat thoughts occur.

Countering Dichotomous (Light Bulb) Thinking	
My Fat Thoughts	*My Counter Statements*
1.	
2.	
3.	
4.	
5.	
6.	
7.	
8.	

Storing Foods (out of Sight, out of Mouth)

The less you see and think about food, the easier it will be to control eating. Where and how you store food can influence what and how much you eat.

Let's examine two approaches to the same problem to illustrate this point. Suppose salted nuts are your passion and you bring home a one-pound bag from Tiny's Nut House. You could make the nuts a constant temptation by keeping them in an open dish, using the classic dodge that, "I need them in case someone drops by."

Another approach would be to keep the nuts out of sight. This would put some effort between the nuts and you. You could lock them in a safe which is stored in your attic behind 24 boxes of old papers and books. In which case would you eat more nuts?

The attic example is far-fetched, but it does show how the accessibility of food can influence whether you eat. Storing food wisely and keeping it out of sight can be helpful. Here are some ways to follow through.

▶ **Hide the high-calorie foods.** High-calorie impulse foods should be stored out of sight. Put the ice cream under the frozen peas and behind the chicken breasts so you won't see it each time you open the door. Store the cookies on a high shelf behind the seldom-used guest dishes, and put the potato chips on a low shelf behind the colander.

This leads back to Antecedents (discussed in Lesson 6). Bringing problem foods in the house and having them available are steps that precede eating. It would, of course, be preferable to intervene at the earliest step and not buy the foods at all. If you do buy the foods, keeping them out of the way is the next logical step.

Keeping food out of sight serves two purposes. If you don't see it, you may not be stimulated to eat. Also, putting some effort between you and the food stops automatic eating and gives you time to change your mind. You can help the cause even more by storing foods in opaque containers. Keeping the brownies in a plastic bowl will make them less tempting than having them in a clear cookie jar.

▶ **Keep healthy snacks available.** Since Sherlock Holmes would now have trouble finding the high-calorie foods in your house, you can use the space vacated by goodies to store healthy foods. If you get an urge to eat, reach for the celery, carrot sticks, raisins, apples, cauliflower, vegetable soup, and oranges.

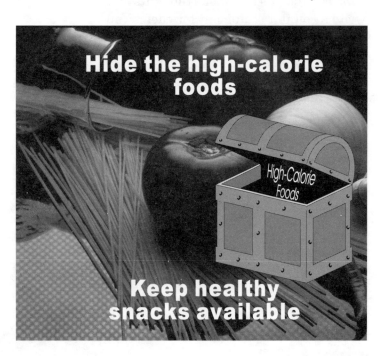
Hide the high-calorie foods

Keep healthy snacks available

The Importance of Protein

Protein is a popular topic of conversation. We hear about high-protein diets and low-protein diets. We know about liquid protein, protein bread, and protein supplements. What is this fuss about? Protein is the most abundant material in the body aside from water. It has many functions and is found in all cells. It plays many roles:

► Protein is contained in hemoglobin, which carries oxygen in the blood.

► Protein is related to DNA (deoxyribonucleic acid), which provides the genes with the code to transmit heredity.

► Protein is used to build muscle and all other body tissue.

► Protein is an important part of insulin, which regulates blood sugar.

► Protein is used to build the enzymes that digest our food.

What Is Protein?

Proteins are built from approximately 20 amino acids which are put together in long chains. Protein can be synthesized or manufactured by the body, but only if the *essential* amino acids are present at the same time. Of the 20 different amino acids, nine are considered *essential* and cannot be made by the body. Therefore, they must be provided in the foods that we eat. The protein our body uses best contains these amino acids. The 11 *nonessential* amino acids can be synthesized by the body, but only if the building blocks are present. These building blocks include the nine essential amino acids, nitrogen, and calories.

You may have heard about *high-quality* and *low-quality* proteins. When the dangers of the liquid protein diet be-

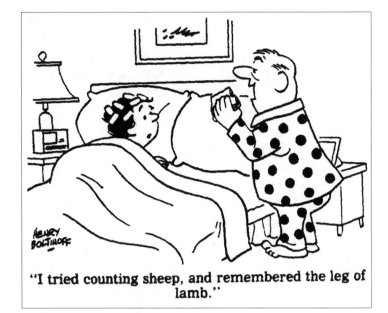

"I tried counting sheep, and remembered the leg of lamb."

came clear in the mid and late 1970s, the use of low-quality protein in the liquid formulas was cited as one of the hazards. High-quality proteins are those the body can use to function properly, because they contain all of the essential amino acids. Low-quality proteins have one or more essential amino acids missing.

Sources of Protein

Meat and dairy products contain high-quality proteins and do not have to be supplemented with other proteins since they contain all nine of the essential amino acids. Plant proteins usually lack one or more of the essential amino acids, but can provide adequate amounts of the essential and nonessential amino acids. Vegetarian diets can provide adequate protein if the sources are reasonably varied and the caloric intake is enough to meet the individual's energy needs.

Eating a variety of legumes and grains will provide high-quality protein. Legumes include dried peas and beans, such as black-eyed peas, chick peas (garbanzo beans), kidney beans, lentils, lima beans, navy beans, and soybeans. Soy protein has been shown to be nutritionally equivalent in protein value to proteins of animal origin. Nuts are also in this category, but they contain high amounts of fat. Grains include barley, corn, oats, rice, sesame seeds, sunflower seeds, and wheat.

Protein rarely exists by itself (egg whites or albumin is the exception) and is most often accompanied with mixtures of fat in foods like meat, fish, poultry, and milk products. Protein contains four (4) calories per gram; this is the same caloric content by weight as carbohydrates. One ounce (28 grams) of lean meat, fish, or poultry contains approximately seven (7) grams of protein and three (3) grams of fat (a total of 55 calories), whereas protein foods with higher fat content provide as much as 70–120 calories per ounce and 5–10 grams of fat per ounce.

How Much Protein Should You Eat?

Some health experts believe that Americans eat too much protein and that reduction would be desirable. A major benefit would be a reduction in total fat since the most popular protein foods (meat, fish, and poultry) also provide significant amounts of fat. We must remember, however, that protein in the diet is essential. Recommended amounts of protein range from 10–15 percent of total calories or approximately 50–75 grams of protein per day for adults. To see how your daily protein intake fits the guidelines for a healthy diet, multiply your target calorie level by 15 percent, the maximum recommended protein calories per day. For example, if your target caloric intake is 1200, 1200 x .15 = 180. Since there are 4 calories in every gram of protein, divide 180 by 4; 180 ÷ 4 = 45. You know that you need to eat about 45 grams of protein daily to meet the government's recommended guidelines. For most people, the main source of dietary protein will come from the Meat, Poultry, Fish, Egg, and Nut Group of the Food Guide Pyramid.

The Meat, Poultry, Fish, Eggs, and Nut Group

The food items in this group include meat, poultry, fish, dry beans, eggs, and nuts. Meat, poultry, and fish provide good sources of protein, B vitamins, iron, and zinc. Dry beans, eggs, and nuts are similar to meats in providing protein and most vitamins and minerals.

How Much Is a Serving?

As a general rule, two to three ounces of cooked lean meat, poultry, or fish count as one serving from the Meat and Protein Group. A three-ounce piece of meat is about the size of an average hamburger, or the amount of meat on a medium chicken breast half. For other foods in this group, count ½ cup of cooked dry beans, two tablespoons of peanut butter, or one egg as one ounce of meat (i.e., ⅓ of a serving). As an example, six ounces for the day (two servings) may come from:

- ► 1 egg (counts as 1 oz of lean meat) for breakfast;

- ► 2 oz of sliced turkey in a sandwich at lunch;

- ► 3 oz cooked lean hamburger for dinner.

How Many Servings?

The Food Guide Pyramid suggests two to three servings per day from the Meat and Protein Group. The total from all servings should be the equivalent of between five and seven ounces of cooked lean meat, poultry, or fish per day. The chart on the following page shows items from this food group.

Meat, Poultry, Fish, Dry Beans, Eggs, and Nuts

Description	Calories	Protein (g)	Carb. (g)	Fat (g)
Beef:				
Chuck arm, lean braised (3 oz)	191	28.0	0	7.9
Ground, lean broiled (3 oz)	231	21.0	0	15.7
Round, lean broiled (3 oz)	204	23.0	0	11.6
Sirloin, lean broiled (3 oz)	229	23.5	0	14.3
Chicken:				
Dark, w skin roasted (3 oz)	215	22.0	0	13.4
Dark, w/o skin roasted (3 oz)	174	23.3	0	8.3
Light, w skin roasted (3 oz)	189	24.7	0	9.2
Light, w/o skin roasted (3 oz)	147	26.3	0	3.8
Fish:				
Flounder/sole, baked (3 oz)	173	25.7	0	7.0
Haddock, baked (3 oz)	95	20.6	0	.8
Lobster, steamed (3 oz)	83	17.4	1.1	.5
Shrimp, breaded & fried (3 oz)	206	18.2	9.8	10.4
Shrimp, boiled (3 oz)	84	17.8	.0	.9
Trout, baked (3 oz)	129	22.4	.0	3.7
Tuna, canned in water (3 oz)	111	25.1	.0	.4
Pork:				
Chop, lean center broiled (3 oz)	190	16.0	0	13.0
Ham, cured roasted (3 oz)	239	17.4	0	18.2
Loin, lean braised (3 oz)	266	25.3	0	17.5
Black-eye peas, boiled (1½ cup)	297	19.8	53.3	1.4
Chick-peas, boiled (1½ cup)	403	21.8	67.5	6.5
Great northern beans, boiled (1½ cup)	315	22.2	55.9	1.2
Kidney beans, boiled (1½ cup)	338	23.1	60.6	1.4
Lima beans, boiled (1½ cup)	326	22.0	58.9	1.1
Navy beans, boiled (1½ cup)	389	23.7	71.9	1.5
Pink beans, boiled (1½ cup)	378	22.9	70.8	1.2
Pinto beans, boiled (1½ cup)	353	21.0	65.8	1.4
Pigeon peas, boiled (1½ cup)	306	17.1	58.6	.9
Split peas, boiled (1½ cup)	347	24.6	62.1	1.2
Egg, raw whole (3 eggs)	126	10.5	.9	8.4
Peanut butter (6 T)	564	23.1	20.7	48.0
Peanuts, dry roasted (1 cup)	814	23.7	34.7	70.5
Rice, long grain brown (1½ cup)	324	7.5	67.2	2.7
Rice, long grain white (1½ cup)	396	8.3	85.8	.9

Note: Each of the food items listed above counts as one serving. This table should be used as a guide for the foods listed. Since food values vary by brand name it is important to read the food labels for these foods.

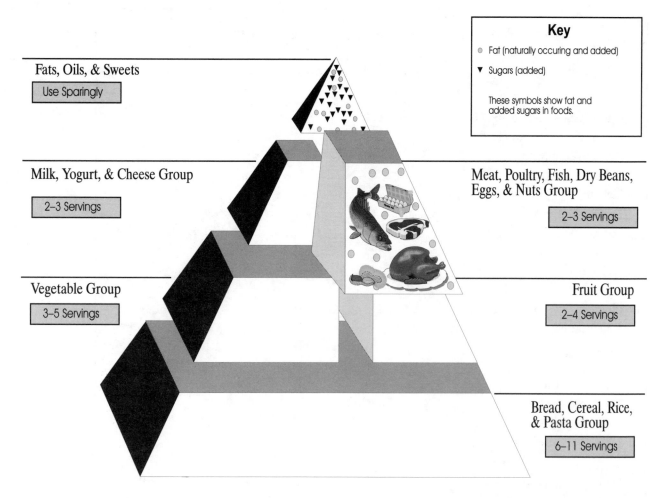

Key

- ○ Fat (naturally occuring and added)
- ▼ Sugars (added)

These symbols show fat and added sugars in foods.

Fats, Oils, & Sweets
Use Sparingly

Milk, Yogurt, & Cheese Group
2–3 Servings

Meat, Poultry, Fish, Dry Beans, Eggs, & Nuts Group
2–3 Servings

Vegetable Group
3–5 Servings

Fruit Group
2–4 Servings

Bread, Cereal, Rice, & Pasta Group
6–11 Servings

Watch out for Fat

As mentioned earlier, the best sources of protein come from animal products, such as dairy, meat, poultry, fish, and eggs. However, these food sources can be high in saturated fat and cholesterol. These tips will help reduce fat in your diet:

- ➤ Choose lean meat, fish, poultry without skin, dry beans, and peas. These foods are the choices that are lowest in dietary fat.

- ➤ Prepare meats in low-fat ways; trim away all the visible fat and boil, roast, or broil these foods instead of frying them.

- ➤ Eat egg yolks sparingly—they are high in cholesterol. Use only one yolk per person in egg dishes and make larger portions by adding extra egg whites.

- ➤ Remember, nuts and seeds are high in fat, so they should be eaten in moderation.

- ➤ For beef, roasts and steaks of round, loin, sirloin, and chuck arm are lean choices.

- ➤ For pork, roasts and chops of tenderloin, center loin, and ham are the leaner choices.

- ➤ For veal, all cuts are generally lean, except for ground veal.

- ➤ Lamb roasts and chops of leg, loin, and fore shanks provide the lean cuts.

- ➤ Fish and shellfish are generally low in fat; however, those canned or marinated in oil are higher.

- ➤ For chicken and turkey, both light and dark meat are lean choices provided the skin has been removed.

Setting Personal Goals

As you set your personal goals for this lesson, consider a focus on attitudes. The internal attitude traps and light bulb thinking trip up lots of people, so see if the material in these sections applies to you. Are there traps your mind sets for you, so that you know in advance you will have problems in certain situations? For instance, if you eat more than you think you should, do you get depressed, say you have no willpower, or think you have seen a definite signal that your control is slipping away? You can then build some counter thoughts. Have some thoughts ready in advance, so you can use them when needed.

Make a sweep through your house and hide the high-calorie foods. Replace them with nutritious foods. Focus this week on the amount of protein you eat and check to make sure you are eating the appropriate number of servings from the Meat Group of the Food Guide Pyramid.

What are the other goals you would like to set? These could be a continuation of goals you set in earlier weeks, or could be new. The purpose is to give you something to strive for in areas that are important to you.

Self-Assessment Questionnaire

Lesson 12

T F 57. Keeping high-calorie foods stored out of sight can decrease impulsive eating.

T F 58. Fat thoughts can hinder a person's efforts to lose weight.

T F 59. Light bulb or dichotomous thinking refers to your own bright ideas about losing weight.

T F 60. The only way to get high-quality protein in your diet is to eat foods from the Meat, Poultry, Fish, Dry Beans, Eggs, & Nuts Group of The Food Guide Pyramid.

T F 61. A diet very high in protein will facilitate weight loss.

(Answers in appendix C)

Monitoring Form—Lesson 12

Today's Date:

Time	Food and Amount	Calories
	Total Daily Calories	

	Personal Goals This Week	*Always*	*Sometimes*	*Never*
1.	Counter the internal attitude traps			
2.	Counter dichotomous thinking			
3.	Hide high-calorie foods			
4.	Keep healthy foods in sight			
5.	My diet has _____ grams of protein			
6.	Eat less than _____ calories each day			

Medication Taken Today ❑ Yes ❑ No	*Physical Activity*	*Minutes*
Milk, yogurt, and cheese ❑ ❑ ❑		
Meat, poultry, etc. ❑ ❑ ❑		
Fruits ❑ ❑ ❑ ❑		
Vegetables ❑ ❑ ❑ ❑ ❑		
Breads, cereals, etc. ❑ ❑ ❑ ❑ ❑ ❑ ❑ ❑ ❑		

Lesson 13

We will begin this lesson with further discussion of the **A** (Attitudes) part of LEARN. Being successful with a program combining medication with lifestyle change requires a certain mind-set. Many people expect too much of the medication and too little of themselves, so we will show you how to strike a balance. We will also discuss the "impossible dream" that some people have, and will then cover creative ways of serving and dispensing food. To cover the N (Nutrition) part of LEARN, we'll continue our journey down the Food Guide Pyramid and talk about carbohydrates and vegetables. There is a lot to say, so let's get moving!

Medication and Your Rate of Weight Loss

People taking MERIDIA or any weight loss medication will usually experience their greatest weight loss in the first six months on the medication. The rate and total amount of weight loss, however, varies widely across people. Some lose quickly and then slow down, others lose in a steady way, and others are late bloomers—they do not lose much early in the program and then something seizes them and the weight loss starts. You may have a different pattern of weight loss entirely.

Do not be alarmed or discouraged if your weight loss has slowed down. This is common. Weight loss often slows after the first three to four months. You will probably continue to lose slowly if you take MERIDIA and keep changing your eating and exercise habits. But try to adjust your expectations so you will not be disappointed. Your priority will shift over time from losing weight to maintaining what you have lost. Remember that even modest weight losses can improve health. They can also make you feel good about yourself, if you take pride in what you have done. It is essential to not dismiss important achievements.

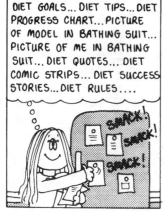
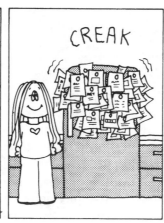
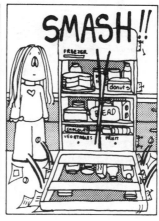
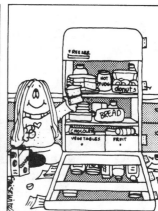

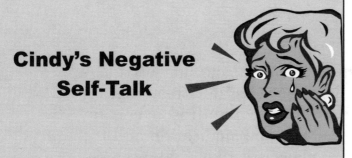

Cindy's Negative Self-Talk

"I knew I wouldn't make it to my goal."

"What good is this 15-pound weight loss when I still have 30 pounds to go?"

"I can only accept myself when I reach my ideal weight."

"The program isn't working anymore."

"I'm just sick that I'm not losing more weight."

Meet Cindy

A person we know named Cindy went through a lot of self-doubt at about this stage of the program. She was discouraged because she wasn't losing more weight and was questioning whether she should keep trying. She was on the verge of giving up. When we asked what type of thoughts she was having, she came up with what you see here in the accompanying chart titled Cindy's Negative Self-Talk.

After some discussion, Cindy came up with more positive ways of looking at things. This helped her get back on the track, to take credit for progress she had made, and to emphasize a realistic, attainable set of expectations. Now look at what Cindy was saying to herself in the chart titled Cindy's More Positive Self-Talk (see next page).

Think of your weight like a turnstile that moves in only one direction. Losing weight is like the turnstile moving forward. Wouldn't it be nice if your weight were like the turnstile in that it never moves in the opposite direction? With the right self-management skills, you can have more confidence that your weight will not bounce back up.

Now, of course, expecting a perfect turnstile is unrealistic, because no person who has lost has a perfectly stable weight. You can expect some weight fluctuation, created in part by fluctuations in your control over eating and activity. One thing that characterizes successful maintainers is that they set an upper limit on how much they allow their weight to increase (usually three to five pounds) before they take corrective action. Hence, the turnstile will move mainly in one direction (weight loss) and will accept a little backward movement, but only to a limited degree before the brakes are applied.

Think of the progress you have made. Any weight you have lost is a positive development. Also, remember our discussion on the Quality of Life. We can measure progress with much more than the scale. Our first order of business is to be sure that these changes are permanent. Therefore, if your weight loss has slowed, pay attention to all you have achieved rather than what you have left to do. Losing more weight is possible for a great many people, so you might find yourself charging ahead, but if not, keep your head high and keep the weight off! Take a few moments to write down the progress you have made since starting the program and all the positive things you have changed. Also, write down all the positive reasons you can think of to maintain changes you have already made and to continue your program. We have provided a table below so that you can take a few minutes now, before continuing with this lesson, to write your thoughts down. So, sharpen your pencil and write your thoughts down.

Impossible Dream Thinking

Along with Dichotomous Thinking, Impossible Dream Thinking ranks high as an attitude barrier to losing weight. This type of thinking occurs when you fantasize or dream about impossible accomplishments. You might have 100 pounds to lose on Thanksgiving and fantasize wearing a size nine to the office Christmas party.

Before you turn the page and skip to the next section, let us assure you that most people are not aware of these thoughts. Yet, after some reflection, most see them clearly. Maybe a few more examples will bring this home.

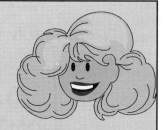

Cindy's More Positive Self-Talk

"A reasonable goal is for me to lose 5–10 percent of my starting weight. I'm actually doing pretty well."

"The 15-pound loss is a big thing for me, and even if I lose no more, I'm a lot better off carrying 15 fewer pounds."

"I don't expect myself to be perfect in other areas of my life. It would be great to be at my ideal weight, but I'll be happier if I focus on being at a 'better' weight rather than a 'best' weight."

"The medication helped me with losing weight. Now it's helping me maintain what I have lost."

"I still might lose more, but right now I don't want to get discouraged. A good goal for me is to keep off the weight I have lost."

Progress I've Made	Positive Things I've Changed	Reasons I Should Maintain the Changes

Oh please, scale, say that I'm down to 110, so I'll look really good and I'll meet someone, and we'll fall in love and get married and I'll be happy for the rest of my life...

SIPRESS

Impossible Dream thinking occurs when you daydream about how wonderful life will be after weight loss. It is common for those losing weight to imagine an improved marriage, better job, wonderful social life, intimate relationships, and other happy endings to their struggle to lose weight. These things may be possible, but it is unlikely that weight loss alone will make them happen.

This type of thinking also occurs when you imagine succeeding at a program without hard work. When most begin a program and fantasize about the future, they do not picture pain and puffing from exercise and the agony of passing up chocolate mousse.

It does no harm to hope for the best and aspire to improve your life. However, weight loss will usually not make a bad marriage good and will not shoot you to the top of the corporate ladder. Getting your weight down can actually be a disappointing experience if the fantasy is not fulfilled. This is what happened with one of our clients, Audrey.

Audrey was one of our first overweight clients. She was 28 years old and was working on an advanced degree in chemistry. She had been heavy since childhood and had been in no serious relationships. She was lonely and yearned to settle down with a stable and loving partner.

Audrey lost weight rapidly and seemed happy about her progress. She spoke often, but in a joking way, about how she would meet the person of her dreams when she got thin. We would easily spot it now, but at the time we did not realize how serious she was about this fantasy. When she reached her goal, she became steadily more depressed because no spectacular romance evolved. It was clear that there were problems other than weight that prevented the relationships from developing, but Audrey saw weight loss as her salvation. Fortunately, we worked with Audrey on these problems, and she did eventually find the romance she was seeking.

This is a dramatic example of Impossible Dream Thinking. This specific case may not parallel your situation, but think honestly about whether you are harboring impossible dreams.

For many people losing weight, life does change in dramatic and positive ways. We hope this happens for you and that what you hope will happen actually occurs. Please remember, however, that weight loss may not automatically change your life.

Here are four ways to deal with Impossible Dream thinking. They can help keep your spirits high.

▶ **Counter the dreams**. Pinpoint your Impossible Dreams and counter them with more rational expectations. Methods for developing counter statements were discussed

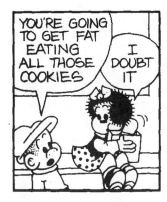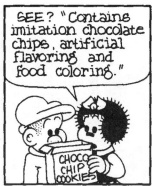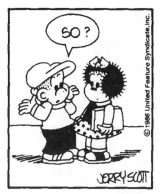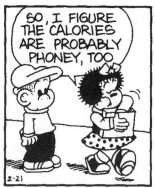

in Lesson 12 in the section on Dichotomous Thinking.

▶ **Set short-term goals.** Concern yourself with what you will do today and tomorrow, not what life will be like when you lose weight. This gives you many chances to experience success because you will be making small accomplishments in route to a larger goal. It will also prevent unrealistic fantasies from dominating your thoughts.

▶ **Focus on behavior, not weight.** Remember that your behavior must change before weight can change, so give yourself credit for following the program. You will have something to feel good about every day and will not be so discouraged by weight setbacks.

▶ **Set flexible goals.** If your goals don't work, set new ones. If you vowed to walk three miles each day but cannot, walk one or two miles every other day and work your way up. This puts the focus on short-term changes in behavior, so Impossible Dream Thinking will fade to the background.

Serving and Dispensing Food

Here are five questions we like to ask to determine whether a person reacts to the site, smell, or thought of food.

❶ Do you feel like eating dessert when it looks appetizing even after eating a large meal?

❷ Is there always room for something you like?

❸ Do you get excited by a buffet?

❹ If you drive by a bakery or fast food place and smell the food, do you want to eat regardless of when you ate last?

❺ Do you feel like eating when you see a picture of a delicious dessert in a magazine?

If you answer "yes" to these questions, you may be high in externality. This means you are sensitive to external cues or signals, namely the sight, smell, or suggestion of food. If this describes you, join the crowd. There are millions like you, both heavy and thin. It can be very helpful for you to reduce your exposure to food. If this description does not fit you, read on anyway. These techniques may help you corral your desire to overeat.

The methods you learned earlier for buying and storing food were designed to reduce exposure to food. We have been moving forward in the sequence of antecedents. We began with the first step (shopping). We then moved a step closer to eating (storing food). We will now move even closer by discussing serving and dispensing food.

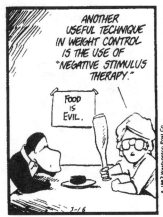 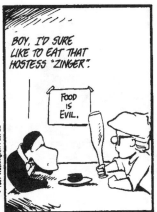 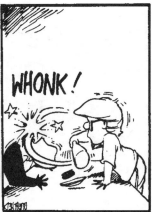 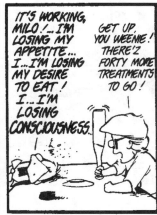

We will describe several techniques for storing food. All follow from a general principle, which is to interrupt the sequence of events associated with eating. Some techniques will apply to you more than others. You can use the principle to develop techniques of your own.

The following techniques are designed to help you control eating when your exposure to food cues is at its peak. The aim is to minimize your contact with these cues.

► **Remove serving dishes from the table.** After first servings have been made, remove the food dishes from the table. Having the food handy is asking for trouble. If the food dishes are in another room or on another table, you can *think* before taking more. This does not prohibit you from having seconds, but it does interrupt the automatic eating that occurs when your plate is a magnet for anything left on the serving dishes.

► **Leave the table after eating.** This may sound anti-social, but some people are helped by leaving the table after dinner. This reduces the time you are exposed to food and to the circumstances of eating. If you finish long before the others, you may be eating too fast, and slowing down would help. If not, perhaps the others can retire to another room with you for the post-meal chat. This technique can work in concert with the previous suggestion to remove serving dishes from the table. If *all* the dishes are gone, it is not necessary to leave the table because exposure to food signals will be low. If food remains, bid the table farewell and depart for safer surroundings.

► **Serve and eat one portion at a time.** Make and serve yourself only one portion of food. If you want two pieces of toast, make one and eat it before making another. If you want a container of yogurt, put half in a bowl and return for the second half if you still want it. You might find yourself passing up the second portion because you are no longer hungry. Here again is a chance to interrupt that automatic eating. This can also help you separate hunger from habit. Because you have eaten one container of yogurt every morning for 10 years does not mean your body is hungry for that amount every day.

► **Follow the five-minute rule.** Wait five minutes before going back for extra helpings. This will help you slow the rate of eating and will give you time to decide how much food you really need.

► **Avoid being a food dispenser.** Are you the gatekeeper of food in your house? Do the kids get their snacks from you? Do you prepare all the food? This is a disadvantage because your routine brings you in contact with food many times each day.

Drop the job of being a food dispenser. Have the children pack their own lunches if possible. Your spouse can manage snacks without you and may be willing to help even more by taking on some of the responsibility you have for distributing food.

Carbohydrates and Your Diet

We promised earlier that we would discuss carbohydrates in this lesson. So, let's get to it. People like to blame carbohydrates for everything. Some people on weight loss programs say that carbohydrates excite the binge center in their brain, and parents blame sugar when their kids misbehave. There is much talk about simple and complex carbohydrates, carbohydrate craving, and low-carbohydrate diets. You may be puzzled by all this, so let's clear the air.

What are Carbohydrates?

Stated in technical terms, carbohydrates are a combination of hydrogen, oxygen, and carbon atoms, which assemble to make simple sugars, complex sugars, or starches. These sugars provide energy to the body. Complex sugars must first be broken down by the body into simple sugars to be utilized. This is why simple sugars (like sucrose) enter the body's energy supply more quickly than the complex sugars or starches in vegetables or cereals.

There are many sources of the simple sugars and starches. Simple sugars consist mainly of sucrose (table sugar), fructose (in fruit and honey), and lactose (in

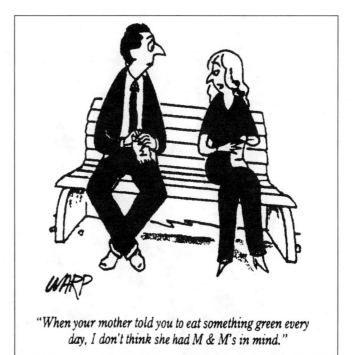

"When your mother told you to eat something green every day, I don't think she had M & M's in mind."

milk). The starches are in foods like cereals, pasta, rice, breads, and vegetables.

Carbohydrates, like protein, provide four calories per gram. In contrast, fat has more than twice the calories per gram. The major part of our diet is carbohydrate, and it is easy to eat too much. Many of the carbohydrate foods we eat are of poor nutritional value and contain only calories from sugar. They are a poor source of nutrition, hence the term *empty calories*. Foods like these are prime candidates for elimination or reduction for individuals trying to lose or maintain weight.

In order for the diet to provide an adequate balance of nutrients, an adult should have approximately 165–180 grams of carbohydrate per day (based on a diet of 1200 calories). This would total from 660–720 calories (140–150 grams at 4 calories per gram). Adults are advised to have 55–60 percent of their total calories in carbohydrates.

The Food Guide Pyramid

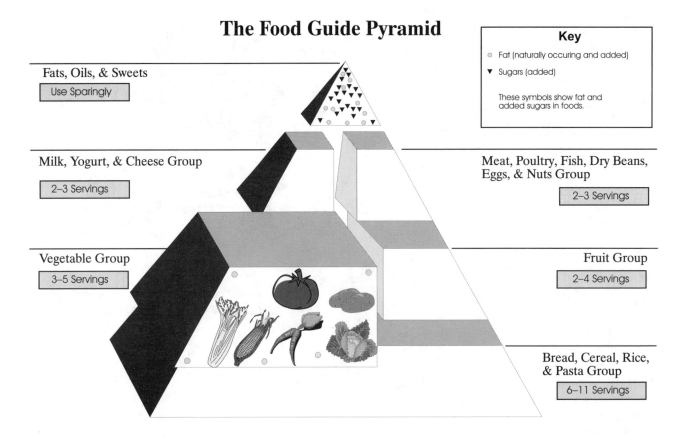

Key

○ Fat (naturally occuring and added)

▼ Sugars (added)

These symbols show fat and added sugars in foods.

Fats, Oils, & Sweets
Use Sparingly

Milk, Yogurt, & Cheese Group
2–3 Servings

Meat, Poultry, Fish, Dry Beans, Eggs, & Nuts Group
2–3 Servings

Vegetable Group
3–5 Servings

Fruit Group
2–4 Servings

Bread, Cereal, Rice, & Pasta Group
6–11 Servings

What does all this jargon mean? Carbohydrates are essential in the diet and are not necessarily bad. In fact, most people should increase their intake of complex carbohydrates. Starches should not have the bad rap they receive. People consider potatoes fattening because they are high in starch, yet potatoes are reasonable to eat because of their nutrition. The amount eaten is usually the problem, along with the goodies that adorn some of these foods. For example, sour cream and butter, which are mainly fat, rapidly increase the caloric intake involved in eating an innocent potato.

It is unwise to follow a low-carbohydrate diet except under medical supervision. Some popular diets which restrict carbohydrate to less than 100 grams per day make it very difficult to maintain adequate nutrition. A sensible plan with 55–60 percent of your calories from carbohydrates is best.

Try to be on the lookout for simple sugars in your diet. These tend to come from foods with many calories and little nutrition. Examples are crackers, doughnuts, pastries, soft drinks, candy, and so forth.

These simple sugars stimulate insulin release. Since insulin is related to hunger, you will feel hungry in less time with simple sugars than with complex sugars. Moving away from candy and other sweet foods, toward vegetables and other complex carbohydrates, is a wise decision.

Vegetables

Description	Calories	Protein (g)	Carb. (g)	Fat (g)
Asparagus, boiled (½ cup)	22	2.3	4.0	.3
Beets, boiled (½ cup)	26	.9	5.7	.0
Broccoli, boiled (½ cup)	23	2.3	4.3	.2
Brussels Sprouts (½ cup)	30	2.0	6.8	.4
Cabbage, raw (1 cup)	16	.8	1.6	.2
Carrots, boiled (½ cup)	35	.9	8.2	.1
Cauliflower, boiled (½ cup)	15	1.2	2.9	.1
Celery, raw (½ cup diced)	11	.4	2.6	.1
Corn—yellow, boiled (½ cup)	89	2.7	20.6	1.1
Cucumber, raw (½ cup diced)	7	.3	1.5	.1
Eggplant, raw (½ cup pieces)	11	.5	2.6	.0
Green beans, boiled (½ cup)	22	1.2	4.9	.2
Lettuce, raw (1 cup)	10	.8	2.0	.2
Lima beans, boiled (½ cup)	109	7.4	21.2	.3
Mixed vegetables, canned (½ cup)	39	2.1	7.6	.2
Mushrooms, boiled (½ cup pieces)	21	1.7	4.0	.4
Okra, boiled (½ cup slices)	25	1.5	5.8	.1
Onion rings, frozen (7 rings)	285	3.7	26.7	18.7
Peas, green, boiled (½ cup)	67	4.6	12.5	.2
Potato, canned w/o skin (½ cup)	54	1.3	12.3	.2
Potato, French fried (10 pieces)	158	2.0	20.0	8.3
Potato, hash brown (½ cup)	163	1.9	16.6	10.9
Potato, mashed (½ cup)	111	2.0	17.5	4.4
Potato, scalloped (½ cup)	105	3.5	13.2	4.5
Squash—zucchini, boiled (½ cup)	14	.6	3.5	.1
Sweet potato, boiled (½ cup)	172	2.7	39.8	.5

Note: Each of the food items listed above counts as one serving. This table should be used as a guide for the foods listed. Since food values vary by brand name it is important to read the food labels for these foods.

Carbohydrates and Extra Calorie Burning

For many years, a simple statement ruled in the minds of experts—"A calorie is a calorie." The feeling was that calories are handled in the same way by the body no matter where they came from. If you ate 3500 calories of oat bran and tofu, you would gain the same weight as you would by eating the same calories from a triple cheeseburger and onion rings. No longer.

The body has an easier time converting fat calories to body fat than it does converting carbohydrate calories. Between 20–25 percent more energy is required for the body to handle carbohydrate than to handle fat. As an example, let's say you eat 100 calories of a high-fat food like butter. On another day, you eat 100 calories of a food high in complex carbohydrates, like a whole grain cereal. Your body will use 20–25 percent more calories to metabolize the carbohydrate. Therefore, the calories from fat and carbohydrate are not equal once they enter your body.

This is good news. Foods high in complex carbohydrates are good to eat for health reasons, and you will burn more calories when you eat them. Many people report that it is much easier to lose weight when they cut back on fat and eat more fruits, vegetables, and grains. With this in mind, let's look at the Vegetable Group of the Food Guide Pyramid.

Vegetables in Your Diet

Do you remember your mother saying to you, "Eat your vegetables, they're good for you"? Mom was right, vegetables are good for you. In fact, both fruits and vegetables are so important in the diet that the Food Guide Pyramid breaks them into separate groups.

Vegetables are an excellent source of Vitamins A and C, and folate. In addition, they provide minerals, including iron and magnesium, and as we mentioned earlier, they are an excellent source of carbohydrates. Vegetables are

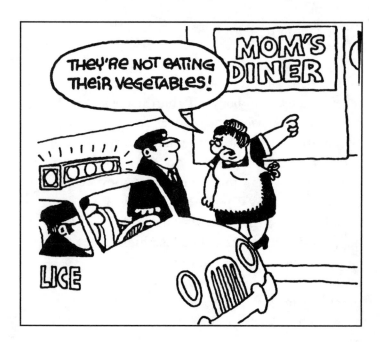

also naturally low in dietary fat. This is good news for people losing weight.

Most Americans fall short in their consumption of vegetables, perhaps because adding produce to their diet is inconvenient, time-consuming, or boring. Vegetables may not appeal to everyone's palate, especially in the ways they are usually prepared, but they are an important ingredient to a healthy and low-fat diet.

How Many Servings?

The suggested number of daily servings is three to five. This may sound like a lot, but it is actually less than you may think. For instance, just one-half cup of boiled green beans, one medium carrot, two stalks of celery, or half of a broccoli spear make one serving.

How Much Is a Serving?

As a general rule, the following will serve as a simple guide to help you include the right amount of vegetables in your daily diet:

- ► 1 cup of raw leafy vegetables
- ► ½ cup of other vegetables, cooked or chopped raw
- ► ¾ cup of vegetable juice

The chart on the previous page may help you to better understand the portion size of a serving. The foods listed count as a single serving.

Serving Tips

There are a large variety of vegetables for you to choose from in our food supply. With a little creativity and planning, vegetables can become a fun and enjoyable part of your everyday diet. Here are some serving tips that you may find helpful:

Fresh vegetables make excellent snacks that you can easily take with you to work, school, or simply enjoy around the house. Celery, carrots, cauliflower, green peppers, cucumbers, and broccoli are good choices.

Steaming vegetables can also be fun and can add variety to your meals. Best of all, it is easy to do and does not leave a big mess. While steaming the vegetables, you can add herbs or other seasonings to enhance flavor, or serve the steamed vegetables with a splash of lemon.

Think of creative ways to add vegetables to the foods you already eat and enjoy. Adding a slice of tomato, two large leaves of lettuce or spinach, and a pickle on the side turns a sandwich into a meal that includes one serving of vegetables.

When you eat fast-food, be creative. Most fast-food establishments now offer vegetable alternatives to French fries. Try a garden salad or baked potato next time. But be careful with dressings and toppings—make sure they are low-fat. Remember to watch those *hidden* calories.

Reevaluating Your Quality of Life

After each four lessons in *The LEARN Program*, we reintroduce the Quality of

Life issue. Why? Because your life and how you feel about yourself may be the most important topic of all, and because many people tend to overlook some very important changes they have made.

Let's take self-esteem as an example. Is there any greater gift than self-esteem? If you are feeling better about yourself, feel like you have more control over your destiny, and feel that you are conquering some problems you thought would get the best of you, you have made great progress. It is our pleasurable task to help point this out to you and to be certain you don't let the occasion slip by without celebrating.

We provide on the previous page the Quality of Life Self-Assessment. Complete it and compare your responses with those from earlier ones (Orientation, Lesson 5—page 66, and Lesson 9—page 117). See if you are ahead of where you were when you started the program.

Setting Personal Goals

Taking stock of your progress *thus far* is a good place to start with setting personal goals. Are you pleased with the changes you have made? What can you do to insure that you maintain what you have accomplished? These are the activities and ways of thinking from which you can set personal goals.

If you are not making the progress you'd like, assuming you have reasonable expectations, how can you kick into a higher gear? You might need some additional help or support. This might come from a professional like a therapist or dietitian, or from a self-help group like Overeaters Anonymous or TOPS (Take Off Pounds Sensibly). Joining a health club, or buying some exercise tapes, or

making a plan to exercise with a friend might help. People get motivated in various ways. The ticket to success is finding which way works for you, and then making sure you do it! Focus this week on eating the right number of servings from the Vegetable Group.

Self-Assessment Questionnaire

Lesson 13

T F 62. It is best to take all of what you will eat in one serving so you will not need additional helpings.

T F 63. Impossible Dream Thinking is having fantasies and images about weight loss, life as a thin person, etc.

T F 64. Carbohydrates are not as important as other nutrients, and they should make up only about 30 percent of your daily diet.

T F 65. The Food Guide Pyramid suggests three to five servings each day from the Vegetable Group.

T F 66. It is important for me to appreciate the hard work I am doing to change my behavior and not give all the credit for weight loss to the medication.

T F 67. I should expect to lose about the same amount of weight as the weeks go on, as long as I take my medication as prescribed.

(Answers in Appendix C)

Monitoring Form—Lesson 13

Today's Date:

Time	Food and Amount	Calories
	Total Daily Calories	

Personal Goals This Week	*Always*	*Sometimes*	*Never*
1. Remove serving dishes from table			
2. Leave table after eating			
3. Avoid dispensing food			
4. Watch out for Impossible Dream Thinking			
5. My diet has _____ grams of carbohydrate			
6. Eat less than _____ calories each day			

Medication Taken Today ❏ Yes ❏ No	*Physical Activity*	*Minutes*
Milk, yogurt, and cheese ❏ ❏ ❏		
Meat, poultry, etc. ❏ ❏ ❏		
Fruits ❏ ❏ ❏ ❏		
Vegetables ❏ ❏ ❏ ❏ ❏		
Breads, cereals, etc. ❏ ❏ ❏ ❏ ❏ ❏ ❏ ❏ ❏		

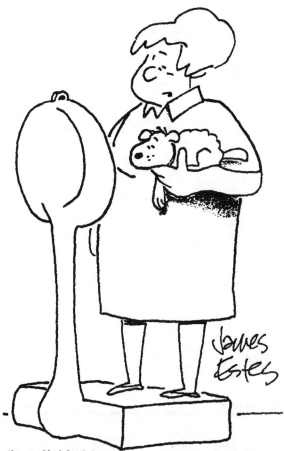

"250 divided by two — that's 125 apiece
. . . I'm doing great, Muffin, but you
have a weight problem."

Lesson 14

We begin with a discussion of how to expand a program of regular physical activity. We have spoken mainly of walking thus far, but there are many other activities you might like to try. Having several activities available increases the chance that being active will be fun, and having fun is one key to making physical activity a permanent part of your life. We will also give you advice on dealing with a support partner, and will cover fruits, another key element of a balanced diet.

Selecting and Starting a Programmed Activity

You may recall from Lesson 10 that there is much good news about physical activity. Its benefits are beyond impressive. Regular physical activity, even in moderate amounts, is one of the most powerful means at your disposal to reduce risk for heart disease and other serious illnesses. Being active can put more life into every step you take, give you more energy, make you feel better about your body, and improve your mood. Best of all it can really help you lose weight and maintain the loss. We suggest you read the section on activity from Lesson 10 to get the full rationale.

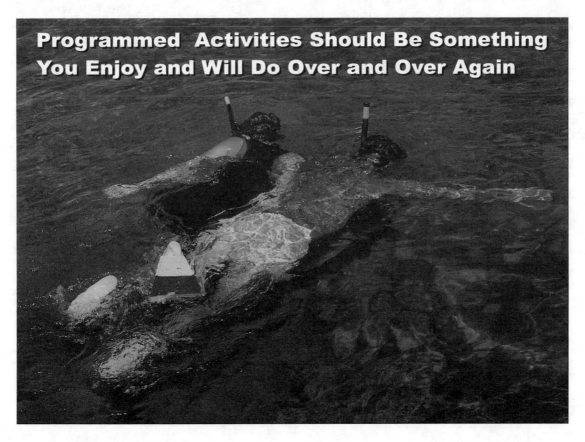

Programmed Activities Should Be Something You Enjoy and Will Do Over and Over Again

If you know that activity is good, and would like to do more, then we need to look at what gets in the way and what might be done. What often gets in the way is embarrassment, being timid about exercise, thinking that you couldn't possibly do as much as necessary, and practical issues such as time. We have given you enough ammunition throughout this program to challenge and defeat each of these obstacles. It's a great time to rise above the barriers and start the activity. Here's how to do it.

Choosing the Best Activity

There are many activities to choose from. Several possibilities will be discussed below. There are four factors to consider in making your decision.

▶ **Select something you can do.** Consider your current physical condition when choosing an activity. Basketball is strenuous and is not advisable if you are not in tip-top condition. Pick something where you can move at your own pace. Walking, cycling, and swimming are good examples.

▶ **Select something you would like to do.** Hiking may be something that always caught your fancy, so go ahead and try. If you are turned off by swimming, don't do it just because you think you should. It helps to like the activities you choose.

▶ **Select a solo or social activity.** We covered this earlier in our discussion of walking. In your choice of an activity, consider whether you would like to exercise alone (jogging, swimming, cycling) or with other people (tennis, golf, aerobics class). If you are a social person, having others around can be an incentive to participate.

▶ **Do not be embarrassed.** This is easier said than done. Many heavy people avoid exercise completely, or avoid it when they can be seen by others. They are embarrassed about their bodies, their clothes, and their poor physical condition. Try to put this aside. Take a deep breath, and ask yourself which is more important, avoiding embarrassment or losing weight.

A Helpful Tip

Let us pass along a tip drawn from our own experience. We exercise regularly and try to have a number of activities to choose from. We run, ride a bike, play tennis, and do strength training. Mixing up these activities provides us with choice and variety, both of which help minimize boredom. We can watch TV, listen to music, or both while doing some of these things, so we sometimes save the exercise when we know there is something we might like to see on the television.

Most people can probably find more than one activity as a possibility. If an outside activity is not possible, then an inside alternative might fit the bill. The key is whether you will still be active

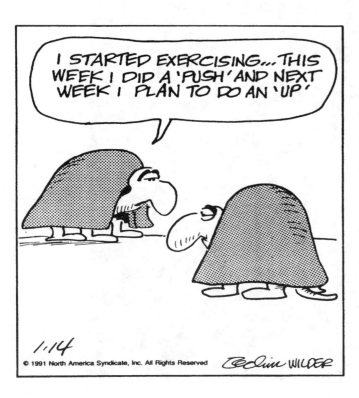

I STARTED EXERCISING... THIS WEEK I DID A 'PUSH' AND NEXT WEEK I PLAN TO DO AN 'UP'

1·14

WILDER

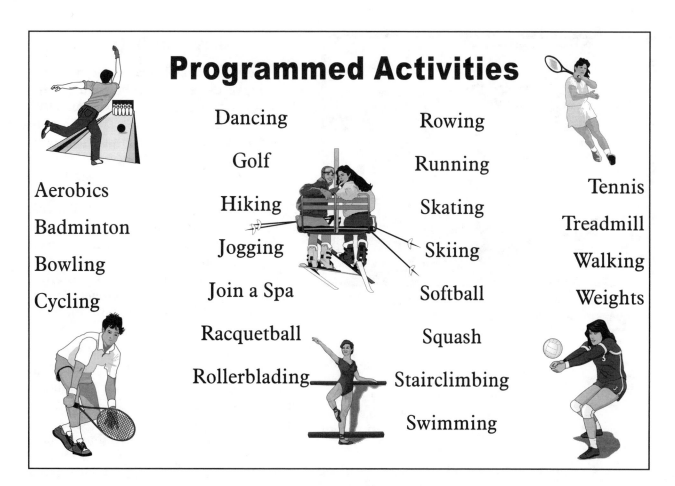

Programmed Activities

Aerobics
Badminton
Bowling
Cycling

Dancing
Golf
Hiking
Jogging
Join a Spa
Racquetball
Rollerblading

Rowing
Running
Skating
Skiing
Softball
Squash
Stairclimbing
Swimming

Tennis
Treadmill
Walking
Weights

months or years from now. Whether this occurs depends in large part on whether you enjoy it, and whether you enjoy it may depend on variety and the presence of other interesting things.

Warming up and Cooling Down

It is important to warm up before exercise and to cool down afterwards. This will help stretch your muscles to avoid strains and pulls. It will also help your heart and circulatory system make the transition from rest to exercise and then back to rest. You should warm up and cool down at least five minutes for a 30-minute bout of exercise.

In general, a good warm-up for most activities is the same activity performed at lower intensity. Walking slowly is a good warm-up for brisk walking, and brisk walking can serve as a warm-up for running. Here are several additional exercises to warm up. Please note that some exercises may be problematic if you have certain conditions. Trunk twists may create difficulty if you have back problems. Check with your physician or a sports medicine specialist if you have such problems.

- ▶ **Trunk Twists.** Stand with your feet shoulder width apart. Extend your arms to the side so they are horizontal. Twist your trunk to the right as if you are trying to look over your right shoulder. Then reverse directions and move your trunk so your left arm extends to your right. This exercise should be done slowly or as a held stretch to avoid jerking of the muscles.

- ▶ **Toe Touches.** Stand with your feet a little more than shoulder width apart. Bend at the waist, and slowly attempt to touch your toes with your fingertips. Keep your knees bent and do not bounce the upper body. Hold the stretch

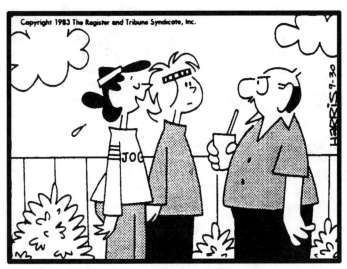

"Stanley exercises religiously. Does one push-up and thanks God it didn't kill him."

Cardiovascular Training

Exercise physiologists have done extensive research to show how much exercise is necessary to improve cardiovascular condition. This refers to the efficiency of your heart, blood vessels, and general circulatory and respiratory systems. From this research was born a formula known to millions of people. This three-part formula deals with *how much, how often,* and *how long* you must exercise to get this training effect. Keep in mind that this formula for cardiovascular training is much different than the activity needed to reach a moderate level of fitness as we discussed in Lesson 10.

This is what aerobics is all about. An activity is *aerobic* if the body uses large amounts of oxygen (i.e., if the heart, lungs, and blood vessels are working hard). As a result of this hard work, these parts of the body become conditioned. This conditioning is associated with greater life expectancy, lowered risk of heart disease, and other positive effects.

What about the F.I.T Approach?

The question then is "How much and what type of activity should I do?" The answer to this question comes from the American College of Sports Medicine (ACSM), an authoritative organization of professionals in exercise physiology and sports medicine.

The ACSM has published a position paper entitled, "The Recommended Quantity and Quality of Exercise for Developing and Maintaining Cardiorespiratory and Muscular Fitness in Adults." *Cardiorespiratory* fitness refers to the condition of your heart (cardio) and lungs (respiratory).

The ACSM document focuses on the F.I.T. principle (Frequency, Intensity,

for a few seconds. Return to the standing position and then repeat. If you have back problems, the sit-and-reach exercise may present fewer difficulties.

▶ **Sit-and-Reach.** Sit on the floor with your legs straight out in front of you. Slowly reach to touch your toes, and hold the reach for a few seconds. As with the toe touches, keeping the legs bent is important to avoid strain on the knees and back.

▶ **Arm Circles.** In the standing position, hold your arms out to the side of your body in a horizontal position. Roll your arms up, back, and then down to produce backward circles.

When you begin your programmed activity, be it cycling, swimming, walking, or anything, begin slowly and gradually increase your pace. To end your exercise session, gradually decrease the pace, and then finish with some combination of the exercises described above. The warming up and cooling down activities are worth the little extra time they take. They can prevent nagging injuries that could keep you away from exercise for a long time.

and Time). These are important for cardiovascular conditioning, while frequency and the number of repetitions is important for increasing muscular strength. There are five main components to the ACSM guidelines:

❶ Frequency of Training
Exercising 3–5 days per week is recommended.

❷ Intensity of Training
During a bout of exercise, your heart rate should be 60–90 percent of maximum. You can estimate your maximum heart rate by subtracting your age from 220. For instance, for a person who is 40 years old, maximum heart rate would be 180 beats per minute (220–40). During a workout, this person would want the heart to beat 108–162 times per minute (this is 60–90 percent of the maximum of 180 beats per minute).

❸ Duration of Training
The recommended duration of activity is 20–60 minutes of continuous aerobic activity. High intensity activities require less duration. The ACSM notes that total fitness can be attained with longer duration programs, and that lower intensity exercise over a longer time is easier to sustain.

❹ Type of Activity
Recommended activities are those that use large muscle groups, are rhythmic and aerobic, and can be maintained continuously. Examples are walking, hiking, running, jogging, cycling, cross country skiing, dancing, skipping rope, rowing, swimming, stair climbing, skating, and endurance game activities.

❺ Resistance Training
To improve muscle strength, 8–12 repetitions of 8–10 exercises that focus on the major muscle groups are recommended for a minimum of two days per week.

If you are sufficiently fit to focus on these issues, these guidelines should be helpful. If not, it is important to emphasize small and gradual changes in physical activity, remembering that any activity is helpful.

Do You Need This?

It takes vigorous activity to get your heart rate to this target zone of 60–90 percent of maximum. Keeping it there for 20 minutes can be difficult for some people. Take your pulse the next time you go for a walk. Use the procedure described in Lesson 7 to take your pulse, except take the pulse immediately after you stop walking. Count the beats in 10 seconds, then multiply by six for the number of beats per minute. The level is probably below the 60–90 percent demanded by the formula.

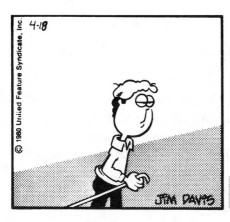
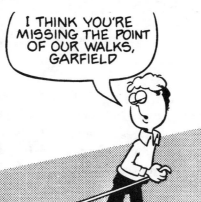
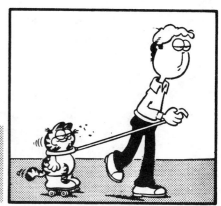

The important question is, "Do you need to do this much?" The answer is "yes" if you want to get the training effect. The answer is an emphatic "no" if you are exercising to boost your weight loss or to reach the moderate level of fitness discussed in Lesson 10. Any exercise is better than no exercise. Low levels of activity can help, so you may be best off ignoring the formula. We presented it here to clarify the numbers that are widely cited. Exercise in any amount carries many benefits, so do not be discouraged if you do not meet the standards set by the formula.

It is also essential to remember that the high level of exercise needed to improve cardiorespiratory fitness is not necessary to lower risk. You may recall information from the Blair study (see the graph on page 123) showing that the greatest benefit to health occurs between people in the least fit (completely sedentary) and the next group (people who are only moderately active). Hence, we must match our activity to our goals, and to improve health and lose weight, small amounts of physical activity may be very helpful.

Remember to be cautious when beginning an exercise program. Guidelines for deciding whether you need medical screening are listed in Lesson 4 (page 53). Review the guidelines and consult a physician if these or any other factors suggest any problems. Most people without a specific health problem can safely begin a program of at least brisk walking.

It is essential that you warm up and cool down before and after exercise. The body does not like abrupt changes, so you must warm up to prepare it for vigorous activity and cool down in the transition from exercise to rest. You may want to review the section about warming up and cooling down that we presented earlier in this lesson.

Danger! An Exercise Threshold Attitude

Many people on weight-loss programs labor under the insidious influence of a dangerous attitude—the exercise threshold. They feel they must do a magic amount of exercise for it to have any value. One client asked us, "Is it enough that I walked around the block after dinner last night?" Implicit in the word "enough" is that exercising below this threshold has no value. You must banish this concept from your mind!

The threshold concept was born from the cardiovascular training idea discussed above. If you will forgive us for stating it again—*any exercise is better than no exercise*. Walking around the block is not as impressive as running a marathon, but it's a far sight better than watching reruns of *Gilligan's Island* and munching on corn chips. If you walk two blocks, it is better than one block, but not as good as three blocks. Do anything to be active. Remember, small amounts of exercise add up, so do not feel you must strain to accomplish some arbitrary level.

Something for Your Partner to Read

In earlier lessons, we discussed ways to select a partner and to ask for help. One way to help your partner help you is to make specific suggestions. We have often encountered partners who ask for guidance on what they can do. Most are genuinely interested in helping and need only suggestions.

This section is written for *you and your partner*. Have your partner read it and then discuss the material together. Decide on concrete ways your partner can help, and implement these right away.

Partners can model good eating habits. A partner may help you immensely by doing what you are trying to accomplish. Eating slowly is a good example. A partner can exercise with you, can help keep food out of sight, and can display a positive attitude. This will remind you to do the same and will be a visible sign that your partner is trying to help.

Partners can praise your efforts. A pat on the back and a few kind words can go a long way. Your partner should not wait for weight loss to occur to be kind to you, and should not focus just on weight. When you make positive changes in eating or exercise, your partner can acknowledge it with supportive comments. By waiting only for changes in your weight, your partner misses many opportunities to help.

Partners can help with the weigh-in. Not everyone on a program will want a partner to know his or her weight, but if the relationship can tolerate this knowledge, having your partner present at a regular weigh-in can help. This gives your partner an idea of how you are doing. You may like this additional motivation. The partner must be forewarned, however, that weight loss will not occur every week, and if the weigh-ins are more frequent than once per week, fluid shifts will give false indications about your progress in the program.

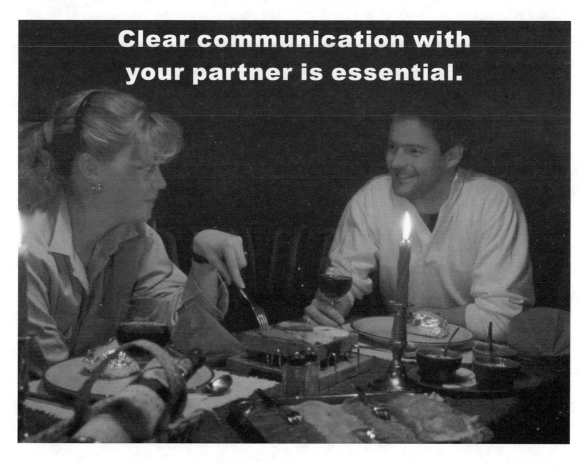

Clear communication with your partner is essential.

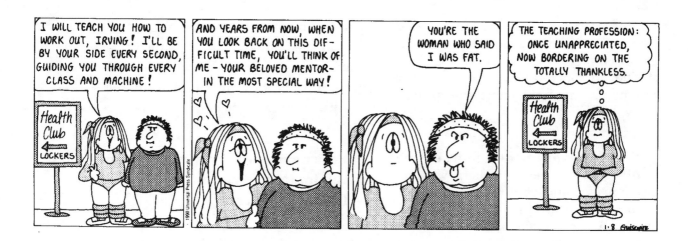

Partners can be rewarded in return. We explained earlier that the person in the program must be kind to the partner in exchange for the partner's support. This is a basic rule of relationships. In fact, many people feel better knowing that they are doing something nice for their partner. We also explained how you should be frank with your partner in asking for support and should be specific in these requests. These same rules apply to the partner. Your partner should tell you in specific terms what he or she can do to be nice. An example of a specific request might be, "I would like you to go to the movies with me once each week."

Ways to Increase Fruit in Your Diet

Fruit and fruit juices are an important ingredient of a well-balanced diet. Fruits are naturally low in sodium and dietary fat, and they are an excellent source of fiber and carbohydrate. They provide generous amounts of Vitamins A and C and potassium. Vitamin A is essential for the growth of teeth, skin, and bones, and it is important for good vision.

Most Americans fall short in their daily consumption of fruits. This is particularly true of children and adolescents. When this happens, the body suffers from a lack of important vitamins, minerals, and fiber. Here are some tips that may help you add fruit to your diet.

Breakfast

Breakfast is an important meal—one that should not be skipped. This is a good opportunity to have a serving of fruit. Six ounces of fruit juice is a good way to start the day. But be careful to make sure you are drinking 100 percent fruit juice. Many of the fruit drinks, ades, and punches on the market contain only a small percentage of actual fruit juice and have a lot of added sugar.

If you have cereal for breakfast, top it off with fresh fruit instead of sugar. Strawberries, blueberries, bananas, and grapes are smart choices and take little time to prepare. If you are in a rush, take the fruit with you. Keep fresh oranges, bananas, kiwifruit, apples, peaches, or pears available to take with you.

Snacks

Fruit makes a good snack—whether in the morning, afternoon, or evening. Canned juices are also convenient and easy to take with you when you are on the go. Instead of a soda or cup of coffee,

The Food Guide Pyramid

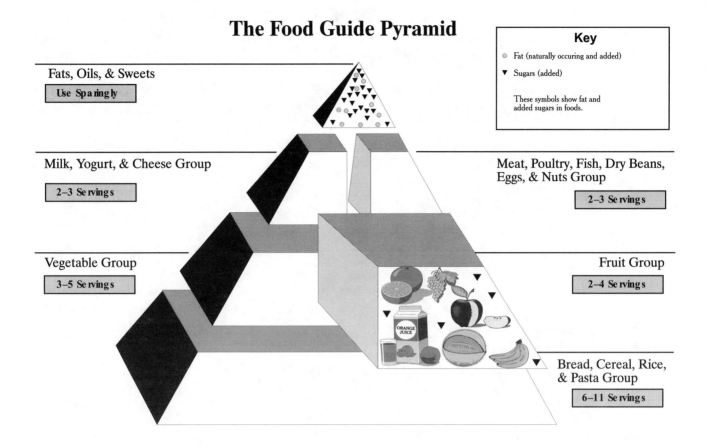

Key

- ○ Fat (naturally occuring and added)
- ▼ Sugars (added)

These symbols show fat and added sugars in foods.

Fats, Oils, & Sweets

Use Sparingly

Milk, Yogurt, & Cheese Group

2–3 Servings

Meat, Poultry, Fish, Dry Beans, Eggs, & Nuts Group

2–3 Servings

Vegetable Group

3–5 Servings

Fruit Group

2–4 Servings

Bread, Cereal, Rice, & Pasta Group

6–11 Servings

drink fruit juice. If you don't have fresh fruit available for a snack, canned fruit will do fine, but watch out for the heavy syrup and added sugars.

Lunch

If you take your lunch to work or school, include some fresh or canned fruit. Fruit is a healthy substitute for dessert. If you eat out, it is still possible to have some fruit. Many restaurants now offer fresh fruit as an appetizer or for dessert, but there are still some that do not offer fruit on the menu. If fruit is not available, ask for fruit juice.

Dinner

Dinner time is a good opportunity to review your fruit intake for the day. If you missed a serving or two during the day, add a glass of fruit juice to your evening menu. Fresh fruit can also be in-cluded with your meal (e.g., a fruit salad) or as a dessert.

How Many Servings?

The Food Guide Pyramid suggests two to four servings per day from the Fruit Group. This is less than you may think and should not be difficult to in-clude in your daily diet.

How Much Is a Serving?

Servings from the Fruit Group are relatively easy to remember. The chart above includes food items that count as a single serving. As a general rule, the fol-lowing count as one serving:

- ► 1 medium apple, orange, banana, peach, or pear
- ► ½ cup of chopped, cooked, or canned fruit
- ► 1 cup of small berries
- ► ¾ cup or 6 oz of fruit juice

Fruits

Description	Calories	Protein (g)	Carb. (g)	Fat (g)
Apple, w/skin (1 med)	81	.3	21.1	.5
Apple juice (6 oz)	87	.15	21.8	.2
Applesauce, sweetened (½ cup)	97	.2	25.5	.2
Apricots (4 med)	68	2.0	15.7	.5
Apricot nectar, canned (6 oz)	106	.7	27.1	.2
Banana (1 med)	105	1.2	26.7	.6
Blackberries, raw (1 cup)	74	1.0	18.4	.6
Blueberries, raw (1 cup)	82	1.0	20.5	.6
Cantaloupe, raw (1 cup)	57	1.4	13.4	.4
Casaba melon, raw (1 cup)	45	1.5	10.5	.2
Cherries, raw (10 med)	49	.8	11.3	.7
Dates, dried (10 med)	228	1.6	61.0	.4
Figs, raw (3 med)	111	1.2	28.8	.6
Fruit cocktail, in water (½ cup)	40	.5	10.4	.1
Grapefruit, raw, pink (½ med)	37	.7	9.5	.1
Grapefruit juice, fresh (6 oz)	72	.9	17.0	.2
Grapes, raw (½ cup)	29	.3	7.9	.2
Grape juice (6 oz)	116	.8	28.4	.2
Honeydew melon, raw (½ cup)	66	1.6	15.4	.6
Kiwifruit, raw (1 med)	46	.8	11.3	.3
Mandarin oranges (½ cup)	46	.8	11.9	.0
Mango, raw (1 med)	135	1.1	35.2	.6
Nectarine, raw (1 med)	67	1.3	16.0	.6
Orange, raw (1 med)	65	1.4	16.3	.1
Orange juice, fresh (6 oz)	83	1.3	19.4	.4
Papaya, raw (1 med)	117	1.9	29.8	.4
Peach, raw (1 med)	37	.6	9.7	.1
Peach, in light syrup (½ cup)	68	.6	18.3	.1
Peach nectar (6 oz)	101	.5	26.0	.1
Pear, raw (1 med)	98	.7	25.1	.7
Pear, canned in light syrup (½ cup)	72	.3	19.1	.1
Pear nectar (6 oz)	112	.2	29.6	.0
Pineapple, raw (½ cup pieces)	38	.3	9.6	.4
Pineapple juice (6 oz)	103	.8	25.4	.2
Raspberries, raw (1 cup)	61	1.1	14.2	.7
Strawberries, raw (1 cup)	45	.9	10.5	.6
Watermelon, raw (1 cup)	50	1.0	11.5	.7

Note: Each of the food items listed above counts as one serving. This table should be used as a guide for the foods listed. Since food values vary by size and brand name it is important to read the food labels for these foods.

Selection Hints

In most parts of the country, certain fruits are seasonal which makes it necessary to choose from a variety of different fruits. Variety is important because different fruits provide different amounts of important nutrients. The following tips may be helpful in your selection:

► Choose citrus fruits, melons, and berries regularly—these are rich in Vitamin C.

► Choose fresh fruits as often as you can—they do not have added sugars and other preservatives. Try to avoid fruits that are canned or frozen in heavy syrups and sweetened fruit juices—you'll save many unwanted calories this way.

Choose fruit juices that are pure fruit juice and that do not contain large amounts of added water and sugars.

Setting Personal Goals

As is true with each lesson, we urge you to pick one or more specific and attainable goals and to do your best to meet them. This is a good time to think about physical activity and to have goals that can lead to a regular program of activity. You may not like being physically active, at least for now, but liking may come with time. Remember that activity is associated with long-term success, so being active improves your chances of conquering weight and eating problems. Also for this week, check to see if you are continuing to eat the appropriate number of servings from the food groups of the Food Guide Pyramid we covered in earlier lessons. And for this week, focus extra effort to make sure you are eating the appropriate number of servings from the Fruit Group.

We have left blank the first two lines under the column "Personal Goals This Week" on this week's Monitoring Form. Put in your own personal goals.

Self-Assessment Questionnaire

Lesson 14

T F 68. Warming up and stretching before exercise is to strengthen your muscles.

T F 69. To get a cardiovascular training effect, there must be the right combination of frequency, intensity, and time.

T F 70. If a partner is working with you to lose weight, it is important to reward him or her for the help they provide.

T F 71. Fruits, vegetables, and cereals tend to be high in fiber.

T F 72. Most Americans eat plenty of fruits and should not worry about increasing their daily intake.

(Answers in Appendix C)

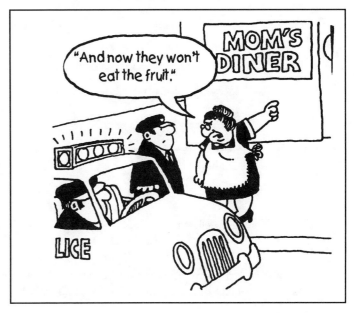

Monitoring Form—Lesson 14

Today's Date:

Time	Food and Amount	Calories
	Total Daily Calories	

Personal Goals This Week	Always	Sometimes	Never
1.			
2.			
3. Participate in Programmed Activity			
4. Eat daily servings from the Fruit Group			
5. My diet has _____ grams of carbohydrate			
6. Eat less than _____ calories each day			

Medication Taken Today ❑ Yes ❑ No	Physical Activity	Minutes
Milk, yogurt, and cheese ❑ ❑ ❑		
Meat, poultry, etc. ❑ ❑ ❑		
Fruits ❑ ❑ ❑ ❑		
Vegetables ❑ ❑ ❑ ❑ ❑		
Breads, cereals, etc. ❑ ❑ ❑ ❑ ❑ ❑ ❑ ❑ ❑ ❑		

Lesson 15

In Lesson 14 we spoke in detail about the wisdom of regular physical activity. We suggested some new attitudes that might help you be more active. The key is to do something regularly. This is probably more important than the type and amount of activity you do. These good feelings can spill over into all other aspects of your program and will help with things like making good food choices. We continue our discussion of programmed activity in this lesson. Finally, we come to the last tier in the Food Guide Pyramid, namely the Bread, Cereal, Rice, and Pasta Group.

Follow-Up on Programmed Activity

Each time you are active provides an opportunity to reinforce positive changes in your life, to feel virtuous, and to be reminded about your good effort. Regular bouts of activity can contribute, but so can little things you do spontaneously. Doing a little extra walking, using an extra flight of stairs, or anything else you do to move more, no matter how modest, should "count" in your mind as exercise. This gives you many, many occasions to feel like you are accomplishing something.

Have you been able to establish a program of activity? This is a place to try really hard. Some people find it easy to be active, but others struggle. But struggle they do, and in the end, any activity they do will be helpful.

More on Activity

We are now in Lesson 15 and have covered much of the introductory information on both lifestyle and routine activity. Much has been said about the importance and benefits of regular activity.

Are You Being More Active?

By this time in the program, our hope is that everybody is exercising daily. If

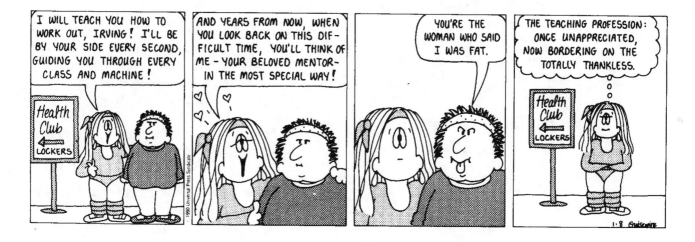

this is possible for you, make it your goal, and do your best to make some time for exercise each day. Of course, missing a day here and there does not mean you have failed in your program. Daily activity is, however, a nice goal to strive for.

Look back over your Monitoring Forms, and see if your level of exercise has changed. Have you found something you like? Do you use this exercise regularly? Does the exercise help you stick to your eating plan and lose weight?

If you are having trouble with the exercise, read over the exercise sections in the earlier lessons. Let us remind you that people who are still exercising a year or two after they enter a program tend to be the ones who have lost weight and kept it off.

There are several good reasons why many people resist exercise. For some people the exercise is difficult to manage physically, and for others, strong negative feelings about sports and exercise present a psychological barrier. One common problem is a busy life and the difficulty in budgeting time each day to be physically activity.

These are all understandable reasons not to exercise. We hope you find the reasons in favor of exercise to be more compelling. It could mean a great deal to you, both now and in the future.

Consider this a pep talk. We really do feel that exercise is important, and we would like to do whatever is possible to encourage you to be active.

Matching Your Activity to Your Goals

In the previous lessons we have discussed various reasons to be active. Some people aim to improve their cardiovascular fitness and choose aerobic ac-

tivities. Some want to increase strength and improve their physique, so they work out with machines or use free weights. Others want to use the exercise to speed weight loss, so they do whatever they can to keep moving, usually with walking or jogging. Each type of activity is valuable, but for different purposes.

By now you have a good idea about what you hope to accomplish with exercise. The table presented on the next page entitled "The Benefits of Various Exercises" shows the strong and weak points of different activities. This may be helpful as you match your exercise to your goals.

It is apparent from the table that the activities useful for controlling body weight also earn high marks for cardiovascular fitness. This is because the movement activities like jogging and cycling require effort (calories) for a sustained time and also give the heart a workout.

Remember, however, that cardiovascular fitness improves only when the right combination of frequency, intensity, and duration are present (see Lesson 14). To utter once again the most oft-repeated sentence in this book: Any exercise is better than no exercise!

The Myth of Spot Reducing

Many people would need a computer to count the number of sit-ups they have done to tighten the tummy, leg exercises to trim the thighs, and contortions of the neck to wipe out a double chin. The trouble is, these things don't work, yet millions still fall for slick advertisements or books that promise ways of reducing specific parts of the body.

Where your body stores fat depends on genetic and hormonal factors. Women tend to store fat below the waist, on their

The Benefits of Various Exercises

	Developing Cardiovascular Fitness	Developing Strength	Muscular Endurance	Developing Flexibility	Controlling Body Fat
Archery[1]	1	2	1	1	1
Badminton[1]	2	1	2	2	2
Baseball[1]	1	1	1	1	1
Basketball—					
half court[1,2]	2	1	2	1	2
vigorous[1,2]	4	1	3	1	4
Bowling[1]	1	1	1	1	1
Canoeing[1]	2	1	2	1	2
Fencing[2]	2	2	3	2	2
Football[2]	2	3	2	1	2
Golf (walking)[1]	2	1	1	2	2
Gymnastics[2]	2	4	4	4	2
Handball[1,2]	3–4	1	3	1	3–4
Horseback Riding[1]	1	1	1	1	1
Judo/Karate[1,2]	1	2	2	2	1
Mountain Climbing[1,2]	3	3	3	1	3
Pool/Billiards[1]	1	1	1	1	1
Racquetball[1,2]	3–4	1	3	1	3–4
Rowing, Crew	4	2	4	1	4
Sailing[1]	1	1	1	1	1
Skating—					
ice[1,2]	2–3	1	3	1	2–3
roller[1,2]	2–3	1	2	1	2–3
Skiing—					
cross-country[1,2]	4	2	3	1	4
downhill[1,2]	1	2	2	1	1
Soccer[2]	4	2	3	2	4
Softball[1,2]	1	1	1	1	1
Surfing[1,2]	2	1	3	2	2
Table Tennis[1]	1	1	1	1	1
Tennis[1,2]	2–3	1	2	1	2–3
Volleyball[1,2]	2	2	1	1	2
Waterskiing[1,2]	2	2	2	1	2

[1] Indicates lifetime sport.

[2] Indicates fitness needed to prevent injury.

4 = Excellent   3 = Good   2 = Fair   1 = Poor

Adapted from C.B. Corbin and R. Lindsey, *Fitness for Life (3rd ed.).* New York: Scott, Foresman & Co., 1993.

The Food Guide Pyramid

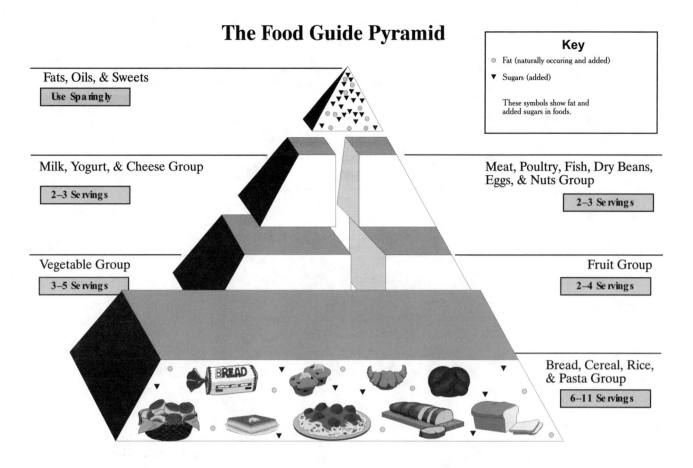

Key

○ Fat (naturally occuring and added)

▼ Sugars (added)

These symbols show fat and added sugars in foods.

Fats, Oils, & Sweets
Use Sparingly

Milk, Yogurt, & Cheese Group
2–3 Servings

Meat, Poultry, Fish, Dry Beans, Eggs, & Nuts Group
2–3 Servings

Vegetable Group
3–5 Servings

Fruit Group
2–4 Servings

Bread, Cereal, Rice, & Pasta Group
6–11 Servings

hips, thighs, and buttocks. When they become heavy, they also store it above the waist. Men tend to store fat above the waist, in the abdomen. When you lose weight, your body burns fat, but you have little control over where it happens.

Exercises will help you with muscle tone. This can improve appearance somewhat. Doing the sit-ups will tighten the muscles in your abdomen and will help you look a little less flabby, but they cannot force your body to take fat from there.

Breads, Cereals, Rice, and Pasta in Your Diet

Here we are, at the last tier of the Food Guide Pyramid. Over the last few weeks we have covered a lot of material on nutrition and on helping improve your diet. By now, you should feel very familiar with the Food Guide Pyramid.

Foods from this group of the pyramid are good sources of complex carbohydrates. These foods are good sources of low-fat energy and provide essential vitamins, minerals, and fiber. Foods from this group should make up the largest part of your daily diet. It is important, however, to watch out for the hidden fats and calories in some of these foods. Bread, cookies, and pastries, for example, typically include sugar and butter, oil, or margarine. Remember, it is easy to eat many calories from this food group and not get good nutrition. Making wise food choices from this group is important.

Bread, Cereal, Rice, and Pasta

Description	Calories	Protein (g)	Carb. (g)	Fat (g)
Bread, wheat (1 slice)	61	2.3	11.3	1.0
Bread, white (1 slice)	64	2.0	11.7	.9
Bagel (½)	82	3.0	15.5	.7
Cereal, cheerios (1 oz)	111	1.4	19.6	1.8
Cereal, corn flakes (1 oz)	110	2.0	25.0	1.0
Cookies, chocolate chip (2 med)	99	1.1	14.6	4.4
Cookies, oatmeal (2 med)	124	1.6	17.8	5.2
Danish, 1 small (1 oz)	125	2.0	13.5	7.5
English muffin, plain (½)	68	2.3	13.1	.6
Pancakes, 4 in. diameter (1)	62	1.9	9.2	1.9
Pasta, enriched cooked (½ cup)	100	3.3	18.7	1.2
Pie, fruit, 2—crust, 8 in. (1/12 piece)	116	.9	18.3	4.6
Rice, enriched cooked (½ cup)	141	1.2	21.5	6.0

Selection Hints

The following guidelines will help you to make good choices from the Bread, Cereal, Rice, and Pasta Group:

Dietary fiber is important for good health, and foods from this food group are good sources of fiber. Choose several servings a day from whole grains, which are found in whole-wheat breads and whole-grain cereals.

Foods that contain low amounts of fat and simple sugars are the best choices for a healthy diet. Choose foods made with small amounts of sugars and fats. These food items include bread, English muffins, rice, and pasta.

Some foods from this group that are made from flour are typically high in fat and sugars. These include cookies, pastries, croissants, doughnuts, and cakes. Keep these foods to a minimum and use fat and sugar substitutes when possible.

Spreads and toppings can add many unwanted calories to the foods in this group while providing little nutrition.

The best advice is to leave these items off or to at least use low-calorie or low-fat toppings, spreads, and sauces.

Most pasta stuffings and sauces use butter or margarine. Use only half of the recipe amount. If milk or cream is called for, use low-fat milk.

If pasta sauces or stuffings call for meat, use lean meat. Trim away any visible fat before cooking, and drain all oil before including in your sauce or stuffing.

How Much Is a Serving?

Servings from this group are simple to remember. As a general rule, the following count as a single serving:

- ▶ 1 slice of bread
- ▶ 1 oz of ready-to-eat cereal
- ▶ ½ cup of cooked cereal, rice, or pasta

How Many Servings?

The Food Guide Pyramid suggests 6 to 11 servings each day from the Bread, Cereal, Rice, and Pasta Group. While this may sound like a lot, remember that foods from this group should be the largest part of your daily diet. The chart here includes foods that count as a single serving.

Breakfast Cereal: The Good, the Bad, the Sugar Coated

Most of us grew up eating cereals for breakfast. The experience included not only the cereal, but reading the box, twisting and tilting the box in all directions to beat our brothers and sisters to the free prize, and saving box tops and proofs of purchase for the wonderful toys we could buy.

Today's marketing of breakfast cereals is clever indeed. Cereals are associated with cartoon characters and sports figures. The manufacturers are sensitive to our nutrition-conscious culture and to the bad rap given to sugar-coated cereals. Witness, for example, how some old favorites have changed names. *Sugar Smacks* are now *Honey Smacks*, *Super Sugar Crisp* is now *Super Golden Crisp*, and *Sugar Frosted Flakes* are now simply *Frosted Flakes*. Some cereals of questionable nutritional value are advertised on television as "part of a nutritious breakfast." The nutritious breakfast they show includes foods like juice, milk, muffins, fruit, and the like, so we suppose one could replace the cereal with a rock and make the same claim.

Breakfast plays an important role in your daily diet. One characteristic common to overweight persons is that they seldom eat breakfast. As they lose weight, many resume eating breakfast. Since cereal is part of the usual breakfast picture, the listing in the cereal table on the following page may be helpful in choosing a cereal with both calories and healthy eating in mind. The ratings have been adapted from an article in *Consumer Reports* magazine published in October, 1996. If you are interested in even more information, we urge you to read the article itself.

Cereals can be good sources of fiber and other nutrients, because the basic grains from which cereals are made (oats, wheat, corn, etc.) contain many nutrients for the calories. However, cereals differ greatly in nutritional value. Some have as much as 16 grams (three teaspoons) of sugar in every serving, so more than half the weight of the cereal is sugar.

The article in *Consumer Reports* points to cereals as "best choices" if each serving has five grams or more of fiber, five grams or less of sugar, and three

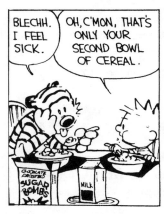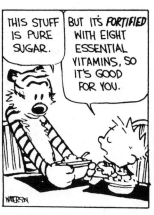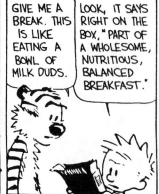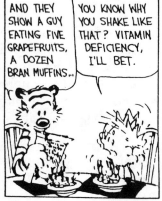

A Nutrition Scorecard for Cereals

The cereals below represent nutritious and not-as-nutritious choices based on the *Consumer Reports* comparison of more than 100 top-sellers. All are national brands; similar store brands should have similar nutrition. Note that cereal ingredients change fairly often. If you're concerned about nutrition, check a cereal's label before buying.

Best Choices
High fiber, very low sugar, low fat
(A serving from this list has 5 grams or more of fiber, 5 grams or less of sugar, and 3 grams or less of fat.)

General Mills Fiber One

Kellogg's All-Bran Extra Fiber

Kellogg's All-Bran Original

Nabisco Shredded Wheat (regular, spoon-size, and wheat 'n bran)

Ralston Wheat Chex

Other Choices
Very low sugar, low fat
(A serving from this list has 5 grams or less of sugar, 3 grams or less of fat, and 0 to 4 grams of fiber.)

General Mills Kix

General Mills Cheerios

General Mills Total Corn Flakes

General Mills Total Whole Grain

General Mills Wheaties

Health Valley Honey Clusters & Flakes with Apples & Cinnamon

Kellogg's Corn Flakes

Kellogg's Crispix

Kellogg's Rice Krispies

Kellogg's Product 19

Kellogg's Special K

Ralston Rice Chex

Ralston Corn Chex

Other Choices
High fiber, low fat
(A serving from this list has 5 grams or more of fiber, 3 grams or less of fat, and 6 to 20 grams of sugar.)

Familia Original Recipe Swiss Muesli

Kellogg's Bran Buds

Kellogg's Complete Bran Flakes

Kellogg's Frosted Mini-Wheats

Healthy Choice Multi-Grain Squares

Healthy Choice Raisin Squares

Nabisco Frosted Wheat Bites and 100% Bran

Post Fruit & Fibre Dates, Raisins, Walnuts

Post Grape-Nuts

Post Premium Bran Flakes

Ralston Multi Bran Chex

Raisin Brans (from various manufacturers)

Plenty of fat
(A serving has more than 3 grams of fat.)

General Mills Cinnamon Toast Crunch

General Mills Raisin Nut Bran

Kellogg's Cracklin Oat Bran

Post Banana Nut Crunch

Kellogg's Blueberry Morning

Kellogg's Great Grains Raisin, Date, Pecan

Quaker 100% Natural Oats, Honey & Raisins

Little Fiber, Plenty of Sugar
(A serving has less than a gram of fiber and at least 10 grams [2 teaspoons] of sugar.)

General Mills Cocoa Puffs

General Mills Reese's Peanut Butter Puffs

General Mills Trix

Kellogg's Cocoa Krispies

Kellogg's Frosted Flakes

Kellogg's Pop-Tarts

Post Cocoa Pebbles

Post Fruity Pebbles

Post Honey-Comb

Post Waffle Crisp

Ralston Cookie-Crisp Chocolate Chip

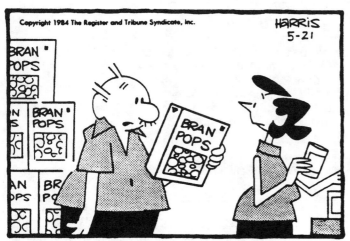

HARRIS
5-21

"It's a new idea in high-fiber breakfast foods. When the cereal is gone, you eat the box!"

grams or less of fat. The authors point out that some cereals that sound healthy may have fat and sugar in surprisingly high amounts. Raisin Nut Bran, Quaker 100 percent Natural Oats, and Blueberry Morning cereals have more than three grams of fat per serving, and Cracklin' Oat Bran has a whopping eight grams of fat per serving, including three grams of saturated fat. Some cereals have less than one gram of fiber per serving and 10 grams or more of sugar (e.g., Cocoa Puffs, Cocoa Pebbles, Trix, Frosted Flakes, Fruity Pebbles). It pays to look at the labels, not the name of the cereal.

Setting Personal Goals

Think about setting a personal goal for physical activity. A good (and attainable) goal is to use every opportunity to be active in your day-to-day routine. Use stairs whenever you can, park further from your destination than you might otherwise, stand rather than sit, avoid shortcuts, and do anything to get more movement into your life.

It can also help to set a specific goal for a regular form of exercise such as walking, jogging, cycling, swimming, etc. The goal you set might be to increase the number of days you engage in this activity or the number of minutes you do the activity. Keeping a chart or graph of your activity can be a nice way to remind yourself of your progress. And, as we say in each lesson, keep up the goal setting for the changes you feel are most important. Review your Monitoring Forms for the past week to see if you are continuing to eat the right amount of servings from the four food groups we have discussed in prior lessons. This week, focus on eating the appropriate number of servings from the Bread, Cereal, Rice, and Pasta Groups.

Self-Assessment Questionnnaire

Lesson 15

T F 73. Exercise can be difficult for many individuals, and may present a psychological barrier to some.

T F 74. No exercise can help you lose fat in specific parts of the body.

T F 75. Foods from the Bread, Cereal, Rice, and Pasta Group are a good source of complex carbohydrates but may contain hidden fat.

T F 76. One characteristic common to overweight persons is that they seldom eat breakfast.

(Answers in Appendix C)

Monitoring Form—Lesson 15

Today's Date:

Time	Food and Amount	Calories
	Total Daily Calories	

Personal Goals This Week	*Always*	*Sometimes*	*Never*
1.			
2.			
3. Increased Activity			
4. Eat daily servings from the Bread & Cereal Group			
5. My diet has _____ grams of carbohydrate			
6. Eat less than _____ calories each day			

Medication Taken Today ❑ Yes ❑ No	*Physical Activity*	*Minutes*
Milk, yogurt, and cheese ❑ ❑ ❑		
Meat, poultry, etc. ❑ ❑ ❑		
Fruits ❑ ❑ ❑ ❑		
Vegetables ❑ ❑ ❑ ❑ ❑		
Breads, cereals, etc. ❑ ❑ ❑ ❑ ❑ ❑ ❑ ❑ ❑ ❑		

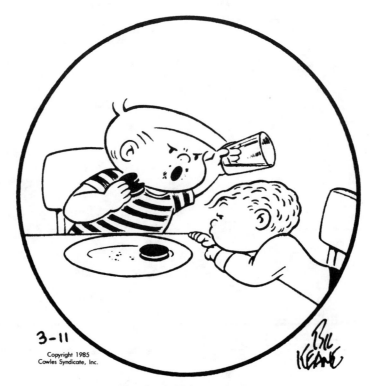

"Go ahead. Make my day."

Lesson 16

We are at a point where it makes sense to take stock of where you stand and to make a plan for launching into the next phase of your program. We will look back over the important issues that have been covered thus far, gaze into the future, and think about ways to make changes that can be truly permanent. Part of this process involves becoming friends with your body, an issue we will cover in detail. We also note that this lesson marks the transition from weekly to monthly lessons. You will read Lesson 17 next week but Lesson 18 a month later and Lesson 19 a month after that.

Taking Stock of Your Progress

If you have been reading one lesson each week, you are almost four months into the program. This is an important landmark. Four months is a long time, so you deserve credit for working hard this long. Many people give up before this point; you may have done so in the past yourself. So, persistence pays off.

What also pays off is being a student of your life circumstances. If you understand the circumstances that prompt you to eat well and be active, and the circumstances that make you eat more and be inactive, you are poised to act. Acting means having a plan so that you place yourself in the circumstances where you

can cope in a constructive way. Let's take stock of where you are with each part of The LEARN Program.

Your Lifestyle Achievements

A key concept we introduced in Lesson 6 dealt with the ABC's (Antecedents, Behaviors, and Consequences). This is a scheme for thinking about the events that occur before, during, and after eating. This is a great time to reapply that scheme to your eating and activity patterns.

You have confronted many situations in which you were and were not successful at sticking with your program. Can you think about what precedes situations in which you have trouble (the antecedents)? For many people, negative

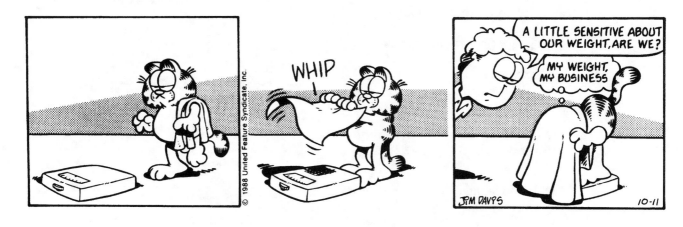

189

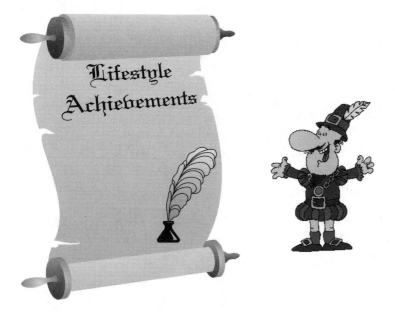

Lifestyle Achievements

feelings such as anger, loneliness, depression, or jealousy make a person want to eat. The time of day might matter, or whether other people are eating in your presence. Can you develop a plan to change the situations that promote eating? Think also about changing the behavior itself (your eating) or the consequences (such as your reaction to making a mistake). Then you can implement the ABC plan to its fullest.

Which lifestyle changes are most important to you? Is it eating slowly, sticking with an eating schedule, keeping tempting foods out of the home, keeping a food diary, or one of the other techniques we discussed? If it works, use it. But go beyond this to understand why it works. Then you can develop additional means for remaining in charge.

Your Exercise Achievements

A great deal has been said about physical activity thus far in the program. Let's review a few of the key points.

❶ Being physically active is one of the strongest predictors of long-term success at weight control.

❷ Physical activity has benefits far beyond weight control. It is associ-

ated with reduced risk of a number of serious diseases, including heart disease. People who are active live longer than those who are not.

❸ It is now known that rigorous activity is not necessary to derive health benefits from physical activity.

❹ Several bouts of activity during the day are as good as one long bout.

❺ The best type of activity is something you enjoy, and hence will continue doing over the long-term.

❻ *Anything* you do to be active, no matter how small, should "count" in your mind as activity. This makes you feel like an "exerciser" and increases your opportunity to feel like you are making progress.

We have spoken thus far about why activity is linked to weight control (Lesson 3), starting an activity program (Lesson 4), fine-tuning a walking program

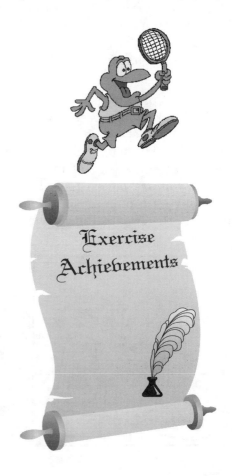

Exercise Achievements

My Commitment to Be Physically Active

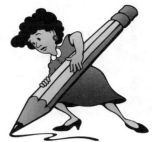

1. I will _____

2. I will _____

3. I will _____

4. I will _____

5. I will _____

(Lesson 5), continuing your walking and lifestyle activity (Lesson 7), making physical activity count (Lesson 8), how you can increase activities in your day-to-day routine (Lesson 10), how to select a programmed activity (Lesson 14), and more. Reread this material to help get inspired, and then find ways in your day-to-day routine to be more active, along with ways you can schedule activity to occur on a regular basis. Declare in the space above what you intend to do.

Your Attitude Achievements

It comes as no accident that the A (Attitudes) is at the center of LEARN. How we think is central to who we are as people. How we think affects how we feel, and our thoughts and feelings are key drivers of our behavior. Eating and exercise are behaviors, so thinking right goes a long way toward acting right.

If you accept the proposition that attitudes are key, then you are in a good position to spot helpful and unhelpful thoughts and to develop ways to think positively. By thinking positively we do not mean you should love everyone, ex-

pect world peace, and put smiley faces where you sign your name. We mean interpreting your progress in a realistic way, having positive but realistic expectations, recovering from lapses, and thinking about your weight, your eating, and your body in a constructive way.

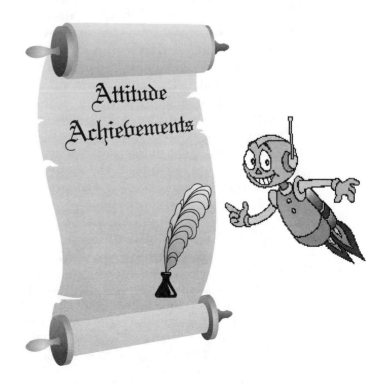

Some Thoughts that Get in My Way	Some Better Thoughts that Will Help Me
_____	_____
_____	_____
_____	_____
_____	_____
_____	_____
_____	_____

Think back on your experience of the last few months. You should be able to remember thoughts that have hurt or helped your cause. They might relate to how you thought about your rate of weight loss, how you felt when you had setbacks, or how much confidence you had in coping with difficult situations. Write down in the space we provide above some positive and negative thoughts. When you have identified the helpful, positive thoughts, practice them. The negative thoughts have probably occurred many hundreds of times over many years, so to counter them will require work. The more you repeat the new thoughts to yourself, the more real they will become, even if the process seems artificial to start with.

Your Relationship Achievements

Support from others can be a real asset. Not everyone wants or needs this support, but if used the right way, it can make a real difference for some people. In Lesson 7 we discussed how to decide whether you would benefit from support (remember our distinction between social and solo dieters?).

You may want go back and read the information on Relationships in Lessons 7, 8, and 14 to ask again whether you are the type of person who would benefit from support, and if so, what you can do to get and keep support from others. Also, it's not an all-or-none matter. You might not need support under ordinary circumstances, but want to call for it in a pinch. Let's say you start to slip off the program, or you feel your control is threatened because of some upsetting events in your life. Support can often be used as crisis intervention.

There are formal ways to get support, if you feel they might help. Overeaters Anonymous provides a great deal of support, to the point where you can have a sponsor you can call day or night. Other programs can provide support from group meetings or from a leader or counselor, and of course, support can come from a professional like a psychologist or dietitian.

Your Nutrition Achievements

As with the other LEARN components, awareness in the nutrition area is important. You can go a long way toward correct nutrition if you use common sense, eat a variety of foods, and follow some plan like the Food Guide Pyramid. The two key issues to remember are a balanced diet and calorie control.

Calorie control is necessary for weight loss and maintenance. By now you should know the calories in most foods and should be pretty good at estimating portion sizes. If the calories you take in are less than what your body burns, you will lose weight. If you eat more than you need, you will gain. Eat the exact amount the body needs, and your weight will be stable. It sounds simple, and it is.

Eating a balanced diet is necessary for good health. You could have a low calorie intake and lose weight, but still eat a terrible diet. The weight loss is gratifying, but you will pay a price in energy level and the general condition of your body. You can eat a balanced diet *and* keep the calories low. This satisfies your need for both weight control and good health.

There is no magic in nutrition. We can offer an iron-clad guarantee you will continue to see diet books, magazine articles, and the like that promise some new discovery. Some will tell you to eat lots of some nutrients (like protein or carbohydrate) and little of others. Others will say that the time at which you eat foods makes a difference, or that certain foods have special fat-burning qualities. Many of these are old diet plans with a new huckster and new hype.

What is common to most of these is that they promise what people want to

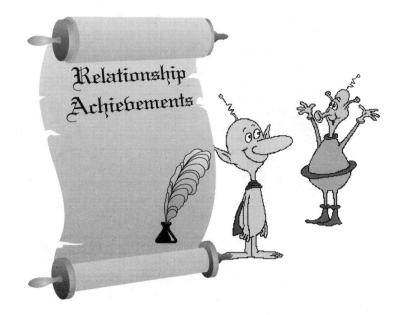

hear—a new solution and something that sounds like magic. They may spin a rationale that sounds good, talking about insulin, hormones, brain chemicals, and things like food addiction and carbohydrate craving. When you get lucky, you will find a plan that won't hurt you. Some might hurt you. Think of how many such plans you have read or heard about in your lifetime. How many could you name? Where are they now? How much would you be willing to bet that any of the ones that are popular now will still be around in a year or two? If they

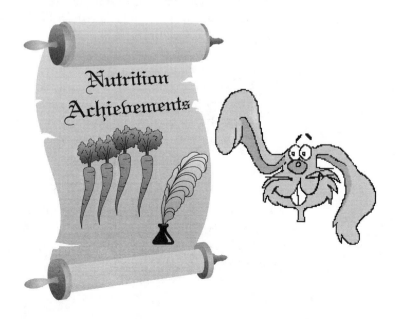

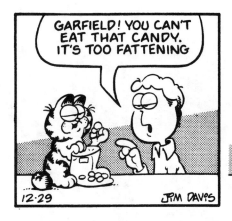
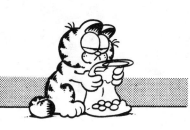
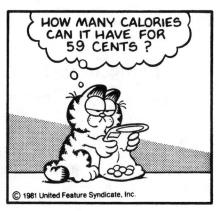

worked, they'd be around forever and everyone in the world would want a copy. None is likely to help you more than following the Food Guide Pyramid.

Are you eating a balanced diet? Are you able to keep your calories where you'd like on most days? You can expect better and worse days, so remember that what counts is how these balance out and how you do over a longer period, say a week or a month.

Your Body and Your Self-Esteem

How we feel about our bodies can be central to how we feel about ourselves. Our view of our own body is called body image, and unfortunately, body image is negative in most people, especially women, and especially people who are overweight. This is not surprising considering the enormous pressure in our society to be thin and for women to be valued for how they look rather than for who they are as people. Many, many people internalize these social norms, find a major difference between the way they look and the way they think they should look, and then hurt themselves emotionally as a result. It really isn't fair, because the social norms present an ideal that is unrealistic and not even healthy.

Let's look at how this might work for a young woman; we'll call her Ann. As Ann approaches puberty, she is full of energy, is athletic, enjoys being active, has fun, and takes pleasure in what her body can do for her. Yet, she is increasingly aware of the need to be thin. She is not prepared for this pressure to be so intense at the very time puberty causes her body to deposit more fat. Instead of accepting and enjoying the changes in her body, she feels her body is betraying her. Natural processes like eating and exercise become a battleground. She must restrict what she eats and must now exercise, not for fun, but for the purpose of losing weight. Ann may enter into a fight with her own body that will never end.

As Ann enters her 20s and then passes the 30, 40, and 50 year benchmarks, two things are likely to happen. One is that she will be dissatisfied with her body. She will overlook its virtues—that it allows her to be active, to move places, and to feel sensual. Instead she will focus on the disparity between ideal and actual and will feel it is her fault that she does not look perfect.

The second event is that Ann will let her body image have too much impact on her self-esteem. Our self-esteem is made up of how we evaluate ourselves on many dimensions (as a parent, child, brother or sister, employer or employee, friend, etc.). Our looks influence us all, but for

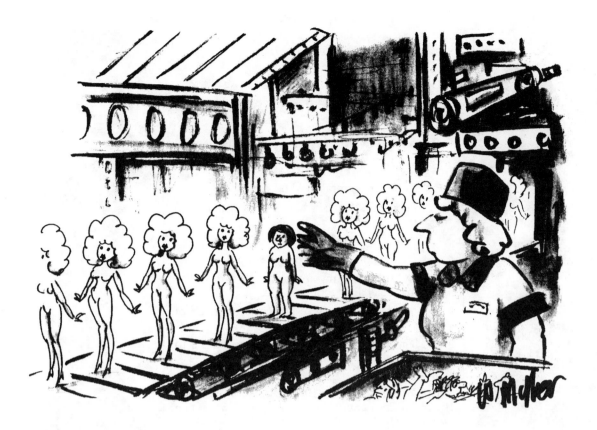

some people, appearance creeps to the heart of self-esteem. It can crowd out other positive influences, so that no matter how good we are at other things, there is always this looming matter of how we look.

Having a Positive Body Image

Having a positive view of our body, no matter how imperfect, is really important. If you dislike how you look, and accept society's unrealistic beauty standards, you will be unhappy with what you accomplish in this program or any other. The risk is that you will make very positive changes in eating, activity, and weight, but feel you are still far from your goal, and therefore will despair over your lack of success. This is a setup for disappointment, frustration, and giving up.

An excellent book on this topic written for the general public is by Dr. Thomas F. Cash and is called *What Do You See*

When You Look in the Mirror?: Helping Yourself to a Positive Body Image. This is published by Bantam Books and can be purchased or ordered in a bookstore. The book contains many good ideas for evaluating how we feel about our bodies, how this affects how we feel about ourselves in general, and how we can respond.

In his book, Cash discusses fundamental assumptions people make about their appearance and their lives. Some of these are shown in the table on the next page entitled, "Faulty Assumptions About Appearance."

These assumptions lead to overestimation of how appearance governs one's life and to overemphasis on changing appearance to improve well-being. With these assumptions, which are very common, a person is always dissatisfied and no weight loss is enough.

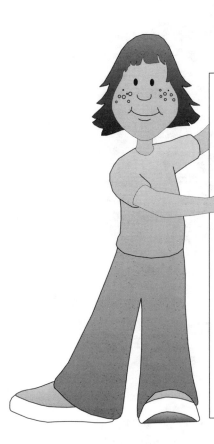
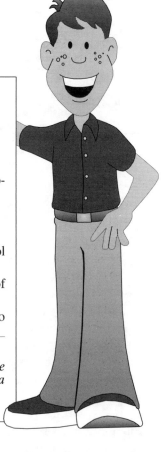

Faulty Assumptions About Appearance

1. Looks are central to who I am.

2. People first notice what is wrong with my appearance.

3. Appearance reflects the inner person.

4. If I look different, I could be happier.

5. By controlling my appearance, I can control my social and emotional life.

6. My appearance is responsible for much of what has happened to me.

7. The only way I could ever like my looks is to change the way I look.

Adapted from Cash T. (1995). *What Do You See When You Look in the Mirror?: Helping Yourself to a Positive Body Image.* New York: Bantam Books.

So, what can we do to be happier about the way we look? The book by Cash includes exercises and means for evaluating whether your body image is changing. Here are some ideas that may be helpful.

➤ **Get accustomed to seeing our bodies.** Most people who do not like their bodies do everything they can to avoid looking at them. Mirrors, especially full-length mirrors, store windows, and other places are avoided. Stop avoiding and find a way to believe that your body can be your friend.

➤ **Challenge the faulty assumptions about appearance and life.** To equate appearance with happiness is to give the body much more power than it deserves. You can be a smashing success at many things in life (most notably being a good person) irrespective of appearance. Appearance is only one aspect of our lives.

➤ **Confront what is realistic for us as individuals.** Given what you have looked like during your adult life, given how your parents looked, and given how difficult it might be for you to lose to an "ideal" weight, be candid, and consider how you might "realistically" look. Perhaps you can do more, but perhaps not.

➤ **Uncouple body image from self-esteem.** The assumption that how you look is who you are can be very damaging.

➤ **Focus on how your body is a gift.** The body can do many fine things for us. It allows us to live, to move, to accomplish what we'd like, not to mention how good it feels when we relax, work out, and engage in sensual activities with another person. The body gives us many gifts of living, and therefore is a gift itself. If we focus on the virtues of our bodies, it becomes less an adversary. Being friends with your body is central to your long-term happiness.

None of these will be easy because how you feel about yourself is the product of years and years of experiences, thoughts, attitudes, and feelings. Just vowing to be happier with the way we look is not enough. We must challenge the faulty assumptions constantly. We must make a concerted effort to reward ourselves for looking good, and then practice this new way of thinking for days, weeks, and months. It takes a lot to undo the powerful messages we have been exposed to, so please keep at it. You deserve to feel good about yourself, no matter what you weigh.

More about Dietary Fat

Counting Grams of Fat

As we discussed earlier in this program, there are many reasons why dietary fat is a central issue in a weight-management program. Among the reasons are that fat has many calories and that fat intake is related to risk of heart disease and some cancers. For these reasons, some nutrition experts recommend that individuals keep a record of their grams of fat intake, in addition to or in lieu of counting calories.

Whether one counts fat or calories depends on the aim of dietary change. If the purpose of the diet is to reduce the risk for chronic disease, counting fat grams would be sensible. If weight control is the issue, counting calories is the reasonable choice. A diet high in fat is typically high in calories, and vice-versa,

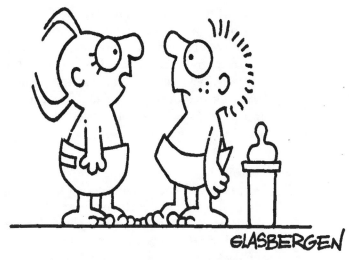

"Be honest with me . . . do disposable diapers make my hips look too big?"

but there are exceptions. For instance, one could drink 25 cans of Coca Cola each day, take in little fat, and still gain weight because of the high sugar content.

Some individuals who use this program choose to record grams of fat as well as calories. Because fat intake is so important, we have provided the grams of fat as well as calorie values in The Calorie Guide (Appendix F) and in many tables throughout this book. Feel free to record fat grams if you wish, but remember that it is essential to keep an accurate record of your calorie intake.

Reduced Fat Foods

The food companies have been working hard to develop products with less fat. The enormous popularity of reduced sugar items such as diet soft drinks has led to a frantic search for ways to preserve the taste of foods while lowering the amount of nutrients that may contribute to health problems.

More and more we will see food items that are reduced in fat. Some will have other nutrients replace the fat, and fat substitutes will be more common. For the most part, we believe these are positive developments as they will allow people to enjoy some of the foods they like but with fewer calories and grams of fat. One risk lies in the way people interpret and then make use of terms like "low fat."

Low fat does not mean low calorie. In fact, many of the low-fat cookies now on the market have nearly as many calories as the cookies they hope to replace. True, if one is destined to eat a certain number of cookies, then it would be better to have the reduced-fat versions, but we cannot assume this will cut calories. Some people feel that because a food seems healthy they can eat more of it. So, if you encounter cookies, crackers, and other foods that are reduced in fat, be certain to check the calories. For some people,

the marketing of these products has had a paradoxical effect—people feel they can eat more and, thus, they increase their calorie intake.

High-Risk Situations— Triggers for Eating

By now you should be a scholar of your eating and activity behaviors. What are your triggers for eating? Talking to your mother-in-law may do it, as might being bored at home, or having your spouse eat ice cream in front of you. It could be a trying day at work, a fight with someone, or fear about money matters. Most people have well-defined triggers. What are yours?

This is where the concept of high-risk situations becomes so important. Throughout the program, you will learn methods for avoiding or coping with situations that spell trouble. Identifying these situations, or triggers, is the first step. What you learn from the Monitoring Forms and from your own study of yourself will provide valuable information as you continue with the program. You can learn to predict the situations that increase your risk and to plot your course accordingly.

Do you remember the Expanded Food Diary you kept in Lessons 3, 4, and 5? Look back and review your diaries during this time. Triggers are typically a mix of the factors that you included in your Expanded Food Diary. Given the right time, feelings, and other circumstances, eating is hard to resist. There may be positive pressure, like offers of food from friends, or negative pressure, like feeling upset. Once the trigger loosens a person's control, it is difficult to stop.

My Eating Triggers

Trigger 1:

Trigger 2:

Trigger 3:

Trigger 4:

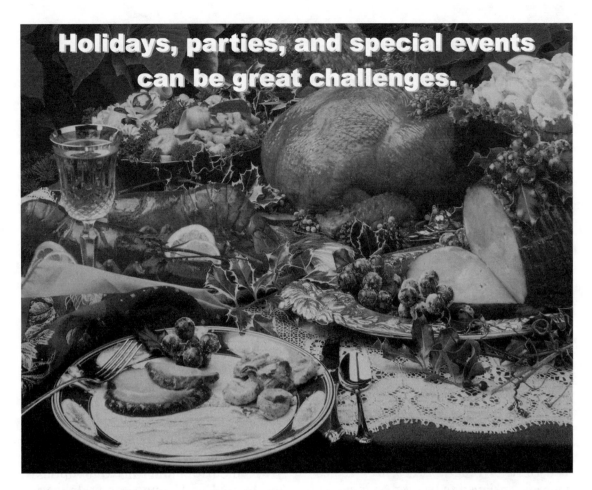

Holidays, parties, and special events can be great challenges.

Make a list of your four main triggers in the spaces provided on the previous page. Remember these, as there will be many suggestions later about how to counter them. A common source of difficulty for most people are parties, holidays, and special events.

A Note about Parties, Holidays, and Special Events

Many people find that their greatest challenge lies in how they handle holidays, parties, and special events. Loads of tempting food is usually available, hosts want and expect you to eat, and let's face it, celebrating just doesn't seem the same when you have to forego the special foods. Eating out at restaurants can be similarly challenging.

There are ways of being clever that can help you enjoy yourself while keeping control. Since we face so many of these events during a year, being prepared with the necessary skills can be a big help. We deal with these issues in detail in Lesson 24 in the section called "Holidays, Parties, and Special Events," and in Lesson 20 in the section on "Eating Away from Home." Feel free to read these sections as needed to help with problems you may anticipate.

Continuing Your Medication

MERIDIA is a medication that can help with both weight loss and with weight maintenance. Some people who take medication and lose weight, regain their lost weight when they stop taking medication. This is not a sign that the medication does not work. Precisely the opposite, it shows that the medication does work. We will discuss this further in Lesson 18.

You might have stopped your medication by now, may still be taking it and losing, or may still be taking it and holding steady. You and your doctor can decide what is best for you, but you may very well find that staying on the medicine is helpful to your long-term success. We will discuss this more in Lesson 18.

Transition from Weekly to Monthly Lessons

As we mentioned in the beginning of The LEARN Program, the first 16 lessons are designed to be used on a weekly basis. If you have followed the program in this way, you have read a lesson each week and could anticipate new material a week later. After Lesson 16 we make an important transition—from weekly to monthly lessons. Lesson 16 is your last weekly lesson. Next week you will begin Lesson 17 which will be your first monthly lesson. Lesson 17 will take you through weeks 17–20 of the program. The total series of lessons is to span a one-year period. This underscores our commitment to long-term, permanent change. The lessons will correspond to weeks in the program according to the chart on the next page.

Why do we make this transition? It is time to think about settling into a routine in which changes that seemed novel in the beginning become automatic and permanent with time. This requires practice and patience. It requires inte-

grating the changes into your life in a way that you can live with and enjoy.

Practicing new habits requires more than a week, so we now plan a month between lessons so you can get as much practice as possible and fine-tune the changes you'd like to make. You may read the lessons on a more rapid timetable if you'd like, but it is still advisable to take a month to work on the changes in each lesson and then move on to the next lesson. And, when the year is over, we're not done even then. We will then discuss *The LEARN Program Weight Maintenance and Stabilization Guide*.

Looking Ahead

With all we have said and done, it is hard to believe there is much more to cover. In fact, there is more in each of the five areas of The LEARN Program. Among the topics we will cover are: dealing with pressures to eat; nutrition topics like fiber, reading food labels, and vitamins; stress and eating; and preparing to deal with long-term stabilization of eating and activity changes.

Setting Personal Goals

As we think of personal goals, it can be helpful to return to the past. By the past, we mean the early lessons in which we discussed some of the fundamental recommendations of this program. Keeping your Monitoring Form is an example. We know people who have been filling out Monitoring Forms for 20 years and more. Others keep the Forms in reserve and start using them if they feel their weight and eating are showing signs of slipping. You can remember how the Monitoring Form was useful in giving you feedback on what you eat, so it is a good policy to keep it until you feel your changes are truly permanent and even then, have it available if you need it.

LEARN Program Lessons and Corresponding Program Weeks

LEARN Program Lesson	Corresponding Program Weeks
16	16
17	17–20
18	21–24
19	25–28
20	29–32
21	33–36
22	37–40
23	41–44
24	45–48
Commencement Lesson	49–52

Scan the early lessons and you will find other suggestions that have worked for you, and then set up your personal goals.

Our specific suggestion is to take at least three of the five LEARN areas, and select one or more goals in each that you feel are crucial for you. We will suggest a similar process toward the end of this program, so this is a good time to begin thinking in this way. You will notice on the Monitoring Form for this lesson that we have left blank the first two lines of the "Personal Goals for This Week." This is not an oversight on our part, but an opportunity for you to decide what *your* goals are for the upcoming week. Fill in the blanks at the beginning of each week with goals you want to achieve.

Self-Assessment Questionnaire

Lesson 16

T F 77. The best kind of exercise is rigorous enough to build muscle, which in turn speeds up metabolism.

T F 78. Many people internalize society's unrealistic standards for beauty, weight, and shape, and are likely to have a negative body image.

T F 79. It is possible to weigh more than the ideal, and even be fairly heavy, and still have good self-esteem and reasonable body image.

T F 80. Medication can be as important to weight maintenance as it is to weight loss.

(Answers in Appendix C)

Monitoring Form—Lesson 16

Today's Date:

Time	Food and Amount	Calories
	Total Daily Calories	

Personal Goals This Week	*Always*	*Sometimes*	*Never*
1.			
2.			
3. Have a positive body image			
4. Take my medication			
5. Eat less than _____ grams of fat each day			
6. Eat less than _____ calories each day			

		Physical Activity	Minutes
Medication Taken Today	❑ Yes ❑ No	*Physical Activity*	*Minutes*
Milk, yogurt, and cheese	❑ ❑ ❑		
Meat, poultry, etc.	❑ ❑ ❑		
Fruits	❑ ❑ ❑ ❑		
Vegetables	❑ ❑ ❑ ❑ ❑		
Breads, cereals, etc.	❑ ❑ ❑ ❑ ❑ ❑ ❑ ❑ ❑		

Lesson 17

Welcome to Lesson 17. It will take you through the next four weeks of your program (weeks 17–20). You can read the remaining eight lessons in The LEARN Program at monthly intervals—one each month—at the end of which time you will have completed one full year.

Lesson 17 is a place where we raise the potentially touchy but important issue of family relationships. We will also discuss how to deal with pressures to eat from other people. This is another place where the "R" (Relationships) part of The LEARN Program can be helpful, because offers and even demands to eat from others can be difficult to resist. We then move to a new category of Attitudes—the "imperatives." Under Nutrition, we will talk more about water soluble vitamins and look closely at food labels. With these things in mind, let's move on.

For You and Your Family to Read

Some time ago, one of us (Dr. Brownell) traveled to Argentina and was invited to speak before a large meeting of a group called FAMALCO in Buenos Aires. Loosely translated, FAMALCO stands for "Families Anonymous of Relatives Fighting Against Obesity." This group was an outgrowth of ALCO, a large, nationwide, self-help group for obesity patterned after Alcoholics Anonymous (AA), much the way Overeaters Anonymous in North America is patterned after AA. FAMALCO is similar in nature to AL-ANON, which is for families of alcoholics. The innovative nature of FAMALCO was inspiring. It is unfortunate that no such group exists in our country. We would like to share what can be learned from this experience with you and your family, *so please ask your family to read this.*

The FAMALCO meeting began with moving testimonials from husbands, wives, children, and parents of people struggling with their weight. Some of the family members expressed sorrow about the weight problem, while others related dismay, sympathy, anger, and hostility. One thing common to all was the pain, suffering, and frustration experienced by both the overweight person and the family. FAMALCO allowed the

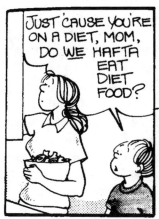
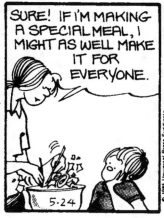
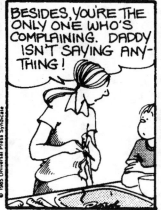
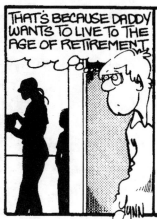

family members to discuss these issues with others in the same situation and provided many opportunities for the families to learn new ways to help the family member and to help themselves.

This meeting reinforced our belief that families can be a great resource for a person losing weight, but that harmony between the individual and the family requires a special effort from both parties. Communication is the first step. The burden falls to the person losing weight to express how he or she feels and how the family can help. This is difficult sometimes when the person resents the family's response to his or her weight. However, you must talk, express, and communicate.

The same responsibility applies to the family. The overweight person may have only a superficial knowledge of how the family feels. When the family finally expresses its feelings, the individual is likely to be relieved because the cards are on the table. This permits open discussion, positive communication, and suggestions from the person losing weight and the family about how they might help each other. We now recom-

mend that the family and you read the section in Lesson 8 on "Communicating with Your Partner." The guidelines presented there can be used to begin and sustain the communication.

When I (Dr. Brownell) completed my lecture before FAMALCO, the audience responded with a warm, loud ovation. I assured the audience that I had learned at least as much from them as they had learned from me. I was even more certain of this when I listened to the speaker following me, Dr. Alberto Cormillot.

Dr. Alberto Cormillot is a prominent physician and public official in Buenos Aires, known all over Argentina for his work on weight loss. He developed a comprehensive approach to overweight that would rival any in the world. In his talk, Dr. Cormillot listed a number of things the family should or should not do. They are as relevant in our country as they are in his.

Things the Family Should Avoid

▶ **Do not hide food from the person losing weight.** He or she will find it and feel resentful.

▶ **Do not threaten.** Behavior is best changed with a soft touch, not coercion, so be nice.

▶ **Do not avoid social situations because of the person's weight.** This will batter the self-esteem of the family member losing weight and will breed resentment in the family.

▶ **Do not expect perfection or 100 percent recovery.** Weight problems are something a person learns to control, not cure. There will be periods of misery, weight gain, and overeating. The individual's achievements should be appreciated and the setbacks met with compassion.

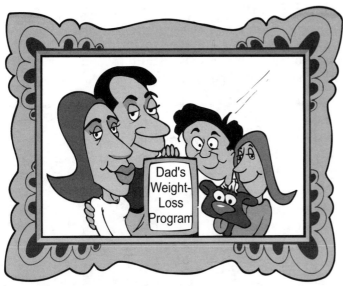

Families can be a great resource for a person losing weight.

- **Do not lecture, criticize, or reprimand.** These rarely help. The person needs to feel better, not worse.

- **Do not play the role of victim or martyr.** Overweight has many causes, both psychological and physiological. It is unfair for the family to blame the overweight family member and to feel victimized. Support and encouragement will do more than guilt and shame.

Things the Family Can Do

- **Keep a positive attitude.** This sounds trite, but can be very important. It is not easy to be upbeat and encouraging when a program grinds on for months and months. Extra effort from the family can make life much easier for the person losing weight.

- **Talk with others in your situation.** Being in a family where a weight problem exists generates strong feelings in the family members. It can help to talk about these with others who deal with the same issues. Many good ideas can be generated from this process.

- **Keep the home and family relaxed.** This will permit the person on a program to pay attention to the task at hand, changing eating and exercise habits.

- **Learn to ignore and forgive lapses.** The family can react many ways to mistakes, bouts of weight gain, and binges. The person losing weight feels bad when these occur, so it is best for the family to adopt a hands-off policy and to forgive and forget.

- **Ask the person losing weight how you can help.** The best way to learn how to help is to ask. Family members are sometimes surprised by what the individual wants.

- **Exercise with the person on a program.** This is a wonderful and healthy way to spend time together. If only a daily walk, this provides time to talk and can help the person with the program.

- **Develop new interests with the family member losing weight.** There are so many things in life to enjoy, and developing new interests can be good for everybody. Individuals losing weight sometimes feel they are embarking on a new life. New activities can involve the family in this process.

To summarize this section for the family, there are many ways the family can help the person losing weight. It begins with communication and proceeds to the things listed above. Both the family and the individual are responsible for making these happen.

Dealing with Pressures to Eat

A major challenge for individuals on weight loss programs is to cope with pressure to eat. Friends, relatives, and strangers—some well-meaning and some not, can make it difficult to lose weight by encouraging you to eat. There are a number of reasons for this.

- **They may be uncomfortable eating in front of you**. People agonize about eating when another person is not. They offer food to be polite, even though they know the offer won't be accepted. You can tell them that you do not feel uncomfortable and that they should eat if they wish.

- **They may be jealous of your success.** Others with weight problems may be jealous of your success. Thin people may also be jealous that you are accomplishing

Pressures to Eat are Challenging

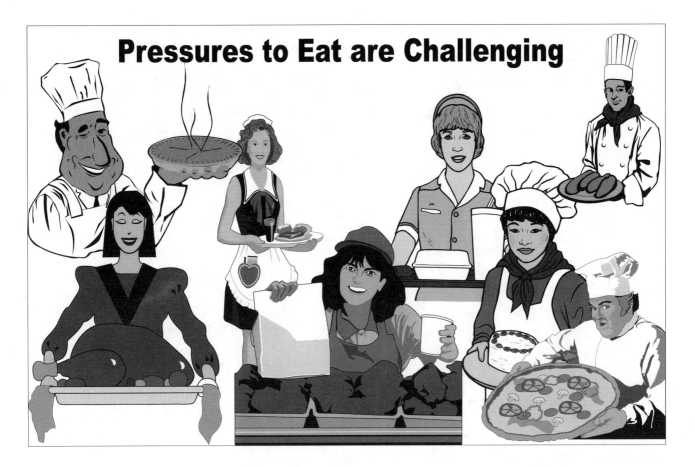

something and are proud of your achievement. This is their problem, so don't let it become yours by agreeing to eat.

► **They may not want you to succeed.** This is rare, but it spells trouble for the person on a program. You can spot it in acts of sabotage. The person may develop a sudden craving for your favorite food or may say demoralizing things like, "You have always failed before and will fail again." There are several reasons why another person would act this way, but we do not want to launch into a lengthy psychological analysis. You are best off ignoring these comments. Confronting the person rarely helps and can make the situation worse. Again, this is their problem, so don't let it influence you. If they offer you food or encourage you to eat, refuse in a polite way, but be sure to refuse.

The person will get the message and will quit trying.

► **They think you are starving.** These people can imagine themselves in your shoes and are certain they would be ravenous. Since so many people associate food with love, encouraging you to eat is one way to show concern. Assure them that you are fine and that they can help by ignoring your diet and by not offering you food.

► **They want to test your determination.** They may want to tease you or to see how serious you are about your program. It seems cruel, but it happens. Show them just how serious you can be.

Be Polite, but Be Firm

When you get pressures to eat, stand up for yourself and refuse. Avoid being aggressive or insulting, even if you suspect evil motives. The polite approach

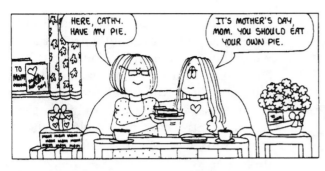

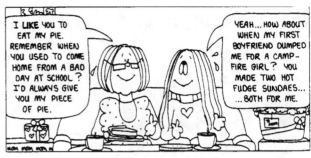

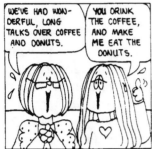

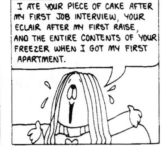

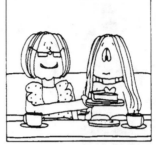

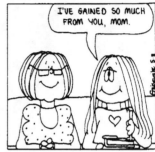

works best. After a few polite refusals, most people will learn that their pressures will not work and will quit pestering you.

If Aunt Irma offers you fudge, you might say, "Gee Irma, I love your fudge, but I'm not very hungry." If your husband stops to get ice cream with you in the car, say "I hope you enjoy it, but I really don't want the calories." If a co-worker says, "Let's go out and get something fattening for lunch," you can reply with, "I'm struggling to avoid those foods, so I'd better not go. If we can go to a place with a salad bar, I'll be glad to join you."

If you have trouble being assertive, try to predict the situations in which you might be pressured to eat. Plan a response, and practice it so you arrive prepared to be polite and firm.

Another Attitude Trap: Imperatives

Imperatives are words that imply urgency and no room for error. Examples of imperative words are "always," "must," and "never." If you are like most people, your vocabulary may be peppered with imperatives. Using these words can pave the path to trouble. Here are some examples from our clients.

- ▶ "I will *never* eat more than 1200 calories."
- ▶ "I *must never* eat cookie dough ice cream again."
- ▶ "I will eat a salad for lunch *every* day."
- ▶ "I will *always* say no when Vicki offers me coffee cake."
- ▶ "I must *always* control my cravings for sweets."
- ▶ "Chocolate is my downfall, so I will avoid it *always*."
- ▶ "I will exercise *every* day."
- ▶ "I must have *perfect* control of my eating."
- ▶ "I will *always* control the moods that make me eat."

These thoughts can float around in your mind waiting to take pot shots at your control. If you exceed your calorie level some day, you can recover from the extra calories if your control stays intact. However, the imperatives can get a clean

Watch out for those ATTITUDE traps

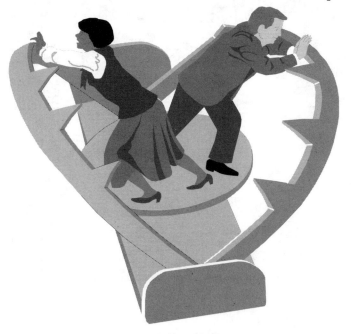

crave peanuts, wonder how they would taste, and fantasize about a peanut feast when the program ends. You might then eat some peanuts, either because you are offered some or you break down and buy them. Feeling like a failure might then weaken control even further and dichotomous thinking can lead to *falling off* your program.

Try to find imperatives in your vocabulary. What do you expect of yourself, and how can you banish words like *never* and *always* from your internal conversations? Replace the imperatives with language that allows some room for error and flexibility. Remember, there is no such thing as a perfect person.

Below are some examples of common imperative statements and some methods to counter them. These may apply to you in one way or another, but if they do not, you can use them as examples to form your own methods of dealing with the imperatives. Once again, being prepared can make you ready to deal with most difficult situations.

The imperatives are habits just like other behaviors and attitudes. To develop a new habit, practice is the key. It seems funny to practice thinking a cer-

shot at you if your mind cranks out thoughts like, "I should never eat more than I'm told." When this happens, you may be a goner. Disappointment occurs, and one can lose sight of positive accomplishments because of a few mistakes.

Individuals who feel they should avoid certain foods are especially likely to fall prey to the imperatives. If you forbid yourself peanuts, you will be fine for a week or two. You may then start to

Imperative and Counter Statements *(examples)*	
Imperative Statement	**Counter Statement**
I will never eat candy bars.	I will do my best to eat fewer candy bars, but if I have one, it is a sign to increase my control, not to let down.
I will never get depressed because it makes me eat.	Everybody feels down at times. If I get depressed, I must think of reacting with something other than eating—walking may be a good choice.
I will exercise every day.	This is my goal, and I will do my best to reach it. When I can't, I will try harder the next day.

tain way, but it really works. Once you know what attitudes give you trouble, you can gradually weaken their ability to influence you by replacing them with positive approaches.

More about Water Soluble Vitamins

In Lesson 10, we introduced the topic of vitamins and discussed the difference between water soluble and fat soluble vitamins. Let's look closer at the water soluble vitamins.

Vitamin C: Good or Bad?

No matter what we hear, people continue to think that vitamin C helps to cure and prevent colds. It has been ascribed other wondrous qualities as well. We recently read reports of a study where vitamin C had been used with cancer patients, as the vitamin advocates recommend. It did no better than a placebo. The advocates claim that the dosage was faulty. It is difficult for the public to make wise decisions when the scientists cannot agree. So, what do we do about vitamin C?

The Recommended Daily Allowance (RDA) for vitamin C is 60 mg, which is relatively easy to consume just by eating a balanced diet. This much vitamin C is contained in one serving of citrus fruit. Why then, do people take much larger doses than suggested? The vitamin pushers recommend that we take not two

or three times the RDA, but 100 or 1000 times the amount. Does it help?

Vitamin C (ascorbic acid) is used by the body for teeth, bones, cells, and blood vessels. It is absolutely essential for health. Vitamin C can be obtained from citrus fruits, berries, fruit juices, green vegetables, tomatoes, cabbage, and potatoes.

Studies have been done on the use of large amounts of vitamin C in hopes it will cure various illnesses. As with the cancer study we mentioned above, these studies typically show no advantage for taking more than recommended. This has been shown most convincingly with the common cold. Still, people cling to the hope it will help, and may send the nearest family member scurrying to the store for orange juice when they get the sniffles.

Since so many people take so much vitamin C, we must be concerned about possible dangers. Fortunately, vitamin C is water soluble. Excessive amounts, for the most part, are excreted through the urine, so your body only uses what it needs. However, there is some evidence that vitamin C can build up in body tissue when large doses are taken.

B Complex Vitamins

The B complex vitamins are also water soluble. This complex includes vitamin B_1 (thiamine), vitamin B_2 (riboflavin), niacin, vitamin B_6, and vitamin B_{12}. Each serves a different purpose and has different recommended amounts for healthy functioning.

Vitamin B$_1$ is necessary for the heart and nervous system because of its role in carbohydrate metabolism. It is available in enriched cereals, bread and other flour products, fish, meat, liver, milk, poultry, and whole grain cereals. Vitamin B$_2$ is important in carbohydrate metabolism and tissue repair. It is necessary for the skin and prevents light sensitivity in the eyes. It is available in leafy green vegetables, lean meat, liver, milk, eggs, and dried yeast.

Niacin is important for the metabolism and absorption of carbohydrate, so it plays a key role in converting food to usable energy. It is available in enriched cereals and bread, eggs, lean meats, liver, and dried yeast.

Vitamins B$_6$ and B$_{12}$ are becoming more popular in health food stores. Vitamin B$_6$ is used for metabolism of protein, carbohydrate, and fat, and is available in many foods, including chicken, fish, liver, whole grain cereals, and egg yolks. Vitamin B$_{12}$ helps prevent anemia and aids in the work of the nervous system. It is found in lean meat, liver, kidney, milk, salt water fish, and oysters.

As with vitamin C, the B complex vitamins are being hawked in health food stores and nutrition centers for all sorts of ills. Most people get enough of the B vitamins from normal eating. There are some conditions for which additional B vitamins are needed, but these should be diagnosed by a physician, not a store clerk. Since these vitamins are water soluble, extra amounts will be excreted, so your money goes just where the extra vitamins end up.

What about Multiple Vitamins?

It is reasonable to take a well-formulated multiple vitamin if you are concerned about getting enough vitamins and minerals in your diet. Check the label to see what percentage of the RDA's they provide, and do not exceed 100 percent. Remember though, chances are that you need no supplements if you eat a balanced diet.

Don't be confused by the fancy sounding vitamins at your store. There is no advantage to natural vitamins (another health-food ploy). The store brand generic vitamins are as good as the more expensive brand names.

Buy a multiple vitamin, which should contain the basic vitamins and minerals you need. Also, be cautious of vitamins that are supposed to help with things like stress. If you think you have some special vitamin deficiency, consult a dietitian or physician.

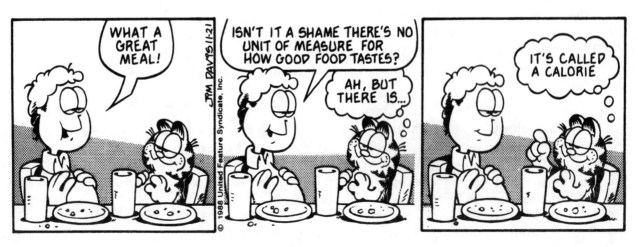

210

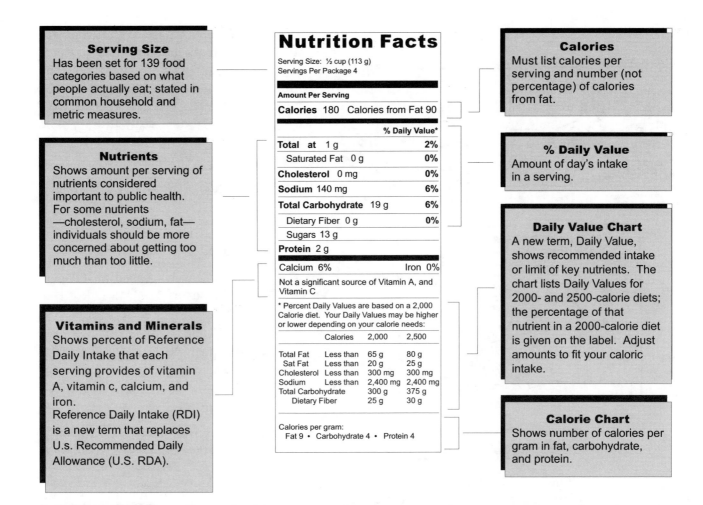

Serving Size
Has been set for 139 food categories based on what people actually eat; stated in common household and metric measures.

Nutrients
Shows amount per serving of nutrients considered important to public health. For some nutrients —cholesterol, sodium, fat— individuals should be more concerned about getting too much than too little.

Vitamins and Minerals
Shows percent of Reference Daily Intake that each serving provides of vitamin A, vitamin c, calcium, and iron.
Reference Daily Intake (RDI) is a new term that replaces U.s. Recommended Daily Allowance (U.S. RDA).

Nutrition Facts
Serving Size: ½ cup (113 g)
Servings Per Package 4

Amount Per Serving

Calories 180   Calories from Fat 90

	% Daily Value*
Total at 1 g	2%
Saturated Fat 0 g	0%
Cholesterol 0 mg	0%
Sodium 140 mg	6%
Total Carbohydrate 19 g	6%
Dietary Fiber 0 g	0%
Sugars 13 g	
Protein 2 g	

Calcium 6%	Iron 0%

Not a significant source of Vitamin A, and Vitamin C

* Percent Daily Values are based on a 2,000 Calorie diet. Your Daily Values may be higher or lower depending on your calorie needs:

		Calories	2,000	2,500
Total Fat	Less than		65 g	80 g
Sat Fat	Less than		20 g	25 g
Cholesterol	Less than		300 mg	300 mg
Sodium	Less than		2,400 mg	2,400 mg
Total Carbohydrate			300 g	375 g
Dietary Fiber			25 g	30 g

Calories per gram:
Fat 9 • Carbohydrate 4 • Protein 4

Calories
Must list calories per serving and number (not percentage) of calories from fat.

% Daily Value
Amount of day's intake in a serving.

Daily Value Chart
A new term, Daily Value, shows recommended intake or limit of key nutrients. The chart lists Daily Values for 2000- and 2500-calorie diets; the percentage of that nutrient in a 2000-calorie diet is given on the label. Adjust amounts to fit your caloric intake.

Calorie Chart
Shows number of calories per gram in fat, carbohydrate, and protein.

Reading Food Labels

By now it should be apparent that one of the keys to eating right for weight loss is portion control (i.e., calories). Learning how to use and apply a calorie guide such as Appendix F in this manual is one way you can control the number of calories you eat each day. Another helpful tool is the food label. The U.S. government has passed legislation requiring almost all food products to include a standardized labeling system. Food labels can be very helpful, and you should know what they mean for you. The following discussion will help you understand how to read and use food labels.

Food label reform was enacted in 1990 to serve three primary purposes. The first is to help Americans choose a more healthful diet. The second is to decrease the confusion about advertising descriptors and other misleading information that has prevailed for years. Finally, the new labeling requirements offer an incentive for food companies to improve the nutritional quality of their products.

Under the new regulations, most foods now require nutrition labeling. Nutrition information is voluntary for many raw foods, including the 20 most frequently eaten fresh fruits and vegetables and raw fish. Although currently voluntary, the Nutrition Labeling and Education Act of 1990 (NLEA) states that if voluntary compliance is insufficient, nutrition information for such raw foods may become mandatory.

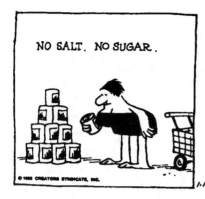

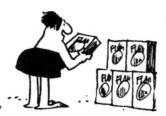

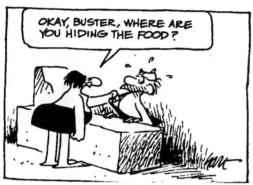

The Nutrition Facts Panel

The new food label includes a revised nutrition acts panel as shown in the diagram on page 211. The heading of the panel includes the new title "Nutrition Facts." This new title alerts consumers that the label meets the requirements of the new regulations. The panel includes certain items that are mandatory and other items that are voluntary. The panel includes new terms that may be unfamiliar to many people. References are made to Daily Values (DV) and comprise two new sets of dietary guidelines: Daily Reference Values (DRVs) and Reference Daily Intakes (RDIs). To help make the new label less confusing, however, only the Daily Reference Value term is used.

Daily Reference Value

Under the new regulations, DRVs have been introduced for those nutrients that contain energy (calories). These include fat, carbohydrate (including fiber), and protein. It is important to under-

stand these percentages so that they are not mistaken as percentages of total calories. The DRVs are based on the number of calories consumed per day. As a common reference, 2000 calories have been established as a daily intake. The DRVs for the energy nutrients are calculated in the following manner:

- ► Fat is based on 30 percent of calories.

- ► Saturated fat is based on 10 percent of calories.

- ► Carbohydrate is based on 60 percent of calories.

- ► Protein is based on 10 percent of calories. The DRV for protein applies only for adults and children over four years of age. Protein for RDIs have been established for special groups.

- ► Fiber is based on 11.5 grams of fiber per 1000 calories.

- ► The DRVs also include sources for some non-energy nutrients, including cholesterol, sodium, and potassium. In addition, the DRVs for fats, cholesterol, and sodium represent the highest limits that are recommended. These values are as follows:

- ► Total fat: less than 65 gm

- ► Saturated fat: less than 20 gm

- ► Cholesterol: less than 300 mg

- ► Sodium: less than 2400 mg

- ► Reference Daily Intakes

The new term Reference Daily Intakes (RDI) replaces the familiar term U.S. Recommended Daily Allowance (U.S. RDA). The values for the new RDIs will remain the same as the old U.S. RDAs, at least for now. The FDA does plan to propose new values for the RDIs sometime in the future.

Ingredients List

The ingredients list of the food is required on the food label. Food components are listed in order by weight from the most to the least.

Take a few minutes to carefully read through the illustration of the food label on page 211. Knowing how to read a food label can save you time in the grocery store aisles and give you a leg up on good nutrition.

A New Weight Change Record

The Weight Change Record we gave you in Lesson 1 (page 28) had spaces to record your weight for the first 16 weeks of the program. You can now retire this form and use the new version we give you in this lesson on page 216. This new form will cover the next 16 weeks of The LEARN Program (this will be months 5–8).

Setting Personal Goals

This is an excellent time to set goals related to relationships. The information for you and your family to read can be an excellent stimulus for discussion. It can open the door for you to express how the family might be most helpful to you. Families do not necessarily understand the weight loss process. Many family members, for example, are surprised by how many months and even years are required for permanent changes in eating and activity habits to occur. Keep alert for imperatives finding their way to your vocabulary, and remember that they leave no room for error. Remember to record your weight change each week for the next month on the new Weight Change Record. Prac-

tice reading food labels. What information on the label is most important for you? Finally, set goals that are personally relevant for you. What will be most helpful in your program?

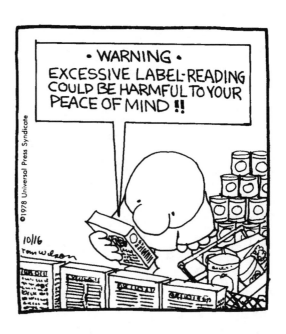

Self-Assessment
Questionnaire

Lesson 17

T F   *81.*   It's not important to involve family members in your weight loss program since behavior changes are all up to you.

T F   *82.*   When someone offers you food, it is best to accept it as a sign of friendship.

T F   *83.*   Imperatives are words like always and never. They leave no room for error.

T F   *84.*   Vitamin B_{12} is the only vitamin for which mega-doses are recommended.

T F   *85.*   The Total Fat listed under the heading "% Daily Value" on the Nutrition Facts Panel of the Food Label indicates the percentage of calories from fat for one serving of the food.

(Answers in Appendix C)

Monitoring Form—Lesson 17

Today's Date:

Time	Food and Amount	Calories
	Total Daily Calories	

Personal Goals This Week	*Always*	*Sometimes*	*Never*
1.			
2.			
3. Communicate with family members			
4. Resist pressures to eat			
5. Read food labels			
6. Eat less than ___ calories each day			

Medication Taken Today ❑ Yes ❑ No	*Physical Activity*	*Minutes*
Milk, yogurt, and cheese ❑ ❑ ❑		
Meat, poultry, etc. ❑ ❑ ❑		
Fruits ❑ ❑ ❑ ❑		
Vegetables ❑ ❑ ❑ ❑ ❑		
Breads, cereals, etc. ❑ ❑ ❑ ❑ ❑ ❑ ❑ ❑ ❑ ❑		

Weight Change Record
(Weeks 17–32)

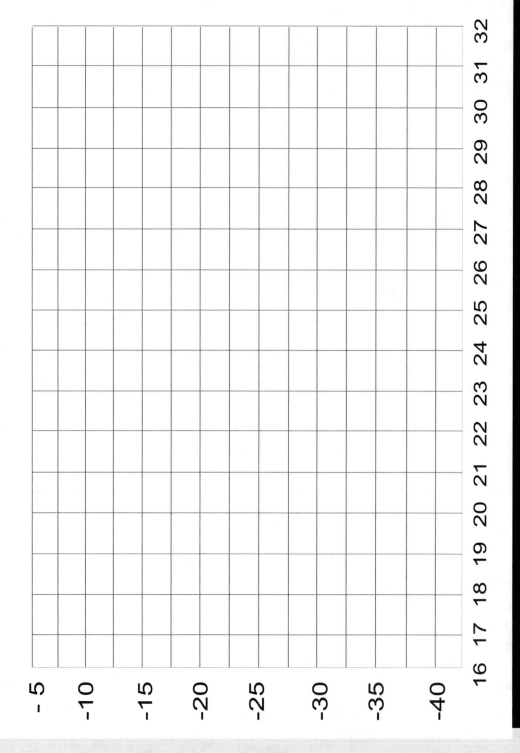

Week

Weight Change (in pounds)

Lesson 18

If you are following The LEARN Program as we planned it, a month has passed since you read Lesson 17. As you start this lesson, you should have completed your fifth month (i.e., 20 weeks) of taking medication and changing your eating and activity habits. Congratulations! This lesson will take you through the next four weeks of the program (weeks 21–25).

Quality of Life Assessment

Plan to begin each of your monthly lessons with a brief checkup to gauge your progress. Start by completing the Quality of Life Self-Assessment on the following page. This is the same quiz you completed on previous occasions.

What areas of your life are you most satisfied with now? We would be surprised if you do not have more energy, a more positive mood, greater mobility, and fewer health complications. Think about how remarkable this is. In just five months, you have achieved some impressive benefits. Compare your current responses to those before the program. This exercise will remind you just how much you have changed. Sometimes people lose sight of their accomplishments. We won't let you forget yours!

For those areas in which you are not more satisfied, what can you do to improve things? We suggest that you identify one area and start there. For instance, if you are not satisfied with your leisure and recreational activities, identify a concrete goal that you would like to achieve. It should be something specific such as reading for 30 minutes a day, going for a bike ride with friends on the weekend, or decorating the downstairs bathroom. Make a specific plan concerning what you will do, when, and

with whom. That's the best way to get new behaviors going. The table on page 219 may help you identify specific areas and a specific plan of action.

Eating and Activity Habits

Have you been keeping records of your food intake and physical activity? If so, here's your chance to study your behavior. Carefully review your Monitoring Form for the past week and identify your approximate daily caloric intake, your typical times of eating, and any situations that gave you trouble. As we discussed in Lesson 16, your Monitoring Form is the key to identifying high-risk situations and learning how to prevent them. In addition, be sure to identify

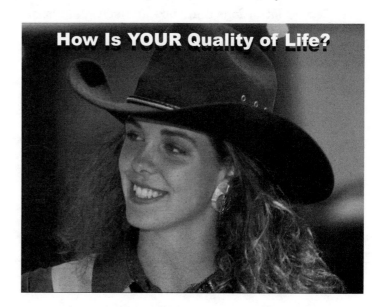

How Is YOUR Quality of Life?

Quality of Life Self-Assessment

Please use the following scale to rate how satisfied you feel now about different aspects of your daily life. Choose any number from this list (1 to 9) and indicate your choice on the questions below.

1 = Extremely Dissatisfied

2 = Very Dissatisfied

3 = Moderately Dissatisfied

4 = Somewhat Dissatisfied

5 = Neutral

6 = Somewhat Satisfied

7 = Moderately Satisfied

8 = Very Satisfied

9 = Extremely Satisfied

1. ___ Mood (feelings of sadness, worry, happiness, etc.)
2. ___ Self-esteem
3. ___ Confidence, self-assurance and comfort in social situations
4. ___ Energy and feeling healthy
5. ___ Health problems (diabetes, high blood pressure, etc.)
6. ___ General appearance
7. ___ Social life
8. ___ Leisure and recreational activities
9. ___ Physical mobility and physical activity
10. ___ Eating habits
11. ___ Body image
12. ___ Overall quality of life

situations that you handled well. For example, you may have found new ways to eat out at your favorite restaurant without exceeding your calorie budget. Celebrate these successes. You can also review your Monitoring Form to determine the composition of your diet, in terms of the amounts of carbohydrate, protein, and fat you ate.

Physical Activity

We hope you are continuing to enjoy your daily activity program. By now, your walking program should feel as familiar to you as your favorite old coat. Review your Monitoring Forms to see how many times you walked or participated in other activities during the past month. You'll probably be amazed at how much you're doing as compared to before the program. If you have not been as active as you had planned, what stopped you? Often, it's as simple as getting out of the habit, as a result of a vacation, business travel, or illness. Resolve today to pick up where you left off. Stop feeling guilty and worrying about the fact that you haven't exercised. That's a waste of energy. Exercise today, even if only for five minutes. The first step is the hardest. After that, you'll be burning up the sidewalk again!

Quality of Life Improvement Worksheet

	Area to Improve	How to Improve	When to Improve
1.	_____	_____	_____
2.	_____	_____	_____
3.	_____	_____	_____
4.	_____	_____	_____
5.	_____	_____	_____
6.	_____	_____	_____

To Record or Not to Record

You may not be keeping daily records of your food intake or physical activity at this point in the program. This is your decision. Some people find that they are very successful without recording daily; they continue to eat a low-fat diet and walk daily. They occasionally keep a three-day diary to get a snapshot of their eating and activity habits or keep records during the holidays, when everyone struggles to maintain a healthy lifestyle. We think this approach can work. So, if you're happy with your progress and are not keeping daily diaries, the diet police are not going to arrest you! Relax!

We do, however, think that it is important to keep records when you have trouble with your eating and exercise. Your Monitoring Form will serve as a compass or road map by which to get your bearings. In such situations, the sooner you start recording, the sooner you will feel better about your behavior and yourself. Of course, the paradox here is that the times you'll benefit most from keeping a diary (when you're hav-

ing trouble) are the times you'll least want to. Try it and see if keeping a diary doesn't help relieve "upset" feelings after overeating, gaining a pound, or missing several days of exercise.

A Challenge

If you have not been diligent in keeping your Monitoring Form lately, consider making a strong commitment to yourself to do so over the next week and review it carefully. At the end of the week, ask yourself these questions:

❶ Is my daily calorie intake where it should be?

❷ Is my diet balanced—am I eating the appropriate number of servings from the five food groups of the Food Guide Pyramid?

❸ Is my daily intake of fat less than 30 percent of my total calorie intake?

❹ Are there patterns that may lead me to eat inappropriately?

❺ Are my thoughts about my weight control and health positive?

❻ Am I getting at least 30 minutes of physical activity on most days?

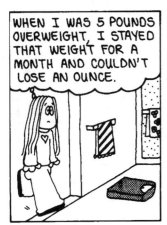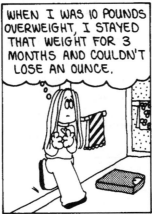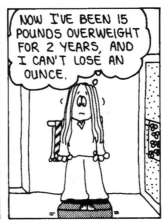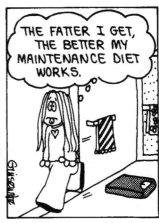

❼ Is there room to increase my physical activity?

❽ Are there other activities I can do to help increase my activity or make it more enjoyable?

Weight Loss

Let's review your Weight Change Record at the end of this month. The first thing you are likely to notice is that your rate of weight loss has slowed substantially since the early part of the program. You may have continued to lose a small amount of weight or you may have hit a plateau. You may be wondering how we know this. It's because weight loss always slows dramatically after the first three to four months, regardless of the treatment approach used. We have observed this occurrence with behavior modification, very-low-calorie diets, higher calorie diets, exercise, surgical interventions and hypnosis, in addition to the medications that we have studied. A slower weight loss after the first three to four months appears to be one of the first laws of nature!

The second law of nature is that this slowdown can be frustrating and perplexing! You may feel that you are working just as hard at weight control today as you did the first day of the program. It doesn't seem fair that your efforts are not rewarded accordingly. And it's not fair.

What can you do about this slower rate of weight loss? Three things:

❶ Understand it,

❷ Focus on your accomplishments, and

❸ Keep up your efforts.

Understand it

Your weight loss has slowed, in part, because you are now a smaller person and require fewer calories to maintain basic bodily functions such as your heart rate, breathing, temperature of 98.6 degrees, and so on. These basic functions comprise your resting metabolic rate, which we discussed in Lesson 3 in the section on "The Benefits of Exercise." As you lose weight, your resting metabolic rate decreases. Smaller bodies generally require fewer calories than larger ones, just as small cars usually burn less gas than big ones.

Let's say that before the program, your body burned 2000 calories a day. If you consumed 1500 calories a day, you would have a deficit of 500 calories a day or 3500 calories a week (7 x 500 = 3500). Since a pound of fat contains approximately 3500 calories, you would lose about one pound a week. Now, after five months, let's say that your body burns only 1750 calories a day because you are a smaller person. If you eat the same 1500-calorie-a-day diet that you did at the start of the program, you will now have a deficit of only 250 calories a day or 1750 a week (250 x 7 = 1750). Do the math and you'll see that you should lose a half pound a week now, rather than a pound.

Your body has a number of other intricate mechanisms that slow the rate of weight loss. These were originally designed to protect us from starvation, a constant threat to our survival until the modern era. Now these same biological mechanisms, combined with our more sedentary lifestyle and abundance of food, appear to limit weight loss in some people to about 10 to 15 percent of initial weight.

Focus on Your Accomplishments

This is where we hope that you can change the focus of your efforts from trying to subdue a body (that maybe defended like Fort Knox) to instead recognizing and enjoying all that you have accomplished. Again, see how your quality of life, health, and fitness have improved. Look at all the things that you can do now that you could not five

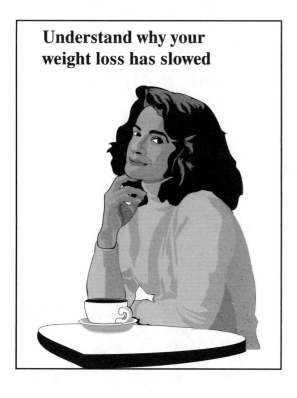

Understand why your weight loss has slowed

months ago. These are the true measures of success, not some arbitrary number on your bathroom scale or looking like the anorectic teenager who adorns the covers of fashion magazines. If your preoccupation with reaching some "fantasy figure" is preventing you from enjoying and feeling proud of your weight loss, we encourage you to reread the section on body image in Lesson 16. Remember, people come in all shapes and sizes; one size does not fit all.

Your ability to celebrate the weight loss that you have achieved is a sign of your self-esteem and self-worth. It is an indication that you know what is truly important—that you have a healthier, fitter, and more active body. Fashions come and go, whether it's skirt lengths, tie widths, or body shapes themselves (remember Twiggy?). Isn't it nice to know that you have taken care of the most important thing—your health and well-being?

The alternative is to remain fixed on reaching a weight that defies your hard work and sincere efforts. This is a classic recipe for frustration—thinking that if "I only work hard enough, I can weigh whatever I want." Unfortunately, your body has not agreed to this deal, any more than it has agreed that you can increase your height by three inches through hard work.

Keep up Your Efforts

Focusing on what you have achieved, rather than on what you have not, will keep your spirits and motivation high. Feeling proud that you reached your initial weight loss goal of 10 percent will propel you forward to continue your healthy eating and activity habits. These new habits will help you maintain your improved health.

Does this mean that you will never lose more weight? No, not at all. Many of

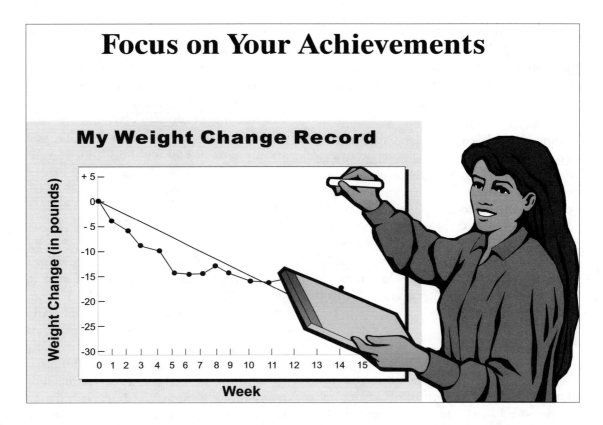

Focus on Your Achievements

My Weight Change Record

Weight Change (in pounds) vs **Week**

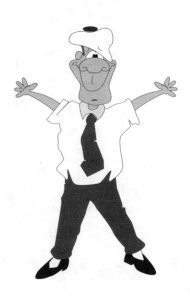

our clients have gone on to lose more after reducing by approximately 10 percent during the first four to six months and then remaining weight stable for a while. But we cannot predict whether or when you will lose more and don't want you to get stuck on this so that you can't enjoy the weight loss you have already achieved. Perhaps the best course is to continue to practice your new eating and activity habits to maintain your improved health and fitness. Over the long-term, your body will settle on the appropriate weight.

The Role of Medication

About this time some people wonder whether MERIDIA is still working. Their weight loss has slowed, and they sometimes feel that the medication does not control their appetite as well as it did earlier. If the medication is still working, why don't they keep losing weight? These are important questions.

MERIDIA works during the first four to six months to help people lose weight. After this time, it can help them keep the weight off. These are two very different but equally important functions. Of the two, we think the medication's assistance in maintaining weight loss is

Keep up Your Efforts

probably the more important. This is because there are many ways of losing 10 percent of initial body weight but very few ways of keeping it off. Weight loss medications have been shown in several studies to be associated with better maintenance of weight loss than treatment by diet and exercise used without medication. In a recent study, people treated by diet and exercise, combined with weight loss medications (not MERIDIA), kept off about 11 percent of body weight after three years of treatment. People treated by diet and exercise alone typically maintain a loss of only about 3 percent of initial weight after three years.

So, don't make the mistake of thinking that MERIDIA isn't working because your weight loss has slowed or even stopped. The medication may be working to help you keep the weight off.

Continue taking your medication every morning as you have for the past five months, unless your doctor has advised you otherwise.

Long-Term Use

People frequently ask how long they should take MERIDIA if it is helping to maintain their weight loss. Discuss this question with your doctor. Together you can decide what is right for you. Some experts feel that, with appropriate persons, weight loss medications can be used long-term, in the same manner as medications to treat hypertension and other medical conditions. Overweight, for many people, is a serious and chronic problem. If a weight loss medication is safe and helps to reduce excess weight and its associated health complications, it may be worth considering long-term use and discussing the issue with your doctor. However, the safety and efficacy of MERIDIA as demonstrated in double-blind, placebo-controlled trials has not been determined beyond one year.

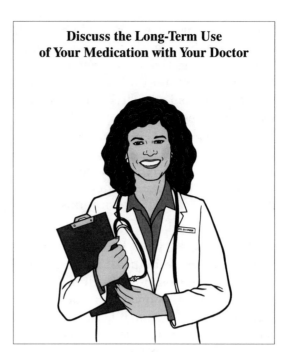

Discuss the Long-Term Use of Your Medication with Your Doctor

Some people may think it is a sign of weakness to take medication to control weight. This view assumes that overweight results from lack of will power or caring. A little more self-control is all that's needed. Nothing could be further from the truth in our view, and we hope yours. Overweight can be a serious problem that deserves serious treatment, including the option of medication. People who take medications long-term to control diabetes, high cholesterol, or migraine headaches aren't made to feel guilty about it. You should not have to feel guilty about taking weight loss medication.

More Facts about Vitamins

Do you take vitamins? Chances are the answer is yes. Do you need the vitamins you take? Chances are the answer is no. Pretty bold statement, right?

The amount of money made on vitamins is unbelievable. The amount of fraud and exploitation is intolerable. An example from our own experience shows this. One of us once stopped in a health food store hoping to find some fruit. Upon entering, the owner was prescribing an assortment of vitamins to a woman who had arthritis and heart disease. She seemed to have little money but was willing to risk it on the hope the fellow might be right. What he told her was not only false, but could have harmed her because he was prescribing high doses of fat soluble vitamins.

When asked why he thought this would help the woman, his response was "prove that it doesn't." He felt no burden to show that his advice was safe and effective. He then asked if I (Dr. Brownell) had cancer, diabetes, poor vision, or impotence (!) and pointed to shelves of vitamins that looked like alphabet soup.

This fellow was in his own small business, but similar hoaxes occur nationwide in chain stores. Many malls, shopping centers, and downtown shopping districts have such stores that seem official because of their fancy displays, nice signs, and wholesome appearance. Yet, they sell vitamins and other products most people don't need.

Perhaps some straightforward talk about vitamins will help clarify this confusing situation. Before we tell you what vitamins are and what they do, let us state our beliefs about vitamins and weight loss, a belief shared by every nutrition expert we have consulted:

THERE IS NO EVIDENCE THAT ANY VITAMIN OR COMBINATION OF VITAMINS HELPS PEOPLE LOSE WEIGHT

To review from Lesson 10, vitamins are required for the transformation of energy in the body and for the regulation of metabolism. They do not produce energy themselves, but are crucial to the body's energy process. Some vitamins are needed to form important enzymes and others acts as catalysts (they speed chemical reactions).

There are two main types of vitamins: fat soluble and water soluble. The fat soluble vitamins are vitamins A, D, E, and K. They are absorbed in fat tissue and are not excreted by the body if you take too much. They can be toxic.

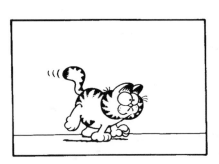
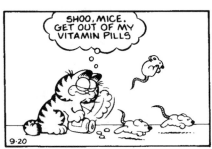
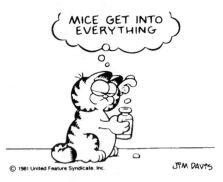

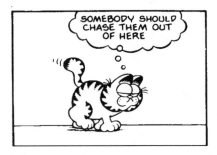
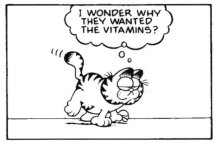
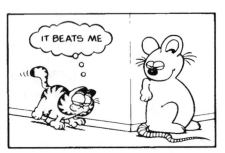

The water soluble vitamins are vitamin C and the B-complex vitamins which include thiamin, riboflavin, and niacin. These are absorbed in the body's water. Excess amounts can usually be excreted through the urine, so taking more than your body needs is wasting money because the vitamins simply pass through.

More information on specific vitamins is given throughout this manual. This includes the functions of each vitamin, their sources in foods, and facts about vitamins and health.

Nutrition experts feel, as a general rule, that most people in developed countries, particularly the U.S., receive adequate vitamins if they eat a balanced diet. Most people need no vitamin supplement at all, much less the mega-doses prescribed by someone with unproven ideas.

Since you are exercising and eating less, taking a multiple vitamin each day will probably not hurt and may help remedy any deficiency created by the change in food intake. But again, if you are careful with the foods you choose, this may not be necessary.

Setting Personal Goals

Make 30 copies of the Monitoring Form for this lesson. Remember, this lesson covers four weeks. At the end of the four weeks, review your Monitoring Forms carefully. Did reviewing these Monitoring Forms reveal any areas that you would like to focus on in the coming month? Perhaps you could record your medication use if you forgot to take your capsules several times last month. Or do you want to concentrate on your eating habits? Increasing your consumption of fruits or fresh vegetables may be a good idea.

We suggest that you pick goals for each of the next four weeks. Write these goals in the section on the Monitoring Form "Personal Goals This Week." Keep a record and find ways to reward yourself when you meet your goals. In addition, plan to weigh yourself and to review your progress *each week* for the next month, before reading Lesson 19. Record your progress each week on the Weight Change Record on page 216. It is perfectly fine to make a copy of this chart for your own personal use. Most people find that it helps to develop a routine for checking on their weight-management skills. Pick a day and time each week that you can devote 15 minutes to reviewing your progress and planning corrective actions for the next week if indicated. If you like, ask a friend or family member to talk with you about your progress. This can be an important motivator and will help you realize what a great job you are doing of taking care of yourself. Congratulations!

Self-Assessment Questionnaire

Lesson 18

T F *86.* It is essential that you continue to record your food intake and physical activity every day—there are no exceptions to this rule.

T F *87.* Weight loss generally slows after the first four to five months of any program, once people have lost approximately 10 percent of their initial weight.

T F *88.* Weight loss medications lose their potency after the first several months. This is evident from the slower rate of weight loss after months four or five.

T F *89.* Fat soluble vitamins give you energy, but water soluble vitamins do not.

(Answers in appendix C)

Monitoring Form—Lesson 18

Today's Date:

Time	Food and Amount	Calories
	Total Daily Calories	

Personal Goals This Week	*Always*	*Sometimes*	*Never*
1.			
2.			
3. Keep Monitoring Forms			
4. Take time to plan weight-management skills			
5. Complete Weight Change Record			
6. Eat less than ___ calories each day			

Medication Taken Today ❑ Yes ❑ No	*Physical Activity*	*Minutes*
Milk, yogurt, and cheese ❑ ❑ ❑		
Meat, poultry, etc. ❑ ❑ ❑		
Fruits ❑ ❑ ❑ ❑		
Vegetables ❑ ❑ ❑ ❑ ❑		
Breads, cereals, etc. ❑ ❑ ❑ ❑ ❑ ❑ ❑ ❑ ❑		

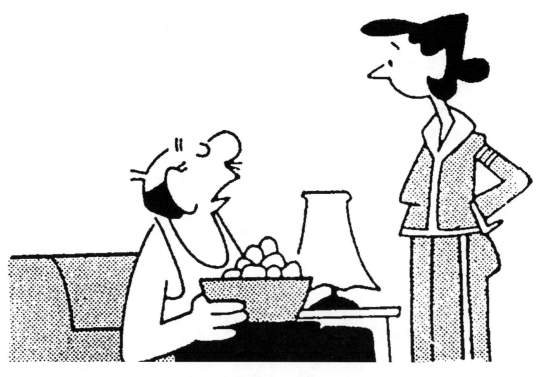

"Stop nagging me about exercise. For your information, opening a bag of chips involves more than 25 different muscles!"

Lesson 19

In this lesson we will take the issue of physical activity to a new level and will discuss jogging and cycling. Remember, you don't have to do anything this strenuous to benefit from activity, but if you fancy yourself doing these things, we'll give you some information on how to proceed. We will also discuss stress and eating, alcohol and weight control, and the role of fiber in a healthy eating plan.

Let's Consider Jogging and Cycling

What a change there has been in society's attitude about exercise, particularly running. As recently as the early 1970s, the longest race in most track meets was two miles, and most people had trouble believing that kooks actually raced for six miles in cross country meets.

Jogging and Running

Now it seems routine for people to brag about doing their 3, 5, 10, or even more miles. The number of people who proclaim themselves runners is staggering. There are running magazines, running clubs, and even running software packages for computers. It is tempting to poke fun at this hysteria and to pass it off as a fad. That would, in our opinion, be a mistake.

Before we discuss running in more detail, let us emphasize again the virtues of brisk walking. Running is fine, but for people who still have many pounds to lose, brisk walking is easier and brings nearly all the benefits. This section is designed to show that running can be helpful to some people, but walking is a fine alternative.

The benefits of running are indisputable. Many positive physical changes occur, as discussed in Lesson 3. However, the psychological advantages are often overlooked. We are not talking about the widely touted runner's high, but about a general sense of accomplishment, self-confidence, well-being, and good feelings.

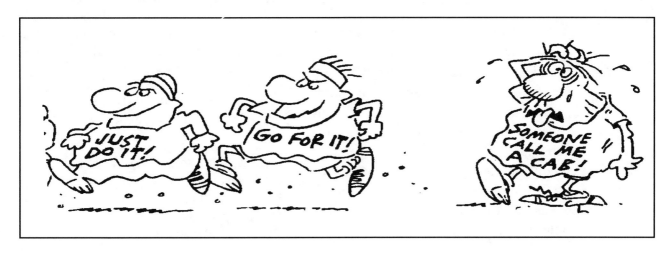

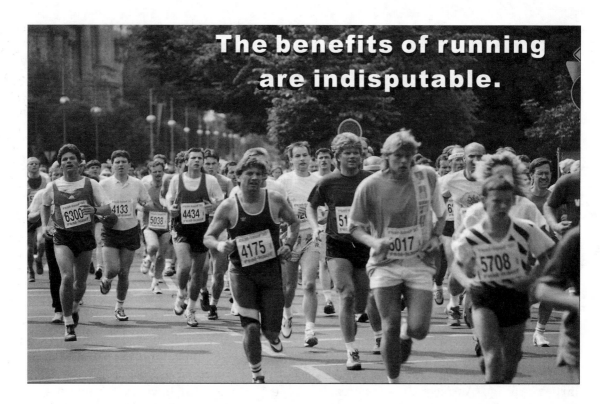

The benefits of running are indisputable.

This psychological advantage may come from running itself, or may simply result from the mastery of something new. At a sports medicine conference one of us (Dr. Brownell) attended in The Netherlands, where I lectured on the psychological benefits of exercise, Dr. John Garrow, an outstanding researcher from England, asked me a telling question. He asked if people would get the same positive effects from something unrelated to exercise, such as learning to play the cello.

Dr. Garrow was questioning whether something inherent to the exercise would be beneficial or whether the effects were due to the excitement of improving at any activity. This is a difficult question to answer. From a practical standpoint, exercise is a good means for producing this mastery because it carries physical benefits as well. After all, it burns more calories than playing the cello!

Cycling

Cycling has the advantages of running, and for some people is more enjoyable. Riding a stationary bicycle indoors or a traditional bike outdoors is good exercise. It spares the knees, ankles, and feet from the pounding they take when running, and is nice for heavy people because weight is supported by the bike. It is an excellent method for burning calories.

If cycling outdoors is feasible for you, give it a try. Cycling to work is terrific when possible. If not, consider buying a stationary bicycle for your home. We each have one and like to alternate between running, cycling, and playing tennis. The cycling is nice in bad weather, and you can do it while watching the news or listening to music.

Running and cycling are not the only exercises, but they are good ones. These activities (along with walking and swimming) are top choices among our clients, so please give them a try. If you are do-

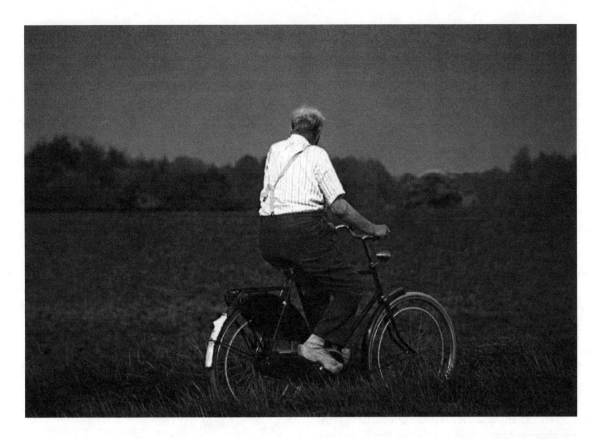

ing something else regularly, stick with it. If you are sporadic in your habits or have not tried anything seriously, consider lacing up the shoes to hit the road or hopping on a bike to sail down the street.

Facts, Fantasies, and Fiber

Over the years, many parents have implored their children to eat more roughage. This basically good advice was about the only attention fiber received until the 1970s, when there was an explosion of interest in the topic. Books and magazines carried fiber diets, and sales of bran cereals increased dramatically. Other high-fiber foods also appeared in the stores. Is this a positive development or is the fiber craze destined to pass with other food fads?

Dietary fiber comes primarily from the tough cell walls of plants. These ma-

terials include cellulose, hemicellulose, lignin, and pectin (which is used by home canners to turn fruit juice to jelly). Fiber is not broken down by digestion like other foods and basically retains its structure during its transit through the digestive system. The strand-like quality of fiber maintains its rigid structure.

Fiber absorbs water during the digestive process. This moisture helps with movement of waste products through the bowel. A brief lesson on digestion should clarify this process.

When you chew and swallow food, both the chewing and saliva begin to break food down into smaller nutrients. Stomach acid continues the process as food moves along, then more digestion continues in the small intestine. Toward the end of the line, waste products combine with water in the large intestine and are eliminated as stools. A stool with much water is larger and softer and moves through the colon more easily. A

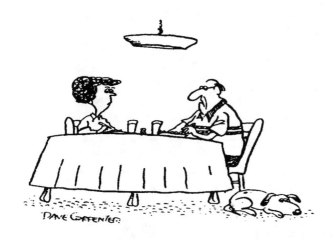

"High fiber, no salt, low cholesterol. No wonder the dog doesn't beg anymore."

verticulitis. This occurs when a bubble or mucous membrane pushes out from inside the intestine. The diet of these Africans averages 25 grams of fiber per day, compared to 6 grams per day for the typical American. Cancer of the colon follows a similar pattern—it occurs rarely in rural Africa and often in industrialized countries. Furthermore, rates for these diseases have increased in the U.S. during this century, during which time fiber intake has decreased dramatically (due to the fiber being refined out of foods and to less reliance on fruits and vegetables).

stool with little moisture is small and hard and creates the discomfort of constipation.

Much of the desirable moisture that facilitates movement of the stools comes from fiber. This is why increased fiber is prescribed for people with problems in the gastrointestinal tract such as diverticulitis, irritable bowel syndrome, and constipation. Some experts claim that fiber also reduces the risk of serious diseases like atherosclerosis and cancer of the colon.

The study of fiber and health gained momentum with the discovery that Africans living in rural settings rarely get di-

Of course, fiber in the diet is only one of many factors which distinguish the rural Africans from us. One such factor is fat in the diet, which has also been linked to disease. There are dozens of nondietary factors (stress, etc.) that might be involved. What does this mean for our diet?

With the current state of science, it is not possible to say that increased fiber in the diet protects against disease, but there are strong hints in this direction. The comparisons between rural and industrialized cultures have now been joined by laboratory studies, so that government agencies like the National Cancer Institute advocate increased fiber in the diet.

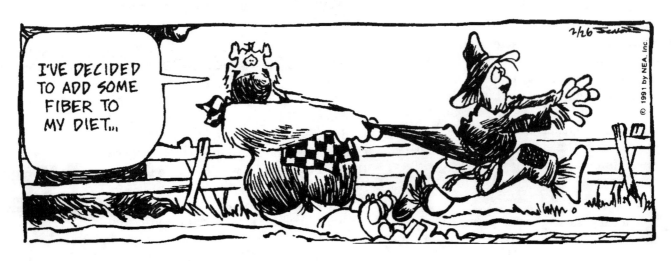

High Fiber Fruits, Vegetables, and Cereals

Fruits

Apples*	Cherries	Oranges	Pineapple
Apricots*	Dried fruit	Peaches*	Plums*
Bananas	Figs	Pears*	Prunes
Berries	Grapefruit		

*with peel

Vegetables

Asparagus	Corn	Mushrooms	Rhubarb
Beans	Eggplant	Okra	Sauerkraut
Broccoli	Endive	Onions	Spinach
Brussel sprouts	Green beans	Parsnips	Squash
Cabbage	Greens, all	Peas	Tomatoes
Carrots	Lettuce	Potatoes	Turnips
Cauliflower	Lima beans	Radishes	Watercress
Celery			

Cereals and Grains

Brans	Oatmeal	Shredded wheat
Brown rice	Puffed wheat	Whole wheat cereal

The average American should increase the fiber in his or her diet. Fiber comes from fruits, vegetables, and cereals. The chart here shows high-fiber foods. The government has not yet established strict guidelines for daily intake of fiber. Most nutritionists suggest that a healthy goal is to aim for an average intake of 25 to 35 grams of fiber each day. Try to increase the number of these foods in your diet. They may help control your appetite, because they do add bulk. They may also have health benefits.

Warning: Alcohol and Calories

As you will see from the table provided on the next page, alcohol is packed with calories. A can of light beer will have 100 calories; the tab for regular beer is 150 calories, about the same as a can of Coke or Pepsi. Mixed drinks and cordials are higher yet. Think of a daiquiri with more than 200 calories and a pina colada over 250.

Some people can have a pretty successful time with weight loss simply by eliminating or greatly reducing their alcohol intake. Many just decide the pleasure they derive from the drinks does not justify all the calories. Remember that you get plenty of calories and no nutrition with alcohol, so if you use up part of your day's allotment of calories with drinks, there will not be much room in the remaining calories to pack in the nutrients you need for healthy living. If the drinks are important to you, use the skills you are learning to help keep the amount under control. Pour small amounts, taste every bit (calories should be tasted, not wasted), be certain to drink only things that are special to you, and don't drink out of habit and continue taking in calories just because you have done so in the past.

Calorie Costs of Alcohol

Beverage	Serving Size (oz)	Calories
Beer or ale	12	140–160
Beer, light	12	100
Bloody Mary	5	116
Bourbon & soda	4	105
Brandy or cognac	1	65–80
Champagne	4	90
Coffee-flavored creme liqueur	1.5	154
Cold Duck	4	120
Cordials and liqueurs, 34 to 72 proof	1	102–125
Creme de Menthe	1.5	186
Daiquiri—with lime	4	222
Distilled spirits:		
Gin, vodka, rum, whiskey; 80 to 100 proof	1.5	95–124
Gin and tonic	7.5	171
Manhattan	2	128
Martini	2.5	156
Pina colada (canned)	4.5	346
Screwdriver	7	174
Sherry	3	125
Tequila sunrise	5.5	89
Tom collins	7.5	121
Vermouth, dry	1	32
Vermouth, sweet	1	45
Wine, dry white	4	79
Wine, red	4	85
Wine, dessert (sweet)	4	181
Wine, light	4	52
Wine, nonalcoholic	6	60
Wine cooler	12	220

Note: The calorie values here are approximations only and may vary depending on a drink's proof, specific sweetness, age, and amount of ice used.

Watch out for all those calories in alcohol

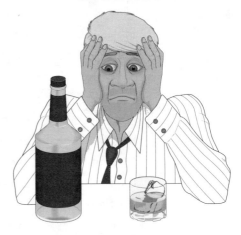

One other factor to be alert for is the "disinhibiting" effect of alcohol. Alcohol releases inhibitions in some people, and they do things they might not do when not drinking. You are working to inhibit your calorie intake, and drinking may make you vulnerable to the "what the heck" phenomenon in which you relax your guard and eat more than you might like.

Stress and Eating

A very interesting (and unexplained) paradox is that stress makes some people eat more and some people eat less. Scientists are working to understand this, but one thing is clear—stress is often cited as a major issue for people who wish to lose weight.

When we discuss the complexity of weight loss with clients in our clinics, the issue of stress arises repeatedly. Some people point to a specific stressful event

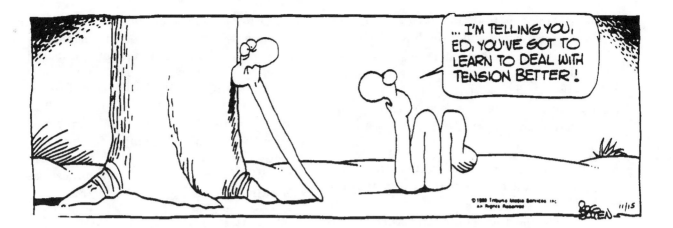

to explain why they gained weight in the first place. Others say that stress makes them want to eat all the time, so they nibble. Still others feel that stress threatens their ability to maintain weight loss and puts them at risk for relapse.

It is no surprise that stress exerts such an important effect on eating. There are clear links between stress and health. Health problems ranging from the common cold to chronic diseases like heart disease, diabetes, and asthma are thought to be affected by stress. It is reasonable to believe that reducing stress would make many people happier and healthier, and that control over eating and weight would be facilitated in the process.

Do you feel that stress influences your eating? Here are some questions to ask yourself:

❶ When you feel pressure to accomplish something, do you feel pulled toward food or pushed away from it?

❷ If you were sitting at a desk working on a project that had to be done quickly, would you want to be eating something?

❸ Do you believe food is something you use to feel better when you are stressed?

❹ Does stress make you eat more?

If you answered "yes" to any of these questions, stress and eating might be linked in important ways. The question then, is what to do about it?

There are two solutions. One is to respond to stress with activities other than eating. Lesson 22 discusses means for developing alternative activities. With a list of such alternatives, you can use the urge to eat as a signal to engage in another activity. Hence, the same stimulus (stress) might exist, but you would not react by eating.

A second solution is to reduce stress. This is an appealing possibility, because stress reduction might affect not only your eating but other areas of your life as well. It may be helpful, therefore, to learn stress management techniques. It would take another book the size of this to provide a complete stress management program, but we can provide a few details about stress and then refer you to materials or programs for more detailed information.

Stress is a fascinating interplay between body, mind, and environment. We each respond to situations in our environment in a unique way. Events that disturb one person mean nothing to another. Some people respond to stress with a racing heart and anger, while others respond with nausea and fear. What is certain is that the ways we think and act are key factors in how we handle stress. Therefore, there are a number of things a person can do to better manage stress. These are skills that you can learn, much as you are learning weight management skills in this program.

We will provide two examples here. The first is the use of relaxation training. Good stress management programs teach specific relaxation skills, so that when stress begins, a person has the ability to halt the process by countering a stress response with relaxation responses. Learning relaxation skills can be very helpful, and can help an individual calm down before an undesirable action occurs (like overeating).

The second example deals with what scientists have called *appraisal*. When an event occurs in our lives, we appraise the situation and then respond. The appraisal determines the response. One person who receives a negative evaluation from a boss might have a negative appraisal, suffer a blow to self-esteem, and feel depressed. Another might blame the boss, get angry, and strike back in some self-defeating way, while yet another might make a more positive appraisal and think of ways to improve work performance. The way we perceive and interpret events is crucial.

Both relaxation training and modifying the appraisal process are part of most stress management programs. So, how do you find one? One possibility is to seek out stress management seminars or training programs. Local hospitals, YMCA's and YWCA's, colleges, and some corporate settings offer stress management programs. Some individuals find they need a formal program in a professional setting, so asking for leads from health professionals you know should be helpful.

Other people do not need a formal program and can use written materials in a very positive way. An excellent guide is a step-by-step manual by Drs. David Barlow and Ronald Rapee entitled *Mastering Stress: A Lifestyle Approach*. The book is published by the American Health Publishing Company (the company that publishes *The Learn Program for Weight Control*). Information can be obtained by calling 1-800-736-7323 or by contacting The LEARN Education Center at the address provided toward the end of this manual.

Setting Personal Goals

Consider jogging and cycling as part of your personal goals. On the nutrition front, do your best to limit alcohol, eat a lot of fiber, and continue to eat the recommended number of servings of fruit from the Food Guide Pyramid. Try to become more aware of your stress level. How do you think stress and eating are related in your life? In addition, think about goals you can set based on your experience thus far in the program. Which behavior or attitude changes are most important for you? Remember that our focus is not just on setting goals, but on setting personal goals.

As a final note, be sure to make 30 copies of the Monitoring Form for this lesson. These forms will be for weeks 25–28 in your program. Be sure to continue to record your weight changes on the Weight Change Record on page 216. Good luck with your next four weeks!

Self-Assessment
Questionnaire

Lesson 19

T F *90.* There are many benefits to jogging and cycling. They are good forms of exercise for people trying to lose weight.

T F *91.* A diet high in fiber may help protect against certain diseases.

T F *92.* A healthy diet should contain between 25 and 35 grams of fiber each day.

T F *93.* Alcohol is not usually a problem for weight control because it has a number of nutrients.

(Answers in Appendix C)

Monitoring Form—Lesson 19

Today's Date:

Time	Food and Amount	Calories
Total Daily Calories		

Personal Goals This Week	*Always*	*Sometimes*	*Never*
1.			
2.			
3. Try jogging or cycling			
4. Monitor daily levels of stress			
5. My diet has _____ grams of fiber			
6. Eat less than _____ calories each day			

Medication Taken Today ❑ Yes ❑ No	*Physical Activity*	*Minutes*
Milk, yogurt, and cheese ❑ ❑ ❑		
Meat, poultry, etc. ❑ ❑ ❑		
Fruits ❑ ❑ ❑ ❑		
Vegetables ❑ ❑ ❑ ❑ ❑		
Breads, cereals, etc. ❑ ❑ ❑ ❑ ❑ ❑ ❑ ❑ ❑		

Lesson 20

If you are using the LEARN lessons on a monthly basis, you should be starting about month seven of your program (or week 29). As you know best, seven months is a long time, and is much longer than most people can stay with weight-loss programs. For this you deserve a big HOORAY! We know how much effort it takes. Since the benefits can be lifelong, and in fact may extend your life, we are really happy for you.

We begin this lesson with a discussion of lifestyle tips to help with eating away from home. We will discuss aerobics and then will cover ways to bring more pleasure to a program partnership. We will also consider fat soluble vitamins.

Eating Away from Home

Trips to restaurants can be a mine field of temptation. The best intentions can crumble when you are enjoying yourself with people who feast on delicious foods. Two aspects of this concern us. The first is how much we eat, but there are methods for keeping eating under control. The second is to control our response to the event.

One trip to a restaurant never torpedoed any weight-control program with its calories alone. An extraordinary meal of 5000 calories could bring only a pound and a half of weight. The *response* to those calories, however, could lead to

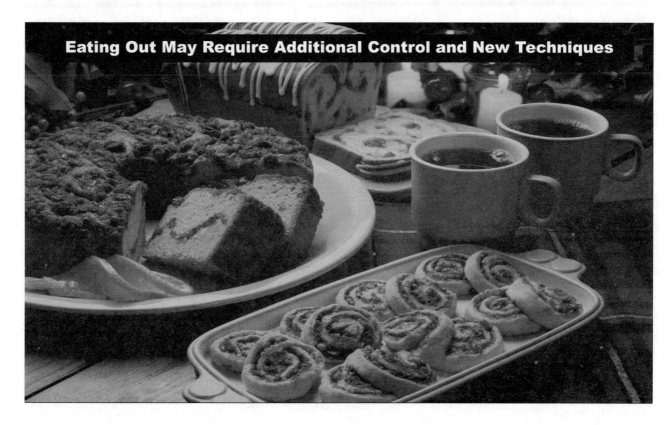

Eating Out May Require Additional Control and New Techniques

trouble. Your attitudes during and after these events are as important as what you eat.

Eating at Restaurants

It is hard to be virtuous at restaurants. This is a real problem for people in business or those whose lifestyle includes eating away from home. What should you do when dessert comes with the meal?

What about a waitress who pours 14 gallons of dressing on your salad? How do you deal with a hot loaf of bread the waiter delivers before the meal even begins? How can you refuse when the dessert cart rolls up like a Brink's truck ready to unload its treasures?

Order à la carte meals. You may be inclined to order full meals because the cost is less than for the sum of its parts. This group plan is a booby trap because you order more than you need simply because the price seems attractive. However, the logic is faulty.

The regular price for a roast beef sandwich might be $5, but for $6 you could get French fries and cole slaw which would normally cost $1 each. The package deal makes sense only if you wanted the other two items anyway. If not, you are saving money you never would have spent. Most of these extras are high-calorie foods like French fries. Order just what you want.

Watch the salad dressing. Since salad dressing is high in fat (oil), eating more than you need really boosts the calories. Ask for salad dressing on the side so you are not at the mercy of a heavy-handed server. Better yet, leave the salad dressing off completely.

If you need dressing, consider bringing your own bottle of low-fat dressing. Many people do this, and unless you're at the White House for an awards banquet, you shouldn't be embarrassed.

Watch for hidden calories. Many foods contain calories that are added in

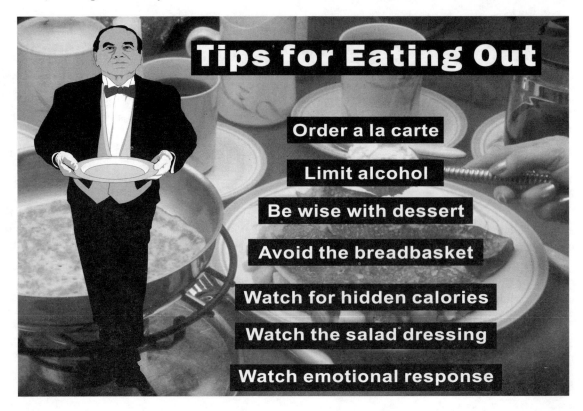

Tips for Eating Out

Order a la carte

Limit alcohol

Be wise with dessert

Avoid the breadbasket

Watch for hidden calories

Watch the salad dressing

Watch emotional response

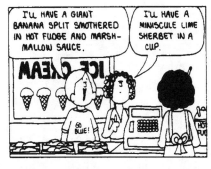
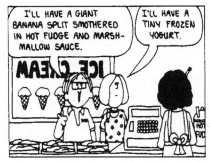
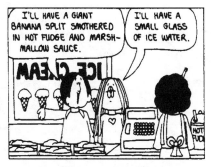
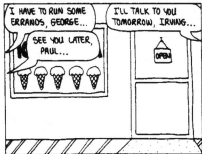
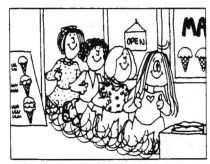
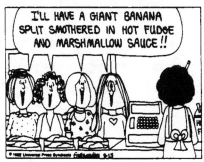

subtle ways. These hidden calories are important to consider. Think about rich sauces added to meats and vegetables in French restaurants, oils added in Italian restaurants, and things breaded and fried in any restaurant. If you cannot guess what is in a dish, ask the waiter or waitress.

Watch alcohol. As we discussed in Lesson 19, alcohol is loaded with calories, and it is easy to consume more than you want in the spirit of being social. This is a real temptation when you sit in the bar area waiting for a table in the restaurant.

When you order alcohol, avoid the hard liquor and sweetened drinks. A jigger of whiskey has 110 calories and a Tom Collins has 180 calories. White wine is a better choice, and better yet is a white wine spritzer. You could also order club soda or tomato juice.

Alcohol generally has *empty* calories. Its sugar brings calories with little or no nutrition. You can estimate the calories in alcohol by remembering that the following drinks have about 100 calories:

- ▶ 12 oz of light beer
- ▶ 8 oz of regular beer
- ▶ 3½ oz of wine
- ▶ 1 shot of liquor

You may want to refer to the chart on page 234 as a reminder of calories in alcohol.

Beware of the breadbasket. Keep an eye out for that wondrous basket. It comes when you are hungry and excited about being at the restaurant. You can refuse the breadbasket, but if one arrives against your will, let it rest across the table. If you are still tempted, imagine there is a mousetrap under the napkin that covers the bread!

There are some people who actually benefit from the breadbasket. They are the ones who use a piece of bread (without butter) to take the edge off their hunger, so that they will eat less higher-calorie foods later in the meal. You might try this approach, but don't use it as an excuse to eat lots of bread and then eat what you would anyway.

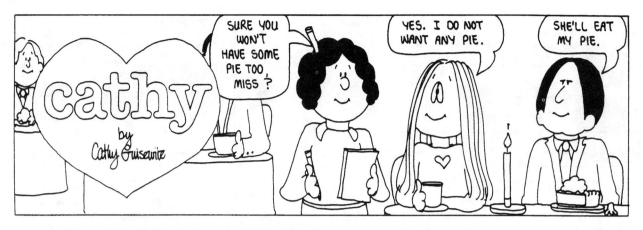

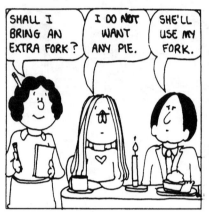

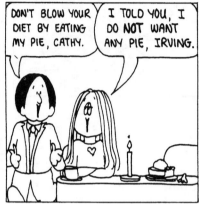

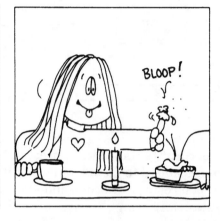

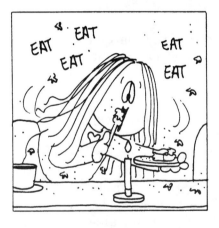

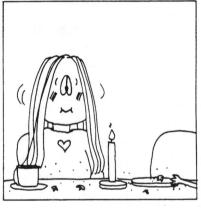

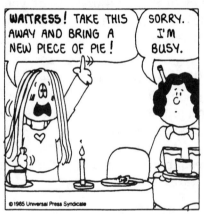

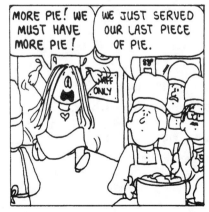

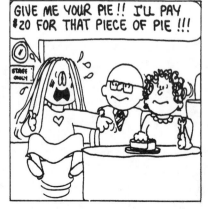

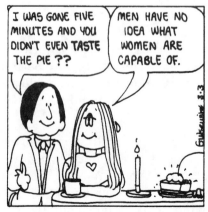

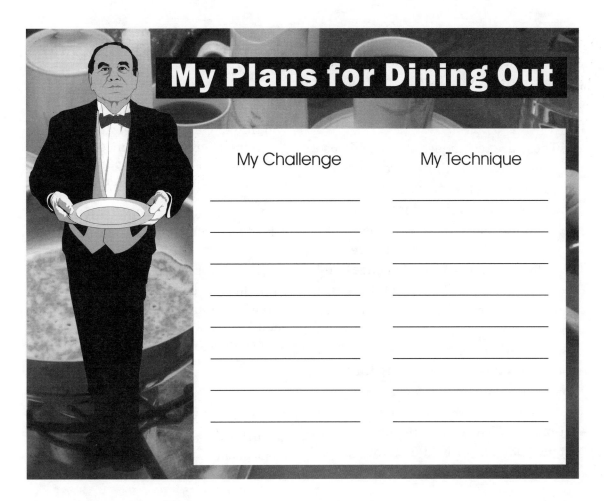

My Plans for Dining Out

My Challenge	My Technique
_____	_____
_____	_____
_____	_____
_____	_____
_____	_____
_____	_____
_____	_____

Bread does *not* have empty calories. It is an important part of your diet—breads and cereals comprise the largest of the five food groups of the Food Guide Pyramid. The purpose of watching the breadbasket is not to cut down on bread, but to avoid eating lots of bread just because it's there.

Be wise with dessert. Do you deserve dessert when you eat out? After all, you don't get special desserts often, so why not enjoy yourself? Ignore this rationalization and get dessert under two conditions:

❶ You are still hungry, or

❷ You have planned it in your day's calories

Think about fresh fruit or gelatin. Both taste good and have far fewer calories than traditional choices.

Engage your partner. Restaurants are a place where your partner can help. This can begin before you arrive for the meal. Some individuals decide with their partners what to order in advance, before their restraint is weakened by the smells and atmosphere of a nice restaurant. Some even have their partner order for them. At the restaurant, the partner can keep the breadbasket in a safe place and can help by not pushing drinks or desserts.

Watch your emotional response. If you eat more than you plan, be careful not to consider it a catastrophe. We have been working to avoid the attitude traps, such as considering some foods *illegal* and setting unrealistic goals of never overeating. If you feel guilty, reread the earlier material, and be prepared to rebound from a bout of overeating by eating less, not more. Do *not* use this as a rationalization to overdo it, but keep these events in perspective and use them as a sign that you can do better the next meal or the next day.

These are techniques that people use to control their eating in restaurants. You may think of others yourself. For example, you might drink extra water to help fill up before the meal comes. We have provided a chart on the previous page for you to list your challenges and techniques that will be helpful for you when dining out. Take a few minutes now to complete the chart. Feel free to make a copy and carry it with you. When you find yourself eating out, take out your chart and review it before going into the restaurant. Also, if you discover additional difficulties, write down techniques that may be helpful in the future. Have fun, but keep control!

Are Aerobics for You?

The answer is probably "No!"—or so you think. We used to feel the same way. We remember when coaches and teachers used calisthenics as punishment or as a way to build character. Push-ups, sit-ups, squat thrusts, and leg lifts ranked somewhere below staying after school on our list of favorite activities.

The situation is much different today. Calisthenics have been replaced with aerobics, slimnastics, Jazzercise®, and the like. This signals not only a change in terminology but a change in the way exercise is viewed. In our opinion, the changes are positive.

When aerobic training became popular, using exercise to build strength took a back seat to improving the condition of the heart. This involves getting the

Aerobics can be done in so many ways that they are suitable for almost everyone.

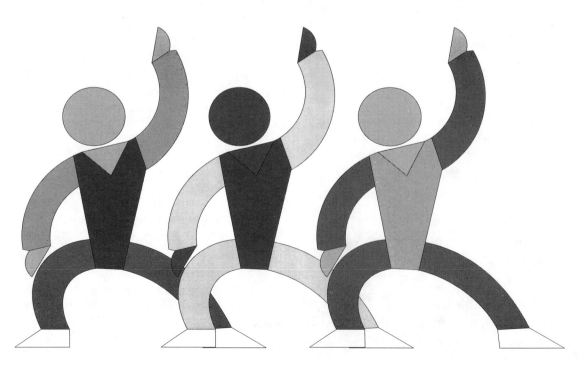

heart rate up and keeping it there. Many different movements can accomplish this, hence the use of dance and other types of movement in aerobics classes. This makes exercise more interesting and more healthy than the calisthenics of old.

Aerobic activities require a large increase in the body's use of oxygen. This is best accomplished by use of large muscle groups, and it involves some form of vigorous and rhythmic movement. Running, cycling, swimming, and rope jumping are examples, but so are dancing to fast music and the other movements you associate with aerobics classes. As we mentioned before, these are the *only* types of exercise that will improve cardiovascular conditioning. They are *not* the only exercises that will help you lose weight, but they are certainly among the best.

Aerobics can be done in so many ways that they are suitable for almost everybody. If you want to do it alone, there are books, TV shows, videotapes, and records. Most of these workout approaches are aerobic in nature. If you would like company, aerobics classes are held at the YMCA, YWCA, exercise centers, and in many companies, churches, and community centers. You can do aerobics at your own pace, even if you are with a group, so don't worry about the shape you're in. There are many excellent books on aerobic exercises. We suggest any of the books by Dr. Kenneth Cooper, which are available in most bookstores. These discuss what to do, how much to do, and how to have fun doing it.

Many people losing weight use more than one form of exercise. This breaks monotony and gives you a chance to do whatever your mood dictates. You might run some days, bicycle other days, and do aerobics on days when a class is scheduled. This allows you to be flexible with your schedule, the weather, and your moods.

Pleasurable Partner Activities

There are many nice things you can do with your partner. These can be used as rewards from you to your partner, from your partner to you, or as a joint bit of pleasure to acknowledge efforts from both of you. The list on the next page gives many possible activities. Some are appropriate for partners in romantic relationships while others are for any partnership.

Share these ideas with your partner and use them for special times. If you are working together as a team, it will be nice to have some fun in addition to the work. Remember that there are many nice partner activities not on the list, so be creative. Add as many ideas to the list as you can.

More about Fat Soluble Vitamins

In Lesson 17 we discussed the water soluble vitamins. In this lesson we will focus on the vitamins that are fat soluble. Vitamins A, D, E, and K are fat soluble. They are stored in fat tissue in the body if consumed in excess. This is why toxic doses are a more important issue with fat soluble than water soluble vitamins. You should be especially wary of people who promote large doses of these four vitamins. As with all vitamins, no more than the Recommended Daily Allowance (RDA) is suggested. Review the chart in Lesson 10 (page 129) for the RDA of all vitamins.

Pleasurable Partner Activities

Take a romantic walk

Go to a concert

Plan a day at the park

Take a nature walk

Send flowers

Pick fresh fruit

Go bowling

Buy a nice wine

Play a new sport

See the city

Send a singing telegram

Plan a mystery weekend

See a movie

Buy cologne or perfume

Get gift certificates

Get a nice plant

Buy a tape or CD

Make Sunday breakfast

Ride bicycles

Go window shopping

Go on a picnic

Get a puppy or a kitten

Send a card

Go to a museum

Get a board game

Buy a new book

Buy a pedometer

Find a fair or festival

Visit a mutual friend

Do your partner's laundry

Write a thank you note

Plan a surprise party

Fix something broken

Balance the checkbook

Watch the sunset

Just sit and enjoy each other

_____   _____

_____   _____

_____   _____

_____   _____

_____   _____

_____   _____

_____   _____

_____   _____

Vitamin A is used for growth of the skin, bones, and teeth and is important in vision. It is found in leafy green vegetables, yellow vegetables, milk, eggs, fortified margarine, liver, and kidney. Vitamin D is crucial for development of bones and teeth, and helps the body use calcium and phosphorus. It is abundant in cod liver oil, and is found in egg yolk, milk, tuna, and salmon.

Vitamin E is useful for the functioning of red blood cells, and helps the body use essential fatty acids. Vitamin E is present in wheat germ, egg yolks, vegetable oils, cereals, and lettuce. Vitamin K is used by the liver in the production of prothrombin. It is found in liver, cabbage, spinach, and kale. The RDA has not yet been established for vitamin K.

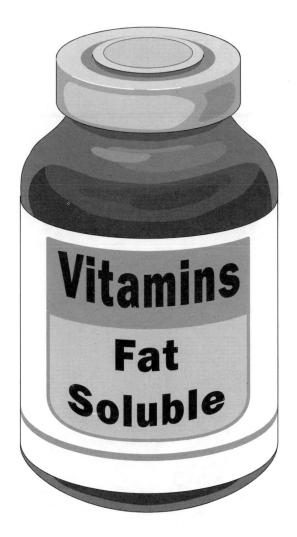

Above all, watch out for bold claims. Taking extra amounts won't do a thing for weight loss and may damage your health.

Setting Personal Goals

We began this lesson with a discussion of techniques for eating away from home. Use these to keep your eating under control. Try aerobic activities as part of your physical fitness routine, and remember all the ways to do aerobic activities: on your own, at the YMCA or YWCA, and at spas, community centers, and places of work. Use the suggestions for partner activities if you are using the partnership approach. Watch to see that you get the vitamins you need, but avoid falling victim to the vitamin hawkers who promise that large doses will cure nearly any ill.

Think also of goals you have carried forward from other lessons. You might believe that keeping the Monitoring Forms, positive thinking, regular walking, or a host of other possibilities are important for you. Find your own personal goals and make these part of your plan.

Self-Assessment Questionnaire

Lesson 20

T F   *94.*   Alcohol can be a problem when eating out because it contains many calories and weakens dietary restraint.

T F   *95.*   Ordering à la carte meals at restaurants helps avoid unwanted calories that come in package meals.

T F   *96.*   Aerobic activities are designed to build strength in the shortest possible time.

T F   *97.*   Vitamin E is associated with virility and may help in the remedy of alcoholism.

(Answers in Appendix C)

Monitoring Form—Lesson 20

Today's Date:

Time	Food and Amount	Calories
	Total Daily Calories	

Personal Goals This Week	Always	Sometimes	Never
1.			
2.			
3.　　Practice techniques for dining out			
4.　　Try aerobic activities			
5.　　Engage in pleasurable partner activities			
6.　　Eat less than _____ calories each day			

Medication Taken Today　❑ Yes　❑ No	Physical Activity	Minutes
Milk, yogurt, and cheese　❑ ❑ ❑		
Meat, poultry, etc.　❑ ❑ ❑		
Fruits　❑ ❑ ❑ ❑		
Vegetables　❑ ❑ ❑ ❑ ❑		
Breads, cereals, etc.　❑ ❑ ❑ ❑ ❑ ❑ ❑ ❑ ❑ ❑		

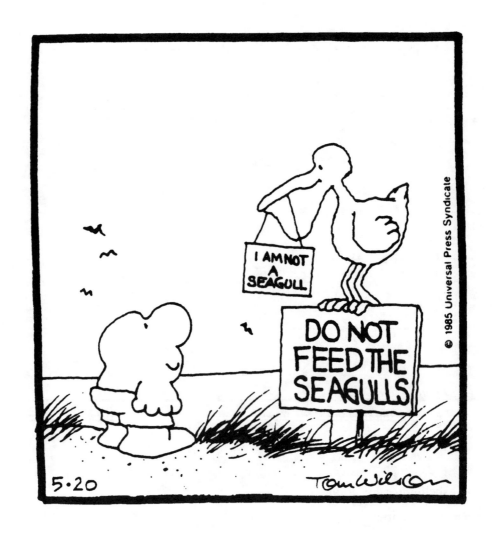

Lesson 21

We have poured through mountains of information over the past 32 weeks together. It is time to integrate this into a practical approach you can use permanently. To do this, we will introduce you to "the Behavior Chain." This gives you a system for deciding which of many techniques to use in a given situation. We will also take a closer look at poultry and fast foods. And if you have been a faithful recorder of your weight change over the past 32 weeks, the Weight Change Record we provided in Lesson 17 should be filled. At the end of this lesson, we provide a new form that will take you into the future. So, if you're ready, let's get started.

Bringing it All Together: The Behavior Chain

We need to organize the information in this program into a logical picture. We have covered ways to identify problem situations, along with techniques (more than 70 by now) to help you control eating and increase exercise. We are still left with an important challenge.

What each person needs is a mental card file or computer database to summon the right technique at the right time in a given situation. For example, if playing a card game (let's say bridge) with your friends is a high-risk situation,

you could look in your file under "Playing Bridge" for a list of techniques. The card in your file would list different aspects of this situation that would determine its degree of risk. These aspects might be who the friends are, whether they serve food, how hungry you are, how well your program has been going, and so forth. Then when a situation arises, perhaps the arrival of potato chips and dip, your card would list several responses.

The Behavior Chain is the path to this process. It is a method for breaking eating episodes into discrete parts. When you examine each part, ideas emerge for stopping eating in its tracks. The ideas that follow can truly increase your understanding of eating.

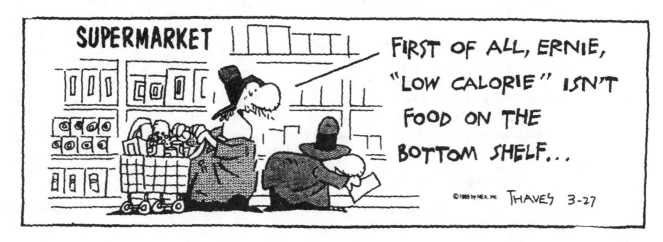

SUPERMARKET

FIRST OF ALL, ERNIE, "LOW CALORIE" ISN'T FOOD ON THE BOTTOM SHELF...

© 1985 by NEA, Inc. THAVES 3-27

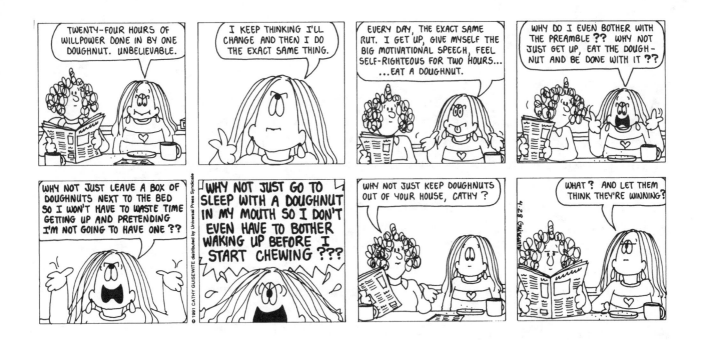

A Chain and its Links

We can view eating as a chain of events that contains many links. The links string together like an ordinary chain. We can use a familiar phrase: *A chain is only as strong as its weakest link.* The good news is that you want to break this chain, so attacking at the weakest link is ideal.

If we return to the example of playing bridge with friends, eating the potato chips resides at the end of a long chain. Preceding it were links like having the chips available, going to the card game hungry, having friends offer the food, and so forth. The chain could be broken at any of these points.

Each act of eating can be viewed with the chain in mind. Once you identify the links in your chain, you can spot the best link to break and how to break it. The more links you break, and the earlier in the chain you break them, the easier it will be to control eating.

A Sample Behavior Chain

Let's illustrate the chain concept with the example of Laura. In her chain,

Laura ate 10 cookies, felt guilty, and then ate even more. Laura's eating occurred in a chain which included many links before the eating and several links after the eating. We could help Laura control her cookie intake by analyzing this chain. Remember that this is an example to illustrate the *principle* of a chain. Think about how this concept applies to your situation.

Laura's chain began when she bought the cookies. She was home on Saturday afternoon and was tired and bored. She got the urge to eat and then ate the 10 cookies while watching TV. She felt guilty and ate more cookies later. We can find 12 links in Laura's chain. These are shown in the figure displayed on page 253.

These are the twelve steps to Laura's dilemma. It started when (1) Laura bought the cookies. She then (2) left the cookies on the counter where they were plainly visible. She was (3) home on Saturday afternoon, which she knows from experience is a high-risk time and place for overeating.

Sample Behavior Chain

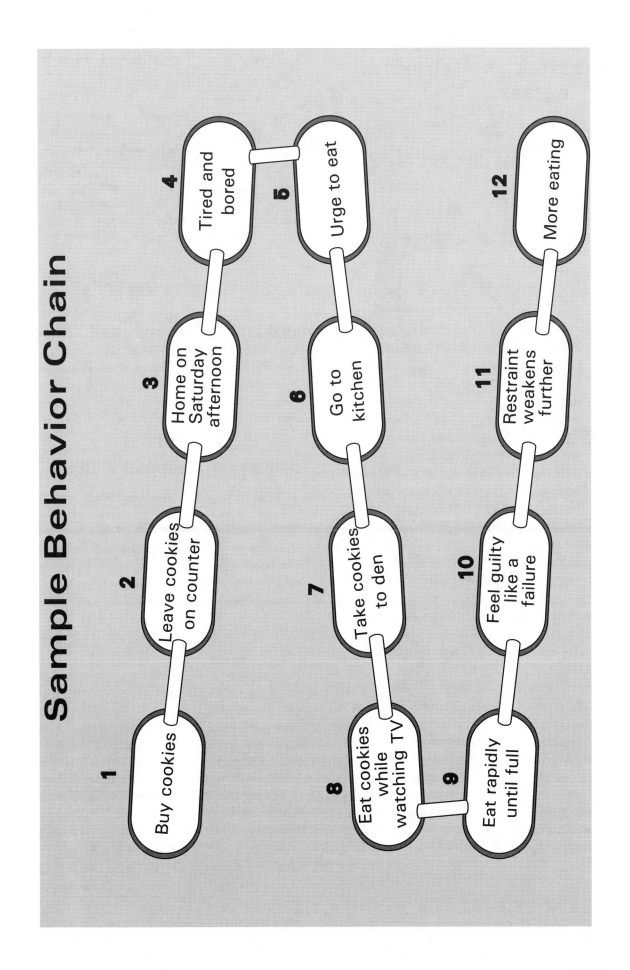

1 Buy cookies

2 Leave cookies on counter

3 Home on Saturday afternoon

4 Tired and bored

5 Urge to eat

6 Go to kitchen

7 Take cookies to den

8 Eat cookies while watching TV

9 Eat rapidly until full

10 Feel guilty like a failure

11 Restraint weakens further

12 More eating

You can break the chain at the weakest link.

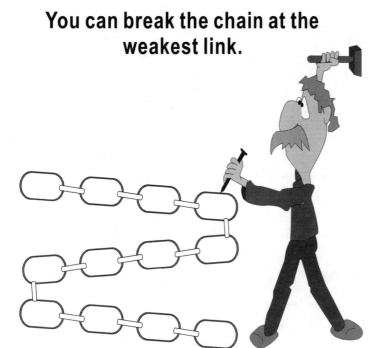

She was (4) tired and bored. She (5) felt an urge to eat and (6) went to the kitchen. She (7) took the cookies to the den and (8) ate them while watching TV. She (9) ate rapidly until she felt full, then (10) felt guilty and like a failure. This (11) weakened her restraint further until (12) she ate even more cookies.

Is Laura an innocent victim of an inevitable chain, or can she do something to interrupt it at a critical point? As you probably guessed, Laura has many options for interrupting the chain. Before we discuss these, think of your own lifestyle and the eating habits you have. How do they exist as chains, and what are the links in the chains?

Take some time now to draw a picture of an eating chain that applies to you. Use the blank chain provided on page 256 to fill in the details. You can use Laura's chain as an example, but make the situation specific to you. Pick a high-risk situation that really gives you trouble. Examples might be arriving home from work, watching television in the evening, feeling depressed or lonely, etc.

Your chain can contain fewer links or more than the blank chain permits, but try to include each important detail. You will see how the links are inextricably tied together to form a sequence of events that is hard to stop once it gets started. If you come armed with techniques for dismantling the chain, you will increase your control.

Interrupting the Chain

Your mind was probably buzzing with ideas as we were discussing Laura's eating chain and as you were writing your own chain. We can use Laura's chain for an example of how a chain might be broken. Some of the possible ways Laura might interrupt her chain are shown in the table on the next page.

Analyzing Your Eating Chain

This chain concept could be a key part of your program. If you can analyze your eating according to the chain notion, you can devise many ways to get control. Contrast this with the common approach which relies solely on willpower once the chain is advanced and food beckons.

Now we can go to work on *your* chain. Look at each of the links in the chain and write down at least two ways the chain could be broken at each link. With Laura's chain, we listed 34 ways to break at least one link. Use the information you have learned in the program to think of *link-breaking techniques*. You might refresh your memory on techniques by referring back to the Monitoring Forms from previous weeks.

There are several things to remember when listing these techniques. The first is to concentrate on the weakest links. For instance, if eating ice cream is the final link in your chain, it might be easier

Breaking the Links in
Laura's Behavior Chain

Link	Link-Breaking Techniques
Buy cookies	Shop from a list Shop on a full stomach Shop with a partner Have a partner do your shopping Buy cookie mix (needs baking)
Cookies on counter	Store in opaque container Freeze cookies Store in inaccessible place
Home during high-risk	Go shopping Schedule programmed activity Plan an enjoyable activity
Tired and bored	Exercise Get more sleep
Urge to eat	List of alternatives to eating Wait five minutes; urge may pass Separate hunger from cravings
Go to kitchen	Use alternative activities Get some exercise Leave house Low-calorie foods available
Take cookies to den	Eat in one place
Eat while watching TV	Do nothing else while eating
Eat rapidly until full	Put food down between bites Pause during eating Serve one cookie at a time Stop automatic eating
Feel guilty, like a failure	Watch dichotomous thinking Banish imperatives Set realistic goals Plan adaptive response
Restraint weakens	Resolve to increase control Read LEARN Manual for ideas
More eating	Examine chain, use techniques Watch attitude traps

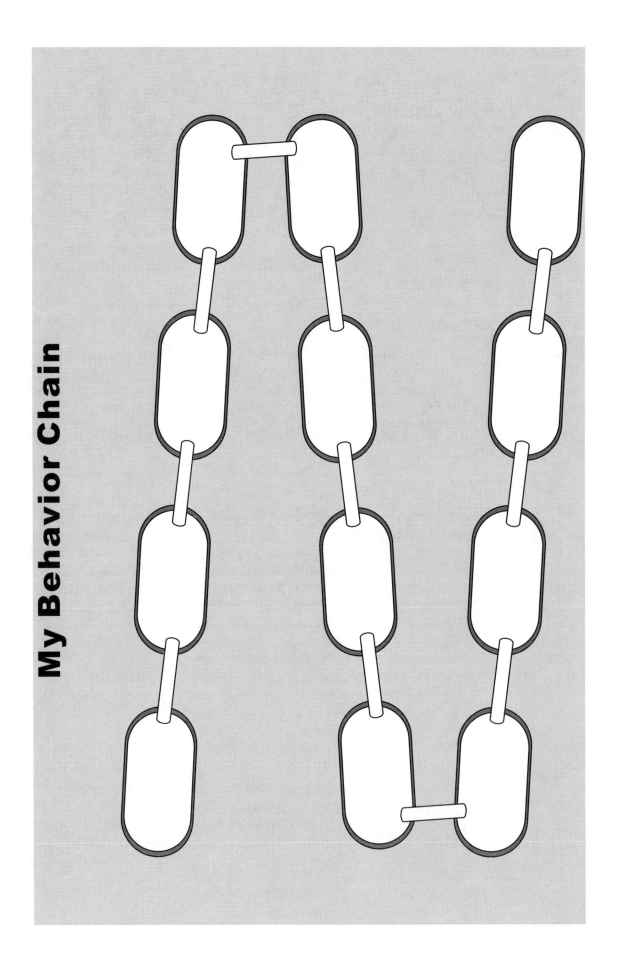

to avoid buying the ice cream initially than to count on willpower when confronted by the food. This leads to the second point, which is to interrupt the chain as early as possible. This does not diminish the importance of interrupting the steps late in the chain, but starting early in the chain gives you more links to work with.

We know what happens when we read things where the author asks us to fill something out. We usually think it's not worth the effort and we read ahead. You may feel that you need not go through this exercise, and you might be correct. Remember, however, that the act of writing these things down will make you think and analyze your high-risk situations like never before.

Using the Stairs

Climbing stairs is a handy way to increase your exercise. It is an ideal way to work extra activity into your lifestyle. It is an efficient way of burning calories. As you may know, climbing stairs burns more calories per minute than almost any activity. Its major virtue, however, is its ready availability. Most of us have several opportunities each day to use stairs. Stairs may be in our home, at work, and in stores. Let's see if we can exploit this opportunity.

People are willing to increase their use of stairs, but rarely think of it. This was shown in a study we did with several colleagues at the University of Pennsylvania. We had observers measure the use of stairs in three public places where stairs and escalators were adjacent: a shopping mall in Philadelphia called the Gallery, a commuter train station, and a bus terminal. Our observers patiently recorded whether 40,000 people used the stairs or escalators.

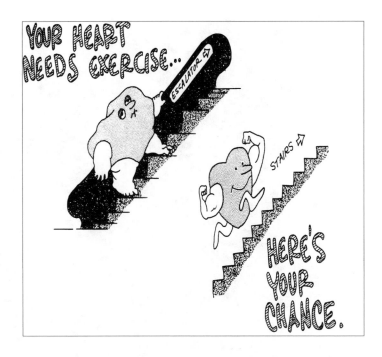

The results were quite informative. Only 5 percent of people used the stairs. For every five normal-weight people who used the stairs, only one heavy person did, which meant that only 1 percent of heavy people used the stairs. People would avoid the stairs even when they had to wait in a crowd to go up the escalator.

We then stationed a sign encouraging people to use the stairs at the base of the stairs and escalators. The sign carried the figure shown here and was designed for us by Tony Auth, the Pulitzer Prize winning political cartoonist of the *Philadelphia Inquirer*. The sign made a big impact. It nearly tripled the number of people using the stairs, and increased the number of overweight people using the stairs by sevenfold. It appeared that people were willing to use the stairs if reminded to do so.

Here is a bit more encouragement. Studies in England and the U.S. were done to investigate the link between exercise and life span (longevity). People who exercised regularly lived longer than those who were sedentary. The

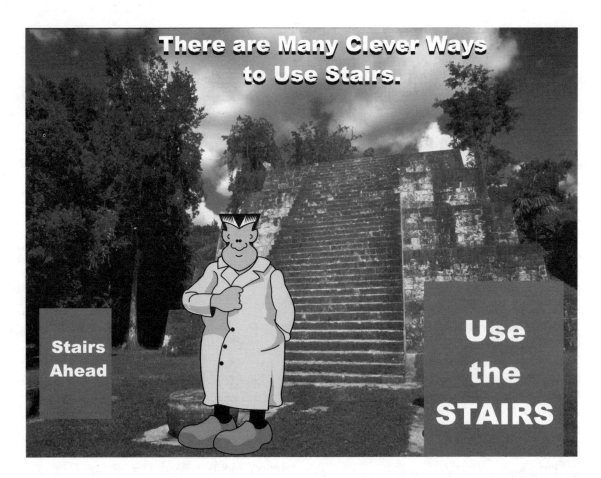

There are Many Clever Ways to Use Stairs.

Stairs Ahead

Use the STAIRS

U.S. study, done by Dr. Ralph Paffenbarger from Stanford University, found that people who climbed only 50 stairs (not flights) or more each day had reduced risk of heart attack.

The value of using the stairs is not well known, but some people are regular stair climbers and are proud of it. Our study with the stairs and escalators was reported in many newspapers because of a wire service article. We received letters from all over the country from people who had been climbing the stairs for years for their exercise program. Some even reported running in a race, which is up the stairs of the Empire State Building! This is way beyond what we have in mind for people losing weight, so let's examine ways to use the stairs sensibly.

There are many clever ways to use stairs. At work, try the bathroom and water cooler on another floor. This will add several trips. Use the stairs at a mall in lieu of an escalator. If you work on the 9th floor of a building, take the elevator part way up and walk the remaining flights. Walk down all the flights. Use the stairs whenever possible at home. Walk to a different floor to make a phone call or to use the bathroom. Whatever you can do will add up.

Poultry: Better than Red Meat?

An article by Bonnie Liebman in the *Nutrition Action Healthletter* provided some interesting facts about poultry. In only 20 years, the intake of chicken in the U.S. has doubled and of turkey has risen by two-thirds. This is a positive development because poultry can be helpful in reducing the intake of saturated fat.

The fact that poultry consumption increased so dramatically was not lost on the beef and pork industries, and difficult though it is to believe, both are attempting to convince the public that their product is like chicken. You may hear ads stating that beef has no more cholesterol than chicken. This is not novel news, because beef is not particularly high in cholesterol. It does, however, have much more saturated fat than chicken, and saturated fat is a worse culprit than dietary cholesterol in raising blood cholesterol. The YGSN (You've Got Some Nerve) award has to go to the campaign by the pork industry to characterize pork as the *other white meat*. This seems a direct attempt to make pork seem like chicken (pork has at least twice the saturated fat of chicken and turkey), and to distance pork from *red meat* (pork has at least as much fat as beef).

Calories and Fat in Poultry

(per 4 oz roasted portion)

Type of Poultry	Calories	Fat (g)
Duck, with skin	384	36.5
Duck, without skin	229	14.5
Goose, with skin	348	28.5
Goose, without skin	271	16.5
Turkey, light, with skin	187	6.0
Turkey, light, without skin	160	1.5
Chicken, light, with skin	253	14.0
Chicken, light, without skin	197	6.0
Chicken, dark, with skin	288	20.5
Chicken, dark, without skin	234	12.5
Ground turkey (3 oz)	191	12.5
Chicken hot dog	116	10.0
Turkey bologna (2 oz)	114	9.0

Note: Figures in table abstracted from Liebman, B. CSPI's Poultry Primer. Nutrition Action Healthletter, November 1986. Their source for calorie and fat information was USDA Handbook #8-5, #8-10, #8-13.

Birds differ in the amount of fat they provide. The leanest poultry is turkey. After poultry is cooked and skinned, chicken has double or triple the fat of turkey, and duck and goose have 50 percent more fat than chicken. The calories and amount of fat in various forms of poultry are in the table here. As Liebman points out in her article, averages can be deceiving, because some cuts of red meat and some parts of poultry can have more or less fat than the average. In general, however, turkey breast without the skin has relatively little fat, and chicken has about half the fat of lean red meats.

When preparing poultry, several factors should be considered. First, removing the skin reduces fat by about 50 percent. Second, fat intake is increased greatly when chicken is battered and fried, because the batter soaks up fat. A fried chicken breast from Kentucky Fried Chicken can have two or three times the fat of a roasted breast (even with the skin on). Finally, think of creative ways to use turkey and chicken in salads with fruits, pasta, and other foods. This can make for some innovative dishes. The cookbooks listed in Lesson 9 provide many ideas for making interesting dishes from these foods.

Fast Food

Fast food restaurants are part of the American landscape. In 1970, there were 30,000 fast food outlets, rising to 140,000 by 1980. In 1995, there were 11,400 McDonald's alone, with three new McDonald's opening every day. Within a 15-minute drive of where I (Dr. Brownell) live in Connecticut, I bet I could find 25 fast-food restaurants, and ocean occupies half of the available

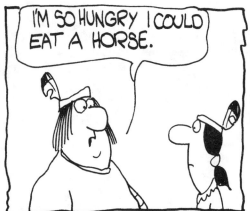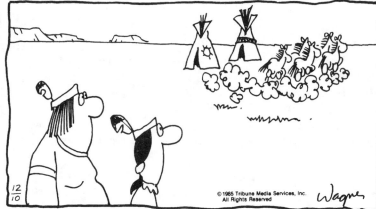

space! In addition to McDonald's, I would find Burger Kings, Kentucky Fried Chickens, Wendy's, Popeye's, and heaven knows what else. And with 24-hour service, breakfast, and drive-through windows, convenience has reached new levels. If you can believe it, 7 percent of the American population eats at McDonald's each day.

The world of fast food has undergone many interesting, and in a few cases, positive changes. Chicken has found its way onto the menu, but in some cases in better form than others (broiled chicken vs. chicken nuggets). Healthier oils are being used to cook French fries in some places, yet people are consuming fries (and therefore fat and calories) in record amounts. Some developments, such as drive-through windows and package deals (value meals), very likely increase the number of customers and amount eaten per customer.

The table shown in Appendix E lists foods from a number of the major fast-food chains and shows the values for calories, fat, carbohydrate, and protein. The foods vary widely in their nutritional value. Foods from these restaurants can be high in saturated fat, sodium, cholesterol, and calories, and low in calcium, vitamins A and D, and fiber. Soft drinks such as Coca Cola and Pepsi are not listed in the table. Calorie values for soft drinks are listed in the Calorie Guide in Appendix F.

The news is not all bad, however. One can walk into some fast food chains and escape with a reasonable meal. We hope the figures shown in the fast food table will be helpful in accomplishing this.

A Review of Your Quality of Life

As we have asked before, we'd like you to complete the Quality of Life Self-Assessment and to compare your scores with those from when you began the program (page 11). See whether changes have occurred in each area.

We emphasize again that there are many ways your life might improve from the changes you are making. The weight loss, improved diet, and increased physical activity can each lead to changes in how you feel about different aspects of your life. We draw your attention to these periodically to show how there are multiple arenas in which to judge how you are doing. Having more energy, being in a better mood, or having more self-confidence are nice changes in a person's life, so we hope you feel good about feeling better!

Quality of Life Self-Assessment

Please use the following scale to rate how satisfied you feel now about different aspects of your daily life. Choose any number from this list (1 to 9) and indicate your choice on the questions below

1 = Extremely Dissatisfied

2 = Very Dissatisfied

3 = Moderately Dissatisfied

4 = Somewhat Dissatisfied

5 = Neutral

6 = Somewhat Satisfied

7 = Moderately Satisfied

8 = Very Satisfied

9 = Extremely Satisfied

1. ___ Mood (feelings of sadness, worry, happiness, etc.)
2. ___ Self-esteem
3. ___ Confidence, self-assurance and comfort in social situations
4. ___ Energy and feeling healthy
5. ___ Health problems (diabetes, high blood pressure, etc.)
6. ___ General appearance
7. ___ Social life
8. ___ Leisure and recreational activities
9. ___ Physical mobility and physical activity
10. ___ Eating habits
11. ___ Body image
12. ___ Overall quality of life

Setting Personal Goals

Much of this lesson focused on the Behavior Chain. Be sure to fill out the blank chain in this lesson and devise plans to break as many links as possible. Use this idea of the Behavior Chain in analyzing your high-risk situations and in planning in advance for countering pressures to eat. It may be useful to draw out more than one chain to help with your most difficult situations. For your exercise, see if there are ways to work extra stair climbing into your lifestyle. Continue monitoring your intake of the recommended number of servings from the five food groups of the Food Guide Pyramid.

As has been the case in previous lessons, we urge you to select goals that are specific to you. Goals that you have learned from experience motivate you in important areas should be a constant part of your weight-control landscape.

Self-Assessment

Questionnaire

Lesson 21

T F 98. Once the eating chain begins, it is not possible to stop
because the links are so
strong.

T F 99. A Behavior Chain, like any
chain, is only as strong as its
weakest links.

T F 100. It is best to interrupt an eating chain at one of its last
links when you know what
foods confront you.

T F 101. Using stairs is a convenient
and accessible way for many
people to increase activity.

(Answers in Appendix C)

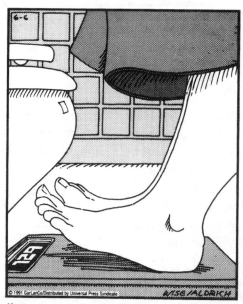

If you stand on the scale just so, you weigh less.

Monitoring Form—Lesson 21

Today's Date:

Time	Food and Amount	Calories
	Total Daily Calories	

Personal Goals This Week	*Always*	*Sometimes*	*Never*
1.			
2.			
3. Sketch your behavior chains			
4. Increase use of stairs			
5. Eat daily servings from the five food groups			
6. Eat less than _____ calories each day			

Medication Taken Today ❑ Yes ❑ No	*Physical Activity*	*Minutes*
Milk, yogurt, and cheese ❑ ❑ ❑		
Meat, poultry, etc. ❑ ❑ ❑		
Fruits ❑ ❑ ❑ ❑		
Vegetables ❑ ❑ ❑ ❑ ❑		
Breads, cereals, etc. ❑ ❑ ❑ ❑ ❑ ❑ ❑ ❑ ❑		

Weight Change Record
(Weeks 17–32)

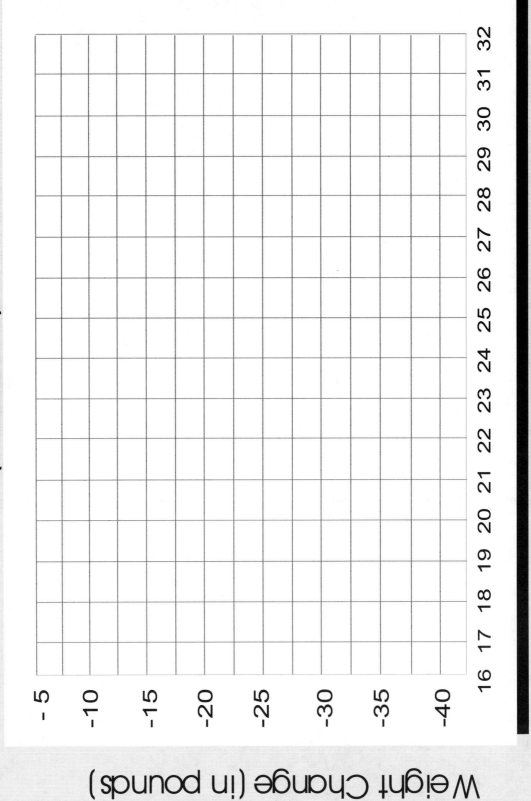

Weight Change (in pounds)

Week

Lesson 22

This lesson begins the last three of the program. If you are following the program as it was designed, this lesson will cover weeks 37–40 of your program. In many ways, these last lessons together may be our most important because we turn our attention to permanent maintenance of weight loss. Central to this are three terms: *lapse, relapse, and collapse.* These will be discussed, as will methods to handle urges to eat.

Preventing Lapse, Relapse, and Collapse

Far too often, a minor slip propels a person to misery. The guilt from a slip makes a person susceptible to more slips and can ultimately lead to loss of all control. This is a gloomy picture, but good news is around the corner! There *are* ways to turn the tables.

Maintenance of weight loss may be the greatest challenge facing overweight persons. Losing weight is difficult enough, but keeping it off ranks up there in difficulty with winning the lottery and finding a compassionate auditor from the Internal Revenue Service. Most overweight people have lost and regained weight many times, so something must be done to interrupt these cycles. The trick is to prevent slips from occurring and to respond constructively when they do occur.

Everyone makes mistakes. Some bounce back and use the slip as a signal to increase control. It is common, however, for the slip to cause a negative emotional reaction (guilt and despair) which builds until all control is lost.

There are two paths to success. The first is to avoid or prevent slips and mistakes and the second is to respond to slips with coping techniques that put *you* in control. We will cover each path separately. In this lesson, we will work on preventing slips, and in Lesson 23 we will emphasize recovering from slips.

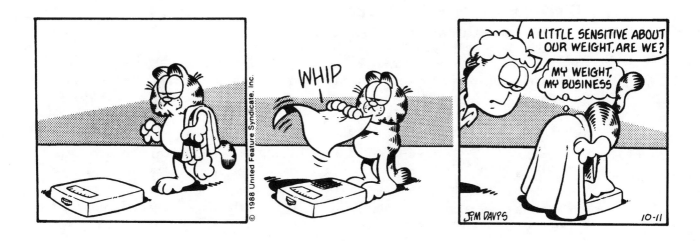

265

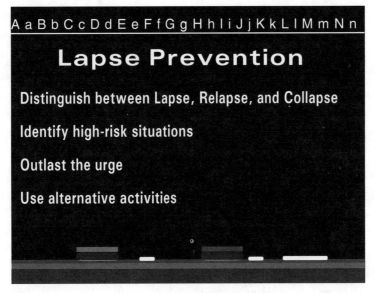

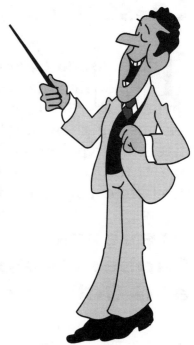

Lapse Prevention

Distinguish between Lapse, Relapse, and Collapse

Identify high-risk situations

Outlast the urge

Use alternative activities

Much of our discussion on this topic is drawn from the excellent work of Dr. G. Alan Marlatt and Dr. Judith Gordon, both psychologists from the University of Washington. They have studied the situations associated with relapse in overweight persons, alcoholics, smokers, drug addicts, and compulsive gamblers. They have also proposed methods for preventing relapse. Their work is described in a classic book entitled *Relapse Prevention* (Guilford Press, New York, 1985—call 1-800-736-7323 for ordering).

Distinguishing Lapse, Relapse, and Collapse

We have used several terms to describe deviating from your weight control plan: mistake, lapse, slip, error, etc. Relapse implies something different and collapse is yet another matter. We fuss with these words because the terms we use can be important.

In recovering alcoholics, one slip or lapse is considered by many to be a re-lapse (i.e., "one drink a drunk"). The same is thought by some to be true for people who stop smoking. Having a single cigarette begins an inevitable path to relapse. However, there is abundant evidence that this is not true.

Many recovering alcoholics have had at least one drink since their reformation, and it is a rare ex-smoker who has not had a cigarette. Yet, they recover from their lapses and prevent a relapse. The same is unquestionably true with overweight individuals.

A *lapse* is a slight error or slip, the first instance of backsliding. It is a discrete event like eating a *forbidden* food, exceeding a calorie level, or gaining weight. *Relapse* occurs when lapses string together and the person returns to his or her former state. When relapse is complete and there is little hope of reversing the negative trend, *collapse* has occurred.

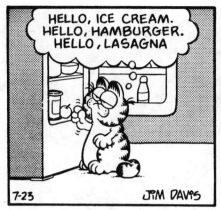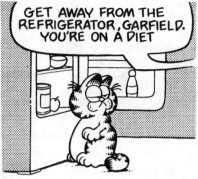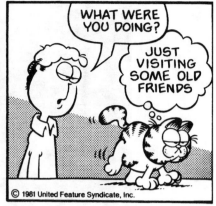

The most important message is that

A LAPSE MUST NOT ALWAYS LEAD TO RELAPSE

The person who can view a lapse for what it is, an unfortunate but temporary problem, is prepared to respond positively to life's inevitable setbacks.

Identifying Urges and High-Risk Situations

The concepts of *urge* and *high-risk situations* were introduced earlier in the program. Distinguishing cravings (urges) from hunger was discussed in Lesson 9, conquering cravings was also covered in Lesson 9, and the Behavior Chain was introduced in Lesson 21. These were all leading to the point we face now, the need to spot trouble before it occurs. Urges can now become a signal for corrective action.

Let's look back over what you have learned. You know much more about your eating than before, so let's take advantage of that information. Think carefully about when you are most likely to find your eating threatened. Is it when you have certain feelings, like loneliness or frustration? Is it when you have to deal with some person? Is it when you feel bad about your life and your weight? Is it when someone offers you food? Look back over your Monitoring Forms and your weight loss experience to identify these situations.

Now that you are a pro at identifying urges and high-risk situations, let's plan ahead. We will learn a technique called *outlasting the urges* and will learn to use alternatives to eating when the high-risk situations arise. These become our armor when we are barraged with temptation.

Outlasting the Urges

It is possible to prevent a lapse by dealing with urges. We title this section *Outlasting the Urges* because an urge will usually go away if you just wait it out. This is easier said than done sometimes, but the rewards are high when you succeed.

Dr. G. Alan Marlatt, the psychologist mentioned previously, feels that an urge can be compared to a wave building in the ocean and then breaking on the beach. Conquering the urges is like surfing. A wave begins small, builds to a crest, breaks, and then subsides. Urges follow a similar course. They usually build gently to their strongest point, weaken, and then gradually fade away.

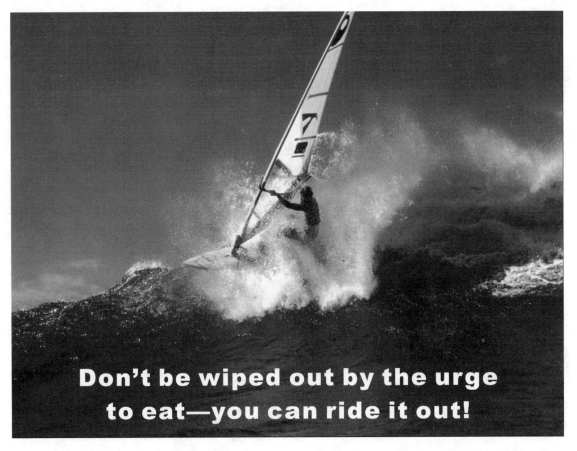

Don't be wiped out by the urge to eat—you can ride it out!

The wave analogy is much different than the way people usually think about urges. Some people feel that an urge builds and builds and will create havoc unless it is gratified by eating. Actually, gratifying an urge by eating makes urges stronger and more frequent. In contrast, letting the urge pass, like the wave rolling in, will weaken it. If you can outlast enough of the urges, they will fade to obscurity.

The image of *urge surfing* is a good one. Pretend you are learning to surf. As the wave rolls in, you can battle it and be wiped out, or you can maintain your balance and ride the wave until it subsides.

Being a good urge surfer involves identifying the urges early in their development and then readying your skills to ride the wave. If the wave is upon you at full strength before you recognize it, you may wipe out no matter how well you surf. If you recognize the wave early, but cannot surf, you will also wipe out. Therefore, both parts are important—early recognition and skills to cope with the urges.

Simply waiting for the urge to pass can be all you'll need, but not always. Some urges and high-risk situations are stronger than others, so techniques other than waiting are necessary. One such technique is the use of alternative activities.

Using Alternative Activities

The principle of using alternative activities is simple. When you get the urge, do something else. If you use urges as a signal for positive activity, eating will become less rewarding and the old associations between urges and eating will diminish. When you see food, think about food, or feel hungry because you are lonely, eating is simply a habit created by an association. We can make new associations.

Incompatible Activities to Eating

Walk the Dog	Play a Board Game
File Coupons	Ride a Bike
Go to a Movie	Brush Your Teeth
Call a Friend	Read This Manual!
Shop for Plants	Frame Some Pictures
Take a Shower	Refinish Furniture
Listen to Music	Play Music
Take a Drive	Knit a Sweater
Read a Romantic Book	Work in a Garden
Read a Mystery Book	Visit a Museum
Go to the Zoo	Buy a Gift
Buy a New Magazine	Plan a Vacation
Kiss Somebody	Paint a Picture
Wash the Car	Buy Tickets
Kiss Somebody Again	Work on a Hobby
Write a Letter	Visit a Neighbor
Get Some Exercise	Donate to Charity
Look at Photo Album	Imagine Being More Fit

My Alternatives to Eating

1. _____

2. _____

3. _____

4. _____

5. _____

6. _____

7. _____

8. _____

9. _____

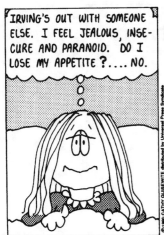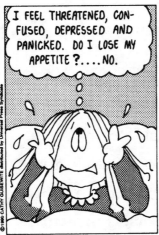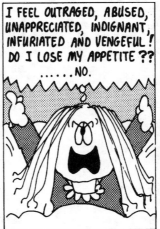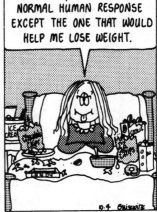

When you recognize urges, think of an activity that is incompatible with eating. For instance, typing a letter and jumping rope are incompatible—both cannot be done at once, unless you are Rubber Man. If you were addicted to typing and agreed to jump rope each time you got the urge to type, the strength of your addiction would fade.

This same approach can work with eating. One cannot play the tuba and eat, so tuba practice would be a good alternative to eating. You might think of more practical methods that would involve activities you enjoy.

Making a List, Checking it Twice

Make a list of activities you could use when you are tempted to eat. The list should contain more than one activity so you have several choices. If you vow to consult the list when you want to eat, your control can improve. Make certain the list contains enjoyable activities so you will actually do them in lieu of eating.

The list provided on the previous page contains ideas for incompatible activi-

ties. Some can be done at home, others take you out of the house. Some take little time while others are more involved. Many are examples from my clients. Do they give you more ideas?

Now that you have ideas from the list, it is time to establish your own list. Write out the activities that would make good alternatives for you. Add as many activities as you can. They should be both enjoyable and feasible. Some may require planning and the right timing, like going to a movie. Others should be available at a moment's notice so you can spring into action when an urge hits.

Try consulting the list when you get the urge to eat. If you can distract yourself for even a few minutes, the urge to eat can fade and your control can increase. Studies have shown that hunger comes and goes during the day, so not succumbing the instant an urge hits can give you precious time to think. Do your best to ride the wave!

Hard Work at the Office

Most people think that working in an office is the perfect setting for getting flabby. Wrong! Certain office activities require great effort. The table below

270

shows just how strenuous life in the office can be.

Setting Personal Goals

There are several activities for your assignment. The first is to distinguish lapse from relapse, and the second is to identify high-risk situations. This information forms the basis for the next two parts of the assignment—to outlast the urges and to use alternative activities to eating. Finally, recheck your diet to make sure you are eating enough fiber. Review the information on fiber in Lesson 19 if you need to.

As you think back over the months you have been in the program, take a moment to review the changes you feel are most important. What are the keys to your success? Use these to establish your personal goals.

Office Calories

Activity	Calories
Throwing in the towel	0
Beating around the bush	35
Bending over backwards	75
Hitting the nail on the head	75
Dragging your heels	90
Tooting your own horn	100
Flirting at the water cooler	150
Avoiding the boss	175
Jumping to conclusions	200
Passing the buck	300
Making mountains out of molehills	400
Running around in circles	450
Climbing the walls	500

Self-Assessment Questionnaire

Lesson 22

T F 102. When a person lapses, relapse is close behind be-
cause nothing can interrupt
the negative cycle of lapses
and out-of-control eating.

T F 103. It helps to have a list of alternatives to eating for use
when urges strike.

T F 104. The emphasis on fiber may
be dangerous because fiber
is indigestible material that
can harm the intestinal system.

(Answers in Appendix C)

Monitoring Form—Lesson 22

Today's Date:

Time	Food and Amount	Calories
Total Daily Calories		

Personal Goals This Week	Always	Sometimes	Never
1.			
2.			
3. Identify high risks			
4. Outlast urges			
5. My diet has _____ grams of fiber			
6. Eat less than _____ calories each day			

Medication Taken Today ❑ Yes ❑ No	*Physical Activity*	*Minutes*
Milk, yogurt, and cheese ❑ ❑ ❑		
Meat, poultry, etc. ❑ ❑ ❑		
Fruits ❑ ❑ ❑ ❑		
Vegetables ❑ ❑ ❑ ❑ ❑		
Breads, cereals, etc. ❑ ❑ ❑ ❑ ❑ ❑ ❑ ❑ ❑ ❑		

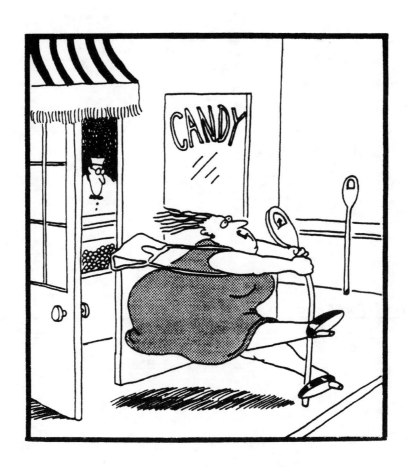

Lesson 23

We hope you had a great month. You are now ready for Lesson 23, which covers weeks 41–44 in your program. In Lesson 22, we noted two ways to keep the reins on urges and to prevent the common journey from lapse to relapse to collapse. One path, preventing lapses, can be attained by avoiding high risk situations and by using alternative activities to short-circuit the urges. This lesson will focus on the second path—to cope with lapses once they occur. We will also cover the role of cholesterol in the diet.

Coping with Lapse and Preventing Relapse

Lapses are inevitable. By this point in the program, most people losing weight have experienced peaks of joy and valleys of distress. It is the rare person who has not eaten some high-calorie foods, overeaten at a special event or holiday gathering, or resorted to favorite foods when times got tough. The issue is not so much *whether* the lapses occur, but the person's *reaction* after they occur.

An example might elucidate this. Two friends, Judy and Joan, were both on a weight-loss program and attended a wedding. Both overate at the buffet, to the tune of 2000 calories. Judy did it on shrimp and steak, whereas Joan fixed her attention on bread and desserts. The extra 2000 calories should not sink their weight loss efforts because the calories amount to less than a pound of weight. Judy and Joan, however, reacted quite differently to the 2000 calorie lapse.

Judy felt guilty about the wedding episode and told herself, "I blew my eating plan." She then thought, "What the heck, I blew it already, I might as well enjoy myself." She ate more when she got home, felt guilty the next day, and continued the overeating for five days. Joan, on the other hand, felt bad about the 2000 calorie lapse, but responded in a more constructive manner. She reflected on what happened and planned accordingly. She increased her walking an ex-

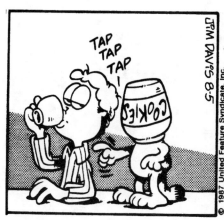 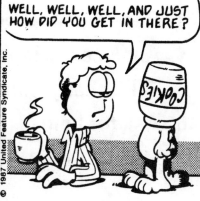 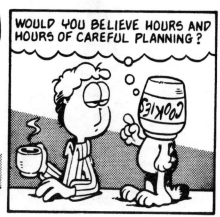

tra 15 minutes for the next four days and cut back on her calorie intake.

Six Steps to Gaining Control

How can we learn from Joan and master our lapses? Following six specific steps can be a big help. These are adapted from the work of Dr. G. Alan Marlatt mentioned in Lesson 22.

❶ **Step 1: Stop, look, and listen.** A lapse is a signal of impending danger, like a train signal and the crossing gates. Stop what you are doing, especially if the lapse has started, and examine the situation. What is occurring? Why is a lapse in progress? Consider removing yourself to a safe location where you won't be tempted and where you can think in a rational manner.

❷ **Step 2: Stay calm.** If you get anxious or blame yourself for the lapse, the situation may get worse. You may conclude that you are a hopeless binge eater and that control is impossible. Coming to these conclusions is easy when you get all worked up. Try to separate yourself from the situation, and view it as an objective observer would—that one lapse does not prove failure. Keeping a cool head makes the following steps easier.

❸ **Step 3: Renew your weight-loss vows.** Take a minute to remind yourself of how far you have come, the progress you have made, and how sad it would be if one lapse canceled out all your hard work. Restate your program goals and renew the vows you made when dieting began.

❹ **Step 4: Analyze the lapse situation.** Instead of blaming yourself for letting go, use the situation to learn what places you at risk. Do certain feelings create the risk? Is it the presence of food, other eating, other activities, etc.? Did you do anything to defend against the urge? Did it work? Why or why not? What thoughts did you have?

Mastering a Lapse

1. Stop, look, and listen
2. Stay calm
3. Renew your program vows
4. Analyze the lapse situation
5. Take charge immediately
6. Ask for help

Step 5: Take charge immediately. Leap into action with your planned techniques. Leave the house, feed the remaining food to the disposal, or do whatever works for you. The alternative activities you listed in Lesson 22 will be a good place to start. Don't wait, and be decisive. Waiting is an excuse for letting go even more. Jump on that lapse like a dog on a bone! Remember that it is usually easier to get control if you leave the situation.

Step 6: Ask for help. Partners, friends, coworkers, and others can be a real source of support. You might review the material on Relationships from earlier lessons where we discussed who to ask for help, how to ask, and how to respond if help is given. If you could really use support during lapses, don't be shy about asking for help.

These six steps are easy to remember. You can even write them on a small card to keep in your wallet or purse. Using them, however, will require some effort.

Becoming a Forest Ranger

Consider yourself a Forest Ranger on the lookout for fires. Your job is to prevent fires and to put them out quickly if they start. Your lapses are like the fires. You will try to prevent them, but when they do flare up, extinguish them immediately. Occasionally a fire may seem out of control, but don't lose the forest!!

Let's develop this idea of the Forest Ranger a bit further. Your job is to take control over your eating, exercise, and weight. The Ranger's job is to keep control over the forest. The Ranger must do everything possible to prevent fires from breaking out. Since fires may be difficult to control once they start, the Ranger believes in "an ounce of prevention..." Prevention is also important for you. You

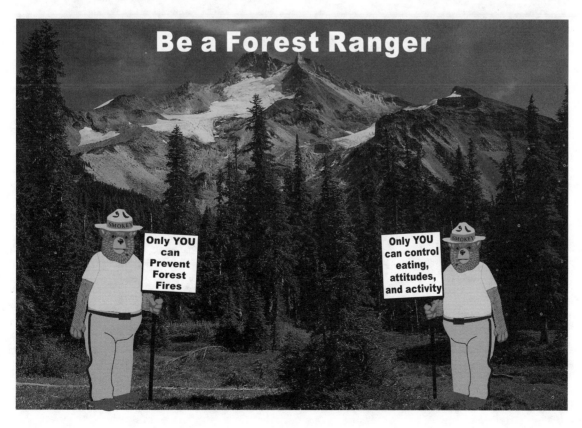

have learned dozens of ways to take control of your eating so that lapses will not occur. As you know, the key is to be prepared for high-risk situations, to plan in advance, and to keep the right attitude.

The Forest Ranger's second task is to stop the spread of fires once they do occur. The Ranger's ability to do this will determine whether the forest is spared or destroyed. A lapse in your eating is like the fire that breaks out. Whether you bounce back and spare your diet, or let the mistake destroy the progress you have made (lapse, relapse, then collapse) depends on your ability to use the techniques described here.

Please remember the dual tasks that confront both you and the Forest Ranger. You are concerned with both prevention and with crisis management. Identify the situations where you are most likely to confront problems. Then plan to use both your prevention techniques and the constructive methods you have learned to deal with lapses.

These are the ways to prevent lapses and to stop lapses dead in their tracks. The information here and in Lesson 22 is, in our opinion, crucial for long-term success. We will review it in the next lesson. Please refer back to these lessons if you find yourself in trouble. This dual approach of preventing problems and of coping with problems when they do arise allows you to hit temptations from two angles.

Life on Chutes and Ladders

There is a well-known children's board game called "Chutes and Ladders," known formerly as "Snakes and Ladders." Many adults remember the

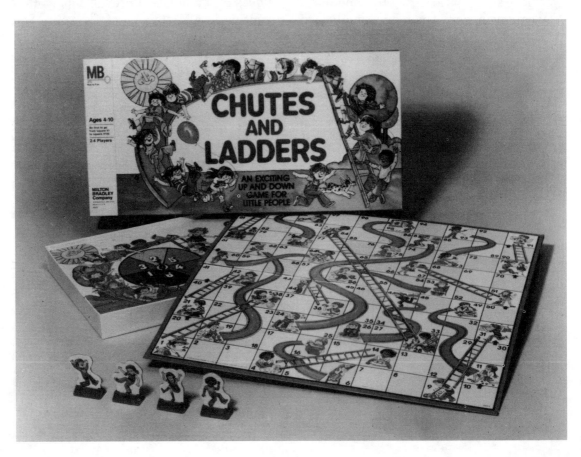

game from their own childhood or from playing with their children. The basic idea behind the game provides a good moral to remember as we discuss lapse, relapse, and collapse.

In Chutes and Ladders, players use a spinner to advance over the 100 spaces on the board. At some points there are ladders which advance a player by many spaces. At other points, there are chutes that can send the player back many spaces. For example, a player who lands on space nine is shown cutting the lawn for his parents. For his effort, he can advance to space 31, which shows the boy going to the circus. A player landing on space 95 is greeted by a picture of a boy who hits a baseball through a window. His transgression sends him back to space 75 where he is emptying his piggy bank.

Sometimes playing Chutes and Ladders goes without a hitch. You land on the ladders and avoid the chutes. Other times the chutes seem to draw you like a magnet. However, even under the worst of circumstances, a player can reach the top of the board and win the game.

Let's say that the Milton Bradley Company made Chutes and Ladders relevant to the situations faced by individuals controlling their weight. One might advance up a ladder by eating under control at a buffet, but might slide down a chute by eating 400 peanuts at Happy Hour. Jogging would qualify one for a ladder and would speed the person toward the ultimate goal. Eating 15 of Cousin Clara's Cocoa Cremeballs would definitely hasten one's descent down a chute.

There are several points to remember from our hypothetical game of Chutes and Ladders. The first is that making progress up the ladders can always be interrupted by a chute. Even a program

Use skills and motivation to help propel you up the ladder of success.

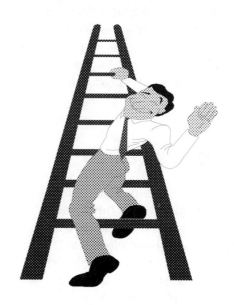

that goes smoothly for weeks can be stymied by setbacks. However, even the longest fall down a chute can be remedied by heading back up the board, hopefully with the aid of a few ladders. If you have the skills and the motivation to control eating and increase exercise, you will be poised to take advantage of the ladders and will advance more quickly.

Weight control, like life, has both chutes and ladders. Being prepared for this fact is half the battle. The other half is having the right attitude and behaviors to remain optimistic when trouble occurs, and to have skills in hand to rebound from lapses. Think now of the situations that can send you down a chute and plan some prevention strategies. Think also of the situations that can propel you up a ladder, then make them happen!

When children play Chutes and Ladders, landing on a chute can be discouraging. He or she may want to quit playing because the immediate setback overwhelms the knowledge that things might get better (there might be a ladder ahead). The immediate bad feelings created by a dietary mistake can make individuals want to quit. It is crucial to remember that life has its chutes, particularly when you're working hard to control your weight. Look ahead for the ladder, and by all means, keep playing the game.

Cholesterol

Cholesterol is a waxy substance necessary for the body's functioning. It can be manufactured by the body or can be eaten in food. High blood levels of cholesterol are related to risk for heart disease, and the blood level of cholesterol is determined in part by what you eat.

Cholesterol is carried in the bloodstream by something called lipoproteins. Some of the cholesterol is deposited on the walls of the arteries as fatty streaks. When these deposits build they form a fibrous plaque which makes the wall of the artery less able to adjust to blood flow. If the artery narrows enough to stop or seriously restrict the flow of blood, vital tissue can be deprived and die. The result is a heart attack if the coronary arteries are involved or a stroke if the blocked arteries supply the brain.

Knowing your own cholesterol level can be important. The National Cholesterol Education Program, a nationwide effort of the National Institutes of Health, suggests that the desirable level of blood cholesterol is below 200 mg/dl. The range from 200–239 mg/dl is considered borderline, and above 240 mg/dl is considered high. Where you fall in these categories will indicate how often blood cholesterol should be checked, the degree to which diet should be changed, and whether special advice from a physician

is necessary. It is advisable, therefore, to have your cholesterol level checked.

You may have heard talk about different types of cholesterol, particularly HDL (high density lipoprotein) cholesterol and LDL (low density lipoprotein) cholesterol. HDL is thought to protect against heart disease, so higher levels are better. LDL has the opposite effect, so lower levels are better. Scientists are learning more about how diet and exercise can be used to raise HDL and lower LDL but it appears that the same methods used to lower total cholesterol will have beneficial effects on HDL and LDL.

To help control blood cholesterol, it is important to limit the amount of fat and cholesterol ingested, and to be sensitive to the type of fat you eat. Saturated fat from animal sources (fats from beef, lamb, pork, ham, butter, cream, whole milk, cheese) and saturated fat from vegetable sources (coconut oil, palm oil, cocoa butter) should be limited. It is desirable to limit saturated fats and to replace them with polyunsaturated fats, which usually come from vegetable oils.

The table on the next page may be helpful in guiding you in choosing foods low in cholesterol. It is important to remember that reducing saturated fat in the diet can have an even more powerful effect in lowering blood cholesterol than can reducing dietary cholesterol. Information on fat is provided in earlier lessons.

Setting Personal Goals

The main priority for this lesson is to use the six steps to deal with lapses. It is easy to remember the steps if you write them down on a card and keep them handy, perhaps in your wallet or purse.

Cholesterol Content of Common Foods

Food	Quantity	Cholesterol (mg)
Dairy Products		
Skim milk	1 cup (8.6 oz)	5
Buttermilk from skim	1 cup (8.6 oz)	5
Low-fat milk (1% fat)	1 cup (8.6 oz)	15
Whole milk (4%)	1 cup (8.7 oz)	34
Ice milk, soft serve	1 cup (6.2 oz)	35
Cream, half & half	1T (0.5 oz)	6
Whipping cream	1T (0.5 oz)	20
Butter	1T (0.5 oz)	29–35
Rich ice cream (16% fat)	1 cup (5.2 oz)	84
Low-fat cottage cheese	4 oz	6
Low-fat yogurt, vanilla/plain	8 oz	11–18
Swiss cheese	1 oz	28
Cheddar cheese	1 oz	28
Cream cheese	1 oz	31
American cheese	1 oz	41
Meats and Poultry		
Bacon, fried and drained	2 slices (0.8 oz)	12
Bologna	1 slice (1.3 oz)	14
Boiled ham	1 oz	15
Hog dog	1 (1.6 oz)	29
Pork chop, broiled, lean	4 oz	100
Roast turkey, light meat	4 oz	87
Fried chicken	4 oz fried in veg. oil	90–103
Ham roast, lean only	4 oz	100
Beef pot roast, lean only	4 oz	103
Sirloin steak, lean only	4 oz	103
Ground beef, broiled	4 oz	107
Roast turkey, dark meat	4 oz	115
Egg, large, poached	1 (1.7 oz)	242
Egg, scrambled in veg. oil	1 (2.3 oz)	263
Beef or calf liver, fried	4 oz	297
Chicken liver, simmered	4 oz	846
Fish and Seafood		
Canned salmon	4 oz	40
Clams, raw	4 (3 oz)	42
Cod	4 oz	57
Scallops, steamed	4 oz	60
Rainbow trout, fresh	4 oz	62
Canned tuna, oil pack	4 oz	63
Halibut steak, broiled	4 oz	68
Lobster	4 oz	96
Canned crab	4 oz	116
Shrimp	4 oz	170

Note: **Figures adapted from** *The Dictionary of Sodium, Fats, and Cholesterol* **by Barbara Kraus, New York: Putnam, 1974.**

This way you will be prepared, so if trouble comes your way, you can whip out the card and put the brakes on any temptation.

As we recommend in each lesson, you can supplement the goals we have listed above with goals that are personal to you. These could include any technique we have recommended, or something we have not discussed but you feel is important. The key is that the goal is meaningful for you.

Self-Assessment Questionnaire

Lesson 23

T F 105. Getting nervous or anxious during a lapse is helpful because anxiety interferes with appetite and allows you to remove yourself from temptation.

T F 106. When dealing with a lapse, it is best to move quickly and decisively before control erodes even further.

T F 107. For controlling your blood cholesterol, it is important to limit intake of saturated fat.

(Answers in Appendix C)

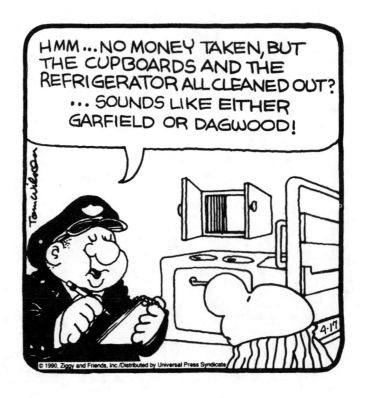

Monitoring Form—Lesson 23

Today's Date:

Time	Food and Amount	Calories
	Total Daily Calories	

Personal Goals This Week	*Always*	*Sometimes*	*Never*
1.			
2.			
3. Use the six steps to cope with relapses			
4. Be a Forest Ranger			
5. Use alternative activities to eating			
6. Eat less than _____ calories each day			

Medication Taken Today ❑ Yes ❑ No	*Physical Activity*	*Minutes*
Milk, yogurt, and cheese ❑ ❑ ❑		
Meat, poultry, etc. ❑ ❑ ❑		
Fruits ❑ ❑ ❑ ❑		
Vegetables ❑ ❑ ❑ ❑ ❑		
Breads, cereals, etc. ❑ ❑ ❑ ❑ ❑ ❑ ❑ ❑ ❑		

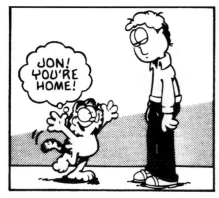
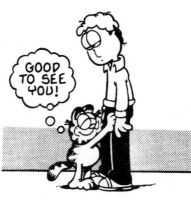
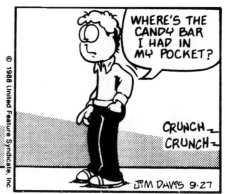

Lesson 24

There are now two lessons remaining in The LEARN Program, this and the graduation (commencement) lesson. There are still important areas to cover. In this lesson, we will discuss material in the lifestyle and nutrition areas. We will deal with special events and holidays, and with the role of minerals in the diet. We will also introduce a lifestyle factor of major importance, the Master Monitoring Form. Let's forge ahead!

As described in the next lesson, one of us (Dr. Brownell) has written *The LEARN Weight Maintenance and Stabilization Guide*. It is a companion to The LEARN Program and is to be used as The LEARN Program ends. It is a step-by-step guide for maintaining your weight loss and possibly losing more. This guide was written in response to hundreds of requests for something dealing specifically with what to do after an initial program ends. The guide can be obtained by calling The LEARN Education Center (1–800–736–7323) or writing to the address provided at the end of this book.

The Master Monitoring Form

There has been a Monitoring Form for each lesson in this program. You have recorded food intake and changes in the five LEARN areas (lifestyle, exercise, attitudes, relationships, and nutrition). This sets the stage for the Master Monitoring Form.

The Master Monitoring Form is similar to the forms you have seen throughout the program. It is unusual, in that it has blank spaces where techniques have been listed in other lessons. The aim is for you to list the techniques which best suit *your* needs. The new form appears toward the end of this lesson.

Keeping records is usually rated as one of the most important aspects of the program. Many clients continue to keep the records for years. Whether you do this or not depends on how long it takes for your new habits to become permanent. We recommend strongly that you complete the records, in some form, for at least eight more weeks. If you have stopped keeping the forms, you might

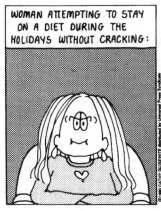

WOMAN ATTEMPTING TO STAY ON A DIET DURING THE HOLIDAYS WITHOUT CRACKING:

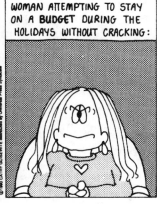

WOMAN ATTEMPTING TO STAY ON A **BUDGET** DURING THE HOLIDAYS WITHOUT CRACKING:

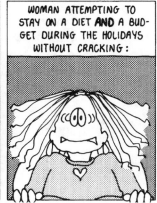

WOMAN ATTEMPTING TO STAY ON A DIET **AND** A BUDGET DURING THE HOLIDAYS WITHOUT CRACKING:

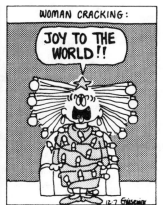

WOMAN CRACKING:

JOY TO THE WORLD!!

What LEARN techniques are most important to you?

start again to see if the process would still be helpful.

The Master Monitoring Form contains the same standard sections for recording eating and physical activity (on the left side and the bottom right side, respectively). The top right part, where the techniques have been listed, is blank. You can complete this part of the form with the techniques you consider most important.

We cannot predict what these techniques will be. For one person it will be to eat slowly, for another it will be to end dichotomous thinking, for another to do aerobic exercise at least four times a week, and for another to keep food out of sight.

These are only examples of the large list of techniques you have learned. Think back over your experiences and decide which techniques are necessary for you. The Master List of Techniques

(Appendix A) described below will be helpful for this task.

When you have arrived at your list of key behaviors, enter them on your Master Monitoring Form. Make photocopies and use them as long as needed. Recording your food intake and your exercise is so important that we have not made these optional. When you add the behaviors we mentioned, your form will be complete.

We are beginning with the Master Monitoring Form in this lesson, so we have the opportunity to discuss your experience with it in the final lesson. Try to start right away, so you will have this experience under your belt for the Commencement Lesson.

Using the Master List of Techniques (Appendix A)

Appendix A contains a summary list of all the techniques we introduced in the program. Use this to review your progress and to determine which techniques were most important to you. Some techniques almost certainly did not apply. If you do no food shopping, the techniques in this area were not relevant. Focus on those most pertinent for you. They may be the techniques you struggled with most, which is one sign that the habits they targeted are difficult to change.

Go through the list of techniques in Appendix A, and circle the ones that are most important in your attempts to lose weight. These are not necessarily the behaviors that are easiest for you. They should be the ones that are the keys to your future success. Circle any behavior you feel fits this bill. Think back care-

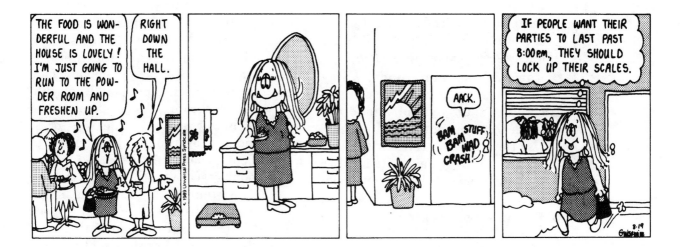

fully over your experience with earlier parts of the program, and consider programs you have been on in the past. Circle the behaviors that help you control your eating and increase your exercise.

Now that you have circled the important behaviors, it is time to narrow the list. You would like to end up with 5–10 behaviors that will be the final entries for your Master Monitoring Form. Having too few techniques can make you miss opportunities to change your habits, and having too many makes record keeping too complex. It is fine to modify the list as your habits change, but for now, this list should be your marching orders to yourself.

Holidays, Parties, and Special Events

Do you get stuffed more than the turkey on Thanksgiving? Do you love the salted nuts people offer at parties? Do you feel obligated to eat when a host or hostess prepares an elegant meal? There are several ways to deal with these special occasions.

Holidays, parties, and special occasions can be a problem because eating is encouraged. Not only does temptation abound, but everyone else is eating, the food is good, there may be social pressure to "try some of this," and it is natural to let go when celebrating. The trick is to be prepared and to avoid the anxiety that comes from trying to diet and celebrate at the same time.

One common mistake is for individuals on weight control programs to vow to eat nothing at the event. This is a real setup, because they either feel guilty when they eat or feel deprived when they don't. You can enjoy yourself and still keep your virtue. Here are five methods for having fun and keeping the reins on uncontrolled eating.

❶ **Plan ahead.** Think about the event before you go. Try to anticipate both the food you will face and the actions of other people. Think about your own desires to eat and the external pressures from others. Have a general idea of what you will eat. You can call ahead and ask what will be served. You can make a tentative list of what you will eat and add up the calories. How does it fit with your day's calorie goal?

❷ **Eat something before you go.** Don't go starved to a special event. Everything will look good, and you will forget that you only want to sample special foods. Have a salad, carrot sticks, cauliflower, or other low-calorie food before you go.

❸ **Eat only special foods.** Stay away from the potato chips, crackers, dip, nuts, bread and other foods that you can have any time. Use the chance to try new foods or foods you rarely have. Remember to make the best use of your calories.

❹ **Be the slowest eater.** Keep your eye on others and be the slowest eater at the event. Be the last to start and the last to finish. You will enjoy the food more and will feel satisfied with less. Pay attention to the texture, smell, and subtleties of taste. This will halt the rapid and automatic eating that brings so many calories.

❺ **Keep a proper perspective.** If you do eat more than you intend, keep a positive attitude. Don't turn an event into more than it really is—just another day with meals and calories. In the scheme of a month or year's worth of eating, what can one day mean? One day's indiscretion should not ruin any program. There are plenty of formerly heavy people who occasionally overdo it. Their trick is to bounce back. As we stated before, your reaction to the eating is more important than the eating itself. Your attitudes are central to your ability to control your eating both during and after the event.

The National Walking Movement

People are walking here, there, almost everywhere. The movement has been bolstered by the discovery that walking can be fun, can be done in the most interesting places, and can be done

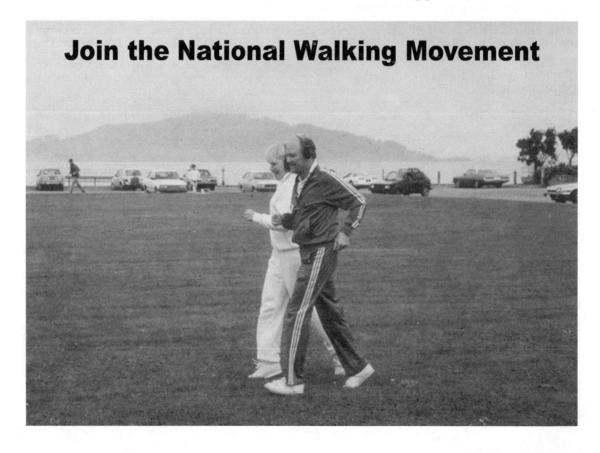
Join the National Walking Movement

Resources for Walkers

American Volkssport Association
1001 Pat Booker Road, Suite 101
Universal City, Texas 78148
(210) 659–2112

Can send you a list of walking clubs in your area. An annual membership ($20 per individual and $25 for families) includes a subscription to *American Wanderer*.

Prevention Walking Club
Rodale Press
Box 6099
Emmaus, PA 18099
(800) 666-1216

Included as a separate section in *Prevention Magazine* dealing with all aspects of walking. Annual subscription $17.94.

Walkabout International
835 Fifth Avenue, Room 407
San Diego, CA 92101
(619) 231–7463

Club with chapters in various cities. Organizes & publishes information about walks.

Walking Magazine
9–11 Harcourt St.
Boston, MA 02116
(617) 266–3322

Bimonthly commercial magazine about walking. $14.95 per year for subscription.

Walking Handbook
The Cooper Institute for Aerobics Research
12330 Preston Road
Dallas, Texas 75230
(800) 635–7050

Forty-page handbook on all aspects of walking. $6.95 per copy (plus postage).

---

with a group of similarly minded people. There is also increasing knowledge about the health benefits of walking. Dr. Ralph Paffenbarger of Stanford University studied 17,000 college alumni as they reached middle and later years. Men who walked briskly nine or more miles each week had 21 percent lower risk of death from heart disease than men who walked less than three miles each week.

The popularity of walking has led Americans to do what they do best, organize. There are walking clubs, walking trails, walking magazines, special walking shoes, and even a clearinghouse for information on walking. Information on these aspects of walking can be a real resource for the person losing or controlling their weight. It can help insure that walking is done correctly and that the experience can turn from drudgery to an enriching experience, both socially and physically.

Walking clubs and informal groups have blossomed all over the country. An example is the American Volkssport Association. This group organizes walking events such as a volkswalk, a 6- or 12-mile nontimed walk where the object is to meet people while enjoying exercise.

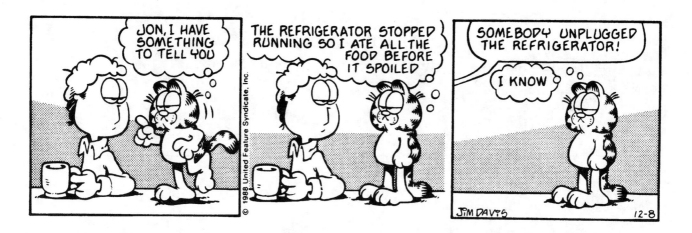

Another example is Walkabout International, a group that began as a small walking club in San Diego and now publishes a schedule listing more than 90 walks each month. Chapters have now formed in different cities. To find resources in your area, the information in the table here may be helpful. Also, check the weekend section of your newspaper for walking events, which may direct you to local clubs. Finally, many road-race events have fun walks attached to them.

More on Minerals

The body contains some 60 different minerals, about 22 of which are essential for life. There are great differences in the amounts of various minerals in the body. An example from the book *Introductory Nutrition* by Dr. Helen Guthrie, from which much of this discussion on minerals is drawn, is that of cobalt and calcium. As mentioned earlier, a deficiency in cobalt (only two parts per trillion of body weight) can be more damaging than a deficiency of calcium (fully 2 percent—two parts per hundred of body weight). The essential minerals are listed in Lesson 10.

Minerals serve to maintain the acid-base balance in the cells, to facilitate many biological reactions, to maintain water balance (sodium and potassium are the key minerals here), to form parts of essential body compounds, to regulate muscle contraction, to transmit nerve impulses, and to aid in growth of body tissue. It is important to consume sufficient amounts of minerals, but excessive amounts can be dangerous.

We will discuss three minerals of particular interest: calcium, sodium, and iron. These are the most frequently discussed minerals, and ones that have important implications for health. For a more detailed discussion of these and the other minerals, refer to the book by Dr. Helen Guthrie mentioned above.

Calcium

Most people think of calcium for its role in formation of bones and teeth. It does play this role, but so do other minerals. Also, this is not the only function of calcium. Approximately 2 percent of the body is calcium, almost all of which is in teeth or bones. An infant's bones are soft and incapable of sustaining much weight. Calcium helps the bones harden, a process called calcification or ossification. Calcium is necessary throughout life to sustain bone strength, but the amount actually needed by the body is often misunderstood. Inadequate calcium early in life makes one more susceptible to osteoporosis (a serious bone disease) in later years. However, there is dispute about how much calcium is needed. Different amounts are necessary during infancy, childhood, pregnancy, adult life, and the later years. The figures range from 540 mg/day for infants to 1200 mg/day for adults. The general RDA for calcium is one gram (1000 mg) per day.

Milk and milk products form the greatest supply of calcium in our diet. People who drink milk and eat milk products usually receive adequate calcium; males are more likely to do this than females. For people who avoid milk products, it is almost impossible to consume enough calcium from other foods to meet dietary standards. In addition to milk products, calcium is available in cereals, beans, some meats, poultry, fish, eggs, fruits, and vegetables.

The two conditions most commonly associated with calcium problems are kidney stones and osteoporosis. The issue of kidney stones is an easy one; there is no evidence that calcium intake is associated with the formation of stones. Osteoporosis is a different matter.

Osteoporosis is the condition of diminished bone mass. It occurs mainly in middle-aged and elderly women and can cause shortened stature, susceptibility to bone fractures, and pain in the lower back. There are multiple causes, but in many cases, calcium and sometimes fluoride supplementation can arrest this destructive process. This is a condition for a physician to monitor, so if you suspect this is an issue for you, speak with a doctor.

Sodium

Sodium is an important mineral which is present mainly in body fluids. It helps regulate fluid balance. Typical intake of sodium is between 3000 and 7000 mg per day, in the form of 7.5 to 18 grams of salt per day. A teaspoon of table salt provides 2000 mg of sodium, so to consume the three to seven grams of sodium daily means eating 1.5 to 4 teaspoons of salt. This seems like a lot, but the average person does it every day!

The suggested *safe and adequate* intake of sodium is 1100 to 3000 mg per day (½ to 1½ teaspoons per day). You can see that this is far below the average intake, so overconsumption of sodium is more a problem than underconsumption.

The sodium we consume comes from two sources: the salt naturally present in foods, and salt added during preparation and serving of food. Some foods, like bacon, are naturally high in sodium. Some foods have salt added in processing, as with some soups. Other foods usually have salt added after preparation (like French fries).

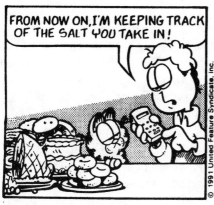
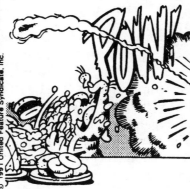
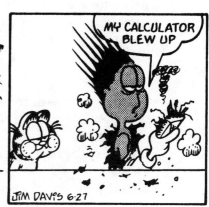

Sodium Content of Foods

Description	mg	Description	mg
Milk, Yogurt, and Cheese		**Fruits**	
Milk, 1 cup	120	Fruit, fresh, frozen, canned, ½ cup	Trace
Yogurt, 8 oz	160		
Natural cheeses, 1½ oz	110–450	**Bread, Cereal, Rice, and Pasta**	
Processed cheeses, 2 oz	800	Cooked cereal, rice, pasta, unsalted, ½ cup	Trace
		Ready-to-eat cereal, 1 oz	100–360
Meat, Poultry, Fish, etc.		Bread, 1 slice	110–175
Fresh meat, poultry, fish, 3 oz	Less than 90		
Tuna, canned, water pack, 3 oz	300	**Miscellaneous**	
Bologna, 2 oz	580	Salad dressing, 1T	75–220
Ham, lean, roasted, 3 oz	1,020	Peanuts, roasted in oil, salted, 1 oz	120
		Potato chips, salted, 1 oz	130
Vegetables		Ketchup, mustard, steak sauce, 1T	130–230
Vegetables, fresh, or frozen (cooked), ½ cup	Less than 70	Corn chips, salted, 1 oz	235
Vegetables, canned or frozen with sauce, ½ cup	140–460	Dill pickle, 1 medium	930
Tomato juice, canned, ¾ cup	660	Soy sauce, 1T	1,030
Vegetable soup, canned, 1 cup	820	Salt, 1t	2,000

An example of having salt added is the case of potato chips. A potato has only 1 mg of sodium per 100 grams, while the same weight of potato chips has 340–1000 grams. The table above shows the salt content of foods. The table was adapted from the *Home and Garden Bulletin Number 252.*

Sodium has been implicated in hypertension. This is the reason that individuals with high blood pressure are often prescribed a low-sodium diet. It has been recognized recently that increased potassium can lower blood pressure, so a combination of sodium restriction and potassium supplementation may be beneficial for blood pressure control.

It is possible to reduce sodium intake to about 3500 mg per day by limiting the use of table salt and by avoiding foods high in salt. To reduce the level further, to the 2000 mg or so recommended for blood pressure control, a strict diet of foods naturally low in sodium is neces-sary. This means eating very little of foods like canned soups, broth, canned vegetables, olives, cured foods, pickles, and salted foods like potato chips and crackers.

Iron

Compared to calcium and sodium, iron exists in rather small amounts in the body. It is still essential. Iron is found mainly in the blood, but some iron is present in every cell. Its primary function is to facilitate the transfer of oxygen and carbon dioxide among body tissues.

The need for iron varies according to age and sex. For instance, an adult man needs 0.9 to 1.2 mg of iron per day. Adult women require almost twice as much (1.4–2.2 mg/day), and adolescent girls need even more (1.9–3.7 mg/day). Liver is the only food that provides appreciable iron, so adding iron to the diet is often necessary. Much of this is done with food products that are fortified or enriched. Some 30 states require that flour be enriched, so additional iron is available in bread products.

Iron deficiency is not common, but can be serious when it does occur. It can result in anemia, which is a deficiency in the number or quality of red blood cells. Iron supplementation can usually remedy this problem.

Most people receive adequate iron in the diet and do not need supplements to prevent pseudo ailments like *iron poor blood*. People who suspect an iron problem should consult a physician or dietitian.

What does all this information on minerals mean? As with vitamins, most people receive adequate minerals if they eat a carefully chosen, balanced diet. However, there are special groups of people who require mineral supplements. Examples are needs for calcium in elderly women and iron in teenage girls. It is best to get specific advice from someone trained in nutrition.

A Note about Breakfast

We mentioned in an earlier lesson that many overweight people skip breakfast. This happens because they may not feel hungry in the morning, they are in a hurry, or they feel that skipping breakfast is a good way to start off the day by saving calories. Most people who successfully lose weight resume eating breakfast as they lose weight. This prevents the situation where you find yourself famished later in the day. To eat breakfast is consistent with the prevailing wisdom among health experts. There are some recent research findings that further support this view. Researchers at the University of Minnesota gave subjects one of five cereals ranging in fiber content, plus milk and orange juice, for breakfast at 7:30 a.m. At 11:00, the sub-

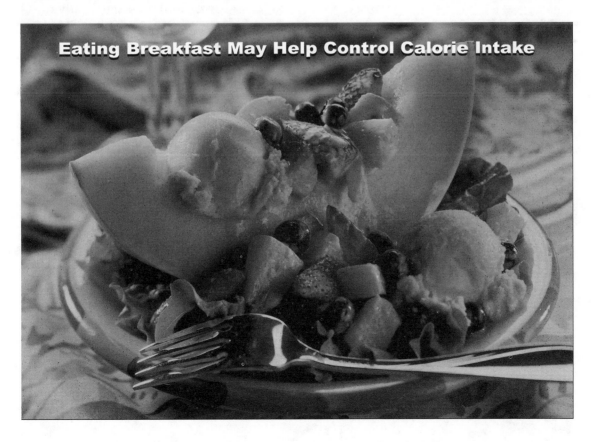

Eating Breakfast May Help Control Calorie Intake

jects were given a buffet lunch, and the amount eaten was carefully recorded. The subjects who had the high-fiber cereals ate fewer calories at lunch than did the people eating the low-fiber cereals. Especially important is that the people eating the high-fiber cereals ate fewer total calories (combining breakfast and lunch) than the subjects with the low-fiber cereals.

Starting the day with breakfast, especially a breakfast high in fiber, may help control calorie intake the rest of the day. In the research study we just described, subjects who ate the high-fiber cereals ate less at lunch even when they felt just as hungry as subjects having the other cereals. So, beginning the day with breakfast will probably help you control your weight. The guide to breakfast cereals in Lesson 15 will give you some guidance about the calorie and fiber content of various cereals. In addition to helping you eat less, the fiber may have positive health consequences.

Indeed, breakfast could be the foundation to developing overall healthy eating habits. This is especially true for children, since many habits learned as children carry over into adulthood. There are many creative ways to make breakfast fun, fast, and easy; it just takes a little planning and dedication. If you are a breakfast-skipper, the breakfast tips that follow may help you incorporate breakfast as an important part of your day. If you are still not convinced, try it for a couple of weeks. The benefits may surprise you.

> **No time?** Try getting up a few minutes earlier—10 minutes will do fine; once you are up and going you will not miss the time. This is plenty of time to have a glass of juice, a bowl of cereal, and some fruit.
> **Still no time?** Plan breakfast around foods that are ready to eat

or take little time to prepare. Examples include canned or fresh fruit, juices, milk, instant breakfast mixes, ready-to-eat cold cereals, yogurt, cheese, bagels, and toast.

> **Take it to go.** If you still find yourself short on time, pack yourself a breakfast-to-go the night before, and eat the following morning when you have a few extra minutes. Try celery stuffed with cheese, fresh or dried fruits, packaged juice or milk, breakfast bars, a bagel, or English muffin.
> **Be creative.** Top cereals with fresh fruit, add jelly or jam to toast, biscuits, or rolls, and add chopped nuts to hot cereals.
> **Not hungry?** Drink some juice, and take something with you for a snack later in the morning. Bread or crackers will do fine. You may wish to add some cheese or fruit. Then drink some milk or water.
> **Plan your breakfast the night before**. Make as much advanced preparation as possible. This way you are not confronted with the decision of what to prepare, and much of your meal can be ready and waiting for you when you wake up.
> **Start a breakfast partnership.** Enjoy the company of your spouse, a child, or a friend. Take turns making healthy breakfast choices. You can also take turns preparing breakfast with a breakfast partner.

Setting Personal Goals

Now is the time to begin keeping the Master Monitoring Form. Select the techniques important to you from the Master List of Techniques (Appendix A) and enter them on the form. We will discuss this in the Commencement Lesson, at which time you can develop a permanent version of the Master Monitoring Form.

You have now had many months of experience with setting personal goals. Therefore, you may wish to list goals on the Master Monitoring Form that are not listed in Appendix A. This is perfectly fine. It is not important that techniques you employ come from us—just that they work. You know best what works for you, and these are what you should enter on the form.

Self-Assessment Questionnaire

Lesson 24

T F 108. Certain techniques are essential for all individuals controlling their weight.

T F 109. Controlling your eating at a special event is easier if you eat something before you go.

T F 110. Iron deficiency is common, and many people need to supplement their eating with additional iron.

T F 111. The average person consumes more than twice the safe and adequate intake of salt each day.

(Answers in Appendix C)

Master Monitoring Form

Today's Date:

Time	Food and Amount	Calories
	Total Daily Calories	

Personal Goals This Week	*Always*	*Sometimes*	*Never*
1.			
2.			
3.			
4.			
5.			
6.			

Medication Taken Today ❏ Yes ❏ No	*Physical Activity*	*Minutes*
Milk, yogurt, and cheese ❏ ❏ ❏		
Meat, poultry, etc. ❏ ❏ ❏		
Fruits ❏ ❏ ❏ ❏		
Vegetables ❏ ❏ ❏ ❏ ❏		
Breads, cereals, etc. ❏ ❏ ❏ ❏ ❏ ❏ ❏ ❏ ❏ ❏		

Commencement Lesson

Here we are, the final lesson of The LEARN Program. We hope you have enjoyed your voyage and have acquired the knowledge and skills to use for permanent weight control. In this lesson we will discuss a few final steps, but will also look ahead to the future. There is more help available whether you want to lose additional weight or would like to maintain and stabilize. Let's finish with a flurry of excitement!

We call this the Commencement Lesson for the same reason colleges use this term to describe graduation ceremonies. Graduation celebrates a special ending, but more important, it signals the beginning (commencement) of a graduate's professional life. We celebrate your completion of this phase of your weight control efforts, and join hands with you as you launch into the next stage.

Interpreting Your Progress

At this stage in the program, individuals have had different experiences and weight losses. Some have done well and attained their goal, and others still have weight to lose. There are those who struggled at times and succeeded at others, but are on their way to a positive outcome. Others struggled throughout and lost no weight at all. Let's reflect on your progress and use it to forge a picture of the future.

Making the transition from the structure of the program to *free living* can be tricky for some people. If you are fearful of this transition or have had difficulty in the past when ending a program, some work in the "A" (Attitudes) part of the LEARN model might help.

Some people who complete programs have an unfortunate way of not taking credit when credit is due. When they do well on a program they attribute their success to the program, but if they flounder, they blame themselves. We hear people say, "Weight Watchers really helped me lose weight" and later say, "The Weight Watchers program was good, I just couldn't stick with it." This attitude can eventually wear away a person's confidence.

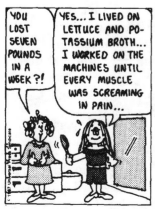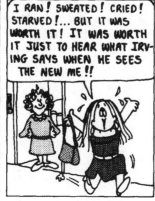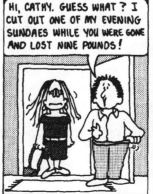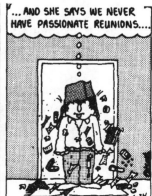

Like a batter on a baseball team, you don't have to hit a home run on every pitch!

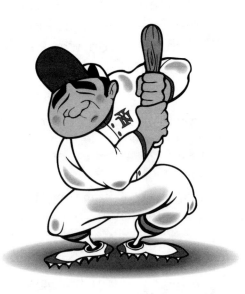

We prefer a different attitude. If you do well on a program, the credit is yours. The program only provides ideas and techniques, but you have the responsibility for implementing them. It is similar to using tools to build a house. Having the right tools can help, but someone has to make the effort to put it all together. Giving the program credit for weight loss is like giving the hammer credit for building the house. When we hear a virtuoso perform a masterpiece on the piano, do we give the piano credit? Whatever you have achieved is yours to boast about. You deserve to feel good and to remember that your efforts were at work. What does this mean?

If you have been responsible for making progress, the progress can continue. If the program has been responsible, it would be natural for you to fall apart. This is not the case, obviously, but beware of the tendency to give the program credit when the credit is yours.

In the past several paragraphs, we have spoken about the program *ending*. Do you notice the contradiction in this idea and the basic concepts of The LEARN Program? A primary thrust of our effort has been to learn new behaviors and habits that can become permanent. In this sense, the program does not end. The key issue is whether you can take away changes that you will live with. If so, we have accomplished part of our mission. If not, try to identify the lessons in the manual that can best facilitate this notion, and then reread the material. The sections on Attitudes are a good place to start.

If you have achieved less than you expected, what can we conclude? Again, the natural tendency is to despair and blame yourself. We do not feel this is fair. Over the course of a lifetime, overweight individuals go through periods of being very motivated and having the strength to try a program, and periods where nothing seems to work and starting a program is a series of false starts.

There are peaks of success and valleys of disappointment, with lots of terrain in-between. Individuals begin programs at many points in these stages. The ones who do best, of course, are those at the peaks. Those at the valleys have trouble. Others fall somewhere in the middle.

For a person who has not done well, we recommend two approaches. The first is to consider waiting until a peak comes along, and then try again. The right timing can be important. The second is to consider trying a different program. This program is not right for everyone, so if something else meets your needs, by all means try it.

Losing weight is like being a batter on a baseball team. You need not hit a home run on every pitch. Even if you strike out, you will have other chances at bat,

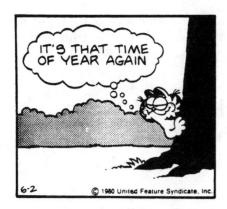
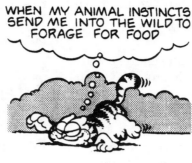
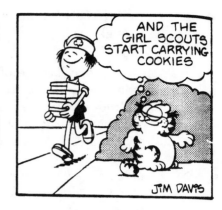

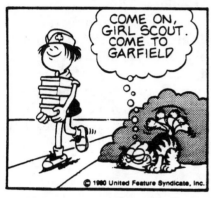
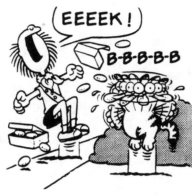
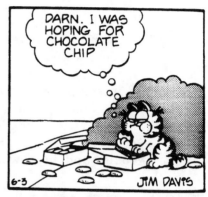

and even if you go hitless in one game, there will be other games. You just want to avoid a prolonged slump! So, keep a positive attitude and keep trying.

Remember Reasonable Weight?

In the very beginning of this program, we discussed the concept of "reasonable weight." Because most people begin programs with expectations of what they will weigh that are based on arbitrary and unrealistic beauty ideals or even on landmarks in their lives (when they got married, finished school, etc.), what should be viewed as terrific progress gets dismissed.

Let us tell a story about Susan. She began a program at 185 pounds saying she wanted to be 125. Susan weighed 125 when she got married but began gaining weight after she had children and had been no less than 150 most of her adult life. In the 52 weeks on the program, Susan lost 25 pounds, and weighed 160. Instead of celebrating the 25 pounds she did lose, she was focused on the remaining weight. How reasonable is it for her to think that 125 is the only acceptable weight?

You may have lost as much weight as you set out to lose, but if not, which is the case with many people, it is important to view what you have done in a positive context. There is no reason to expect perfection—we do not expect the perfect job, the perfect hair, the perfect eyes, the perfect nose—the perfect life. Why, then, are we only satisfied with total weight loss? The answer is that society teaches us that weight is under total control of the individual, and we have ideals that are highly unrealistic. It would be like saying there is only one acceptable eye color and that people with other colors were imperfect and weren't trying hard enough to change who they are.

You may be one of the many people who would like to weigh much less but will not or cannot. The choice, then, is whether to wage a wholesale assault on your self-esteem by feeling there is something wrong, or to accept what is reasonable and feel good about progress you are able to make. You know which path we favor.

A great deal of research has been done on goal setting. It won't surprise you to hear that people get frustrated, disappointed, and even depressed when they do not reach their goals. Goals, therefore, have to be challenging, but not impossible to reach. By setting realistic goals, and by rewarding yourself for

reaching them, your self-esteem will increase and you will be in a much better position to sustain changes you make.

Making Your Habits Permanent

There are several keys to developing permanent habits. *Practice* is one such key. The 25 lessons in this program may not provide enough time for all your habits to change. Eating habits develop over years and years, so we must be patient for the changes to become permanent. By the time a person is 40, at least 40,000 meals have been consumed. This is lots of practice, so new habits may take time.

Another key is *awareness*. Try to remain a student of your eating and exercise habits. Be aware of what stimulates your eating and of methods for turning the tide. The Master Monitoring Form is designed with this in mind.

Examining Your Master Monitoring Form

We introduced the Master Monitoring Form in the last lesson to give you some experience with it. How did it work for you? This seemingly simple step of getting the form in good order can be quite important. It can help you define which techniques are important for you, and can provide feedback on how you are doing. Let's review the procedures for making the form work to your advantage.

As we mentioned in Lesson 24, many clients generally list record keeping as one of the most important aspects of the program. You may remember from the

Record Keeping Can Be a Key in Weight Control

early lessons that record keeping has several virtues. It reminds you of the techniques that can help you lose weight and can give you positive feedback about changes you make. It can also help control eating because there is always some accountability when the record is filled out every day.

You can add or delete techniques from the form you completed in Lesson 24. The Master List of Techniques (Appendix A) shows all the techniques used in the program. Pick the ones most likely to help. This is a good time to refer back to the Behavior Chain you completed in Lesson 21. This showed how trouble can be avoided by interrupting the eating chain at various places. This may give you clues for techniques to add to the Master Monitoring Form.

Don't hesitate to change the Master Monitoring Form in the weeks ahead. A blank form is provided in this lesson. Make as many copies as you need. We recommended in the last lesson that you continue to complete this form for at least eight more weeks. Do it well beyond this point if it will help. We know some people who have kept forms like this for more than 10 years.

Doing a Master Self-Assessment

Appendix B and Appendix C contain the questions and answers for the Master Self-Assessment. These are taken from each lesson in the program. Try doing a Master Self-Assessment by answering the questions after the lessons and comparing your answers to those in Appendix C. You may want to study the manual until you get all the questions correct. Wrong answers can clue you to areas where you need to solidify your knowledge.

A Special Guide for Weight Maintenance

As we mentioned in the previous lesson, we have received many requests from people using The LEARN Program to provide a follow-up guide. Some people wanted help with losing more weight while others wanted information on maintenance and stabilization. Now such a guide is available, *The LEARN Weight Maintenance and Stabilization Guide*. This detailed, step-by-step guide is designed to focus on approaches that are specific to long-term weight control.

The skills necessary to keep weight off are different from those needed to lose weight initially. One must settle into a routine that becomes stable. Long-term motivation and commitment are central to this endeavor, and one must solidify the thoughts, actions, and feelings necessary for permanent changes. The guide is written with just this in mind. It contains practical information drawn from the many suggestions received from people, from research done at our clinics and from many other research centers, and from many years of experience working with people on maintaining weight loss.

Information on obtaining *The LEARN Maintenance and Stabilization Program* is available by calling the LEARN Education Center at 1–800–736–7323, by writing to the address listed at the back of this book, or by the Internet at www.Learneducation.com.

Where to Go from Here

There are a number of options you might consider for losing more weight, for maintaining what you have lost, or for getting back on the right path if you falter. These are just suggestions—you might have better ideas of your own. The key is to have a plan, to know what path you will follow, and to know when the plan should be put into action. Here are some of the things to consider.

Use *The LEARN Weight Maintenance and Stabilization Guide*

This guide, discussed above, has been developed around the issues specific to further weight loss, stabilization and maintenance. It is written in the same tone and spirit as *The LEARN Program* and is meant to be friendly, welcoming, easy-to-use, and optimistic. It deals with issues such as crisis intervention, self-confidence, body image, a flexible eating plan you can maintain, and how to enjoy yourself while still maintaining control. This guide can be ordered by calling 1-800-736-7323.

Use *The LEARN Program* Again

You might start at the beginning and follow the program through as if you were doing it for the first time. Many people do this. It is not a sign that they failed the first time around. Rather, it shows they know what works for them, and they know when to go back to it. An alternative to starting at the beginning is to use sections in the manual that are most pertinent to you at the time. For example, if holidays are throwing you for a loop, you could pay attention to the sections dealing with this topic.

You may want to pay special attention to the goals you set at the end of each lesson (in the Setting Personal Goals section). The aim of this section was to encourage you to find goals that were particularly important for you. Chances are these goals are still important. Focusing on them is a good way to keep your program moving along as you wish.

Consider Medication

A number of leading experts feel that weight loss medications should be considered for use over the long-term, to help people maintain a healthier weight. Therefore, you may still be taking MERIDIA. If not, and you feel medication might be helpful, consult your physician. The two of you are in the best position to judge whether taking medication will be a useful course of action.

Enlist Social Support

If you find your motivation flagging, enlisting a friend or a support partner might be just the thing you need. Two people working together can produce a synergy where each motivates the other and in turn enhances self-motivation. Besides, working with another person on some common goal can really be fun. There is abundant material in this manual on how to identify support people, how to enlist their help, and how to communicate in positive ways to keep the support flowing.

Join a Program

Many commercial and self-help programs are available, each offering different approaches. There is no single best approach, but rather best fits between approaches and individuals. Stated another way, some might be better for you and others better for different people.

If you think a program might help, focus on what the most important features of a program are for you. Do you need a structured meal plan, prepared foods, a place to exercise, support from others in the program, a trained counselor, frequent meetings, convenience, low cost, or other factors important to you? Then think about which program does the best job of meeting your needs.

Some people find programs a great help in special times of need. For in-

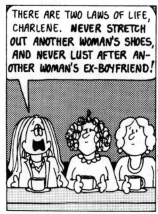 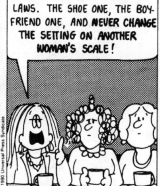 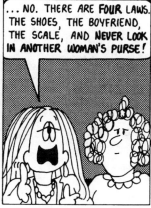 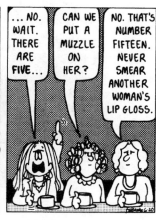

stance, a person might attend Overeaters Anonymous meetings every few months as a "booster" to their program. This is like getting booster shots to keep immunity high after an initial immunization. Another person might rejoin Weight Watchers at the sign of some crisis (they feel control is slipping, or they have regained some weight).

See a Professional

Professionals offer support and expert advice in a number of areas. By now you should have a good sense of areas where you are strong and other areas where you struggle. Let's take compulsive eating (binge eating) as an example. Many people find that their compulsive eating gets better when following The LEARN Program, but not all. In this case, seeing a psychologist or other health professional to deal with this problem could be a big help. What follows is a list of common problems and suggestions for a professional to see.

➤ For nutrition advice
—see a Registered Dietitian

➤ For medical problems
—see a Physician

➤ For medication
—see a Physician

➤ For compulsive eating
—see a Specialist in eating disorders (Psychologist, Psychiatrist, or Social Worker)

➤ For lack of exercise
—see a Personal Trainer or Exercise Specialist

➤ For life stresses
—see a Psychologist, Psychiatrist, or Social Worker

➤ For depression, anxiety
—see a Psychologist, Psychiatrist, or Social Worker

➤ For relationship problems
—see a Psychologist, Psychiatrist, or Social Worker

➤ For weight control
—see someone with training in exercise, nutrition, or psychology, or a Certified LifeStyle Counselor

Looking at Your Quality of Life

For one final time, we provide our survey on quality of life (see next page). Take a minute to complete it, and then compare your responses to those from the same survey you filled out in the Introduction and Orientation. Have you seen improvements, and in what areas? Are you pleased with the changes?

The Quality of Life Self-Assessment points out several important points. The first is that when a person sets out to lose weight, he or she should ask why. People we ask tell us they want to look better

Quality of Life Self-Assessment

Please use the following scale to rate how satisfied you feel now about different aspects of your daily life. Choose any number from this list (1 to 9) and indicate your choice on the questions below.

1 = Extremely Dissatisfied	6 = Somewhat Satisfied
2 = Very Dissatisfied	7 = Moderately Satisfied
3 = Moderately Dissatisfied	8 = Very Satisfied
4 = Somewhat Dissatisfied	9 = Extremely Satisfied
5 = Neutral	

1. ___ Mood (feelings of sadness, worry, happiness, etc.)
2. ___ Self-esteem
3. ___ Confidence, self-assurance and comfort in social situations
4. ___ Energy and feeling healthy
5. ___ Health problems (diabetes, high blood pressure, etc.)
6. ___ General appearance
7. ___ Social life
8. ___ Leisure and recreational activities
9. ___ Physical mobility and physical activity
10. ___ Eating habits
11. ___ Body image
12. ___ Overall quality of life

(have better body image), have more energy, improve their health, feel better about moving around, etc. It is essential, then, that people look to these areas as ways to judge their performance. As we said several times, the scale is only one index of your success. If a person eats a better diet, and is physically active, many quality of life areas can improve, even if weight does not.

If you made strides in any area of the survey, you deserve to feel good. Improving your day-to-day life is a major accomplishment indeed. As you move on through the months and years, reward yourself for making these changes and remember what advantages you can achieve by healthy eating, physical activity, and weight control.

If you experienced any medical gains, you should feel especially blessed. Changes such as reduced blood pressure and cholesterol, or better control of blood sugar, are terribly important. These can pay off big time.

Our Salute to You!

If you have been following the LEARN lessons as they were designed, it should now be about 11 months (or 48 weeks) since you started the program. By the time you complete this lesson, it will be a year. Let's place this in context. Some people start diets and give up the same day. Others last a few days, perhaps a few weeks, or on rare occasions, a few months. Why?

Many programs are fads, and people find quickly that they are impossible to follow or simply don't work. And let's face it—sticking to any program for a long time is difficult. A person in for the long haul encounters many challenges, will feel deprived, will think "it's not fair when other people can eat all they want," and may get frustrated by slow progress. Hence, many people get off the train before it has reached its final destination.

We salute you for staying with the program! It is a REALLY good sign that you have been able to think of your weight control plan as something that requires persistence and flexibility over the long term. It would be nice if there were some easy solution, but when all is said and done, even with the help of weight loss medications, it comes down to personal effort. We are delighted that you have made the effort and hope that the rewards have been and will continue to be substantial. If we could be there with you right now, we'd be standing side by side giving you a standing ovation!

Ending Where We Began

We can end where we began—with emphasizing the most important principles of all. You may recall that one of the first things we mentioned was a concept called self-efficacy. It tells us that the people most likely to make successful, long-term changes are those with the skills and confidence to do so. You have learned many skills—skills to help you confront difficult situations, to handle setbacks, to make changes you can live

with, and to enjoy the whole process. You hold your weight control future in your hands. Use the skills and you'll do just fine.

You should be confident in your ability. You should not and could not be confident that you will be perfect, or that you will have an easy path to your goal. But, you can be confident that despite bumps in the road, occasional detours, and perhaps even getting lost on occasion, you can find your way back to the road and continue on your important journey.

Give yourself a pep talk when you need it. If you were your own coach, think about what you would need to hear to be most effective, and then inspire yourself in that way. Do whatever you can to be confident that you have the necessary skills, and then use the skills, use the skills, and use them some more. It can work.

A Final Weight Change Record

We leave you with one final Weight Change Record. You will find it on page 307. We have replaced the week number at the bottom of the form with blank lines along with the weight change in pounds. This is so you can start the chart at any point in time.

Saying Farewell

Let us offer our sincere hope that you enjoyed this program and that you are on your way to accomplishing your weight loss goals. It can be a hard struggle, but with the right attitude and new habits, success can be yours. Keep up the spirit!

Finally, please contact us with your ideas and comments about this program.

Success stories are welcome, as are suggestions for improving the program. We pay attention to what we hear and would like to hear from you. Send comments to us at:

American Health Publishing Company
P.O. Box 35328, Dept. 10
Dallas, TX 75235-0328

You may also fax or e-mail your comments to us at the numbers listed in the very beginning of this book.

Good luck!!

Good Luck!

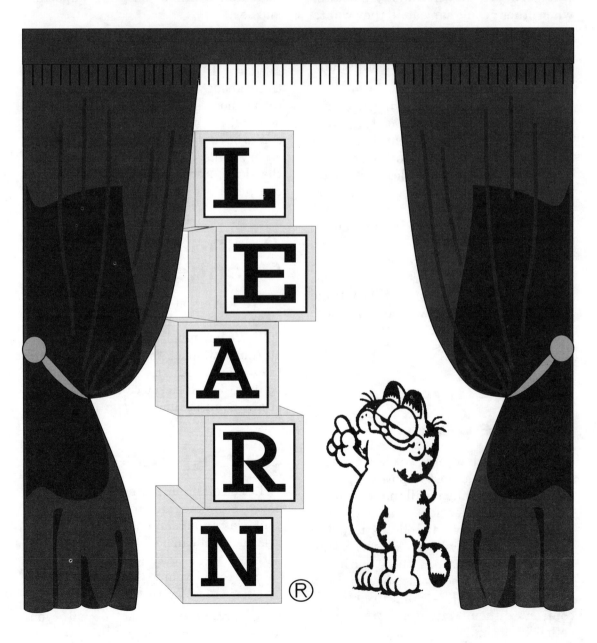

Weight Change Record

Weight Change (in pounds)

Week

307

Master Monitoring Form

Today's Date:

Time	Food and Amount	Calories
	Total Daily Calories	

Personal Goals This Week	*Always*	*Sometimes*	*Never*
1.			
2.			
3.			
4.			
5.			
6.			

Medication Taken Today ❑ Yes ❑ No	*Physical Activity*	*Minutes*
Milk, yogurt, and cheese ❑ ❑ ❑		
Meat, poultry, etc. ❑ ❑ ❑		
Fruits ❑ ❑ ❑ ❑		
Vegetables ❑ ❑ ❑ ❑ ❑		
Breads, cereals, etc. ❑ ❑ ❑ ❑ ❑ ❑ ❑ ❑ ❑		

Appendix A

Master List of Techniques

Lifestyle Techniques

1. Alter the antecedents to eating (the behavior chain) . . . 251
2. Avoid being a food dispenser . . . 157
3. Buy foods that require preparation 137
4. Do not clean your plate 78
5. Do nothing else while eating 77
6. Eat in one place. 78
7. Examine patterns in your eating 34
8. Follow an eating schedule 77
9. Follow the five-minute rule 158
10. Identify triggers for eating 198
11. Identify your behavior chains 254
12. Interrupt your behavior chains . . 254
13. Keep a food diary. 20
14. Keep a weight change record. . . . 22
15. Keep problem foods out of sight. 146
16. Keep healthy foods visible 146
17. Leave the table after eating 158
18. Maximize awareness of eating . . . 20
19. Pause during the meal 90
20. Plan in advance for high-risk situations 267
21. Prepare in advance for special events 287
22. Prevent automatic eating. 34
23. Put your fork down between bites. 89
24. Remove serving dishes from table 158
25. Serve and eat one portion at a time 158
26. Shop from a list 136
27. Shop on a full stomach 136
28. Take medication daily 43
29. Use the ABC approach. 75
30. Use alternatives to eating 268
31. Use techniques for eating away from home 239

Exercise Techniques

32. Always warm up and cool down 169
33. Choose and use a programmed activity 167
34. Counter the exercise threshold concept. 66
35. Experiment with jogging 229
36. Experiment with cycling 230
37. Experiment with aerobics. 244
38. Increase lifestyle activity 103
39. Increase walking 71
40. Keep an exercise diary. 219
41. Know the calorie values of exercise 126
42. Maximize pleasure of walking . . . 70
43. Understand the benefits of exercise. 48
44. Use stairs whenever possible . . . 257
45. Use the pulse test for fitness feedback 92

Attitude Techniques

46. Ban perfectionist attitudes 134
47. Banish imperatives 136
48. Be a Forest Ranger for urges and lapses 277
49. Be aware of high-risk situations. . 267
50. Beware of attitude traps. 143
51. Confront or ignore cravings . . . 114
52. Cope positively with slips and lapses. 275
53. Counter food and weight fantasies 130
54. Counter impossible dream thinking 155
55. Distinguish hunger from cravings 114
56. Distinguish lapse and relapse . . . 266

57. Focus on behavior rather
    than weight 42
58. Outlast urges to eat 267
59. Realize complex causes
    of obesity 97
60. Set realistic goals 116
61. Stop dichotomous thinking 144
62. Use six steps to gain control
    during lapses 275
63. Use the shaping concept for
    habit change 116

Relationship Techniques

64. Do shopping with your partner . . 124
65. Exercise with partner 60
66. Explain your program with
    friends and family. 9
67. Have partner do shopping for you 137
68. Have partner and family
    read this manual 172
69. Identify and select a support person 101
70. Make specific and positive
    requests of partner 102
71. Refuse pressures to eat 205
72. Reward your partner 103
73. Seek additional support 10
74. Tell your partner how to help . . . 102
75. Use pleasurable partner
    activities 245

Nutrition Techniques

76. Be aware of calorie values
    of foods. 239
77. Choose a diet low in fat, saturated
    fat, and cholesterol 36
78. Choose a diet with plenty of
    vegetables, fruits, and grains. . . . 36
79. Consume adequate vitamins 223
80. Deal with pressures to eat 205
81. Determine your target calorie
    level 46
82. Drink alcohol in moderation 36
83. Eat a balanced diet 35
84. Eat a variety of foods 36
85. Eat appropriate servings from the
    five food groups 81
86. Eating away from home 239
87. Follow a balanced diet 35
88. Get adequate carbohydrate
    in your diet. 159
89. Get adequate protein in diet 148
90. Hide high-calorie foods 146
91. Increase complex
    carbohydrates 161
92. Increase fiber in diet 231
93. Keep healthy snacks available . . . 146
94. Know the food guide pyramid . . . 36
95. Limit fat to 30 percent of
    total calories 110
96. Make low-calorie foods appetizing 113
97. Make small dietary changes you
    can live with. 44
98. Read food labels 211
99. Select an eating plan. 38
100. Set a calorie goal. 46
101. Take no more than
    recommended doses of vitamins . 209
102. Use salt in moderation 36
103. Use sugars in moderation 36
104. Watch the calories from
    alcohol 233

Appendix B

Master Self-Assessment

	True	*False*

Lesson 1

1. It is best to call your doctor if you have any questions about the side effects of your medication. _____ _____

2. A good way to be certain to take a medication on schedule is to take it at the same time and place every day. _____ _____

3. People who take weight loss medications don't need to worry about the foods they choose to eat. The medication does all the work. _____ _____

4. Very few people can accurately estimate the quantity and calories of food. _____ _____

5. Record keeping may be the most important aspect of a weight loss program. _____ _____

Lesson 2

6. Automatic eating is common in overweight people and distracts them from the taste of food. _____ _____

7. The Food Diary helps uncover patterns in your eating habits. _____ _____

8. The five food groups are Milk and Yogurt Products, Vegetables, Fruits, Meats and Proteins, and Breads and Cereals. _____ _____

9. Ice cream and several other high-sugar desserts are not allowed in this program. _____ _____

Lesson 3

10. Exercise isn't of much use for weight loss because it burns relatively few calories. _____ _____

11. Exercise can help prevent the loss of muscle tissue during weight loss. _____ _____

12. The calorie is the measure of the amount of fat in food. _____ _____

13. The calorie level necessary to lose weight is the same for all people. _____ _____

Lesson 4

14. Walking one mile burns almost as many calories as running the mile. _____ _____

15. Expensive exercise suits are worth the money because the special materials help the body. _____ _____

16. Everyone should walk with a partner because the company increases pleasure. _____ _____

17. You can identify your triggers and high-risk situations for overeating by keeping a food diary and examining it carefully. _____ _____

18. You should weigh yourself every morning. _____ _____

Lesson 5

19. Weight loss is the best measure of success in The LEARN Program.

20. Most people have difficulty estimating the amounts of food they eat and the calories they consume.   ____   ____

21. Exercise produces large weight losses on a short-term basis.   ____   ____

22. Binge eating is characterized by eating large amounts of food with an accompanying sense of loss of control.   ____   ____

23. Exercise must be strenuous in order to be beneficial.   ____   ____

Lesson 6

24. The ABC approach stands for Alternatives, Behavior, and Consciousness.   ____   ____

25. It can be helpful to develop a militant attitude about the "toxic food environment" we face.   ____   ____

26. By Lesson 6 in this program, nearly everyone has developed a plan of regular, vigorous physical activity.   ____   ____

27. It is helpful to set specific, concrete, and attainable goals at each step of the program.   ____   ____

28. If you eat an equal number of servings from the five food groups of the Food Guide Pyramid, you will have a balanced diet.   ____   ____

29. Eating on a schedule is not advisable because it is too regimented.   ____   ____

Lesson 7

30. Research has shown that social support can be intrusive and does not help with lifestyle changes such as weight loss.   ____   ____

31. Eating rapidly helps you enjoy food more because the taste buds get more stimulation.   ____   ____

32. Pausing during a meal increases food intake because the body digests food and sends out signals to eat more.   ____   ____

33. Your resting pulse will increase as you lose weight and get in better condition.   ____   ____

34. Exercise is not a good predictor of who will keep weight off over the long-run, but the health benefits are reason enough to do it.   ____   ____

Lesson 8

35. Discovering the psychological roots of your weight problem is the most important factor in weight reduction.   ____   ____

36. All overweight people have an excessive number of fat cells.   ____   ____

37. There is no such thing as a slow or underactive metabolism.   ____   ____

38. You should tell your program partner in specific terms how he or she can help.   ____   ____

39. It is important to reinforce your partner for helping you.   ____   ____

Lesson 9

40. Since too much dietary fat has been linked to heart disease and other health-related risks, it's best to eliminate all fat from your diet.   ____ ____

41. The recommended daily intake of dietary fat is 30 percent or less of total calories.   ____ ____

42. One gram of fat contains more than twice the calories of one gram of carbohydrate or protein.   ____ ____

43. Saturated fat is usually solid at room temperature and is found only in animal foods, such as meats and dairy products made from whole milk or cream.   ____ ____

44. Since all fruits and vegetables have only small amounts of fats, it is not as important to count the amount of fat in these foods as it is to count the dietary fat from meat and dairy products.   ____ ____

45. To conquer food cravings, distraction will be helpful for some people and confirmation will be helpful for other.   ____ ____

46. Shaping refers to encouraging others to help you lose weight.   ____ ____

Lesson 10

47. Most people get enough exercise to realize the many health benefits of an active lifestyle.   ____ ____

48. Exercise must be done in specific amounts for it to aid you with weight loss.   ____ ____

49. Thirty minutes of moderate-intensity physical activity is now recommended for Americans.   ____ ____

50. Climbing stairs requires more energy per minute than many traditional exercises like swimming and jogging.   ____ ____

51. All nutrients that we eat contain calories.   ____ ____

Lesson 11

52. Thoughts and attitudes generally occur out of our control and are automatic when we are confronted by certain situations.   ____ ____

53. When taking medication for weight loss, it is important to appreciate how essential the drug is to your success.   ____ ____

54. It is wise to shop for food when you are hungry to test the new restraint you have learned.   ____ ____

55. Buying foods that require preparation can increase your awareness of eating and help you eat less.   ____ ____

56. The recommended number of daily servings from the Milk, Yogurt, and Cheese Group is two to three.   ____ ____

Lesson 12

57. Keeping high-calorie foods stored out of sight can decrease impulsive eating.   ____ ____

58. Fat thoughts can hinder a person's efforts to lose weight.   ____ ____

True   False

59. Light bulb or dichotomous thinking refers to your own bright ideas about losing weight.   _____   _____

60. The only way to get high-quality protein in your diet is to eat foods from the Meat, Poultry, Fish, Dry Beans, Eggs, & Nuts Group of The Food Guide Pyramid.   _____   _____

61. A diet very high in protein will facilitate weight loss.   _____   _____

Lesson 13

62. It is best to take all of what you will eat in one serving so you will not need additional helpings.   _____   _____

63. Impossible Dream Thinking is having fantasies and images about weight loss, life as a thin person, etc.   _____   _____

64. Carbohydrates are not as important as other nutrients, and they should make up only about 30 percent of your daily diet.   _____   _____

65. The Food Guide Pyramid suggests three to five servings each day from the Vegetable Group.   _____   _____

66. It is important for me to appreciate the hard work I am doing to change my behavior and not give all the credit for weight loss to the medication.   _____   _____

67. I should expect to lose about the same amount of weight as the weeks go on, as long as I take my medication as prescribed.   _____   _____

Lesson 14

68. Warming up and stretching before exercise is to strengthen your muscles.   _____   _____

69. To get a cardiovascular training effect, there must be the right combination of frequency, intensity, and time.   _____   _____

70. If a partner is working with you to lose weight, it is important to reward him or her for the help they provide.   _____   _____

71. Fruits, vegetables, and cereals tend to be high in fiber.   _____   _____

72. Most Americans eat plenty of fruits and should not worry about increasing their daily intake.   _____   _____

Lesson 15

73. Exercise can be difficult for many individuals, and may present a psychological barrier to some.   _____   _____

74. No exercise can help you lose fat in specific parts of the body.   _____   _____

75. Foods from the Bread, Cereal, Rice, and Pasta Group are a good source of complex carbohydrates but may contain hidden fat.   _____   _____

76. One characteristic common to overweight persons is that they seldom eat breakfast.   _____   _____

Lesson 16

77. The best kind of exercise is rigorous enough to build muscle, which in turn speeds up metabolism.   _____   _____

78. Many people internalize society's unrealistic standards for beauty, weight, and shape, and are likely to have a negative body image. _____ _____

79. It is possible to weigh more than the ideal, and even be fairly heavy, and still have good self-esteem and reasonable body image. _____ _____

80. Medication can be as important to weight maintenance as it is to weight loss. _____ _____

Lesson 17

81. It's not important to involve family members in your weight loss program since behavior changes are all up to you. _____ _____

82. When someone offers you food, it is best to accept it as a sign of friendship. _____ _____

83. Imperatives are words like always and never. They leave no room for error. _____ _____

84. Vitamin B$_{12}$ is the only vitamin for which mega-doses are recommended. _____ _____

85. The Total Fat listed under the heading "% Daily Value" on the Nutrition Facts Panel of the Food Label indicates the percentage of calories from fat for one serving of the food. _____ _____

Lesson 18

86. It is essential that you continue to record your food intake and physical activity every day—there are no exceptions to this rule. _____ _____

87. Weight loss generally slows after the first four to five months of any program, once people have lost approximately 10 percent of their initial weight. _____ _____

88. Weight loss medications lose their potency after the first several months. This is evident from the slower rate of weight loss after months four or five. _____ _____

89. Fat soluble vitamins give you energy, but water soluble vitamins do not. _____ _____

Lesson 19

90. There are many benefits to jogging and cycling. They are good forms of exercise for people trying to lose weight. _____ _____

91. A diet high in fiber may help protect against certain diseases. _____ _____

92. A healthy diet should contain between 25 and 35 grams of fiber each day. _____ _____

93. Alcohol is not usually a problem for weight control because it has a number of nutrients. _____ _____

Lesson 20

94. Alcohol can be a problem when eating out because it contains many calories and weakens dietary restraint. _____ _____

95. Ordering à la carte meals at restaurants helps avoid unwanted calories that come in package meals. _____ _____

96. Aerobic activities are designed to build strength in the shortest possible time. _____ _____

True *False*

97. Vitamin E is associated with virility and may help in the remedy of alcoholism. ____ ____

Lesson 21

98. Once the eating chain begins, it is not possible to stop because the links are so strong. ____ ____

99. A Behavior Chain, like any chain, is only as strong as its weakest links. ____ ____

100. It is best to interrupt an eating chain at one of its last links when you know what foods confront you. ____ ____

101. Using stairs is a convenient and accessible way for many people to increase activity. ____ ____

Lesson 22

102. When a person lapses, relapse is close behind because nothing can interrupt the negative cycle of lapses and out-of-control eating. ____ ____

103. It helps to have a list of alternatives to eating for use when urges strike. ____ ____

104. The emphasis on fiber may be dangerous because fiber is indigestible material that can harm the intestinal system. ____ ____

Lesson 23

105. Getting nervous or anxious during a lapse is helpful because anxiety interferes with appetite and allows you to remove yourself from temptation. ____ ____

106. When dealing with a lapse, it is best to move quickly and decisively before control erodes even further. ____ ____

107. For controlling your blood cholesterol, it is important to limit intake of saturated fat. ____ ____

Lesson 24

108. Certain techniques are essential for all individuals controlling their weight. ____ ____

109. Controlling your eating at a special event is easier if you eat something before you go. ____ ____

110. Iron deficiency is common and many people need to supplement their eating with additional iron. ____ ____

111. The average person consumes more than twice the safe and adequate intake of salt each day. ____ ____

Appendix C

Answers for Self-Assessment Questions

Lesson 1

1. True   Your doctor is in the best position to know whether symptoms you experience are due to the medication. Your doctor may be able to change the dose to minimize side-effects and to promote weight loss.

2. True   This helps establish a routine that can be a useful reminder each day.

3. False   The medication is an aid, but the choices of what to eat are yours. Don't forget to take credit when you lose weight—it is your effort that makes the difference.

4. True   One study found that persons losing weight who observed common foods and estimated quantity and calories averaged errors of 60 percent. Therefore, using a calorie guide and scale is important.

5. True   Persons who have lost weight and maintained their loss often report that record keeping was one key to their success.

Lesson 2

6. True   Many overweight people eat without paying attention to all they consume. They miss the taste in much of what they eat.

7. True   The Food Diary helps you discover times, foods, feelings, and activities associated with eating.

8. True   These are the five food groups of the Food Guide Pyramid. In order to have a balanced diet, a variety of foods should be eaten from these groups.

9. False   No foods are prohibited. You can learn to eat any foods in moderation. Making foods illegal only sets up a person for failure.

Lesson 3

10. False   Exercise has many benefits aside from the calories you burn. It is one of the *most* important aspects of weight control.

11. True   Exercise maximizes the loss of fat and can prevent the loss of muscle. Exercise combined with diet is preferable to diet alone for weight loss.

12. False   The calorie is a measure of the energy your body gets from a food. Fat supplies some of these calories in some foods, but so do carbohydrate and protein.

13. False   There are differences in how much weight people lose on the same caloric intake. Some people need to make a greater restriction in caloric intake than do others in order to lose weight.

Lesson 4

14. True   How far you go is more important than how fast you go, so walking is an ideal exercise. Of course, running will get the job done faster!

15. False   Expensive exercise clothes contain no special materials and have no advantage over clothes most people have anyway. Their only advantage is cosmetic.

16. False   Many people do profit from exercising with a partner, but many enjoy doing their exercise alone. It is a matter of individual preference.

17. True   Your food diary will allow you to identify times, places, activities, and other events which are frequently associated with your overeating. Identifying these situations will allow you to intervene appropriately.

18. False   You decide how frequently you should weigh yourself. Some people benefit from daily weighings, but others do not. It is your call.

Lesson 5

19. False   Weight loss is one measure of success. Equally if not more important are improved health, fitness, and quality of life.

20. True — Most people underestimate their daily calorie intake by at least 20 percent. This comes from forgetting to record some of the foods, underestimating their portion sizes, and being unaware of hidden calories in foods.

21. False — Exercise increases weight loss only slightly on a week-to-week basis. The real benefits of exercise are in improving physical and emotional well being, as well as improving the maintenance of weight loss.

22. True — A significant minority of overweight persons suffer from binge eating. The LEARN Program may help with this problem, as may other resources described in Lesson 5.

23. False — The great news about exercise is that short bouts of activity, performed at a comfortable level, will improve your health and fitness. Small amounts of activity add up over the course of the day.

Lesson 6

24. False — The ABC approach stands for Antecedents, Behavior, and Consequences. It shows the importance of what occurs before, during, and after eating.

25. True — Just like many people get angry at tobacco companies trying to peddle their toxic products, it can be helpful to think of food advertisements, restaurants that serve enormous portions, and fast food restaurants with tricks like drive-through windows, package meals, and very large servings of things like fries as an enemy trying to take your money and make you sick. Resist!!!

26. False — Some people take longer than others to become active because new habits take a while to develop. Also, vigorous activity isn't necessarily the goal. If you do vigorous activity, fine, but anything you do to be more active will be helpful.

27. True — Goals help keep you oriented to the areas of greatest importance, and provide a way for you to reward yourself when you make positive changes.

28. False — Different numbers of servings are recommended for each of the five food groups. Refer to Lesson 6 for specific information.

29. False — Eating on a schedule helps define the times you eat so that you minimize the times of the day associated with eating.

Lesson 7

30. False — Considerable research has been done on social support and shows that people who have more support tend to have better health and tend to do better in many areas of life.

31. False — Taste buds catch nothing but a blur if the food shoots past like a rocket. Slowing down can help you enjoy food more.

32. False — Pausing gives the body a chance to signal that enough has been eaten. It can keep you satisfied with less food.

33. False — As your weight declines and you become more fit, your resting heart rate will probably decline, showing that your heart can accomplish its work with fewer beats.

34. False — Exercise is one predictor of who will keep weight off in the long run.

Lesson 8

35. False — Psychological problems are not at the root of all cases of overweight. There is no evidence that uncovering these *causes* helps with weight loss.

36. False — People who have been overweight in childhood may have excessive fat cells, but other overweight persons may not. They have fat cells that are too large.

37. False — There are wide variations in metabolic rate among different people. Some are cursed with a *slow metabolism* and may be prone to easy weight gains in body weight.

38. True — Do not expect your partner to read your mind. Tell your partner exactly what he or she can do to help. Remember, be specific, ask for positive changes, and be nice to your partner in return.

39. True — Relationships are two-way streets. You want your support partner to feel good about helping you, so more help will come your way. Reinforcing him or her for helping is a great way to see that this happens.

Lesson 9

40. False   Fat plays an important role in the body and should not be eliminated from your diet. It is important for good health, however, most people eat too much fat.

41. True   Fat, as a percentage of total calories eaten, should be 30 percent or less of your daily diet.

42. True   One gram of fat contains nine calories while one gram of carbohydrate or protein contain only four calories.

43. False   It is true that saturated fats are generally solid at room temperature, but is not true that saturated fats are found only in animal products. Coconut and palm oils also contain saturated fats.

44. False   It is important to be familiar with the fat content of all foods. Vegetables are usually low in fat, however, nuts are an example of vegetables that are very high in fat.

45. True   One size does not fit all. Different approaches to food cravings will help different people.

46. False   Shaping refers to making gradual progress in a step-by-step fashion so that goals are attainable.

Lesson 10

47. False   Only about 22 percent of the American adult population is active enough to realize health benefits. The rest are either totally sedentary or not active enough.

48. False   This concept of an exercise threshold is a barrier to exercise for many people. Any exercise can help, so do whatever you can.

49. True   Thirty minutes of incremental physical activity over most days (at least five) is now recommended for people to reach a moderate level of physical fitness.

50. True   Climbing stairs is an excellent way to burn calories. However, most people cannot climb stairs for extended periods, so it is best considered a lifestyle activity in which exercise can be added to your daily routine.

51. False   Vitamins, minerals, and water are considered nutrients essential to our bodies, yet, they contain no calories.

Lesson 11

52. False   It can be difficult to change thoughts we have had for years, but with repeated practice, old thoughts can give way to new, constructive, more helpful thoughts.

53. False   Weight loss is due to changes you make. Sure the drug helps, but it is possible to take the drug and lose no weight. Any weight you lose is due to YOUR efforts, and it is YOUR efforts that can persist, whether or not you are taking a drug.

54. False   Shopping on an empty stomach is asking for trouble. You will do less impulse buying if you shop after eating.

55. True   Taking the time to prepare foods will give you a chance to make a determined decision to eat. Many times the food will not be worth the effort, so you can ask yourself how important the eating really is.

56. True   The Food Guide Pyramid recommends two to three servings daily from the Milk, Yogurt, and Cheese Group.

Lesson 12

57. True   Remember the refrigerator battle cry, "Out of Sight, Out of Mouth!"

58. True   Each of us holds internal conversations, and many overweight individuals have fat thoughts. These thoughts and attitudes can greatly hinder weight loss efforts if they are not countered.

59. False   This refers to thinking that you are on or off a program, perfect or terrible with your behavior, and legal or illegal in your eating. This must be replaced with a more rational perspective.

60. False   Eating a variety of legumes and grains will also provide high-quality protein.

61. False   Protein has calories just like the other major nutrients (fats and carbohydrates) and does not have any magical qualities for weight loss. Protein is important to a balanced diet, but the recommended amounts should be enough to help keep you active and healthy.

Lesson 13

62. **False** It is best to take one portion at a time because it gives you time to decide whether you need more. It interrupts automatic eating.

63. **True** These images and fantasies can distract a person from the day-to-day behaviors needed to lose weight, and can lead to serious disappointment when the individual loses weight and significant life issues do not change.

64. **False** Carbohydrates should make up the largest portion of your daily diet (between 55 and 60 percent of total calories). It is important, however, to watch for hidden calories in these foods and to limit the added calories, such as toppings, butter, and dressings.

65. **True** The Food Guide Pyramid suggests between three and five servings each day from the Vegetable Group.

66. **True** The more you attribute your changes to your own efforts, the more confidence you will have to cope with the different challenges you will face.

67. **False** Weight loss is most rapid at the beginning of a program, and after three months or so, the weight loss slows down for some people. There still may be plenty left to lose, but don't expect the same rate of weight loss all along.

Lesson 14

68. **False** The two purposes of stretching and other warm up exercises are to loosen the muscles to avoid strain and to permit the heart and circulatory system to make a gradual transition from rest to hard work. You should warm up and cool down for at least five minutes each time you exercise.

69. **True** These are the three parts of the formula, so if you wish to get a training or aerobic effect, you must do each part in specific amounts.

70. **True** Behavior, even helping behavior, fades away if it is not rewarded (people like to be appreciated). So, if a partner helps you, show your appreciation in creative ways, and the desire to help you will persist.

71. **True** These foods are naturally high in fiber and are good additions to your diet if you wish to increase fiber intake.

72. **False** Most American do not eat the recommended number of servings of fruit on a daily basis. Hence, most people should increase their intake of fruit.

Lesson 15

73. **True** Some people have had negative experiences with exercise and may be reluctant to be active because of embarrassment.

74. **True** Spot reducing is a myth. Your body adds and removes fat according to genetic and hormonal factors. You can reduce fat in general, but you cannot dictate where it will come from.

75. **True** Foods from this group are very high in complex carbohydrates and most people should increase their intake from this food group. Breads, cakes, cookies, etc., however, have hidden calories, and it is important to watch out for these.

76. **True** Many overweight people avoid eating breakfast because they may not be hungry first thing in the morning or because they hope to save calories by not eating. This typically leads to more calories being consumed during the day, however.

Lesson 16

77. **False** There are many kinds of exercise that can help with your weight loss. The best kind is the kind you will do. Doing something rigorous is fine, if you can keep it up, but low-level activities will be better if you can stick with them over the long term.

78. **True** With the "ideal" being extremely thin, shaped, and sculpted, it is virtually impossible for most people to look like they think they should, no matter how much dieting and exercise they do. People deserve to feel good about their bodies, and the first step is to have a *realistic* standard.

79. **True** It's not easy, because society places so much importance on being thin. However, many people uncouple weight from their self-esteem and manage to appreciate their personal qualities and to accept their body for the pleasure it can bring them.

80. True   Studies have shown that medications can be quite helpful for maintaining weight loss. Some experts believe that the most important role of medication is in facilitating long-term weight control.

Lesson 17

81. False   Families can be a great resource for a person losing weight, but that harmony between the individual and the family requires a special effort.

82. False   It is nice to be friendly, but it is more important that you control what you eat. Be polite, but be firm in not yielding to pressure to eat.

83. True   These words are a setup for failure because they represent standards that no person can meet.

84. False   There is no weight loss advantage to taking mega-doses of any vitamin. Sticking with the Recommended Daily Allowances (RDA) is the best policy. This can usually be done by eating a balanced diet, and at most, can be accomplished with a multiple vitamin.

85. False   The amount of total fat listed under the heading "% Daily Value" of the food label represents the amount of a day's intake in a serving, based on a 2000-calorie diet.

Lesson 18

86. False   Recording your eating and exercise behaviors daily is critical when you are losing weight. Many people, however, find that they can record less frequently after the first four to five months and still enjoy excellent weight control. Experiment and see what works for you. You should definitely resume recording when you encounter difficulties.

87. True   Researchers cannot explain exactly why weight loss slows, even when people have more weight to lose. They key is not to interpret this slower rate of weight loss as a sign of failure. Focus on your many accomplishments.

88. False   Don't make the mistake of thinking that medications do not work because you don't continue to lose weight indefinitely. Medications help you lose weight during the first several months and then later help you keep it off. You may be more successful keeping your weight off for one or more years if you remain on medication. Talk with your doctor about this option.

89. False   Vitamins do not contain energy themselves, but aid in the breakdown of other nutrients into energy that the body can use.

Lesson 19

90. True   Jogging and cycling have both psychological and physical benefits. They are ideal for many people who are losing and maintaining weight.

91. True   With the current state of science, it is not possible to say that increased fiber in the diet protects against diseases, but there are strong hints that this may be the case.

92. True   Most nutritionists suggest that a healthy goal is to aim for an average intake of 25 to 35 grams of fiber each day.

93. False   Alcohol is loaded with calories and has no nutrition al all. It also releases inhibitions in some people, including inhibitions that can control eating.

Lesson 20

94. True   Alcohol releases inhibitions and weakens dietary restraint. It contains little nutrition and many calories.

95. True   Package deals, like getting a hamburger, fries, and cole slaw together more cheaply than separately, deliver more food (and calories) than you may want or need. Only get the package if you are sure you want all its components.

96. False   Aerobic activities do little for strength. They increase the body's use of oxygen and improve the condition of your heart. They are valuable for both health and weight loss.

97. False   Unless you are vitamin deficient or have special dietary needs, you probably need no vitamin supplements. A balanced diet usually provides adequate vitamins.

Lesson 21

98. False   People losing weight sometimes feel the chain is out of control, but a chain can be broken by using the right techniques at the proper time in a given situation.

99. True   A behavior chain can be broken at any link. Concentrate on the weakest links, where the chain is easiest to break.

100. False   It can be difficult to interrupt a chain at one of the final links because the momentum created by the earlier links can be powerful. Consider breaking the early links before the process gets rolling.

101. True   Most people have access to stairs, so it is easy to add several flights to your routine.

Lesson 22

102. False   Some people think that a lapse leads to relapse because they feel guilty at any mistake. By using special coping techniques, you can see that a lapse can be a signal to do better, not worse.

103. True   This can provide you with a list of enjoyable activities that can become associated with the signals that are used to stimulate eating.

104. False   Precisely because fiber is indigestible, it facilitates movement of food and waste products through the digestive system. Eating a high-fiber diet may also reduce risk for several chronic diseases.

Lesson 23

105. False   Anxiety makes it hard to think and weakens restraint that might keep eating in check. It is best to stay calm during a lapse so you can make a rational plan for responding.

106. True   The longer you wait during a lapse, the more momentum builds for overeating. Acting swiftly and decisively is the best approach. Consider yourself a Forest Ranger. Your task is to prevent fires and to move quickly when a fire breaks out.

107. True   Saturated fat can raise your cholesterol level, so it is important to control the intake of foods high in cholesterol and foods high in saturated fat.

Lesson 24

108. False   Different people respond to different techniques. It is best to select a small number of techniques that work for you and to focus on them.

109. True   Eating a low-calorie food before you go takes the edge off hunger. This can help you avoid high-calorie foods like chips and nuts, so you can use your calories for special foods you really want.

110. False   Iron deficiency is not common. Most people obtain adequate iron from normal eating and do not need supplements.

111. True   Most experts recommend reductions in salt intake. Excess sodium comes from salt in foods naturally and from the salt we add to food.

Appendix D

Guidelines for Being a Good Group Member

Many programs deal with participants in groups. This is done for an important reason. Members of the group can provide tremendous help to one another. The help may come in the form of encouraging words, a pat on the back, ideas to solve a specific problem, or just the knowledge that others in similar circumstances care about you.

Importance of the Group

From a problem-solving perspective, a group provides a shared experience that can help you develop an effective program. But beyond providing information, group members can provide support and encouragement. Most people losing weight encounter times when their motivation is high and other times when it is difficult to move in the right direction. When you take a detour from your program, the group can help the motivation return. When you are highly motivated yourself, you can encourage someone else in the group who may have trouble.

Good Chemistry and Teamwork

When a group has the right chemistry, it functions like a well-oiled machine. The meetings are enjoyable, informative, and motivational. Each group member receives as much as he or she gives, and all are better off for the effort.

The analogy of a sports team is especially appropriate. Let's take a basketball team, for example. We all know of teams with great individual players, but the team goes nowhere if the players do not work together. One player may have an opportunity to take a shot, but passing to a teammate who has a better shot will help the team. Teams with far less talent win championships by working together and helping one another. This intangible *team spirit* motivates everyone to work harder. Each player receives and gives, and all benefit in the process.

Being a good group member is a responsibility of anyone entering a group. But more than duty, it is the best

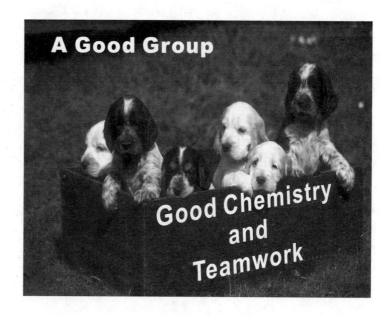

A Good Group

Good Chemistry and Teamwork

way to lose weight. Entering a group with a spirit of cooperation and the willingness to help others will insure that the help comes back to you. In the long run, you emerge the winner.

To be a good group member means following specific guidelines. There are things to do, things to say, and ways to act. The guidelines that follow can make this happen.

Guidelines and Responsibilities

Attend Meetings and Be Punctual

People in a group are responsible for attending meetings, not only for themselves but for others. When a group member misses a meeting, others in the group may worry about the person, may wonder if the absence is a sign of trouble, etc.

There will undoubtedly be times when you question whether you should attend a meeting. You might have overdone it on nacho chips, it may be rainy and miserable outside, or you may have had a difficult time with work or with the kids. These are the times when your program might be most in jeopardy, so it is important to attend the meeting. The group functions best when all attend, so remember that by joining a group you are agreeing to do your level best to make the meetings.

Being on time is another key factor. When you arrive late for a group, you draw attention to yourself, disrupt the proceedings, miss what has happened thus far, and force the group leader to either ignore what you have missed or cover it again. Showing up late, especially if it occurs chronically, is a sign of disrespect for other members of the group.

Sometimes, of course, being late is inevitable. You might have just arrived in town on the flight from Tokyo where you were thinking of acquiring Sony or Toyota. If you live in Arizona, you might have been attacked by the Abominable Cactus. Or you might have some more common reason like a traffic jam, late baby-sitter, or deadlines at the office. These things are understandable, but when you are late when you can help it, we start to worry.

Being late can be a sign of many things. Some people are always late because they fall into the Type A behavior pattern. They are always rushing and want to get in every last bit of activity before departing for the group. Such a person would cringe at sitting around for a few minutes with nothing to do. Our advice is to go ahead and cringe, but be on time.

Sometimes group members are late because they have done poorly and want to avoid speaking with the group leader. Others might be angry at the group leader or dissatisfied with the program or their progress. These things are usually not done on a conscious level, but if you look closely at your reasons for being late, these things may be the driving factors. If you find yourself being late, or wanting to be late, think about the reasons.

Really Listen

Sure, we all listen in a group, but do we really listen? Are you tuned in to what is happening? Do you hear the emotions behind the words that another group member might be using?

It is quite apparent when someone in the group is not listening. Yawning, roll-

It's important to *really listen* and be non-judgmental

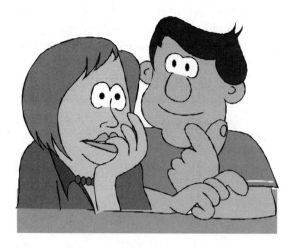

ing the eyes, looking out the window, or daydreaming are giveaways. It is easy to get distracted, especially if what is being discussed is not relevant to you, or if something else important is occupying your thoughts. It takes a real effort to listen carefully.

Being a good listener involves watching the person who is speaking. Do they look like they are expressing some strong emotions? Is the topic a sensitive one? Have you experienced a similar situation or feeling? Have you found some approach helpful with the problem? It is fine to ask questions if you don't understand what the person was saying, and it

is certainly fine to respond with supportive statements or suggestions. It will be nice when others in the group do this for you, so start by really listening.

Be Nonjudgmental

This may sound like psychological jargon, but here is what it means to be nonjudgmental. Sometimes you might feel that what another group member says or does is wrong, silly, or even stupid. There is a tendency to come down on these people or to point out the folly in their ways. The risk lies in being too negative, which can antagonize the person on the other end and make the remaining group members mad at you for being critical.

This does not mean that you are in a group where *everything is wonderful* and no negative emotions can be expressed. It is important to remember that there are different ways of saying things. What others say can be used as an opportunity for growth or an occasion to create bad feelings. The basic concept is for group members to accept one another. In such a climate, people in the group feel free to say things they might otherwise hide for fear of being criticized.

The chart provided below gives some examples of judgmental and nonjudgmental statements. As you can see, the

Being Nonjudgmental

One person says	Judgmental Response	Nonjudgmental Response
I just couldn't exercise this week.	You must be getting lazy.	It's hard to keep motivated to exercise.
I don't think this group is helping.	You are just making excuses.	Can we do something to help?
Others here don't understand me.	You talk too much.	I would like to. What can I do?

nonjudgmental statements are supportive and understanding, and open the door for further discussion. They show others that you care about them and are willing to help.

Be an Active Participant

In any group, some people are more active than others. This is fine, and can reflect differences in personalities. Not everyone has to be chirping away like a magpie to benefit from the group. However, opening up to be an active participant can help both you and the other members of the group.

Being silent in a group sometimes reflects being shy or reserved. In other cases, it shows that a person is angry, resentful, or bored. Whatever the reason, try to speak up when you have something worth saying. If you would like to share some of your own experiences, would like to ask if anyone has a solution to a particular problem you face, or can provide ideas of your own about an issue, speak up. Many times what you have to say will be listened to with all the attention given to a group leader, and you might have ideas that the leader or others in the group do not have.

If you are more the silent type, don't feel pressured to be exceptionally talkative. Not everyone will participate equally or will speak the same amount. When you do have something to offer, please share it with the others.

Share the Air Space

Think of the air in the group room as the territory around an airport. If too many planes enter the air space, the situation becomes dangerously confus-

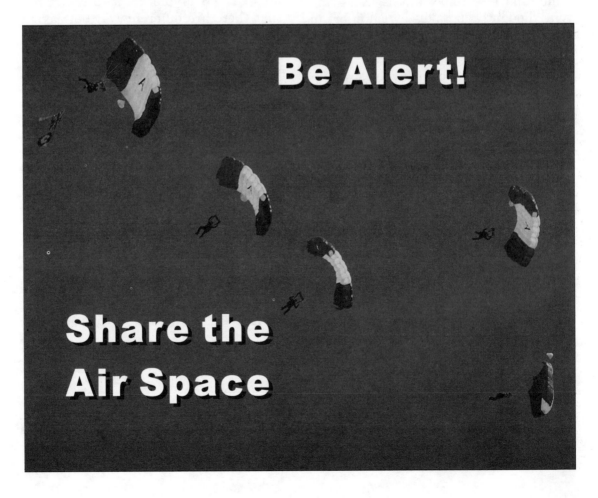

ing. If one jet occupies more than its share of the air space, say by circling in an erratic pattern, it would be tough going for the others.

In a group, there is only so much air space. Only so many voices can be heard and so many things said in the course of a group. For members of the group who are particularly verbal, there can be a tendency to monopolize the conversation and to crowd others from the air space.

Again, not everyone speaks the same amount, so if some people are naturally more active in the group, there is no need to pull in the reins. But if such a person interrupts or always speaks first, there may be a problem with sharing the air space. If the person takes a long time to make a point, or has to say something during every discussion, it may be time to open the air space to others. Look at the way you speak in the group, and see if any of these apply to you. If so, try to pull back and think before speaking. By all means speak up when you have something to say, and say what you feel, but try not to speak just because there is an opportunity.

Be Supportive

One of the fundamental reasons there are groups is for group members to support each other. This can be motivating and encouraging. In fact, sometimes a kind word or a supportive gesture will mean more coming from a fellow group member than the exact same word or gesture coming from the group leader.

Group members should try to be nice, helpful, and understanding. When another group member is troubled by something, do what you can to show that you understand. You can offer moral support by showing that you understand that the person faces a difficult situation. Share similar experiences you might have had, and most of all, give some constructive

suggestions if you can think of ways to help.

In Summary

When you enter a group, you enter a situation in which you can reap impressive rewards. You have the opportunity to not only learn the facts and techniques of the program, but to support and be supported, learn and instruct, help and be helped. This does not happen automatically, so people must be serious about their responsibilities as group members. In so doing, they will benefit from you and you will benefit from them. All will be better off and the long-term result can be permanent weight loss.

Appendix D—Guidelines for Being a Good Group Member

Appendix E

Fast Food Guide

Description	Calories	Pro (g)	Carb (g)	Fat (g)
Arby's				
Roast Beef Sandwiches				
Arby's Melt w/ Cheddar	368	18	36	18
Arby Q	431	22	48	18
Bac 'N' Cheddar Deluxe	539	22	28	34
Beef 'n Cheddar	487	25	40	28
Giant Roast Beef	555	35	43	28
Junior Roast Beef	324	17	35	14
Regular Roast Beef	388	23	33	19
Super Roast Beef	523	25	50	27
Chicken				
Breaded Chicken Fillet	536	28	46	28
Chicken Cordon Bleu	623	38	46	33
Chicken Fingers (2 Pieces)	290	16	20	16
Grilled Chicken BBQ	388	23	47	13
Grilled Chicken Deluxe	430	23	41	20
Roast Chicken Club	546	31	37	31
Roast Chicken Deluxe	433	24	36	22
Roast Chicken Santa Fe	436	29	35	22
Sub Roll Sandwiches				
French Dip	475	30	40	22
Hot Ham 'N' Swiss	500	30	43	23
Italian Sub	675	30	46	36
Philly Beef 'N' Swiss	755	39	48	47
Roast Beef Sub	700	38	44	42
Triple Cheese Melt	720	37	46	45
Turkey Sub	550	31	47	27
Light Menu				
Roast Beef Deluxe	296	18	33	10
Roast Chicken Deluxe	276	20	33	6
Roast Turkey Deluxe	260	20	33	7
Garden Salad	61	3	12	.5
Roast Chicken Salad	149	20	12	2
Side Salad	23	1	4	.3
Other Sandwiches				
Fish Fillet	529	23	50	27
Ham 'n Cheese	359	24	34	14
Ham 'n Cheese Melt	329	20	34	13
Potatoes				
Cheddar Curly Fries	333	5	40	18
Curly Fries	300	4	38	15
French Fries	246	2	30	13
Potato Cakes	204	2	20	12
Baked Potato (Plain)	355	7	82	.3
Baked Potato w/ Margarine and Sour Cream	578	9	85	24
Broccoli 'N' Cheddar Bkd Potato	571	14	89	20
Deluxe Baked Potato	736	19	86	36

Description	Calories	Pro (g)	Carb (g)	Fat (g)
Soups				
Boston Clam Chowder	190	9	18	9
Cream of Broccoli	160	7	15	8
Lumberjack Mixed Vegetable	90	2	10	4
Old Fashion Chicken Noodle	80	6	11	2
Potato w/ Bacon	170	6	23	7
Timberline Chili	220	18	17	10
Wisconsin Cheese	280	10	20	18
Desserts				
Apple Turnover	330	4	48	14
Cherry Turnover	320	4	46	13
Cheesecake (Plain)	320	5	23	23
Chocolate Chip Cookie	125	2	16	6
Chocolate Shake	451	15	76	12
Jamocha Shake	384	15	62	10
Vanilla Shake	360	15	50	12
Butterfinger Polar Swirl	457	15	62	18
Heath Polar Swirl	543	15	76	22
Oreo Polar Swirl	482	15	66	22
Peanut Butter Cup Polar Swirl	517	20	61	24
Snickers Polar Swirl	511	15	73	19
Burger King				
Burgers				
Whopper	640	27	45	39
Whopper w/ Cheese	730	33	46	46
Double Whopper	870	46	45	56
Double Whopper w/ Cheese	960	52	46	63
Whopper Jr. Sandwich	420	21	29	24
Whopper Jr. w/ Cheese	460	23	29	28
Hamburger	330	20	28	15
Cheeseburger	380	23	28	19
Double Cheeseburger	600	41	28	36
Double Cheeseburger w/ Bacon	640	44	28	39
Sandwiches/Side Orders				
BK Big Fish Sandwich	700	26	56	41
BK Broiler Chicken Sandwich	550	30	41	29
Chicken Sandwich	710	26	54	43
Chicken Tenders (8 Piece)	310	21	19	17
Broiled Chicken Salad	200	21	7	10
Garden Salad	100	6	7	5
Side Salad	60	3	4	3
French Fries (Med, Salted)	370	5	43	20
Coated French Fries (Med, Salted)	340	0	43	17
Onion Rings	310	4	41	14
Dutch Apple Pie	300	3	39	15

Fast Food Guide *(continted)*

Description	Calories	Pro (g)	Carb (g)	Fat (g)
Drinks				
Vanilla Shake (Medium)	300	9	53	6
Chocolate Shake (Medium)	320	9	54	7
Chocolate Shake (Medium)	440	10	84	7
Strawberry Shake (Medium)	420	9	83	6
Breakfast				
Croissan'wich w/ Sausage, Egg, and Cheese	600	22	25	46
Biscuit w/ Sausage	590	16	41	40
Biscuit w/ Bacon, Egg, Cheese	510	19	39	31
French Toast Sticks	500	4	60	27
Hash Browns	220	2	25	12

Dairy Queen

Description	Calories	Pro (g)	Carb (g)	Fat (g)
Burgers/Sandwiches/Side Orders				
Homestyle Hamburger	290	17	29	12
Homestyle Cheeseburger	340	20	29	17
Homestyle Double Cheeseburger	540	35	30	31
Homestyle DD Hamburger	440	30	29	22
Homestyle DD Cheeseburger	540	36	31	31
Homestyle Bacon Double Cheeseburger	610	41	31	36
Homestyle Ultimate Burger	670	40	29	43
Hot Dog	240	9	19	14
Cheese Dog	290	12	20	28
Chili Dog	280	12	21	16
Chili 'N' Cheese Dog	330	14	22	21
Fish Fillet Sandwich	370	16	39	16
Fish Fillet Sandwich w/ Cheese	420	19	40	21
Chicken Breast Fillet	430	24	37	20
Chicken Breast Fillet w/ Cheese	480	27	38	25
Chicken Strip Basket w/ Gravy	860	35	88	42
Chicken Strip Basket w/ BBQ Sauce	810	33	88	37
Grilled Chicken Breast Fillet	310	24	30	10
French Fries, Small	210	3	29	10
French Fries, Regular	300	4	40	14
French Fries, Large	390	5	52	18
Onion Rings	240	4	29	12
Ice Cream and Yogurt				
Vanilla Soft Serve, ½ Cup	140	3	22	4.5
Chocolate Soft Serve, ½ Cup	150	4	225	
Nonfat Frozen Yogurt, ½ Cup	100	3	21	0
Small Vanilla Cone	230	6	38	7
Regular Vanilla Cone	350	8	57	10
Large Vanilla Cone	410	10	65	12
Small Chocolate Cone	240	6	37	8
Regular Chocolate Cone	360	9	56	11
Regular Yogurt Cone	280	9	59	1
Small Chocolate Sundae	290	6	51	7
Regular Chocolate Sundae	410	8	73	10
Regular Cup of Yogurt	230	8	49	.5
Regular Yogurt Strawberry Sundae	300	9	66	.5
Small Misty Slush	220	0	56	0

Description	Calories	Pro (g)	Carb (g)	Fat (g)
Regular Misty Slush	290	0	74	0
Strawberry Misty Cooler	190	0	49	0
Small Chocolate Malt	650	15	111	16
Regular Chocolate Malt	880	19	153	22
Small Chocolate Shake	560	13	94	15
Regular Chocolate Shake	770	17	130	20
DQ Sandwich	150	3	24	5
Strawberry Shortcake	430	7	70	14
Banana Split	510	8	96	12
Chocolate Dilly Bar	210	3	21	13
Chocolate Mint Dilly Bar	190	3	20	12
Toffee Dilly Bar w/ Heath Pieces	210	3	24	12
Fudge Nut Bar™	410	8	40	25
Buster Bar	450	10	41	28
Peanut Buster Parfait	730	16	99	31
Small Dipped Cone	340	6	42	17
Regular Dipped Cone	510	9	63	25
Starkiss	80	0	21	0
Caramel & Nut Bar	260	5	32	13
Fudge Bar	50	4	13	0
Vanilla Orange Bar	60	2	17	0
Lemon Freez'r™ ½ Cup	80	0	20	0
Small Butterfinger Blizzard	520	11	80	18
Regular Butterfinger Blizzard	750	16	115	26
Small Chocolate Sandwich Cookie Blizzard	520	10	79	18
Regular Chocolate Sandwich Cookie Blizzard	640	12	97	23
Small Strawberry Blizzard	400	9	66	11
Regular Strawberry Blizzard	570	12	95	16
Small Heath Blizzard	560	10	82	21
Regular Heath Blizzard	820	14	119	33
Small Chocolate Chip Cookie Dough Blizzard	660	12	99	24
Regular Chocolate Chip Cookie Dough Blizzard	950	17	143	36
Small Reeses Peanut Butter Cup Blizzard	590	14	81	24
Regular Reeses Peanut Butter Cup Blizzard	790	19	105	33
Small Strawberry Breeze	320	10	68	.5
Regular Strawberry Breeze	460	13	99	1
Small Heath Breeze	470	11	85	10
Regular Heath Breeze	710	15	123	18
Choice Vanilla Big Scoop	250	4	27	14
Choice Chocolate Big Scoop	250	4	28	14
Strawberry-Banana Pizza, 1/8	180	3	29	6
Heath Treatzza Pizza 1/8 Pizza	180	3	28	7
M&M Treatzza Pizza 1/8 Pizza	190	3	29	7
Peanut Butter Fudge, 1/8 Pizza	220	4	28	10
Frozen Log Cake, 1/8 Cake	280	5	4	39
Frozen 8" Round Cake, 1/8 Cake	340	7	53	12
Frozen 10" Rd Cake, 1/12 Cake	360	7	55	12
Frozen Heart Cake, 1/10 Cake	270	5	41	9
Frozen Sheet Cake, 1/20 Cake	350	7	54	12

Description	Calories	Pro (g)	Carb (g)	Fat (g)
Hardee's				
Breakfast				
Rise 'N' Shine Biscuit	390	6	44	21
Jelly Biscuit	440	6	57	21
Apple Cinnamon 'N' Raisin Biscuit	200	2	30	8
Sausage Biscuit	510	14	44	31
Sausage & Egg Biscuit	630	23	45	40
Bacon & Egg Biscuit	570	22	45	33
Bacon, Egg, & Cheese Biscuit	610	24	45	37
Ham Biscuit	400	9	47	20
Ham, Egg & Cheese Biscuit	540	20	48	30
Country Ham Biscuit	430	15	45	22
Big Country Breakfast (Sausage)	1000	41	62	66
Big Country Breakfast (Bacon)	820	33	62	49
Frisco Breakfast Sandwich (Ham)	500	24	46	25
Regular Hash Rounds	230	3	24	14
Biscuit 'N' Gravy	510	10	55	28
Three Pancakes	280	8	56	2
Ultimate Omelet Biscuit	570	22	45	33
Sandwiches				
Hamburger	270	14	29	11
Cheeseburger	310	16	30	14
The Boss	570	27	42	33
Cravin' Bacon Cheeseburger	690	30	38	46
The Works Burger	530	25	41	30
Mesquite Bacon Cheeseburger	370	19	32	18
Quarter Pound Dbl Cheeseburger	470	27	31	27
Chicken Fillet Sandwich	480	26	54	18
Regular Roast Beef	320	17	26	16
Big Roast Beef Sandwich	460	26	35	24
Grilled Chicken Sandwich	350	25	38	11
Mushroom 'N' Swiss Burger	490	28	39	25
Frisco Burger	720	33	43	46
Hot Ham 'N' Cheese	310	16	34	12
Fisherman's Fillet	560	26	54	27
Fried Chicken/Sides				
Breast	370	29	29	15
Wing	200	10	23	8
Thigh	330	19	30	15
Leg	170	13	15	7
Cole Slaw (4 oz)	240	2	13	20
Mashed Potatoes (4 oz)	70	2	14	0
Gravy (1½ oz)	20	0	3	0
Baked Beans (5 oz)	170	8	32	1
Salads/Fries				
Side Salad	25	1	4	0
Garden Salad	220	12	11	13
Grilled Chicken Salad	150	20	11	3
Fat Free French Dressing	70	0	17	0
Ranch Dressing	290	1	6	29
Thousand Island Dressing	250	1	9	23
French Fries (small)	240	4	33	10
French Fries (medium)	350	5	49	15
French Fries (large)	430	6	59	18
Shakes/Desserts				
Shake (Vanilla)	350	12	65	5
Shake (Chocolate)	370	13	67	5

Description	Calories	Pro (g)	Carb (g)	Fat (g)
Shake (Strawberry)	420	11	83	4
Shake (Peach)	390	10	77	4
Vanilla Cone	170	4	34	2
Chocolate Cone	180	5	34	2
Cool Twist Cone	180	4	34	2
Hot Fudge Sundae	290	7	51	6
Strawberry Sundae	210	5	43	2
Peach Cobbler (6 oz)	310	2	60	7
Big Cookie	280	4	41	12
Jack In The Box				
Breakfast				
Breakfast Jack	300	18	30	12
Pancake Platter	400	13	59	12
Sausage Croissant	670	21	39	48
Scrambled Egg Pocket	430	29	31	21
Sourdough Breakfast Sandwich	380	21	31	20
Supreme Croissant	570	21	39	36
Ultimate Breakfast Sandwich	620	36	39	35
Hash Browns	160	1	14	11
Sandwiches				
Chicken Caesar Sandwich	520	27	44	26
Chicken Fajita Pita	290	24	29	8
Chicken Sandwich	400	20	38	18
Chicken Supreme	620	25	48	36
Grilled Chicken Fillet	430	29	36	19
Spicy Crispy Chicken Sandwich	560	24	55	27
Burgers				
Hamburger	280	13	31	11
Cheeseburger	320	16	32	15
Double Cheeseburger	450	24	35	24
Jumbo Jack	560	26	41	32
Jumbo Jack w/ Cheese	650	31	42	40
Grilled Sourdough Burger	670	32	39	43
Ultimate Cheeseburger	1030	50	30	79
¼ lb. Burger	510	26	39	27
Salads				
Garden Chicken Salad	200	23	8	9
Side Salad	70	4	3	4
Mexican/Teriyaki				
Taco	190	7	15	11
Monster Taco	283	12	22	17
Chicken Teriyaki Bowl	580	28	115	1.5
Sides/Desserts				
Seasoned Curly Fries	360	5	39	20
Small French Fries	220	3	28	11
Regular French Fries	350	4	45	17
Jumbo French Fries	400	5	51	19
Super Scoop French Fries	590	8	76	29
Onion Rings	380	5	38	23
Egg Rolls–3 Piece	440	3	54	24
Egg Rolls–5 Piece	750	5	92	41
Chicken Strips (breaded) 4 Piece	290	25	18	13
Chicken Strips (breaded) 6 Piece	450	39	28	20
Stuffed Jalapenos–7 Piece	420	15	29	27

Fast Food Guide *(continted)*

Description	Calories	Pro (g)	Carb (g)	Fat (g)
Stuffed Jalapenos–10 Piece	600	22	41	39
Bacon & Cheddar Potato Wedges	800	20	49	58
Hot Apple Turnover	350	3	48	19
Cheesecake	310	8	29	18
Chocolate Chop Cookie Dough Cheesecake	360	7	44	18
Carrot Cake	370	3	58	15

Kentucky Fried Chicken

Chicken
Description	Calories	Pro (g)	Carb (g)	Fat (g)
Breast, extra crispy	353	27	15	21
Breast, original recipe	257	26	8	14
Drumstick, extra crispy	173	13	6	11
Drumstick, original recipe	147	14	4	9
Kentucky Nuggets (one)	46	3	3	3
Thigh, extra crispy	371	20	14	27
Thigh, original recipe	278	18	9	20
Wing, extra crispy	218	12	8	16
Wing, original recipe	181	12	6	13

Side Orders
Description	Calories	Pro (g)	Carb (g)	Fat (g)
Baked Beans	105	5	19	1
Buttermilk Biscuit	269	5	32	14
Corn on the Cob	176	5	32	3
Cole Slaw	103	1	12	6
Kentucky Fries	268	5	34	13
Mashed Potatoes & Gravy	62	2	10	2
Potato Salad	141	2	13	9

Long John Silver's

Fish/Seafood
Description	Calories	Pro (g)	Carb (g)	Fat (g)
Large South of the Border	1380	35	167	64
Regular South of the Border	690	18	84	32
Large Classic	1470	35	170	72
Regular Classic	730	18	85	36
Large Ceasar	1460	36	167	73
Regular Ceasar	730	18	83	37
Large Ranch	1460	35	170	72
Regular Ranch	730	18	85	36
Large Cajun	1450	36	170	70
Regular Cajun	730	18	85	35
Batter-Dipped Fish Sandwich	320	17	40	13
Ultimate Fish Sandwich	430	18	44	21
Flavorbaked™ Fish Sandwich	320	23	28	14
Popcorn Fish	290	13	27	14
Flavorbaked Fish (1 Piece)	90	14	1	2.5
Clams	300	11	31	17

Chicken
Description	Calories	Pro (g)	Carb (g)	Fat (g)
Large South of the Border	1370	36	162	64
Regular South of the Border	690	18	81	32
Large Classic	1450	36	165	72
Regular Classic	730	18	83	36
Large Ceasar	1450	37	162	73
Regular Ceasar	730	18	81	37
Large Ranch	1450	36	165	72

Description	Calories	Pro (g)	Carb (g)	Fat (g)
Regular Ranch	730	18	82	36
Large Cajun	1440	37	165	71
Regular Cajun	720	18	83	35
Flavorbaked Chicken	110	19	0	3
Flavorbaked Chicken Sandwich	290	24	27	10
Popcorn Chicken	250	15	17	14
Batter-Dipped Chicken (1 Piece)	120	8	11	6

Shrimp
Description	Calories	Pro (g)	Carb (g)	Fat (g)
Popcorn Shrimp	280	11	27	15
Large South of the Border	1380	32	169	64
Regular South of the Border	690	16	84	32
Large Classic	1460	32	172	72
Regular Classic	730	16	86	36
Large Ceasar	1460	32	169	73
Regular Ceasar	730	16	84	37
Large Ranch	1460	32	171	72
Regular Ranch	720	16	86	35
Large Cajun	1450	32	172	71
Regular Cajun	720	16	86	35
Batter-Dipped Shrimp (1 Piece)	35	1	2	2.5

Side Items
Description	Calories	Pro (g)	Carb (g)	Fat (g)
Fries	250	3	28	15
Cheese Sticks	160	6	12	9
Hushpuppy (1 Piece)	60	1	9	2.5
Corn Cobbette	140	3	19	8
Corn Cobbette (w/out Butter)	80	3	19	.5
Green Beans	30	2	5	.5
Rice Pilaf	140	3	26	3
Coleslaw	140	1	20	6
Baked Potato	210	4	49	0
Side Salad	25	1	4	0

McDonald's

Sandwiches, Fries & Chicken
Description	Calories	Pro (g)	Carb (g)	Fat (g)
Hamburger	270	12	34	10
Cheeseburger	320	15	35	14
Quarter Pounder	430	23	37	21
Quarter Pounder w/ Cheese	530	28	38	30
Big Mac	530	25	47	28
Arch Deluxe	570	29	43	31
Arch Deluxe w/ Bacon	610	33	43	34
Crispy Chicken Deluxe	530	27	47	26
Fish Fillet Deluxe	510	24	59	50
Grilled Chicken Deluxe	330	27	42	6
Small French Fries	210	3	26	10
Large French Fries	450	6	57	22
Super Size French Fries	540	8	68	26
Chicken McNuggets (4 Piece)	190	12	10	11
Chicken McNuggets (6 Piece)	290	18	15	17
Chicken McNuggets (9 Piece)	430	27	23	26

Breakfast & Salad
Description	Calories	Pro (g)	Carb (g)	Fat (g)
Egg McMuffin	290	17	27	12
Sausage McMuffin	360	13	26	23
Sausage McMuffin w/ Egg	440	19	27	28
English Muffin	140	4	25	2

Description	Calories	Pro (g)	Carb (g)	Fat (g)
Sausage Biscuit	430	10	32	29
Sausage Biscuit w/ Egg	510	16	33	35
Bacon, Egg & Cheese Biscuit	440	17	33	26
Biscuit	260	4	32	13
Sausage	170	6	0	16
Scrambled Eggs (2)	160	13	1	11
Hash Browns	130	1	14	8
Hotcakes (plain)	310	9	53	7
Hotcakes (Marg. 2 pats & Syrup)	580	9	100	16
Breakfast Burrito	320	13	23	20
Low-fat Apple Bran Muffin	300	6	61	3
Apple Danish	360	5	51	16
Cheese Danish	410	7	47	22
Cinnamon Roll	400	7	47	20
Garden Salad	35	2	7	0
Grilled Chicken Salad Deluxe	110	21	5	1
Desserts/Shakes				
Vanilla Low-fat Ice Cream Cone	120	4	23	.5
Strawberry Low-fat Ice Cream Sundae	240	6	5	11
Hot Caramel Low-fat Ice Cream Sundae	300	7	62	3
Hot Fudge Sundae	290	8	53	5
Nuts (Sundae)	40	2	2	3.5
Baked Apple Pie	260	3	34	13
Chocolate Chip Cookie	170	2	22	10
McDonaldland Cookies	180	3	32	5
Low-fat Vanilla Shake (small)	340	12	60	5
Low-fat Chocolate Shake (small)	340	12	62	5
Low-fat Strawberry Shake (small)	340	12	61	5

Pizza Hut

Data is based on one slice of medium pizza.

Description	Calories	Pro (g)	Carb (g)	Fat (g)
Cheese				
Thin 'N Crispy Crust	205	11	21	8
Hand Tossed Crust	235	13	29	7
Pan Crust	261	12	28	11
Beef				
Thin 'N Crispy Crust	229	13	21	11
Hand Tossed Crust	260	15	29	9
Pan Crust	286	14	28	13
Ham				
Thin 'N Crispy Crust	184	10	21	7
Hand Tossed Crust	213	12	29	5
Pan Crust	239	11	28	9
Pepperoni				
Thin 'N Crispy Crust	215	11	21	10
Hand Tossed Crust	238	12	29	8
Pan Crust	265	11	28	12
Italian Sausage				
Thin 'N Crispy Crust	236	11	21	12
Hand Tossed Crust	267	13	29	11
Pan Crust	293	12	27	15
Pork Topping				
Thin 'N Crispy Crust	237	12	21	12
Hand Tossed Crust	268	14	29	10

Description	Calories	Pro (g)	Carb (g)	Fat (g)
Pan Crust	294	13	28	14
Meat Lover's				
Thin 'N Crispy Crust	288	15	21	13
Hand Tossed Crust	314	17	29	11
Pan Crust	340	16	28	18
Veggie Lover's				
Thin 'N Crispy Crust	186	9	22	7
Hand Tossed Crust	216	11	30	6
Pan Crust	243	10	29	10
Pepperoni Lover's				
Thin 'N Crispy Crust	289	15	22	16
Hand Tossed Crust	306	16	30	14
Pan Crust	332	15	28	17
Supreme				
Thin 'N Crispy Crust	257	14	21	13
Hand Tossed Crust	284	16	30	12
Pan Crust	311	15	28	15
Super Supreme				
Thin 'N Crispy Crust	270	14	22	14
Hand Tossed Crust	296	16	30	13
Pan Crust	323	15	28	17

Roy Rogers

Description	Calories	Pro (g)	Carb (g)	Fat (g)
Hamburgers & Chicken				
Bacon Cheeseburger	581	32	25	39
Cheeseburger	563	30	28	37
Hamburger	456	24	27	28
RR Bar Burger	611	36	28	39
Roast Beef Sandwich	317	27	29	10
Chicken Breast	412	33	17	24
Chicken Leg	140	12	6	8
Chicken Thigh	296	18	12	20
Chicken Wing	192	11	9	13
Side Orders				
Biscuit	231	4	27	12
Cole Slaw	110	1	11	7
Regular French Fries	268	4	32	14
Potato w/ Bacon & Cheese	397	17	33	22
Potato w/ Broccoli & Cheese	397	14	40	18
Potato w/ Sour Cream & Chives	408	7	48	21
Potato Salad	107	2	11	6
Breakfasts				
Apple Danish	249	5	32	12
Breakfast Crescent w/ Bacon	431	15	26	30
Breakfast Crescent (plain)	401	13	25	27
Breakfast Crescent w/ Sausage	449	20	26	30
Egg & Biscuit Platter w/ Bacon	435	20	22	30
Egg & Biscuit Platter (plain)	394	17	22	27
Pancake Platter w/ Sausage	608	14	72	30

Fast Food Guide (*continued*)

Description	Calories	Pro (g)	Carb (g)	Fat (g)
Taco Bell				
Tacos				
Taco	170	10	11	10
Soft Taco	210	12	20	10
Taco Supreme	220	11	13	13
Soft Taco Supreme	260	13	22	14
Double Decker Taco	340	16	37	15
Double Decker Taco Supreme	390	16	39	18
Steak Soft Taco	200	14	18	7
BLT Soft Taco	340	11	22	23
Kid's Soft Taco Roll-Up	290	16	20	16
Burritos				
Bean Burrito	380	13	55	12
Burrito Supreme	440	19	50	18
Big Beef Burrito Supreme	520	26	52	23
7-Layer Burrito	540	16	65	24
Chili Cheese Burrito	330	14	37	13
Chicken Club Burrito	540	22	43	31
Bacon Cheeseburger Burrito	560	29	43	30
Specialties				
Tostado	300	11	31	14
Mexican Pizza	570	21	41	36
Big Beef MexiMelt	300	16	21	16
Taco Salad w/ Salsa	840	32	62	52
Taco Salad w/ Salsa w/out Shell	420	26	29	21
Cheese Quesadilla	370	16	32	20
Chicken Quesadilla	420	24	33	22
Border Wraps				
Steak Fajita Wrap	460	20	48	21
Chicken Fajita Wrap	460	18	49	21
Veggie Fajita Wrap	420	11	51	19
Steak Fajita Wrap Supreme	510	21	50	25
Chicken Fajita Wrap Supreme	500	19	51	25
Veggie Fajita Wrap Supreme	460	11	53	23
Border Lights				
Light Chicken Burrito	310	18	41	8
Chicken Burrito	400	19	45	16
Light Chicken Burrito Supreme	430	25	52	13
Chicken Burrito Supreme	550	30	50	26
Light Chicken Soft Taco	180	13	21	5
Chicken Soft Taco	250	15	23	11
Light Kid's Chicken Soft Taco	180	13	20	5
Kid's Chicken Soft Taco	240	15	21	11
Nachos & Sides				
Nachos	310	2	34	18
Big Beef Nachos Supreme	430	12	43	24
Nachos Bell Grande	740	16	83	39

Description	Calories	Pro (g)	Carb (g)	Fat (g)
Pintos 'N Cheese	190	9	18	8
Mexican Rice	190	6	20	10
Cinnamon Twists	140	1	19	6

Wendy's

Description	Calories	Pro (g)	Carb (g)	Fat (g)
Sandwiches				
Plain Single	360	25	31	16
Single w/ Everything	420	26	37	20
Big Bacon Classic	570	34	46	29
Jr. Hamburger	270	15	34	10
Jr. Cheeseburger	320	17	34	13
Jr. Bacon Cheeseburger	380	21	34	19
Jr. Cheeseburger Deluxe	360	18	36	16
Kids' Meal Hamburger	270	15	33	10
Kids' Meal Cheeseburger	320	17	33	13
Grilled Chicken Sandwich	310	27	35	8
Breaded Chicken Sandwich	440	28	44	18
Chicken Club Sandwich	470	31	44	20
Spicy Chicken Sandwich	410	28	43	15
Fresh Salads-To-Go				
Caesar Side Salad	110	8	8	5
Deluxe Garden Salad	110	7	10	6
Grilled Chicken Salad	200	25	10	8
Grilled Chicken Caesar Salad	260	28	17	10
Side Salad	60	4	5	3
Taco Salad	590	29	53	30
Soft Breadstick	130	4	24	3
Desserts & Side Orders				
Chocolate Chip Cookie	270	4	38	11
Frosty Dairy Dessert (small)	340	9	57	10
Frosty Dairy Dessert (medium)	460	12	76	13
Frosty Dairy Dessert (large)	570	15	95	17
French Fries (small)	260	3	33	13
French Fries (medium)	380	5	47	19
French Fries (biggie)	460	6	58	23
Plain Baked Potato	310	7	71	0
Bacon & Cheese Baked Potato	540	17	78	18
Broccoli & Cheese Baked Potato	470	9	80	14
Cheese Baked Potato	570	14	78	23
Chili & Cheese Baked Potato	620	20	83	24
Sour Cream & Chives Baked Potato	380	8	74	6
Small Chili	210	15	21	7
Large Chili	310	23	32	10
Dessert				
Brownie	264	3	37	11
Hot Fudge Sundae	337	7	53	13
Strawberry Shortcake	447	10	59	19
Chocolate Shake	358	8	61	10
Vanilla Shake	306	8	45	11

Appendix F

The LEARN Program Calorie Guide

This calorie guide is designed to help you understand the dietary content of the foods you eat. It is not intended to be an all inclusive guide. Other, more complete calorie guides are available in most bookstores. The foods listed here should help you as you go through The LEARN Program.

Calories are listed for average serving sizes whenever possible. You may wish to convert some measurements to others to simplify matters. For example, some beverages are listed in fluid ounces while others are listed in cups. Several measurement equivalents are shown below to help with this task.

The protein, carbohydrate, and fat content of all the foods listed in the Calorie Guide are presented in grams (g). Unfortunately, the nutrient content for all food items were not available at press time, therefore, some of this information may be missing.

Helpful Measures

3t = 1T	= ½ fl oz	
16T = 1 cup	= 8 fl oz	= ½ pint
2 cups = 1 pint	= ½ quart	= ⅛ gallon
1 quart = 2 pints	= ¼ gallon	= .946 liter
1 gallon = 4 quarts	= 3.785 liter	1 liter = 1.057 quarts
1 oz = 28.35 g	1 lb = 16 oz	= 453.59 g

Description	Cal	Pro (g)	Carb (g)	Fat (g)
Alcohol (see Beverages)				
Almonds				
dried (1 oz) *24 nuts*	167	5.7	5.8	14.8
dry roasted (1 oz)	167	4.6	6.9	14.7
oil roasted (1 oz) *22 nuts*	176	5.8	4.5	16.4
Anchovy, raw (3 oz)	111	17.3	.0	4.1
Apples				
raw, w/skin (1 med)	81	.3	21.1	.5
raw, w/o skin (1 med)	72	.2	19.0	.4
boiled, w/o skin (1 cup)	91	.5	23.3	.6
Apple juice, canned (1 cup)	116	.2	29.0	.3
Apple sauce				
canned, unsweetened (½ cup)	53	.2	13.8	.1
canned, sweetened (½ cup)	97	.2	25.5	.2
Apricots				
raw (3 med)	51	1.5	11.8	.4
canned in water (4 halves)	20	.6	4.9	.0
canned in heavy syrup (4 halves)	75	.5	19.3	.1
dried, uncooked (10 halves)	83	1.3	21.6	.2
Apricot nectar, canned (1 cup)	141	.9	36.1	.2
Artichoke, boiled (1 med)	53	2.8	12.4	.2
Artichoke hearts, boiled (½ cup)	37	1.9	8.7	.1
Asparagus				
boiled (½ cup - 6 spears)	22	2.3	4.0	.3
canned (½ cup)	24	2.6	3.0	.8
frozen, boiled (4 spears)	17	1.8	2.9	.3
Avocado (1 med)	306	3.6	12.0	30.0
Bacon				
broiled, pan fried (3 med pieces)	109	5.8	.1	9.4
Canadian, grilled (2 slices)	86	11.3	.6	.4
Bagel (1 med)	163	6.0	30.9	1.4
Baking powder (1 t)	3.	.0	.7	.0
Bamboo shoots, raw (½ cup)	21	2.0	4.0	.2
Banana (1 med)	105	1.2	26.7	.6
Barbecue sauce (1 T)	12	.3	2.0	.3
Bass				
baked (3 oz)	215	17.7	2.3	14.6
stuffed, baked (3 oz)	222	13.9	9.8	13.5
Beans				
green, fresh, boiled (½ cup)	22	1.2	4.9	.2
green, canned (½ cup)	13	.8	3.1	.1
green, frozen, boiled (½ cup)	18	.9	4.2	.1
kidney, boiled (½ cup)	113	7.7	20.2	.4
kidney, canned (½ cup)	104	6.6	19.0	.4
lima, boiled (½ cup)	121	7.3	19.6	.6
lima, canned (½ cup)	96	5.9	17.9	.2
navy, boiled (½ cup)	130	7.9	23.9	.5
navy, canned (½ cup)	148	9.8	26.8	.6
northern, great, boiled (½ cup)	105	7.4	18.6	.4
northern, great, canned (½ cup)	150	9.6	27.6	.5
pinto, canned (½ cup)	93	5.5	17.5	.4
refried, canned (½ cup)	135	7.9	23.4	1.4
white, boiled (½ cup)	125	8.7	22.4	.3
white, canned (½ cup)	153	9.5	28.7	.4
yellow, boiled (½ cup)	127	8.1	22.3	1.0
yellow, canned (½ cup)	180	9.0	30.0	3.0
Bean sprouts, raw (½ cup)	16	1.6	3.1	.1
Beef, cooked (3.5 oz)				
brisket, lean	241	29.4	.0	12.8
chipped, dried	165	29.0	1.4	3.9

Description	Cal	Pro (g)	Carb (g)	Fat (g)
chuck pot roast, lean	231	33.0	.0	10.0
chuck blade roast, lean	270	31.1	.0	15.3
corned beef brisket, cured	251	18.2	.5	19.0
flank steak, lean	244	28.0	.0	13.8
ground, extra lean	250	24.5	.0	16.1
ground, lean	268	23.9	.0	18.3
ground, regular	287	23.0	.0	20.9
porterhouse steak, lean	218	28.2	.0	10.8
rib eye, lean	225	28.0	.0	11.6
round steak, lean	184	28.5	.0	7.0
sirloin steak, lean	208	30.4	.0	8.7
T-bone steak, lean	214	28.1	.0	10.4
Beef stew				
w/ vegetables (1 cup)	218	15.7	15.2	10.5
w/o vegetables, creamed (1 cup)	377	20.1	17.4	25.2
Beer (see Beverages)				
Beets				
boiled (½ cup slices)	26	.9	5.7	.0
canned (½ cup slices)	27	.8	6.1	.1
Beverages (nonalcoholic)				
cider, apple (6 oz)	90	.0	21.0	.0
choc milk, 1% fat (1 cup)	158	8.1	26.1	2.5
choc milk, 2% fat (1 cup)	179	8.0	26.0	5.0
choc milk, whole (1 cup)	208	7.9	25.9	8.5
coffee, black (1 cup)	5	.1	1.1	.0
coffee w/ sugar (1 cup)	35	.1	9.1	.0
coffee w/ sugar & cream (1 cup)	109	.9	10.1	7.6
lemonade, frozen conc (8 oz)	133	.1	34.7	.1
lemonade, from powder (8 oz)	102	.0	26.9	.0
milk, skim (8 oz)	86	8.4	11.9	.4
milk, 1% fat (8 oz)	102	8.0	11.7	2.6
milk, 2% fat (8 oz)	121	8.1	11.7	4.7
milk, whole (8 oz)	150	8.0	11.0	8.0
milk shake, thick vanilla (8 oz)	350	12.1	55.6	9.5
milk shake, thick choc (8 oz)	356	9.2	63.5	8.1
soft drinks (12 oz)				
cola	151	.1	38.5	.1
cola, diet	2	.2	.3	.0
cream soda	191	.0	49.3	.0
eggnog	513	14.6	51.6	28.5
fruit punch	200	.0	49.9	.0
ginger ale	124	.1	31.9	.0
grape soda	161	.0	41.7	.0
orange soda	177	.0	45.8	.0
orange soda, diet	2	.0	.6	.0
root beer	152	.1	39.2	.0
tea, black (1 cup)	3	.0	.5	.0
tea, w/ sugar (1 cup)	33	.1	8.5	.0
tea, w/ sugar & cream (1 cup)	107	.9	9.5	7.6
Beverages (alcoholic)				
beer and ale (12 oz)				
ale	150	1.7	10.0	.0
beer, regular	150	1.1	11.1	.0
beer, light	100	.7	4.8	.0
distilled spirits				
brandy (1 oz)	70	.0	.0	.0
cognac (1 oz)	70	.0	.0	.0
gin, 100 proof (1.5 oz jigger)	124	.0	.0	.0
rum, 100 proof (1.5 oz jigger)	124	.0	.0	.0
vodka, 100 proof (1.5 oz jigger)	124	.0	.0	.0
whiskey, 100 proof (1.5 oz jigger)	124	.0	.0	.0

Description	Cal	Pro (g)	Carb (g)	Fat (g)
liqueurs and cordials (1 oz)				
absinthe	84	.0	.0	.0
anisette	111	.0	.0	.0
Benedictine	112	.0	.0	.0
brandy, fruit	86	.0	.0	.0
Cherry Herring	80	.0	.0	.0
creme de menthe	125	.0	.0	0.1
Drambuie	110	.0	.0	.0
Southern Comfort	120	.0	.0	.0
triple sec	83	.0	.0	.0
mixed drinks				
daiquiri (3.5 oz)	194	.0	7.2	.0
highball, 4 oz	83	.0	.0	.0
Manhattan (3.5 oz cocktail)	224	.0	3.2	.0
martini (3.5 oz cocktail)	218	.0	.3	.0
old fashioned (4 oz)	180	.0	.0	.0
pina colada (6.8 oz can)	525	1.3	61.3	16.9
screwdriver (7 oz)	174	1.2	18.4	.1
tequilla sunrise (5.5 oz)	189	.6	14.7	.2
tom collins (7.5 oz)	121	.1	3.0	.0
whiskey sour (3.5 oz)	144	.2	5.8	.1
wines & wine beverages (3.5 oz)				
sparkling coolers	63	.2	8.8	.2
dessert, dry	130	.2	4.2	.0
dessert, sweet	158	.2	12.3	.0
table, red	74	.2	1.8	.0
table, rose	73	.2	1.5	.0
table, white	70	.1	.8	.0
Biscuits, 1 medium (homemade)	102	2.1	12.8	4.8
Blackberries				
raw (½ cup)	37	.5	9.2	.3
canned, heavy syrup (½ cup)	118	1.7	29.6	.2
frozen, unsweetened (1 cup)	97	1.8	23.7	.7
Blackeyed peas (cowpeas)				
boiled (½ cup)	99	6.6	17.8	4.5
canned (½ cup)	92	5.7	16.4	.7
Blueberries				
raw (½ cup)	41	.5	10.2	.6
canned, heavy syrup (½ cup)	112	.8	28.2	.4
frozen, sweetened (1 cup)	187	.9	50.5	.3
Bluefish, raw (3 oz)	124	14.7	.0	6.8
Bologna (see sausage)				
Bouillon, beef broth (1 cube)	6	.6	.6	.1
Bouillon, chicken broth (1 cube)	9	.7	1.1	.2
Brains, simmered beef (3.5 oz)	160	11.1	.0	12.5
Bran flakes (1 oz)	100	4.0	20.0	1.0
Braunschweiger (see sausage)				
Breads (1 slice or piece)				
bread sticks (2 sticks)	77	2.4	15.1	.6
cinnamon raisin	80	2.0	15.0	1.0
corn	178	3.8	27.5	5.8
cracked wheat	66	2.3	12.5	.9
french	81	2.7	14.8	1.1
hoagie or submarine roll	400	13.0	73.0	7.0
italian	78	2.8	14.9	.6
mixed grain	64	2.5	11.7	.9
oatmeal	71	2.4	13.0	1.2
pita pocket (1 pocket)	106	4.0	20.6	.6
pumpernickel	82	2.9	15.4	.8
raisin	70	2.1	13.2	1.0

Description	Cal	Pro (g)	Carb (g)	Fat (g)
rye	66	2.1	12.0	.9
white	64	2.0	11.7	.9
whole wheat	61	2.3	11.3	1.0
Breadcrumbs (1 cup)	392	12.6	73.4	4.6
Bread pudding (1 cup)	496	14.8	75.3	16.2
Bread stuffing (1 cup)	416	8.8	39.4	25.6
Broccoli				
raw (½ cup chopped)	12	1.3	2.3	.2
boiled (½ cup)	23	2.3	4.3	.2
Brussels sprouts, boiled (½ cup)	30	2.0	6.8	.4
Buns				
cinnamon (1 bun)	179	4.5	36.7	1.9
hot cross	111	2.0	18.0	3.0
Butter (1 T)				
regular	108	.1	.0	12.2
whipped	81	.1	.0	9.2
Cabbage, green				
raw (½ cup shredded)	8	.4	1.9	.1
boiled (½ cup shredded)	16	.7	3.6	.1
Cakes (1/12 of cake)				
angel food, homemade	161	4.8	35.7	0.1
angel food, from mix	126	3.2	28.6	.2
Boston cream pie	207	3.5	34.2	6.5
carrot, from mix	187	1.6	36.1	4.0
cheesecake	257	4.6	24.3	16.3
chocolate chip, from mix	189	1.8	35.6	4.4
coffee cake, from mix	116	2.2	18.9	3.5
cupcake (1 cupcake)	172	2.2	28.4	6.0
cottage pudding	93	1.8	14.7	3.0
devils food, homemade	227	3.4	30.4	11.3
devils food, from mix	312	4.0	53.6	11.3
fruit cake, homemade	163	2.1	25.7	6.6
german chocolate, from mix	250	3.0	36.0	11.0
gingerbread, homemade	267	3.0	35.0	12.9
honey spice, from mix	363	4.2	62.7	11.1
pineapple upside-down	236	2.5	37.4	9.1
pound	142	1.7	14.1	8.9
sponge	188	4.8	35.7	3.1
white	285	4.6	40.9	11.6
yellow	283	4.3	38.9	12.4
Cake icing (½ cup)				
chocolate	518	4.4	92.8	19.2
chocolate fudge	586	3.4	103.8	22.2
white	600	.8	130.2	10.4
Candy				
almond joy (1 oz)	136	1.5	16.4	2.3
baby ruth (2 oz bar)	260	4.0	36.0	12.0
butterfinger (2 oz bar)	260	4.0	38.0	12.0
butterscotch (1 oz)	113	.0	26.9	1.0
candy corn (¼ cup)	182	.1	44.8	1.0
caramels (1 oz)	113	1.1	21.7	2.9
chocolate				
almonds, coated (1 oz)	161	3.5	11.2	12.4
bar (1.65 oz bar)	254	3.8	27.1	14.5
chips (1 oz)	148	1.6	17.8	7.8
cherries, coated (2 pieces)	175	1.0	32.0	4.5
kisses (1.5 oz –9 pieces)	222	3.4	23.7	12.5
milk (1 oz)	147	2.2	16.1	9.2
peanuts, coated (1 oz)	159	4.6	11.1	11.7
semi-sweet (1 oz)	144	1.2	16.2	10.1
sweet (1 oz)	150	1.2	16.4	10.0

Description	Cal	Pro (g)	Carb (g)	Fat (g)
fudge (1 oz)	113	.8	21.3	3.5
gum drops (1 oz)	98	.0	24.8	0.2
hard (1 oz)	109	.0	27.6	.3
jelly beans (1 oz)	104	.0	26.4	.1
life savers, all flavors (1 piece)	9.1	.0	3.0	.0
marshmallow (1 large)	19	.1	4.8	.0
mints (3 cup)	100	.0	24.7	.6
peanut brittle (1 oz)	119	1.6	23.0	2.9
peanut butter chips (1.5 oz)	228	8.9	19.3	12.8
peanut butter cups (1.8 oz)	281	6.4	25.9	16.7
Cantaloupe, raw (1 cup)	57	1.4	13.4	.4
Carrots				
raw (1 med)	31	.7	7.3	.1
boiled (½ cup slices)	35	.9	8.2	.1
canned (½ cup slices)	17	.5	4.0	.1
Carrot juice, canned (1 cup)	97	2.3	22.8	.4
Casaba melon, raw (1 cup)	45	1.5	10.5	.2
Cashew nuts				
dry roasted (1 oz)	163	4.4	9.3	13.2
oil roasted (1 oz)	163	4.6	8.1	13.7
Catfish				
channel, raw (3 oz)	99	15.5	.0	3.6
breaded & fried (3 oz)	194	15.4	6.8	11.3
Catsup *(see ketchup)*				
Cauliflower				
raw (½ cup slices)	12	1.0	2.5	.1
boiled (½ cup slices)	15	1.2	2.9	.1
Caviar, black & red (1 T)	42	3.9	.6	2.9
Celery				
raw, 1 stalk (7.5" long)	6	.3	1.5	.1
boiled (½ cup diced)	11	.4	2.6	.1
Cereals (1 oz)				
all-bran (⅓ cup)	71	4.0	21.1	.5
almond delight (¾ cup)	110	2.1	23.0	1.6
alpha bits (1 cup)	110	2.3	24.1	.7
booberry (1 cup)	110	1.0	24.0	1.0
bran, 100% (½ cup)	76	3.5	20.7	1.4
bran chex (⅔ cup)	90	2.9	23.0	.7
bran flakes (¾ cup)	93	3.6	22.2	.5
cap'n crunch (¾ cup)	121	1.4	22.9	2.6
cheerios (⅓ cup)	111	4.3	19.6	1.8
cinnamon toast crunch (¾ cup)	120	1.0	23.0	3.0
cocoa krispies (¾ cup)	110	1.5	25.2	.4
coco puffs (1 cup)	110	1.0	25.0	.1
corn chex (1 cup)	110	2.0	25.0	.2
corn flakes (1 cup)	110	2.0	25.0	.1
cream of rice, cooked (¾ cup)	95	1.6	21.1	.1
cream of wheat, cooked (¾ cup)	100	2.9	20.8	.4
farina, cooked (¾ cup)	87	2.5	18.5	.1
froot loops (1 cup)	111	1.7	25.0	.5
frosted mini-wheats (4 biscuits)	102	2.9	23.4	.3
golden grahams (¾ cup)	109	1.6	24.1	1.1
granola (3 cup)	138	3.5	15.6	7.7
grape-nuts (⅞ cup)	104	2.8	22.7	.8
honey comb (1⅓ cups)	110	1.4	25.4	.3
honey nut cheerios (¾ cup)	107	3.1	22.8	.7
kix (1½ cups)	110	2.5	23.4	.7
life (⅔ cup)	111	5.2	18.6	1.8
lucky charms (1 cup)	110	2.6	23.2	1.1
malt-o-meal, cooked (¾ cup)	92	2.6	19.4	.2

Description	Cal	Pro (g)	Carb (g)	Fat (g)
maypo, cooked (¾ cup)	128	4.4	23.9	1.8
oatmeal, cooked (¾ cup)	109	4.6	18.4	1.9
product 19 (¾ cup)	108	2.8	23.5	.2
puffed rice (2 cups)	114	1.8	25.6	.2
puffed wheat (2 cups)	104	4.2	22.6	.4
rice chex (1⅛ cups)	110	1.7	25.0	.3
rice krispies (1 cup)	112	1.9	24.8	.2
shredded wheat (4 biscuits)	102	3.1	22.6	.6
special K (1⅓ cups)	111	5.6	21.3	.1
sugar frosted flakes (¾ cups)	108	1.4	25.7	.1
sugar smacks (¾ cup)	106	2.0	24.7	.5
super sugar crisp (7/8 cup)	106	1.8	25.6	.3
total (1 cup)	100	2.8	22.3	.6
trix (1 cup)	109	1.5	25.2	.4
wheat chex (⅔ cup)	100	2.9	23.0	.7
wheaties (1 cup)	99	2.7	22.6	.5
Cheese (1 oz)				
american, processed	106	6.3	.5	8.9
blue	100	6.1	.7	8.2
brick	105	6.6	.8	8.4
camembert, domestic	85	5.6	.1	6.9
cheddar	114	7.1	.4	9.4
colby	112	6.7	.7	9.1
cottage, creamed	30	3.5	.8	1.3
cream cheese (2 T)	99	2.1	.8	9.9
edam	101	7.1	.4	7.9
fontina	110	7.3	.4	8.8
gouda	101	7.1	.6	7.8
gruyere	117	8.5	.1	9.2
limburger	93	5.7	.1	7.7
monterey	106	6.9	.2	8.6
mozzarella	80	5.5	.6	6.1
muenster	104	6.6	.3	8.5
neufchatel	74	2.8	.8	6.6
parmesan, grated (1 T)	23	2.1	.2	1.5
parmesan, hard	111	10.1	.9	7.3
pimento, processed	106	6.3	.5	8.8
provolone	100	7.3	.6	7.6
ricotta, part skim (½ cup)	171	14.1	6.4	9.8
romano	110	9.0	1.0	7.6
roquefort	105	6.1	.6	8.7
swiss	107	8.1	1.0	7.8
velveeta	84	5.2	2.2	6.1
Cherries				
raw (10 cherries)	49	.8	11.3	.7
sour, canned in syrup (½ cup)	116	.9	29.8	.1
sour, canned in water (½ cup)	43	.9	10.9	.1
sweet, canned in syrup (½ cup)	107	.8	27.4	.2
sweet, canned in water (½ cup)	57	1.0	14.6	.2
Chewing gum (1 piece)	10	.0	2.0	.0
Chicken, (3.5 oz)				
dark, fried w/ skin	285	27.2	4.1	16.9
dark, fried w/o skin	239	29.0	2.6	11.6
dark, roasted w/ skin	253	26.0	0.0	15.8
dark, roasted w/o skin	205	27.4	.0	9.7
light, fried w/ skin	246	30.5	1.8	12.1
light, fried w/o skin	192	32.8	.4	5.5
light, roasted w/ skin	222	29.0	.0	10.9
light, roasted w/o skin	173	30.9	.0	4.5

Description	Cal	Pro (g)	Carb (g)	Fat (g)
parts, w/ skin				
breast, fried (½ breast)	218	31.2	1.6	8.7
breast, roasted (½ breast)	193	29.2	.0	7.6
drumstick, fried (1 drumstick)	120	13.2	.8	6.7
drumstick, roasted (1 drumstick)	112	14.1	.0	5.8
thigh, fried (1 thigh)	162	16.6	2.0	9.3
thigh, roasted (1 thigh)	153	15.5	.0	9.6
wing, fried (1 wing)	103	8.4	.8	7.1
wing, roasted (1 wing)	99	9.1	.0	6.6
Chicken a la king, homemade (1 c)	468	27.4	12.3	34.3
Chicken fricassee, homemade (1 c)	386	36.7	7.4	22.3
Chicken pot pie, homemade (1 slice)	545	23.4	42.5	31.3
Chickpeas (garbanzo beans)				
boiled (½ cup)	135	7.2	22.5	2.2
canned (½ cup)	143	5.9	27.2	1.4
Chili/chili con carne				
with beans (1 cup)	286	14.6	30.4	14.0
without beans (1 cup)	412	15.4	12.1	33.5
Chili powder (1 t)	8	.3	1.4	.4
Chocolate (see candy)				
Chocolate syrup (2 T)	82	.7	22.1	.3
Chop suey (1 cup)	300	26.0	12.8	17.0
Chow mein, chicken (1 cup)	255	31.0	10.0	10.0
Cider (see beverages)				
Clams				
raw (3 oz)	63	10.9	2.2	.8
steamers (3 oz)	126	21.7	4.4	1.7
breaded & fried (3 oz)	171	12.1	8.8	9.5
Clam sauce (4 oz)				
red sauce	81	3.6	9.3	3.2
white sauce	121	4.5	4.2	9.6
Cocoa (see beverages)				
Coconut, dried (1 oz)	187	2.0	6.7	18.3
Codfish				
raw (3 oz)	70	15.1	.0	.6
broiled (3 oz)	89	19.4	.0	.7
frozen & breaded (3 oz)	174	12.0	6.0	12.0
Coffee (see beverages)				
Cola (see beverages)				
Cold cuts (see sausage)				
Coleslaw (½ cup)	42	.8	7.5	1.6
Collards, boiled (1 cup chopped)	27	2.1	5.0	.3
Cookies				
animal crackers (10 pieces)	112	1.7	20.8	2.4
apple newtons (2 cookies)	147	1.3	28.0	2.7
applesauce raisin (2 cookies)	140	2.0	17.0	8.0
brownies w/ nuts (2" square)	97	1.3	10.2	6.3
butter (10 cookies)	229	3.1	35.5	8.5
cherry newtons (2 cookies)	147	1.3	26.7	2.7
chocolate chip (1 cookie)	46	.5	6.4	2.7
choc fudge sandwich (3 cookies)	150	2.0	19.0	7.0
choc coated grahams (2 cookies)	124	1.4	17.6	6.2
choc & cream sandwich (1 cookie)	49	.5	7.1	2.1
fig bar (1 bar)	53	.5	10.6	1.0
fig newtons (2 cookies)	100	1.0	20.0	2.0
gingersnaps (1 cookie)	34	.3	4.7	1.6
ladyfingers (2 ladyfingers)	79	1.7	14.2	1.7
macaroon (2 cookies)	181	2.0	25.1	8.8
marshmallow sandwich (4)	120	1.0	22.0	3.0
molasses (1 cookie)	137	2.0	24.7	3.4

Description	Cal	Pro (g)	Carb (g)	Fat (g)
nilla wafers (7 cookies)	130	1.1	21.0	4.0
nutter butter peanut butter (2)	140	3.0	18.0	6.0
oatmeal (1 cookie)	62	.8	8.9	2.6
oatmeal raisin (4 cookies)	235	3.2	38.2	8.0
oreo (3 cookies)	140	1.0	20.0	6.0
peanut butter (1 cookie)	50	.8	5.9	2.6
shortbread (1 cookie)	42	.5	4.9	2.3
sugar (2 cookies)	71	1.0	10.9	2.7
sugar wafers (2 cookies)	92	.9	13.9	3.7
vanilla wafers (5 cookies)	92	1.1	14.9	3.2
Cooking oil (see oils)				
Corn, grits				
dry (1 cup)	579	13.7	124.2	1.8
cooked (1 cup)	146	3.5	31.4	.5
Corn, yellow				
boiled (½ cup)	89	2.7	20.6	1.1
canned, cream style (½ cup)	93	2.2	23.2	.5
canned, vacuum pack (½ cup)	83	2.5	20.4	.5
Cornbread (see breads)				
Corn muffins (see muffins)				
Corn oil (see oil)				
Cornstarch (1 T)	30	.0	7.2	.0
Cornsyrup (see syrup)				
Cottage cheese (see cheese)				
Crab				
raw (3 oz)	71	15.6	.0	.5
canned (3 oz)	84	17.4	.0	1.0
steamed (3 oz)	87	17.2	.0	1.5
Crackers				
cheese (5 crackers)	81	1.4	7.8	4.9
graham (2 squares)	60	1.0	10.8	1.5
oyster (10 crackers)	33	.7	5.3	1.0
ritz (4 crackers)	70	1.0	9.0	4.0
ry-krisp (3 large square)	40	1.5	13.0	.2
saltines (2 crackers)	26	.6	4.4	.6
soda (10 crackers)	125	2.6	20.1	3.7
triscuit (3 crackers)	60	1.0	10.0	2.0
wheat thins (8 crackers)	70	1.0	9.0	3.0
zwieback (1 piece)	30	.7	5.2	.6
Cranberries, raw (1 cup)	46	.4	12.1	.2
Cranberry juice, canned (1 cup)	147	.1	37.7	.1
Cranberry sauce, jelled (½ cup)	209	.3	53.7	.2
Crayfish				
raw (3 oz)	76	15.9	.0	.9
steamed (3 oz)	97	20.3	.0	1.2
Cream & cream substitutes				
creamer, non-dairy liquid (½ oz)	22	.0	2.1	1.6
creamer, non-dairy powder (1 t)	11	.1	1.1	.7
half & half (1 T)	20	.4	.6	1.7
heavy whipping (1 T)	52	.3	.4	5.6
light (1 T)	29	.4	.6	2.9
light whipping (1 T)	44	.3	.4	4.6
medium, 25% fat (1 T)	37	.4	.5	3.8
sour, cultured (1 oz)	52	.8	1.0	5.0
sour, half & half cultured (1 oz)	40	.8	1.2	3.6
sour, imitation (1 oz)	59	.7	1.9	5.5
Cream puff w/ filling (1 cream puff)	303	8.5	26.7	18.1
Cucumber (½ cup slices)	7	.3	1.5	.1
Custard, baked (1 cup)	305	14.3	29.4	14.6
Dates, pitted (10 dates)	228	1.6	61.0	.4

Description	Cal	Pro (g)	Carb (g)	Fat (g)
Dips (1 oz)				
bacon	71	1.0	2.0	6.0
blue cheese	100	6.1	.7	8.2
clam	67	1.0	3.0	5.0
onion	70	1.0	2.0	6.0
Doughnuts (1 doughnut)				
cake	105	1.3	12.2	5.8
chocolate coated	130	1.0	14.0	8.0
glazed old fashioned	310	3.0	34.0	18.0
powdered sugar	110	1.0	15.0	5.0
raised / yeast	176	2.7	16.0	11.3
Duck, roasted (3.5 oz)				
w/ skin	337	19.0	.0	28.4
w/o skin	201	23.5	.0	11.2
Eggs				
boiled, hard/soft (1 large)	79	6.1	.6	5.6
fried (1 large)	83	5.4	.5	6.4
omelette, plain (1 large)	95	6.0	1.4	7.1
poached (1 large)	79	6.0	.6	5.6
scrambled w/ milk & fat (1 large)	95	6.0	1.4	7.1
white, fresh/frozen (1 large)	16	3.4	.4	.0
whole, fresh/frozen (1 large)	79	6.1	.6	5.6
yolk, fresh (1 large)	63	2.8	.0	5.6
Eggnog (see beverages)				
Eggplant				
raw (½ cup pieces)	11	.5	2.6	.0
boiled (½ cup)	13	.4	3.2	.1
Farina (see cereals)				
Figs				
raw (1 med)	37	.4	9.6	.2
dried (10 figs)	477	5.7	122.2	2.2
Fish (see individual kinds)				
Fish fillets, frozen				
batter-dipped (3 oz)	180	10.0	15.0	10.0
Fish sticks, frozen				
1 stick (about 1 oz)	76	4.4	6.7	3.4
batter-dipped (3 oz)	165	7.5	11.2	11.2
Flounder / sole				
raw (3.5 oz)	68	14.9	.0	.5
baked (3.5 oz)	202	30.0	.0	8.2
frozen, breaded (3.5 oz)	210	10.5	10.5	14.0
Flour				
enriched, 1 cup	455	12.9	95.4	1.2
wheat, 1 cup sifted	400	15.0	80.0	2.0
Frankfurters (see sausage)				
French toast, 1 slice	150	5.0	11.0	9.0
Frog legs, 3.5 oz	73	16.1	.0	0.3
Frostings (see cake icing)				
Frozen custard (see ice cream)				
Fruit (see individual listing)				
Fruit cocktail				
canned, water pack (½ cup)	40	.5	10.4	.1
canned, heavy syrup (½ cup)	93	.5	24.2	.1
canned, juice pack (½ cup)	56	.6	14.7	.0
Garbanzo beans (see chickpeas)				
Garlic, raw (3 cloves)	13	.6	3.0	.1
Gelatin				
plain, 1 pkt	25	6.0	.0	.0
fruit flavors, ½ cup	80	2.0	19.0	.0
diet, ½ cup	8	2.0	.0	.0

Description	Cal	Pro (g)	Carb (g)	Fat (g)
Gin (see beverages)				
Ginger ale (see beverages)				
Gingerbread (see cakes)				
Ginger root, raw (¼ cup)	17	.4	3.6	.2
Granola bar, (.8 oz bar)	109	2.0	16.0	4.0
Grape juice, canned (1 cup)	155	1.0	37.0	.2
Grapefruit				
raw, pink & red (½ cup)	43	.6	11.1	.1
raw, white (½ cup)	42	1.0	10.5	.1
canned, juice pack (½ cup)	44	.7	11.2	.1
Grapefruit juice, canned (1 cup)	96	1.2	22.7	.2
Grapes (1 cup)	57	.5	14.2	.5
Gravy (½ cup)				
beef	62	44	5.6	1.4
chicken	94	2.2	6.4	6.8
mushroom	60	1.6	6.6	3.2
Grits (see corn grits)				
Gum (see chewing gum)				
Haddock				
raw (3 oz)	74	16.1	.0	.6
broiled (3 oz)	95	20.6	.0	.8
smoked (3 oz)	99	21.4	.0	.8
Halibut				
raw (3 oz)	93	17.7	.0	2.0
broiled (3 oz)	119	22.7	.0	2.5
frozen, batter—dipped (3 oz)	195	7.5	11.2	11.2
Ham (see pork)				
Hamburger (see beef, ground)				
Hash, corned beef (see beef)				
Herbs	0	.0	.0	.0
Herring, atlantic				
raw (3 oz)	135	15.3	.0	7.8
baked, broiled (4 oz)	230	26.1	.0	13.1
pickled (4 oz)	297	16.1	10.9	20.4
Hollandaise sauce, ½ cup	119	2.4	6.9	9.9
Hominy, canned				
white (½ cup)	69	1.0	15.0	.4
yellow (½ cup)	64	1.3	13.9	.3
Honey, 1 T	60	.0	16.0	.0
Honeydew melon, raw (½ cup)	66	1.6	15.4	.6
Horseradish, 1 T	10	.0	1.0	.0
Ice cream (½ cup)				
chocolate	280	5.0	35.0	14.0
strawberry	230	4.0	20.0	15.0
vanilla	270	5.0	26.0	17.0
French, vanilla	189	3.5	19.1	11.3
sherbet, orange	135	1.1	29.4	1.9
Ice cream bar, vanilla w/choc (3 fl oz)	320	1.0	34.0	20.0
Ice cream cone, plain	60	1.0	11.0	1.0
Ice cream sandwich (2.7 fl oz)	204	2.2	30.1	8.3
Ice milk, vanilla (½ cup)	92	2.6	14.5	2.8
Ice milk bar	140	3.0	22.0	5.0
Icings (see cake icings)				
Jams, 1 T	53	.0	13.5	.0
Jellies, 1 T	53	.0	13.5	.0
Jello	81	2.0	19.0	.0
sugar free	80	2.0	19.0	.0
Juice (see types)				
Kale, boiled (½ cup chopped)	21	1.2	3.7	.3
Ketchup, 1 T	16	.2	4.1	.1

Description	Cal	Pro (g)	Carb (g)	Fat (g)
Kiwifruit, raw (1 med)	46	.8	11.3	.3
Knockwurst (see sausage)				
Kumquats, raw (1 med)	12	.2	3.1	.0
Lamb (3 oz)				
leg, roasted, lean	163	24.0	.0	6.6
loin chops, broiled, lean	269	21.4	.0	19.7
Lard, 1 T	115	.0	.0	12.8
Leeks				
raw (½ cup chopped)	32	.8	7.4	.2
boiled (½ cup chopped)	16	.4	4.0	.1
Lemon, raw (1 med)	22	1.3	11.6	.3
Lemonade, 8 oz	80	.0	20.0	.0
Lemon juice				
fresh (1 T)	4	.1	1.3	.0
fresh (1 cup)	60	.9	21.1	.0
Lentils, boiled (1 cup)	231	17.9	39.9	.7
Lettuce (fresh)				
iceberg, raw (3 leaves)	9	.6	1.2	.0
looseleaf, raw (1 cup)	15	1.2	3.0	.3
romaine, raw (1 cup)	8	1.0	1.4	.2
Lima beans (see beans)				
Lime, raw (1 med)	20	.5	7.1	.1
Liver (cooked)				
beef, 4 oz	183	27.6	3.9	5.5
chicken, 4 oz	178	27.6	1.0	6.2
Liverwurst, (see sausage)				
Lobster, steamed (4 oz)	111	23.2	1.5	.7
Lobster Newberg, 1 cup	468	17.2	11.	39.4
Lox (see salmon)				
Luncheon meats (see sausage)				
Macadamia nuts, dried (1 oz)	199	2.43	.9	20.9
Macaroni (cooked)				
shells, small, 1 cup	162	5.5	32.6	.8
spirals, 1 cup	189	6.4	38.0	.9
Macaroni & cheese (1 cup)	420	20.0	50.0	16.0
Mackerel, broiled (3 oz)	223	20.3	.0	15.1
Mandarin oranges, canned				
juice packed (½ cup)	46	.8	11.9	.0
light syrup (½ cup)	76	.6	20.4	.1
Mango, raw (1 med)	135	1.1	35.2	.6
Margarine (1 T)	100	.0	.0	11.0
Marshmallow (see candy)				
Mayonnaise (see salad dressing)				
Meatloaf (see sausage)				
Meats (see beef, lamb, pork)				
Melba toast, 1 slice	25	1.0	6.1	.5
Melons (see types)				
Milk, cow (1 cup)				
whole (3.7% fat)	157	8.0	11.4	8.9
skim	86	8.4	11.9	.4
low fat (2% fat)	121	8.1	11.7	4.7
dry, whole, regular	635	33.7	49.2	34.2
dry, nonfat, regular	435	43.4	62.4	.9
dry, nonfat, instant	326	31.9	47.5	.7
Milk shake (see beverages)				
Molasses, 1 T	60	.0	14.0	.0
Muffins				
blueberry (1.5 oz)	130	2.0	18.0	5.0
bran, raisin (2.5 oz)	190	3.0	30.0	7.0

Description	Cal	Pro (g)	Carb (g)	Fat (g)
corn (2.5 oz)	220	4.0	33.0	8.0
English	130	4.3	25.4	1.3
oat bran (2.75 oz)	180	5.0	27.0	7.0
wheat bran	140	2.0	24.0	4.0
Mushrooms				
raw (½ cup pieces)	9	.7	1.6	.2
boiled (½ cup pieces)	21	1.7	4.0	.4
canned (½ cup pieces)	19	1.5	3.9	.2
Mussels				
raw (3 oz)	73	10.1	3.1	1.9
steamed (3 oz)	147	20.2	6.3	3.8
Mustard, 1 T	14	1.0	1.0	1.0
Mutton (see lamb)				
Nectarine, raw (1 med)	67	1.3	16.0	.6
Noodles, 1 cup				
egg, cooked	212	7.6	39.7	2.4
chow mein, canned	237	3.8	25.9	13.8
Nuts (see individual kinds)				
Nuts, mixed, 1 oz	170	8.0	3.0	14.0
Oat bran				
raw (1 cup)	231	16.3	62.2	6.6
cooked (1 cup)	87	7.0	25.1	1.9
Oatmeal (see cereal)				
Ocean perch				
raw (3 oz)	80	15.8	.0	1.4
broiled (3 oz)	103	20.3	.0	1.8
Oils, all vegetable, 1T	120	.0	.0	14.0
Okra, boiled (½ cup slices)	34	1.9	7.5	.3
Olives, pitted (1 oz)	33	.2	1.8	3.0
Omelette (see eggs)				
Onion				
raw (½ cup)	27	.9	5.9	.2
boiled (½ cup)	29	1.0	6.6	.2
canned (½ cup)	21	1.0	4.5	.1
Onion rings, frozen (7 rings)	285	3.7	26.7	18.7
Oranges				
navel, raw (1 med)	65	1.4	16.6	.1
valencia, raw (1 med)	59	1.3	14.4	.4
Orange juice, fresh (1 cup)	111	1.7	25.8	.5
Oysters				
raw (3 oz) about 6 med	58	5.9	3.3	2.1
steamed (3 oz) about 12 med	117	12.0	6.7	4.2
canned (3 oz)	58	6.0	3.3	2.1
breaded & fried (3 oz)	167	7.5	9.9	10.7
Pancakes, plain (3.6 oz)	183	5.7	36.5	2.4
Papaya, raw (1 med)	117	1.9	29.8	.4
Parsley (¼ cup chopped)	10	.7	2.1	.1
Parsnips, boiled (½ cup)	63	1.0	15.2	.2
Pastries				
cream puff with custard filling	303	8.5	26.7	18.1
Danish, 1 small	161	2.6	18.8	8.8
Peach				
raw (1 med)	37	.6	9.7	.1
canned, heavy syrup (1 cup)	190	1.2	51.0	.3
canned, light syrup (1 cup)	136	1.1	36.5	.1
canned, juice pack (1 cup)	109	1.6	28.7	.1
canned, water pack (1 cup)	58	1.1	14.9	.1
Peach nectar, canned (1 cup)	134	.7	34.7	.1

Description	Cal	Pro (g)	Carb (g)	Fat (g)
Peanuts				
boiled (½ cup)	102	4.3	6.8	7.0
dry roasted (1 oz)	164	6.6	6.0	13.9
oil roasted (1 oz)	165	7.6	5.3	14.0
Peanut butter				
creamy/smooth (1 T)	95	4.6	2.5	8.2
chunk style/crunchy (1 T)	94	3.9	3.5	8.0
Pear				
raw, (1 med)	98	.7	25.1	.7
canned, heavy pack (1 cup)	188	.5	48.9	.3
canned, juice pack (1 cup)	123	.9	32.1	.2
canned, light syrup (1 cup)	144	.5	38.1	.1
canned, water pack (1 cup)	71	.5	19.1	.1
Peas, green				
raw (½ cup)	63	4.2	11.3	.3
boiled (½ cup)	67	4.3	12.5	.2
canned (½ cup)	59	3.8	10.7	.3
frozen (½ cup)	63	4.1	11.4	.2
Pecans				
dried (1 oz)	190	2.2	5.2	19.2
dry roasted (1 oz)	187	2.3	6.3	18.4
oil roasted (1 oz)	195	2.0	4.6	20.2
Peppers, sweet				
raw, chopped (½ cup)	13	.4	3.2	.1
boiled, chopped (½ cup)	19	.6	4.6	.1
canned (½ cup)	13	.6	2.7	.2
Perch (see ocean perch)				
Pickles				
Bread and butter (1 oz)	30	.0	7.0	.0
dill, 1 medium	12	.4	2.7	.1
sweet, 1 large	41	.1	11.1	.1
sweet relish (1 T)	21	.1	5.1	.1
Pies (1/6 pie)				
apple	250	2.0	37.0	11.0
banana cream	180	2.0	21.0	10.0
blueberry	270	3.0	40.0	11.0
Boston cream (see cakes)				
cherry	250	3.0	36.0	11.0
chocolate cream	190	2.0	24.0	10.0
coconut creme	190	2.0	22.0	11.0
custard	200	5.0	28.0	8.0
lemon meringue (1/8 of pie)	210	2.0	38.0	5.0
mince	280	2.0	48.0	9.0
peach	245	3.0	35.0	11.0
pecan (1/8 of pie)	330	3.0	51.0	13.0
pumpkin	200	3.0	29.0	8.0
strawberry cream	170	2.0	20.0	9.0
sweet potato	150	2.0	21.0	7.0
Pie crust, 1/6 of pie shell (1 oz)	130	1.0	12.0	8.0
Pike, northern, broiled (4 oz)	128	28.0	.0	1.0
Pineapple				
raw, (1 cup)	77	.6	19.2	.7
canned, heavy syrup (1 cup)	199	.9	51.5	.3
canned, juice pack (1 cup)	150	1.0	39.2	.2
Pineapple juice (1 cup)	139	.8	34.4	.2
Pistachios, shelled (1 oz)	172	4.2	7.8	15.0
Pizza				
cheese (½ of pie)	270	10.0	28.0	14.0
sausage & cheese (¼ pie)	350	22.0	34.0	14.0

Description	Cal	Pro (g)	Carb (g)	Fat (g)
Plum				
raw (1 med)	36	.5	8.6	.4
canned, heavy syrup (3 plums)	119	.5	30.9	.1
canned, juice pack (3 plums)	55	.5	14.4	.0
Pomegranate, raw (1 med)	104	1.5	26.4	.5
Popcorn				
popped, plain, air popped (1 cup)	30	1.0	6.0	.4
popped in oil, plain (1 oz)	220	3.0	20.0	15.0
microwave (3 cups)	140	2.0	14.0	9.0
Popovers, 1 medium	90	3.5	10.3	3.7
Pork (4 oz)				
bacon (see bacon)				
ham, canned	266	23.8	.4	18.2
ham, cured, roasted	276	24.5	.0	19.0
ham, fresh, roasted	333	28.4	.0	23.5
ham luncheon meat (1 oz)	31	4.7	1.1	.9
ham, spread, deviled (1 T)	35	2.0	.0	3.0
loin, braised	310	37.4	.0	16.6
loin, chops	291	31.7	.0	17.4
spareribs, braised (6.3 oz)	703	51.4	.0	53.6
Pork and beans (½ cup)	133	6.5	25.2	2.0
Potato salad (½ cup)	179	3.4	14.0	10.3
Potatoes				
au gratin, fresh (½ cup)	160	6.2	13.7	9.3
raw, w/o skin (1 med)	88	2.3	20.1	.1
baked, w/ skin (1 med)	220	4.7	51.0	.2
baked, w/o skin (1 med)	145	3.1	33.6	.2
canned, w/o skin (½ cup)	54	1.3	12.3	.2
french fried, (10 pieces)	158	2.0	20.0	8.3
hash brown, fresh (½ cup)	163	1.9	16.6	10.9
mashed, flakes (½ cup)	118	2.0	15.8	5.9
mashed, fresh (½ cup)	111	2.0	17.5	4.4
scalloped, fresh (½ cup)	105	3.5	13.2	4.5
sweet, baked (1 med)	118	2.0	27.7	.1
sweet, boiled (½ cup mashed)	172	2.7	39.8	.5
sweet, candied (1 med)	144	.9	29.3	3.4
sweet, canned (1 cup pieces)	183	3.3	42.3	.4
Potato chips (1 oz)	148	1.8	14.7	10.1
Potato salad (½ cup)	179	3.4	14.0	10.3
Pretzels				
Dutch style (1 oz)	110	3.0	24.0	.0
sticks (1 oz)	110	3.0	22.0	1.0
Prunes				
canned, heavy syrup (5 prunes)	90	.8	23.9	.2
dried (10 prunes)	201	2.2	52.7	.4
dried, cooked (½ cup)	113	1.2	29.8	.2
Prune juice (1 cup)	181	1.6	44.7	.1
Puddings (½ cup)				
banana	150	2.0	24.0	5.0
butterscotch	170	2.0	26.0	7.0
chocolate	170	3.0	28.0	6.0
chocolate-vanilla	170	3.0	28.0	6.0
rice	120	3.0	20.0	3.0
tapioca, vanilla	170	3.0	27.0	4.0
vanilla	180	3.0	28.0	6.0
Pumpkin				
boiled (½ cup mashed)	24	.9	6.0	.1
canned (½ cup mashed)	41	1.3	9.9	.3
Pumpkin seeds, salted (1 oz)	127	5.3	15.3	5.5

Description	Cal	Pro (g)	Carb (g)	Fat (g)
Quail, breast (1 oz)	35	6.4	.0	.8
Quince (1 med)	53	.4	14.1	.1
Rabbit, roasted (4 oz)	175	25.8	.0	7.2
Radishes, raw (10 med)	7	.3	1.6	.2
Raisins				
seedless (½ cup)	227	2.6	59.6	.4
seeded (½ cup)	222	1.9	58.9	.4
Raspberries				
raw (1 cup)	61	1.1	14.2	.7
canned, heavy syrup (½ cup)	117	1.1	29.9	.2
Relish (see pickles)				
Rice				
brown, cooked (1 cup)	232	4.9	49.7	1.2
white, cooked (1 cup)	223	4.1	49.6	.2
wild, raw (1 cup)	565	22.6	120.5	1.1
Rice mixes (commercial)				
beef (½ cup)	152	3.0	25.2	4.1
chicken (½ cup)	153	3.1	25.1	4.2
fried (½ cup)	159	3.2	25.2	4.8
Rockfish, broiled (3 oz)	103	20.4	.0	1.7
Rolls and buns (1 med)				
brown & serve, club	100	3.0	19.0	1.0
dinner, plain	60	2.0	11.0	1.0
French	108	4.2	21.3	1.5
hoagie or submarine	400	13.0	73.0	7.0
hamburger bun	115	4.3	22.0	2.2
hot dog	108	3.7	20.9	2.0
kaiser	184	7.0	35.4	2.9
sweet roll	133	1.8	17.5	6.6
Root beer (see beverages)				
Roughy, orange, raw (3 oz)	107	12.5	.0	6.0
Rum (see beverages)				
Safflower oil (see oil)				
Salad dressings (1 T)				
bleu cheese	77	.7	1.1	8.0
bleu cheese, diet	30	.0	2.0	2.0
Caesar	70	1.0	2.0	7.0
French	67	.1	2.7	6.4
French, diet	18	.0	3.0	1.0
Italian	69	.1	1.5	7.1
Italian, diet	6	.0	1.0	.0
mayonnaise	57	.1	3.5	4.9
Ranch	78	.1	1.1	8.3
Ranch, reduced calorie	16	.0	4.0	.0
Thousand Island	59	.1	2.4	5.6
Thousand Island, reduced calorie	20	.0	3.0	1.0
vinegar and oil	67	.5	2.3	6.5
Salad oil (see oils)				
Salads				
coleslaw (see coleslaw)				
chicken & celery (1 oz)	64	3.0	3.0	5.0
fruit, mixed, canned in water (4 oz)	34	.4	8.9	.1
fruit, mixed, cnd, light syrup (4 oz)	66	.4	17.2	.1
fruit, mxd, cnd, heavy syrup (4 oz)	83	.4	21.7	.1
garden (½ cup)	80	1.5	18.1	.3
gelatin (see gelatin)				
macaroni (½ cup)	200	40	21.0	10.0
potato (see potato salad)				
tuna (4 oz)	212	18.2	10.7	10.5

Description	Cal	Pro (g)	Carb (g)	Fat (g)
Salami (see sausage)				
Salmon, chinook				
raw (3 oz)	153	17.1	.0	8.9
smoked (3 oz)	99	15.5	.0	3.7
Salt	0	.0	.0	.0
Sardines				
canned in soybean oil (2 sardines)	50	5.9	.0	2.8
canned in tomato sauce (1 sardine)	68	6.2	.0	4.6
Sauces and Toppings (1 T)				
barbecue	12	.3	2.0	.3
butterscotch	60	.0	13.0	1.0
cheese (4 oz)	240	5.0	11.0	20.0
chili	24	.9	4.1	1.3
chocolate	50	1.0	11.0	.0
cream, half & half	20	.4	.6	1.7
soy	9	.9	1.5	.0
tartar	70	.0	2.0	7.0
tomato, canned (½ cup)	37	1.6	8.8	.2
Worcestershire	10	.0	2.0	.0
Sauerkraut, canned (½ cup)	22	1.1	5.1.	2
Sausage, cold cuts				
beef (1 link)	75	3.8	.0	6.1
bologna (1-oz slice)	80	4.0	1.0	7.0
Braunschweiger (1 oz)	80	4.0	.0	7.0
brown & serve sausage (1 link)	60	3.5	1.0	4.1
frankfurter (1 link)	160	5.0	2.0	14.0
knockwurst (2 oz)	180	7.0	1.0	16.0
liverwurst (1 oz)	97	4.0	1.0	9.0
meatloaf (4 oz)	200	10.0	8.0	14.0
minced ham (1 oz)	68	4.6	.1	5.3
mortadella (1 oz)	88	4.6	.9	7.2
Polish sausage (1 oz)	92	4.0	.5	8.1
pork sausage, cooked (1 oz)	105	5.6	.3	8.8
salami (1 oz)	119	6.5	.7	9.7
scrapple (1 slice)	65	2.7	4.2	3.7
Scallions (see onions)				
Scallops, raw (3 oz)	75	14.3	2.0	.6
Scrapple (see sausage)				
Sesame seeds, dried kernels (1 T)	47	2.1	.8	4.4
Shad, baked (1 oz)	56	4.8	.0	3.9
Sherbet (see ice cream)				
Shortbread (see cookies)				
Shortcake, strawberry (3 oz)	170	2.0	30.0	5.0
Shortening (1 T)	113	.0	.0	12.8
Shrimp				
raw (3 oz)	90	17.3	.8	1.5
breaded & fried (3 oz)	206	18.2	9.8	10.4
cocktail (4 oz)	113	7.0	19.0	1.0
canned (3 oz)	102	19.6	.9	1.7
steamed (3 oz)	84	17.8	.0	.9
Soft drinks (see beverages)				
Sole (see flounder)				
Soup (commercial, 1 cup)				
asparagus, cream	87	2.3	10.7	4.1
bean	190	9.0	30.9	3.4
bean, black	116	5.6	19.8	.05
beef broth	18	2.0	1.0	.0
beef noodle	84	4.8	9.0	3.1
celery, cream	90	1.7	8.8	5.6
chicken broth	39	4.9	.9	1.4

Description	Cal	Pro (g)	Carb (g)	Fat (g)
chicken, cream	116	3.4	9.3	7.4
chicken, gumbo	56	2.6	8.4	1.4
chicken, noodle	75	4.0	9.4	2.5
chicken with rice	60	3.5	7.2	1.9
chicken vegetable	74	3.6	8.6	2.8
clam chowder, Manhattan	78	4.2	12.2	2.3
clam chowder, New England	95	4.8	12.4	2.9
green pea	164	8.6	26.5	2.9
minestrone	83	4.3	11.2	2.5
mushroom, cream	129	2.3	9.3	9.0
onion	57	3.8	8.2	1.7
split pea with ham	189	10.3	28.0	4.4
tomato	86	2.1	16.6	1.9
turkey noodle	69	3.9	8.6	2.0
vegetable, vegetarian	72	2.1	12.0	1.9
vegetable beef	79	5.6	10.2	1.9
Soybean nuts				
dry roasted (½ cup)	387	34.0	28.1	18.6
roasted (½ cup)	405	30.3	28.9	21.8
roasted & toasted (1 oz)	129	10.5	8.7	6.8
Soybean tofu, raw (½ cup)	183	19.9	5.4	11.0
Soybean oil (see oils)				
Soybeans				
green, boiled (½ cup)	127	11.1	10.0	5.8
mature, boiled (½ cup)	149	14.3	8.5	7.7
Soy sauce (see sauces)				
Spaghetti				
cooked, with egg (4 oz)	149	5.8	28.3	1.2
with meatballs (4 oz)	116	4.4	17.6	4.0
with meat sauce (4 oz)	134	3.9	18.6	5.2
Spanish rice, cooked (1 cup)	90	2.0	20.0	.0
Spices	0	.0	.0	.0
Spinach				
raw (½ cup chopped)	6	.8	1.0	.1
boiled (½ cup)	21	2.7	3.4	.2
canned (½ cup)	25	3.0	3.6	.5
Squash				
acorn, baked (½ cup)	57	1.1	14.9	.1
acorn, boiled (½ cup)	41	.8	10.7	.1
crookneck, boiled (½ cup)	18	.8	3.9	.3
hubbard, boiled (½ cup)	35	1.8	7.6	.4
scallop, boiled (½ cup)	14	.9	3.0	.2
zucchini, raw (½ cup)	9	.8	1.9	.1
zucchini, boiled (½ cup)	14	.6	3.5	.1
Stew (see beef & vegetable stew)				
Strawberries				
raw (1 cup)	61	1.1	14.2	0.7
canned, heavy syrup (½ cup)	117	1.1	29.9	.2
Stuffing, cornbread (1 oz)	110	3.0	22.0	1.0
Sturgeon, cooked (4 oz)	153	23.5	.0	5.9
Succotash				
boiled (½ cup)	111	4.9	23.4	.8
canned (½ cup)	81	3.31	7.9	.6
Sugar (beet or cane)				
brown, packed (1 cup)	821	.0	212.1	.0
granulated (1 cup)	770	.0	199.0	.0
granulated (1 T)	46	.0	11.9	.0
granulated, 1 lump (2 cubes)	19	.0	5.0	.0
granulated, 1 packet (.2 oz)	23	.0	6.0	.0

Description	Cal	Pro (g)	Carb (g)	Fat (g)
powdered (1 cup unsifted)	462	.0	119.4	.0
powdered (1 T unsifted)	31	.0	8.0	.0
Sunflower seeds, hulled				
dried (1 oz)	162	6.5	5.3	14.1
dry roasted (1 oz)	165	5.5	6.8	14.1
oil roasted (1 oz)	175	6.1	4.2	16.3
Sweetpotatoes (see potato)				
Swordfish				
raw (3 oz)	103	16.8	.0	3.4
baked (3 oz)	132	21.6	.0	4.4
Syrups (1 T)				
Chocolate	46	.3	12.4	.2
Corn, light or dark	60	.0	15.0	.0
Maple	50	.0	12.8	.0
Molasses	60	.0	14.0	.2
Sorghum	53	.0	14.0	.0
Tangerine, raw (1 med)	37	.5	9.4	.2
Tapioca (see puddings)				
Tartar sauce (see sauces)				
Tea (see beverages)				
Tomatoes				
green, raw (1 med)	30	1.5	6.3	.3
red, raw (1 med)	24	1.1	5.3	.3
red, boiled (½ cup)	30	1.3	6.8	.3
red, canned (½ cup)	35	1.0	6.0	1.0
red, paste, canned (½ cup)	110	5.0	24.7	1.2
red, stewed (½ cup)	34	1.2	8.3	.2
puree, (½ cup)	51	2.1	12.5	.2
Tomato juice (1 cup)	43	1.9	10.2	.1
Tomato juice, cocktail (1 cup)	51	1.7	12.2	.2
Tomato ketchup (see ketchup)				
Toppings (see candy & sauces)				
Tortilla, flour (7 in. diam.)	80	2.0	14.0	2.0
Trout				
mixed species, raw (3 oz)	126	17.7	.0	5.6
rainbow, raw (3 oz)	100	17.5	.0	2.9
rainbow, baked (3 oz)	129	22.4	.0	3.7
Tuna				
canned in oil, light (3 oz)	169	24.8	.0	7.0
canned in oil, white (3 oz)	158	22.6	.0	6.9
canned in water, light (3 oz)	111	25.1	.0	.4
canned in water, white (3 oz)	116	22.7	.0	2.1
Tuna Salad (see salads)				
Turkey, roasted (4 oz)				
dark, with skin	251	31.2	.0	13.1
dark, without skin	212	32.4	.0	8.2
white, with skin	223	32.4	.0	9.4
white, without skin	178	33.9	.0	3.7
Turnip, boiled (4 oz)	26	1.7	4.9	.3
Turnip greens				
raw (½ cup)	7	.4	1.6	.1
boiled (½ cup)	15	.8	3.1	.2
canned (½ cup)	17	1.6	2.8	.4
Veal, roasted (4 oz)				
ground	195	27.6	.0	8.6
loin	246	28.1	.0	14.0
rib	259	27.2	.0	15.8
Vegetable juice (1 cup)	45	1.4	11.0	.3
Vegetables (see types)				
Vegetables, mixed (½ cup)	39	2.1	7.6	.2

Description	Cal	Pro (g)	Carb (g)	Fat (g)
Vegetable stew (8 oz)	170	5.0	20.0	8.0
Venison, roasted (4 oz)	179	34.3	.0	3.6
Vinegar, white (1 cup)	30	.4	12.0	.4
Vodka (see beverages)				
Waffles (2 pieces)	280	6.0	51.0	6.0
Walnuts, dried (1 oz)	172	6.9	3.4	16.1
Water chestnuts, raw (½ cup)	66	.9	14.8	.1
Watermelon (1 cup)	50	1.0	11.5	.7
Wheat (see cereals, flours)				
Wheat germ, crude (1 cup)	414	26.6	59.6	11.2
Whiskey (see beverages)				
Whitefish				
raw (3 oz)	114	16.2	.0	5.0
baked, stuffed (3.5 oz)	215	15.2	5.8	14.0
smoked (3 oz)	92	19.9	.0	.8
Wine (see beverages)				
Yeast, baker's, dry (.6 oz)	15	2.0	2.0	.0
Yogurt (1 cup)				
plain, skim milk	127	13.0	17.4	.4
plain, whole milk	139	7.9	10.6	7.4
coffee, low-fat	194	11.2	31.3	2.8
strawberry, low-fat	250	9.0	48.0	2.0
vanilla, low-fat	194	11.2	31.3	2.8

Ordering Information

This manual and the other materials distributed through The LEARN Education Center are not available in bookstores. You may write, call, or visit us on the Internet to obtain current pricing and shipping charges. Discounts are available for bulk orders. Below are other materials and services also available.

The LEARN Education Center

The LEARN Education Center was established to respond to the increasing demand for scientifically sound, state-of-the-art publications, training courses and services. The Center is dedicated to the development of health and wellness materials, including audio tapes, newsletters, professional training guides, leadership training programs, and professional counseling services.

For your ordering convenience, a toll free number is available and may be called 24 hours a day. In addition, you can order via our Internet address at www.LearnEducation.com. Payments can be made with a major credit card, check, or money order.

All orders are shipped with 24 hours of receipt, and next day and second day delivery service is available. As you use our publications, we sincerely welcome any comments you may have to improve these materials, and we encourage you to tell us how we are doing.

For ordering or general information, please write or call us at:

The LEARN Education Center
P.O. Box 35328, Dept. 70
Dallas, Texas 75235-0328

Toll free telephone   1-800–736–7323
In Dallas telephone   817–545–4500
Fax   817–545–2211

E-mail address:
     LEARN@LearnEducation.com

Internet address:
     www.LearnEducation.com

The LEARN Institute for LifeStyle Management

The LEARN Institute was established to provide state-of-the-art training programs to health professionals working with overweight clients. The LEARN Institute is the first to offer specific training and certification in the field of weight control. The **LifeStyle Counselor Certification Program** has been developed to provide a comprehensive cross-disciplinary training program to health professionals working in the field of weight and stress management.

Two certifications are currently offered and training is provided in various cities throughout the United States. Certifications currently being offered include:

Certification in Weight Control

Certification in Stress Management

For more detailed information on The LifeStyle Counselor Certification Program or a free brochure call or write to:

The LEARN Institute for
     LifeStyle Management
P.O. Box 35328, Dept. 50
Dallas, Texas 75235-0328

Toll free telephone   1-800–736–7323
In Dallas telephone   817–545–4500
Fax   817–545–2211

E-mail address:
     TheInstitute@LearnEducation.com
Internet address:
     www.LearnEducation.com

The American Association of LifeStyle Counselors

The American Association of LifeStyle Counselors is a nonprofit corporation dedicated to providing its members and the public with the most current, safe, and sound lifestyle-management programs and services. Individuals who complete the LifeStyle Counselor Certification Program become eligible for membership in the American Association of LifeStyle Counselors (AALC). Only members of the AALC can use the title of **Certified LifeStyle Counselor**. If you would like to locate a Certified LifeStyle Counselor in your area you may write, call, or visit the AALC's Internet site as follows:

**The American Association
of LifeStyle Counselors
P.O. Box 35328, Dept. 55
Dallas, Texas 75235-0328**

In Dallas telephone	**817–545–3220**
Fax	**817–545–2211**
E-mail address	**AALC@AALC.com**
Internet address	**www.AALC.com**

Other Materials

Publications currently available from The LEARN Education Center are as follows:

Weight Management

The LEARN Program for Weight Control—7th Edition by Kelly D. Brownell, Ph.D.

The LEARN Program for Weight Control—Medication Edition by Kelly D. Brownell, Ph.D. and Thomas A. Wadden, Ph.D.

The LEARN Program Monitoring Forms

The LEARN Program Cassettes by Kelly D. Brownell, Ph.D.

The LEARN Weight Maintenance and Stabilization Guide by Kelly D. Brownell—Available January, 1998.

The Health & Fitness Club Leader's Guide—Administering A Weight Management Program by Ross Andersen, Ph.D., Kelly D. Brownell, Ph.D., and William L. Haskell, Ph.D.

The LifeStyle Counselor's Guide for Weight Control by Brenda L. Wolfe, Ph.D., et al., eds.

The Weight Control Digest—annual subscription.

Weight Sex & Marriage by Richard B. Stuart, Ph.D. and Barbara Jacobson

Eating Disorders

Binge Eating by Christopher G. Fairburn, M.D. and G. Terence Wilson, Ph.D.

Overcoming Binge Eating by Christopher Fairburn, M.D.

Eating Disorders and Obesity, Kelly D. Brownell, Ph.D. and Christopher G. Fairburn, M.D., eds.

Physical Activity and Exercise

Living with Exercise—by Steven N. Blair, P.E.D.

Stress Management

The LifeStyle Counselor's Guide for Stress Management, by Leslie A. Telfer, Ph.D., et al.

Mastering Stress—A LifeStyle Approach by David H. Barlow, Ph.D. and Ronald M. Rapee, Ph.D.

Mind Over Mood by Dennis Greenberger, Ph.D. and Christine A. Padesky, Ph.D.

Other Materials:

The Balancing Act by Georgia Kostas, M.P.H., R.D.

Body Images—Development, Deviance, and Change by Thomas F. Cash, Ph.D. and Thomas Pruzinsky, Ph.D.

Body Image Therapy—A Program for Self-Directed Change by Thomas F. Cash, Ph.D.

More of What's Cooking by Veronica C. Coronado with Patty Kirk, R.D., L.D.

Motivational Interviewing by William R. Miller and Stephen Rollnick.

About the Authors

Kelly D. Brownell, Ph.D. is an internationally known expert on weight control. He received training at Purdue University, Rutgers University, and Brown University. After serving on the faculty of the University of Pennsylvania School of Medicine for 13 years, he joined the faculty at Yale University, where he is Professor of Psychology, Professor of Epidemiology and Public Health, Director of the Yale Center for Eating and Weight Disorders, and Master of Silliman College. He has written 12 books and more than 200 research papers and book chapters, and holds appointments on 10 editorial boards.

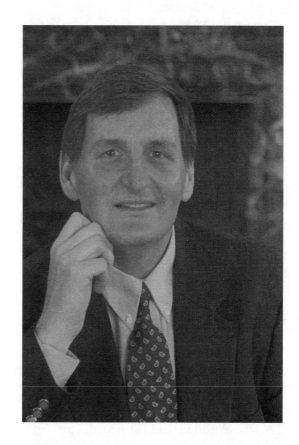

Dr. Brownell has received awards from the American Psychological Association and the New York Academy of Sciences, and has been awarded research grants from the National Institutes of Health, the MacArthur Foundation, and the National Institute of Mental Health. He has been the President of the Society of Behavioral Medicine, the Division of Health Psychology of the American Psychological Association, and the Association for the Advancement of Behavior Therapy. He has been an advisor to the U.S. Navy, American Airlines, Johnson & Johnson and other organizations.

He has appeared on the *Today Show*, *Good Morning America*, *Nova* and *20/20*, and his work has been featured in the *New York Times, Washington Post, Glamour, Redbook, Family Circle, Vogue*, and other publications.

Thomas A. Wadden, Ph.D. received his bachelors degree from Brown University and his doctorate in clinical psychology from the University of North Carolina at Chapel Hill. In 1981, he joined the faculty at the University of Pennsylvania School of Medicine, where he is currently Professor of Psychology and Director of the Weight and Eating Disorders Program. He has written three books and over 150 scientific papers.

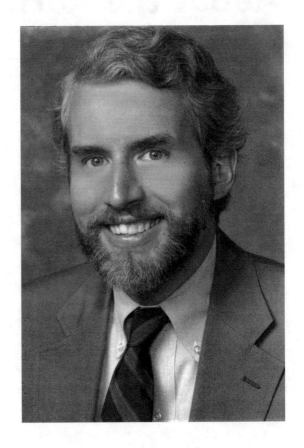

Dr. Wadden is widely regarded for his research on weight control that has investigated approaches including diet, exercise, behavior therapy, social support, and medication. His research is supported by a Research Scientist Development Award from the National Institute of Mental Health, as well as by additional grants from government and industry. He has served as an advisor to the Federal Trade Commission, the Federal Bureau of Investigation, and Shape Up America.

Dr. Wadden has appeared on *Good Morning America,* the *Today Show, 20/20*, and the *NBC Nightly News*. His research has been featured in the *New York Times, Wall Street Journal, Washington Post, Reader's Digest, Prevention,* and other publications.

Foreword

This study focuses on the adjustment challenges facing the textile and clothing industries across the globe. The analytical work was initially suggested during informal consultations between the OECD Trade Committee and civil society organisations. It took two years of extensive discussions in the Working Party of the Trade Committee to deepen understanding of the issues and finalise the study.

Thousands of jobs have been suppressed in the textile and clothing industries, and a considerable restructuring is anticipated with the elimination of quantitative restrictions by the end of 2004, as agreed under the WTO Agreement on Textiles and Clothing. This event is best viewed as part of a longer process of adjustment that has taken place over both the medium term (the phase-out of quantitative restrictions has lasted a decade) and the long term (the textile and clothing industries have long migrated with the industrial evolution of countries). Planning for the post-2004 market, combined with technological developments and evolutionary changes in national policies, has already encouraged a major reordering of patterns in trade and investment. Firms in all countries and segments of the industry will continue to face adjustment challenges.

The end of quantitative restrictions is also causing concern that a few of the larger developing countries may capture a disproportionate share of the economic benefits arising from the quota phase-out. The concerned countries are looking to the ongoing multilateral trade negotiations in the context of the Doha Development Agenda to secure improved market access conditions that can help them minimise their adjustment hardships.

This study reviews the most recent market developments throughout the entire supply chain, from natural fibres to retail distribution. It examines the policy challenges in the fields of trade, labour adjustment, technology and innovation, and other regulatory dimensions that are important determinants of a country's drive towards global integration. It covers adjustment in both developed and developing countries and underscores the vulnerability of suppliers located in small developing and least developed countries that have specialised in the final assembly of clothing products using imported textiles.

The study argues that countries aspiring to maintain an export-led strategy in textiles and clothing need to complement their industrial cluster of expertise in manufacturing by developing their expertise in the higher value-added segments of the supply chain. National suppliers would thus need to place greater emphasis on education and training in services-related skills, such as design, material sourcing, quality control, logistics and retail distribution and to encourage the establishment of joint structures where domestic suppliers can share market knowledge and offer more integrated solutions to prospective buyers.

The study also argues that a key objective of governments is to strengthen the capacity of the private sector to deal effectively with rapid change and growing competition in order to capture the trade opportunities that are being created through improved market access. This involves: supporting the emergence of qualified pools of expertise and the adaptability of the workforce; improving the regulatory environment for essential business services; stimulating collaborative innovation processes in the fields of dissemination and technology transfer; and negotiating improved market access for textile and clothing products, especially by seeking to eliminate remaining obstacles to the establishment of retail distribution systems and distorting production measures.

The preparation of the study has benefited from extensive discussions in the OECD's Trade Committee and its Working Party. The lead drafter of the study was Denis Audet under the supervision of Raed Safadi. The study has also benefited from contributions by Howard Rosen (Chapter 3), Henning Klodt and Dean Spinanger (Chapter 4), and Peter Walkenhorst (Annex A). The authors wish to acknowledge the able statistical assistance provided by Karinne Logez and insightful comments from Jérôme Delarue, Blaise Durand-Réville, Louis Gionet, Hinrich Hormann, Francesco Marchi, Viktor Vollmer and numerous individuals in the Association of German Textile Machinery Manufacturers (VDMA).

The study is published on the responsibility of the Secretary-General of the OECD.

Table of Contents

Foreword 3

Acronyms 9

Executive Summary 11

Chapter 1 Adjustment Challenges in Textiles and Clothing 17

Introduction 17
A typology of the textile and clothing supply chain 19
Adjustment challenges by production segment 19
Policy challenges 29

Chapter 2 Market Developments and Trade Policies 35

Introduction 35
Key trends in production, consumption and trade 36
Trade policy measures 55
Conclusion 73

Chapter 3 Trade-Related Labour Adjustment Policies 93

Introduction 93
International trade and labour adjustment 94
Characteristics of displaced workers 99
Labour market adjustment policies 102
Conclusion 113

Chapter 4 Technology and Innovation 135

Introduction 135
Technology and trade in the textile and clothing industries 135
Insights into technology trends in the textile and clothing industries 142
Innovation systems in OECD countries 147
Conclusion 160

Chapter 5 Business Facilitation 175

Introduction 175
The overarching environment in textiles and clothing 176
Logistical dimensions of the international movement of goods 178
Customs facilitation dimensions 188
Essential business services 194
Other dimensions 199
Conclusion 203

Annex A Literature Review of Quantitative Studies 213

Introduction 213
Quantitative aspects of trade liberalisation in the textile and clothing industries 213
Studies at the global level 218
Studies with a regional focus 222
Conclusion 225

Tables Chapter 2

Table 2.1. Textile and clothing employment in the United States and in the European Union, by production segment, 1970 and 2002. 38

Table 2.2. Productivity and capital intensity in textile and apparel manufacturing in the United States and the European Union... 39

Table 2.3. Employment by size of establishments in the United States and the European Union...... 40

Table 2.4. Distribution of world value added, selected sectors. 47

Table 2.5. Shares of manufacturing value added in selected regions. 48

Table 2.6. State-owned enterprises in China, 2001. 52

Table 2.7. Leading exporters of textiles and clothing, 1990-2002. 54

Table 2.8. Simple average tariffs, selected countries. 57

Table 2.9. Distribution of tariff peaks in textiles and clothing. 58

Table 2.10 Cost competitiveness under outward processing programmes. 62

Table 2.11. Textile and clothing machinery imports, 1994-2002. 65

Table 2.12. LDC utilisation rates of GSP schemes in textiles and clothing, 2001. 67

Table 2.13. US textile and clothing imports under preferential trade arrangements, 2003. 69

Table 2.A1.1. Selected characteristics of textile branches, selected years and countries. 76

Table 2.A1.2. Selected characteristics of clothing branches, selected years and countries. 77

Table 2.A1.3. Leading exporters and importers of textiles, 1980-2002. 78

Table 2.A1.4. Leading exporters and importers of clothing, 1980-2002. 79

Table 2.A1.5. Clothing exports in selected economies, 1980-2002. 80

Table 2.A1.6. OECD textile exports by destination, 1980-2001. 81

Table 2.A1.7. OECD clothing exports by destination, 1980-2001. 82

Table 2.A1.8. OECD textile imports by origin, 1980-2001. 83

Table 2.A1.9. OECD clothing imports by origin, 1980-2001. 84

Table 2.A1.10. Bound tariffs in textiles and clothing, post-Uruguay Round. 85

Table 2.A1.11. Applied tariffs in textile and clothing products, 1996. 86

Tables Chapter 3

Table 3.1. Net job losses in textiles and clothing between 1970 and 2000. 95

Table 3.2. Changes in US employment by sectors, 1974-2000. 96

Table 3.3. Changes in US employment in manufacturing industries, 1974-2000. 96

Table 3.4. Demographic characteristics of displaced workers. 101

Table 3.5. Education characteristics of displaced workers. 101

Table 3.6. Tenure characteristics of displaced workers. 102

Table 3.7. Earnings and replacement rates of displaced workers. 102

Table 3.8. Classification of labour market adjustment policies. 103

Table 3.9. Standardised unemployment rates. 105

Table 3.10. Unemployment insurance provisions. 106

Table 3.11. Brief summary of unemployment insurance programmes in five countries. 107

Table 3.12. Expenditure on training and unemployment compensation, 2000. 108

Table 3.A1.1. Job losses in textiles and clothing in six countries, 1970-2000. 115

Table 3.A1.2. Employment in textiles and clothing, by production segment. 116

Table 3.A2.1. The French unemployment insurance and solidarity scheme. 118

Table 3.A2.2. Unemployment insurance assistance. 119

Table 3.A2.3. Duration of assistance. 120

Table 3.A2.4. Re-employment benefits. 120

Table 3.A2.5. Minimum daily assistance. 121

Table 3.A2.6. Long-term unemployed as a share of total unemployed. 122

Table 3.A2.7. Level of assistance under the Japanese unemployment system. 126
Table 3.A2.8. Benefits for workers under 60 years of age. 126
Table 3.A2.9. Duration of assistance for unemployed who lose their jobs as a result of
            bankruptcy or dismissal 126
Table 3.A2.10. Duration of assistance for unemployed 127
Table 3.A2.11. Amount of unemployment insurance assistance. 127
Table 3.A2.12. Unemployment insurance assistance. 128
Table 3.A2.13. TAA and JAFTA-TAA, 2002 to July 2003. 129
Table 3.A2.14. TAA services by participant. 129
Table 3.A2.15. Profile of TAA and NAFTA-TAA participants, 1999 and 2000. 130

Tables Chapter 4

Table 4.1. Concentration in world machinery and transport equipment exports, 1981-2002 140
Table 4.2. Shares, changes in shares and yearly growth rates for SITC product groups 141
Table 4.3. Germany's employment in manufacturing industries, 1993-2001 145
Table 4.4. Share of textiles and clothing in total manufacturing employment in OECD countries ... 148
Table 4.5. Revealed comparative advantages in textiles and clothing 150
Table 4.6. R&D intensity of OECD countries, 1990-2000. 151
Table 4.7. R&D specialisation and trade performance of textiles and clothing. 152
Table 4.A1. Description of 3-digit SITC (Rev.2) categories in Section 7, Machinery
            and Transport Equipment 2000 163

Tables Chapter 5

Table 5.1. US imports of textiles and clothing by mode of transport, 2003. 179
Table 5.2. Transit, freight and duty cost on US imports of textiles and clothing. 182
Table 5.3. Rail transport in the EU and the United States, 1970-2001 186
Table 5.4. Freight transport in five regions, 2000 186
Table 5.5. Structure of customs tariffs on clothing products. 192
Table 5.6. Structure of customs of tariffs on textile products. 194
Table 5.7. Business telephone charges in OECD countries. 196
Table 5.8. Industrial electricity charges in OECD and non-OECD countries. 198
Table 5.9. Establishments by employment size in the United States and the European Union. 203
Table 5.A1.1. Freight costs by mode of transport for textile and clothing imports in the
            United States, 2003. 206

Tables Annex A

Table A.1. Estimates of MFA quota rents and price premiums for textiles and clothing, 1994 214
Table A.2. Structure of EU pre- and post-Uruguay Round tariffs in the textile and clothing
            industries 214
Table A.3. Annual welfare gains from ATC reforms in the European Union, 1997. 223
Table A.4. Structural characteristics of ATC reform studies 227
Table A.5. Estimates of annual welfare gains from ATC reforms. 228

Charts

Chart 2.1. Schematic representation of production-sharing possibilities 43
Chart 5.1. Transport chain for traded goods in containers. 178

Figures

Figure 3.1. Main phases in labour market adjustment policies and programmes. 104
Figure 3.2. TAA participants by industry, 1975-1999. 109
Figure 4.1. World exports, 1965-2002. 136
Figure 4.2. Total merchandise exports, exports of textile and clothing products and textile
and clothing machinery, 1992-2002. 137
Figure 4.3. Textile and clothing machinery exports to major regions/countries. 137
Figure 4.4a. Working hours per unit output in spinning and weaving from 1750. 138
Figure 4.4b. Working hours per unit output in spinning and weaving from 1925. 139
Figure 5.1. Freight rates per TEU, 2001. 187
Figure 5.2. Average applied tariffs and number of tariff lines for clothing products. 191
Figure 5.3. Average applied tariffs and number of tariff lines for textile products. 193
Figure A.1. Hourly labour costs in the primary textile industry, 1993. 216
Figure A.2. Expected changes in terms of trade after MFA quota removal. 220

Boxes

Box 2.1. Preferential trade arrangements. 60
Box 2.2. A new world blue jeans capital emerged in Mexico with NAFTA. 64
Box 3.1. Job loss from imports: measuring the costs. 100
Box 3.2. Some of the key TAA reforms of 2002. 111
Box 4.1. The essence of globalisation in the textile machinery sector at the micro level. 144
Box 5.1. Adverse impacts of customs delays on textile and clothing production. 190
Box 5.2. Adverse impacts of high electricity costs and unreliable electricity systems on
textile and clothing production in several developing countries. 199

Acronyms

AGOA	African Growth Opportunity Act (US)
AMS	aggregate measure of support
APEC	Asia-Pacific Economic Cooperation Forum
ASEAN	Association of South-east Asian Nations
ATC	Agreement on Textiles and Clothing (WTO)
ATPDEA	Andean Trade Promotion and Drug Eradication Act (US)
CAD	computer-aided design
CAM	computer-assisted methods
CBTPA	Caribbean Basin Trade Partnership Act (US)
CGE	Computable general equilibrium
CLF	clothing, leather and footwear
CNY	Chinese yuan
CPI	Consumer Price Index (US)
EBA	Everything but Arms (EU)
ECA	European Carpet Association
EFTA	European Free Trade Association
ETAP	European Association for Textile Polyolefins
DDA	Doha Development Agenda
FDI	Foreign Direct Investment
FTA	Free Trade Agreement
FTAA	Free Trade Agreement of the Americas
GATS	General Agreement on Trade in Services
GATT	General Agreement on Tariffs and Trade
GSP	General System of Preferences
GTAP	Global Trade Analysis Project
HS	Harmonised System
IAF	International Apparel Federation
IMO	International Maritime Organisation
IMF	International Monetary Fund
ISPS	International Ship and Port Safety Code

ITC	International Trade Commission
ITMA	International Textile Machinery Association
LDC	least developed countries
LTA	Long-Term Arrangement Regarding International Trade in Cotton Textiles
MFA	Multi-Fibre Arrangement
MFN	Most-favoured nation
NAFTA	North American Free Trade Agreement
NIE	newly industrialised economy
OETH	Observatoire Européen du Textile et de l'Habillement
OPP	outward processing programmes
RCA	revealed comparative advantage
ROOs	Rules of origin
RTA	regional trade arrangement
SAARC	South Asian Association for Regional Cooperation
SMEs	small and medium-sized enterprises
SOE	state-owned enterprise
SOLAS	Convention on the Safety of Life at Sea
SSI	small-scale industry (India)
STA	Short-term Arrangement Regarding International Trade in Textiles
TAA	Trade Adjustment Assistance (US)
TBT	Agreement on Technical Barriers to Trade (WTO)
TCM	textile and clothing machinery
TEU	20 foot equivalent unit
TPL	tariff preference-level provisions
UNCTAD	United Nations Conference on Trade and Development
WIA	Workforce Investment Act (US)
WTO	World Trade Organization

Executive Summary

Rules governing world trade in textiles and clothing will change drastically when new regulation is enforced at the end of 2004. Countries will no longer be able to protect their own industries by restricting the quantity of textile and clothing products being imported. The World Trade Organization's (WTO) "Agreement on Textiles and Clothing" (ATC) will challenge the decades of trade restrictions on global suppliers. Considerable adjustments have been made for all those involved in the supply chain: from cotton producers to fashion retailers; and from the least developed countries (LDCs) to the most developed countries. Understandably, there is considerable concern about the emergence of more competitive suppliers in China capturing a disproportionate share of the economic benefits when import restrictions are lifted.

Import restrictions, initially imposed under the Multi-Fibre Arrangement (MFA), fragmented the international supply chain by encouraging the diversity of supplies. This process worked to the disadvantage of the more efficient and quota-constrained suppliers, many of which subcontracted clothing production to low-wage third countries. Hence, the rules benefited the least competitive suppliers, most of them located in small developing countries and LDCs that have specialised in producing clothing products from imported textiles. Such countries are increasingly aware of their vulnerability and are seeking to improve their access to markets within developed countries in order to minimise the expected hardships. However, in developed countries, more than 4 million jobs have already disappeared, as their suppliers have responded to competitive pressures by shifting production towards faster growth products, modernising equipment and adopting new working methods, especially in outsourcing sewing activities to low-wage countries. As of 2005, retail groups in developed countries will have greater liberty in purchasing products on a global basis. The world exports of textile and clothing machinery still originate predominantly from developed countries. On balance, developed countries have considerable interests in these dynamic industries and their interests are better served by an open and liberal multilateral trading environment.

This publication examines the recent market developments in the textile and clothing industries in both developed and developing countries. It highlights the challenges facing governments in the areas of trade policies, labour adjustment, technology and innovation and other regulatory areas that are key determinants of a country's ability to integrate in the world economy. Finally, the publication offers recommendations to assist governments in establishing a coherent policy and regulatory framework to ensure that their industries are ready to meet the adjustment challenges.

Market forces: what are the key developments?

Migration of textile capacity to the most competitive developing countries. Without quantitative import restrictions, there are no trade obstacles to developing stronger clusters of textile expertise in the most competitive developing countries. The recent surge in China's imports of up-to-date textile and clothing equipment bears witness to this trend and points to what will be the future sources of textile and clothing production and exports. The main beneficiaries are the Chinese clothing suppliers that can buy textiles directly from domestic sources and hence meet shorter turnaround delivery requirements. Access to high-quality textiles is considered one of the most important determinants of the competitiveness of clothing suppliers. Other developing countries with both textile and clothing capacity may also be able to prosper in this new competitive environment. As a result, the textile industry in developed countries will face intensified competition in both their export and domestic markets. The migration of textile capacity will nevertheless be influenced by objective competitive factors and will be hampered by the presence of distorting domestic measures and weak domestic infrastructure in several developing countries and LDCs.

The growing importance of the non-clothing applications of textiles or technical textiles. The textile industry is undergoing a major reorientation towards non-clothing applications of textiles, *i.e.* technical textiles, which represent the fastest-growing segment of total textile applications. Technical textiles are often defined as "those textile materials and products manufactured primarily for their technical and performance properties rather than for their aesthetic or decorative characteristics". They are used in many applications, including furniture, automotive, construction, environment, health and hygiene. It is estimated that technical textiles now account for more than half of total textile production. The processes involved in producing technical textiles are human and capital-intensive and, for the moment, concentrated in developed countries.

Time factors and international competitiveness. While low wages can still give developing countries a competitive edge in world markets, time factors now play a far more crucial role in determining international competitiveness. The comparative advantage of developing countries in the assembly process, *i.e.* in low-wage sewing, does not necessarily translate into a comparative advantage in managing the entire supply chain when all services-related dimensions are taken into consideration. Countries that aspire to maintain an export-led strategy in textiles and clothing need to complement their industrial cluster of expertise in manufacturing by developing their expertise in the higher value-added segments of the supply chain. To pursue these avenues, national suppliers need to place greater emphasis on the education and training of services-related skills, such as design, material sourcing, quality control, logistics and retail distribution.

Leadership role of large retail groups. Retail distribution is increasingly dominated by large retail groups in the main consuming countries, where the trend is towards greater product specialisation, brand-name products and market segmentation. These large retail groups collect market information about the latest trends in styles and tastes, and their integration of this information gives them considerable leverage in dealing with suppliers. Nevertheless, offshore suppliers can benefit from working in close co-operation with large retail groups as they learn to: manufacture quality products; apply the buyer's code of conduct; and deliver products in a timely fashion. Developing business relationships between national business clusters and the large retail groups plays an instrumental role in improving the supply chain. For exporting countries seeking to develop their export strategies, nurturing contacts between domestic clusters and large retail groups is a must.

Trade policy: what are the challenges?

Liberal trade and investment policies play a key role in this adjustment process. They can help to restrain price pressures on imported goods and therefore encourage the emergence of firms that are able to compete on domestic and international markets. Trade policies, other than quantitative import restrictions, have had a major impact in developing geographical patterns of trade in textiles and clothing. In particular, eliminating import quotas will increase the appeal of preferential trade arrangements, such as regional trade arrangements and the General System of Preferences (GSP). However, it will also reduce the appeal of outward processing programmes (OPP) under which textile materials are temporarily exported to lower-wage countries and then re-imported as clothing products under preferential provisions.

The challenge for policy makers in developed countries is to draft rules of origin for their preferential arrangements that will mainly benefit LDCs and the small developing countries that are most vulnerable to competition from large and integrated suppliers in China and India. Recognising that there is, at present, virtually no production of high-quality textiles in LDCs, preferential access arrangements in favour of LDCs must take into account that they have to use competitive textiles originating from third countries to compete on export markets. Under these circumstances, it seems inevitable that in providing LDCs with preferential access, there will be some collateral benefits for suppliers of high-quality textiles.

Average tariff protection on textile and clothing imports remains high compared to the protection afforded on manufactured products. In developed countries, the average tariff applied on clothing products is 16.1% versus 6.2% on manufactured products. In developing countries, the average tariffs are 23% and 13.5%, respectively. Moreover, there are considerable differences among developed countries in the level of tariffs applied on textile and clothing imports and in the recurrence of tariff peaks, *i.e.* tariffs exceeding 15%. There are also similar imbalances among developing countries and LDCs.

Labour adjustment: how will countries cope with job losses?

Although trade liberalisation yields economy-wide benefits, opening up markets to international competition puts pressure on labour markets and results in both temporary and permanent hardships for displaced workers. Displaced workers tend to have a low level of education, low skill levels and they are predominantly women and minorities. All these characteristics make it more difficult for workers to adjust to changes in the labour market. Furthermore, it is also difficult to isolate the causes of worker displacement as technological change, productivity gains, increased import competition and shifts in production can all contribute to job losses. Therefore, there is a need for broader programmes aimed at helping the unemployed in general rather than specific programmes designed only for those who lose their jobs because of increased competition in trade-related industries.

The main goal of any labour adjustment programme should be re-employment: either returning to one's previous job or finding a new job as soon as possible and with minimal disruption in earnings. With that objective in mind, countries have used various programmes to train workers and provide job search assistance. The recent introduction in Germany and the United States of "wage insurance" aims at encouraging workers to return to work as soon as possible. Wage insurance is designed for workers whose new wage is lower than their previous wage so as to bridge the income gap between the two wages. Hence, it is hoped that workers will be encouraged to take new jobs sooner. It is also hoped that new employers will provide workers with on-the-job training, which has proven to be more effective and cheaper than government-financed classroom training.

Technology and innovation: what role does it play?

Huge productivity gains were achieved through innovations in the textile industry, but the clothing industry relies on sewing techniques that have barely changed over the last century. Although these industries can be considered to be mature, they use technological innovations that are largely generated in other industries: in chemicals (man-made fibres); and machinery (computer-aided design systems). This study argues that technology transfer between machinery suppliers and users plays a pivotal role in the performance of textile and clothing suppliers. Hence, it is appropriate for governments to encourage the dissemination of advanced technological knowledge in information and communication and take advantage of the opportunities it offers. Governments should also keep in mind that, in the long run, innovative capacities basically depend on the availability of suitable human capital. Therefore, a sound education and qualification system seems much more important for sustainable technical progress than public innovation programmes.

Regulatory frameworks: what else is needed?

Lifting import restrictions will leave countries whose regulatory framework is ill-equipped to deal with international competition exposed and vulnerable. They stand to pay a high price for inefficient domestic regulatory regimes, obsolete infrastructure in essential business services, cumbersome customs procedures and other distorted market structures.

A reliable transport infrastructure and efficient customs procedures complement each other in minimising transit periods for shipments involved in international trade and can make geographically remote locations more internationally competitive. Countries need to assess the logistical costs involved in export markets with a view to: setting up a competition-enhancing environment in various port services; strengthening competition conditions in and between transport modes; addressing the terrorist risks in transport without losing sight of the benefits of frictionless transport systems; and better integrating the enforcement of national laws and regulations, *e.g.* customs procedures, taxation, sanitary and environment protection, with other service providers in ports.

Outdated regulatory frameworks in electricity and telecommunications services act as taxes on textile and clothing suppliers and, more importantly, undermine the capacity of national suppliers to focus production on higher value-added segments of the supply chain that depend on reliable infrastructure to ensure quick market responses. Hence, reliable and up-to-date telecommunications and electricity infrastructures give textile and clothing suppliers a competitive edge.

While it is important to nurture entrepreneurship within small- and medium-sized enterprises (SMEs), there is a danger of distorting investment incentives. This is particularly true where exemptions are offered to small-scale operations that could not otherwise compete with more efficient large-scale operations. Recent work by the OECD in the context of the Bologna Charter on SME Policies has found that education and training are the single most effective means of encouraging entrepreneurship in societies. Above all, the role of government is to pursue a sound and stable macroeconomic environment able to sustain non-inflationary economic growth. There is strong evidence that real economic growth and, in turn, net employment creation are stimulated in an environment of low inflation. The pursuit of sound macroeconomic policies fosters market adjustment to changes in the competitive environment and facilitates the redeployment of affected resources to other productive sectors. The pursuit of government actions at the macroeconomic and microeconomic levels, *i.e.* trade, labour adjustment, innovation, and essential business infrastructure, brings benefits that go well beyond the textile and clothing industries.

Policy recommendations

- Shift the industrial cluster of expertise from manufacturing to the higher value-added segments of the supply chain by placing greater emphasis on education and training of services-related skills, such as design, material sourcing, quality control, logistics and retail distribution.
- Support the emergence of qualified pools of expertise and the adaptability of the workforce.
- Improve the regulatory environment for essential business services.
- Stimulate collaborative innovation processes in the fields of dissemination and technology transfer.
- Negotiate improved market access for textile and clothing products, especially for high-quality textiles.
- Remove remaining obstacles that prevent retail distribution systems and remove production measures that distort markets.

Chapter 1

Adjustment Challenges in Textiles and Clothing

Considerable worldwide restructuring is anticipated following the termination of quantitative restrictions at the end of 2004, as agreed under the WTO Agreement on Textiles and Clothing (ATC). This chapter summarises the key adjustment challenges facing these industries with a view to assist governments in establishing a coherent policy and regulatory framework that facilitates the adjustment of the private sector. This multifaceted process involves: supporting the emergence of qualified pools of expertise and the adaptability of the workforce; improving the regulatory environment for essential business services; stimulating collaborative innovation processes in the fields of dissemination and technology transfer; and negotiating improved market access for textile and clothing products, especially eliminating remaining obstacles to the establishment of retail distribution systems and distorting production measures.

Introduction

The scheduled elimination of quantitative restrictions under the World Trade Organization (WTO) Agreement on Textiles and Clothing (ATC) at the end of 2004 is challenging the global sourcing channels that were formed during decades of trade restrictions and entails considerable adjustments for all stakeholders, especially clothing assemblers in remote, low-wage countries.[1] Given the economic importance of these industries for both developed and developing countries, this study examines the process of adjustment in the textile and clothing industries in the post-ATC period with a view to assisting governments in establishing a coherent policy and regulatory framework to facilitate adjustment in the private sector.

The import quotas initially imposed under the Multi-Fibre Arrangement (MFA) contributed to the international fragmentation of the supply chain by accelerating the diversification of supply. This disadvantaged the more efficient and quota-constrained suppliers, many of which subcontracted clothing assembly to low-wage third countries. Hence, the MFA benefited the least competitive suppliers, most of which were located in small developing countries and in least developed countries (LDCs). Aware of their post-ATC vulnerability, the least competitive countries now seek to improve their access to developed country markets so as to minimise the expected hardships. They are particularly anxious about losing export markets to Chinese exporters and are lobbying for expanded product eligibility under the General System of Preferences (GSP) and other preferential programmes, complemented by more liberal rules of origin to qualify for preferential access.

During the decades of MFA-related quotas, the textile industry did not migrate as fast as the clothing industry to developing country locations. In the post-ATC period, there will be no major obstacles to the emergence of high-quality textile capacity and stronger clusters of expertise in developing countries. Moreover, there will be neither quantitative trade restrictions nor MFA-related guaranteed market access to mask the competitive weaknesses of exporting countries. If countries are to maintain an export-led development strategy in textiles and clothing, these weaknesses must be addressed.

The role now played by textile and clothing production in the industrialisation process of developing countries is far more differentiated than it was a generation ago. While low wages can still give developing countries a competitive edge in world markets, quick turnaround times now play a far more crucial role in determining international competitiveness in the fashion-oriented and ever more time-sensitive textile and clothing markets. The comparative advantage of developing countries in the assembly process, *i.e.* low-wage sewing, does not necessarily translate into a comparative advantage in the management of the entire supply chain when all services-related dimensions are considered. Countries that aspire to maintain an export-led strategy in textiles and clothing need to complement their industrial expertise in manufacturing by developing their expertise in the higher value-added segments of the supply chain. This can be done by upgrading domestic skills in design, material sourcing, quality control, logistics and retail distribution.

For developed countries, the post-ATC environment will have varying effects on different segments of the supply chain. Their textile and clothing suppliers will be exposed to greater competitive pressures. They also host the world's fashion and design hubs. Retail groups in developed countries will have greater liberty to source products globally and to accelerate the expansion of their distribution networks worldwide. Moreover, world exports of textile and clothing machinery originate predominantly in developed countries. On balance, developed countries have multifaceted interests in textile and clothing, and their long-term interests are better served by an open and liberal multilateral trading environment.

Although the prime responsibility for adjustment falls on the firms themselves, governments play a supporting role by establishing a coherent policy and regulatory framework. The objective of such a framework should be to strengthen the private sector's capacity to deal with rapid change and growing competition and to capture the trade opportunities created as a result of improved market access. This involves dismantling trade-distorting production measures, improving the regulatory environment for essential business services, supporting the emergence of qualified pools of expertise and the adaptability of the workforce, negotiating improved market access for textile and clothing products, and eliminating the obstacles to the establishment of retail distribution systems in developing countries.

Liberal trade and investment policies play a key role in this adjustment process. They can help to restrain pressure on the price of imported inputs and thus facilitate the emergence of competitive firms that are able to compete on domestic and international markets. However, liberalisation often encounters serious structural obstacles and imposes temporary hardships on certain segments of the economy. Governments can ease the transition by facilitating the redeployment of affected resources to other productive activities without reverting to costly trade protection and subsidisation measures.

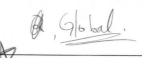

A typology of the textile and clothing supply chain

The textile and clothing industries have distinctive characteristics and involve a large and diversified range of activities that employ a varying mix of labour and capital. For the sake of simplicity, the entire supply chain can be presented as four production segments. The structural adjustment pressures or the drivers of change for each of these segments are discussed below.

Natural fibres. The preparation of natural fibres involves various agricultural activities that are influenced by factor endowments, *i.e.* the quality of land and regional climate and the country's agricultural policies. Various natural fibres are used in the production of textiles, *i.e.* cotton, flax, jute, silk, sisal and wool. Two of them involve animal husbandry, *i.e.* silkworms and sheep herding.

Textiles. The preparation of textile products, from either natural or man-made fibres, involves manufacturing activities in which technological innovations have greatly increased the speed of operations and resulted in huge productivity gains. Non-clothing applications of textiles – the so-called "technical textiles" – are now more important than clothing applications and account for the fastest-growing segment of total textile production in developed countries.

Clothing. The preparation of articles of clothing involves manufacturing activities as well. The clothing sector is also referred to as the "apparel" or "garment" sector. The pre-assembly stage involves designing, grading, marking of patterns and cutting of textiles into individual components. It has been revolutionised through the application of computer-aided design (CAD) and computer-assisted methods (CAM) systems. By contrast, the assembly stage remains highly labour-intensive and involves delicate handling and sewing operations that do not lend themselves to automation. Aside from productivity gains attributable to better needles and more secure fabric-holding techniques, sewing techniques remain basically those of a century ago. This industry is almost unique in its low ratio of capital equipment to labour inputs. However, technological progress in telecommunications and transport networks has made it easier for clothing manufacturers to divide the supply chain on an international basis and to perform the assembly stage in low-wage countries.

Retailing. Retailing activities have changed significantly with the blurring of the traditional boundaries between retailers, brand marketers and manufacturers. Retailers are increasingly involved in global sourcing as lead buyers through a wide variety of organisational channels, such as vertical integration, subcontracting and licensing arrangements. The retail stage has also become increasingly concentrated into large, lean retail organisations that are able to exert considerable influence throughout the supply chain.

Adjustment challenges by production segment

Adjustment in natural fibres

In the post-ATC period, world demand for natural fibres will reflect two opposing consumption trends. In clothing applications, the demand for natural fibres is growing, while in non-clothing applications, the demand for man-made fibres is rising. Hence, the demand for natural fibres is unlikely to exceed the average growth rate of around 2% a year achieved in recent years for the consumption of textiles for clothing applications.

In the post-ATC period, the main drivers of adjustment for natural fibres will be related to the migration of textile capacity to some developing countries and the results of ongoing agricultural negotiations and dispute settlement procedures in the WTO.

Migrating demand for natural fibres

Suppliers of natural fibres will have to accompany the migration of textile capacity to the most competitive developing countries, particularly China and India. These two countries are already strong producers of natural fibres. One implication is that a certain share of world demand for natural fibres that has traditionally gone to developed countries will be redirected to developing countries. Therefore, some production shares of natural fibres in developed countries will have to compete on world markets in terms of quality, delivery and price. It is also expected that access conditions to developing countries will take a more prominent place on the trade policy agenda.

Tariff protection for natural fibres is generally much lower than for finished textiles and clothing products. Moreover, textile-producing countries enforce various duty-remission programmes to improve the cost competitiveness of domestic processing industries. Where high tariffs are levied on natural fibres to protect domestic agricultural producers, the brunt of the costs of protection is ultimately borne by domestic processing industries. In developing countries with predominately labour-intensive agricultural production, the reduction of tariffs on fibres may be difficult to justify for policy makers unless there are clear offsetting labour gains in the processing industries. For least developed countries, like Bangladesh, the prospect of losing employment in clothing manufacturing owing to intensified competition on export markets may worry policy makers and reduce the likelihood of downward tariff adjustment in fibres and/or textiles for fear of exacerbating the employment situation.

WTO agricultural negotiations and dispute settlement

Another challenge for natural fibres relates to the outcome of the ongoing WTO multilateral trade negotiations in agriculture. Under the WTO's Agreement on Agriculture, WTO members have undertaken reduction commitments in respect of market access, domestic support and export subsidy. The negotiations are expected to lead to improved commitments in each of these areas.

Cotton is the principal natural fibre used in clothing applications, and domestic support to cotton production is currently the subject of a formal trade dispute under the WTO dispute settlement procedure. The outcome of this dispute may have a significant impact on the cost competitiveness of fibre producers worldwide. The prospect of a WTO package that may include a meaningful reduction in domestic support and export subsidies could force high-cost producers to rationalise production by adopting more efficient production methods or by shifting production to other crops. As the protracted WTO negotiations in agriculture attest, domestic groups are resisting adjustment towards less protected and distorted markets which would otherwise benefit the processing industries and support economic diversification into higher value-added production segments.

Adjustment in the textile industry

The main drivers of adjustment in the textile industry in the post-ATC period are related to: *i)* the migration of textile capacity to developing countries; *ii)* the adoption of up-to-date equipment by producers; *iii)* the fading attractiveness of outward processing programmes (OPP); and *iv)* the importance of rules of origin to qualify for preferential trade arrangements.

Migration to developing countries

With the imminent demise of the ATC, there will no longer be any trade obstacles to the development of stronger clusters of textile expertise in the most competitive developing countries. The recent surge in China's imports of up-to-date textile and clothing equipment bears witness to this trend and points to what will be the future sources of textile and clothing production and exports.[2] With modern equipment, Chinese textile suppliers are improving their productivity and are increasingly producing export-quality textiles. The main beneficiaries are the Chinese clothing suppliers which can procure their textile inputs directly from domestic sources and hence meet shorter turnaround delivery requirements. Access to high-quality textiles is considered one of the most important determinants of the competitiveness of clothing suppliers. As a result, the textile industry in developed countries will face intensified competition in both their export and domestic markets. The migration of textile capacity will nevertheless be influenced by objective competitive factors and will be hampered by the presence of distorting domestic measures and weak domestic infrastructure in several developing and least developed countries.[3]

The textile industry is also undergoing a major reorientation towards non-clothing applications of textiles, *i.e.* technical textiles, which represent the fastest-growing segment of total textile applications. Technical textiles are often defined as those textile materials and products manufactured primarily for their technical and performance properties rather than for their aesthetic or decorative characteristics. They are used in many applications, including furniture, automotive, health and hygiene, transport, construction and environment. The processes involved in producing technical textiles are human- and physical-capital-intensive and, for the moment, concentrated in developed countries. With the transfer of technology and the expansion of knowledge sharing through global university networks, many developing countries have access to the knowledge base that can allow the technical textiles industries to flourish. Whenever major industries shift to or expand production in developing countries, it is only a matter of time for inputs to be produced there as well.

Shrinking productivity gap

During the twentieth century, improved spinning and weaving equipment led to significant productivity gains. The textile industry has become a capital-intensive industry in which up-to-date equipment plays a crucial role in the competitiveness of firms.[4] Important productivity gains have historically been driven by the symbiotic relationship between competitive textile and clothing industries and a creative textile and clothing machinery (TCM) industry. However, this symbiotic relationship is weakening, as new materials are developed mainly in the chemical industry and new processes are developed in the machinery industry. As a result, the technological competitiveness of textile and clothing firms largely depends on their ability to adopt new products and processes developed outside the textile and clothing industries. Therefore, the major focus of these industries' innovation activities is on technology transfer. With globalised knowledge networks, technology transfer is rapid, and the productivity gap that has differentiated developed and developing countries is expected to shrink since modern equipment can be operated efficiently in the most competitive developing countries.

Throughout the 1980s and the 1990s, the TCM industry in developed countries nevertheless succeeded in maintaining its high share of the world's exports by accompanying the international shift in the demand for capital equipment. The four main exporting countries are Germany, Italy, Japan and Switzerland; together they account for almost two-thirds of industrial countries' exports of machinery. This is due to various factors, including: *i)* industrial consolidation among firms; *ii)* the development of ties between equipment manufacturers in developed and developing countries; *iii)* concentration of production on the high value-added segments of the equipment market; and *iv)* close contacts with equipment users wherever they are located.

Preferential trade arrangements

Trade policies other than MFA-related quotas have also had a major impact on the development of geographical patterns of trade in textiles and clothing. The elimination of import quotas will reduce the attractiveness of outward processing programmes and, conversely, increase the attractiveness of other preferential trade arrangements, such as regional trade arrangements (RTAs) and GSP regimes. The magnitude of economic benefits accruing under these arrangements varies greatly because of their differences in scope and the specificity of the rules of origin that confer preferential access under various arrangements.

The outward processing programmes, or production-sharing programmes, involve the temporary export of textiles or pre-cut fabrics from the OPP-initiator country to low-wage countries for final assembly. The finished articles are then re-imported under preferential provisions. For low-wage countries, the assembly of imported fabrics into clothing is a simple form of industrial activity. OPP eligibility often acts as a booster for these countries' export-oriented strategies by giving them instant access to high-quality inputs and foreign distribution networks. For developed countries, outward processing transactions strengthen the competitive position of domestic suppliers by enabling them to transfer labour–intensive sewing activities to low-wage countries. To make outward processing transactions worthwhile, the cost savings associated with low-wage assembly in offshore centres and tariff reductions must exceed the inherent additional costs of production fragmentation, namely: two-way shipments; longer and larger inventory; and added co–ordination to manage the fragmented supply chain.

Under the MFA-related quota regime, the inherent cost inefficiencies of outward processing transactions were partly masked by the trade-distorting impact of quota allocations. Moreover, outward processing transactions provided a protected market for textiles made in OPP-initiator countries. In 1995, outward processing trade accounted for 15% of the European Union's external trade in textiles; in 1999, it accounted for 24% of total clothing imports by the United States.[5] Since then, the importance of outward processing trade has considerably diminished in the EU owing to the entry into force of several free trade agreements (FTAs) with neighbouring countries that made OPP almost redundant. In a less pronounced way, the importance of outward processing trade for the United States diminished with the implementation of the North American Free Trade Agreement (NAFTA), but OPP eligibility was expanded under the Trade Development Act of 2000 and outward processing trade accounted for 10.9% of US clothing imports in 2003.

Without the trade-distorting impact of quota allocations, the inherent vulnerability of business models developed under OPP is exposed. On the one hand, outward processing transactions remain economically attractive only if the margin of preferential duty exceeds the difference between the OPP-related cost and the logistical cost incurred for competitive suppliers.[6] With distance and time acting as trade barriers, there are no net cost advantages from outward processing transactions involving offshore assembly centres that are either geographically remote from the OPP-initiator country or nearby with poor transport infrastructure.

On the other hand, in certain instances offshore centres will be able to offer lower prices to buyers of clothing products assembled from third-country textiles. This means that the textile industry in OPP-initiator countries will lose its protected OPP textile export markets and will have to adjust to intensified foreign competition in its domestic markets. Moreover, OPP recipients that have gradually developed their expertise are conscious of their vulnerability and are requesting better trade opportunities from developed countries to help them compete with the most competitive suppliers. Most requests concern the negotiation of FTAs with developed countries and/or improved GSP access. In any of those options, improved access will mean more competitive pressure on the domestic textile industry of developed countries.

Trade opportunities under regional trade arrangements

In the post–ATC period, comprehensive RTAs can provide a useful policy framework to underpin the development of a regionally integrated textile and clothing supply chain and to facilitate economic diversification strategies for their members, but they do not necessarily imply competitiveness. While a comprehensive RTA is necessary, it is insufficient to promote trade flows and a qualitative transformation in textile and clothing production. Although production and trade opportunities are created under comprehensive RTAs, certain domestic factors play an instrumental role in reaping trade opportunities. Among these factors are: the ability to attract the right kind of lead retailers, brand marketers and manufacturers; a pre–existing cluster of expertise; a vibrant entrepreneurial environment; and geographical proximity to minimise the transit time of shipments during transport.[7]

Prior to NAFTA, access of Mexican suppliers to US markets was primarily driven by outward processing transactions in which Mexican suppliers merely assembled components imported from the United States. Under NAFTA, the trade rules have changed and all activities of the supply chain, not only sewing, can be performed in Mexico (and in Canada). In the context of NAFTA, Mexico has been able to promote the consolidation of its regional clusters of textile and clothing expertise and to move beyond the simple assembly of imported components, thereby creating backward and forward linkages in the domestic economy. Similarly, the customs union between Turkey and the European Union has paved the way for further integrating the Turkish textile and clothing markets into the larger European markets. However, despite their growing integration with larger regional markets, both Mexico and Turkey are not shielded from the need to adjust to external competitive pressures, as products originating from countries such as China are increasingly competitive in both the EU and NAFTA markets.

Stringent rules of origin for textiles and clothing

Rules of origin (ROOs) are a necessary part of preferential trade arrangements such as GSP in order to ensure that trade preference is granted to products that effectively originate from the beneficiary countries. Similarly, they are a necessary part of FTAs in order to preserve the preferential treatment accorded to member countries and avoid the problem of trade deflection, *i.e.* the entry of imports into the region through the member country whose import tariff is the lowest. There are considerable disparities in the rules of origin applied under various preferential arrangements and in their utilisation rates.[8]

Specific and more stringent rules of origin are often applied for sensitive products, such as textiles and clothing, and make it more difficult for suppliers to ensure the regional content. This creates an incentive for manufacturers to source inputs from regional suppliers and may act as a trade barrier. By limiting the sourcing of inputs from regional partners, ROOs may encourage a vertical integration of the production chain that may not be competitive outside the regional market. A further problem with specific rules of origin is that the determination of regional content for yarns, fabrics and final products that involve multiple components can be so burdensome and costly that suppliers prefer not to use the preferential arrangements.

Several countries have recently improved their GSP regimes by broadening the scope of eligible textile and clothing products and/or offering comprehensive duty-free and quota-free treatment for products originating from the least developed countries.[9] While rules of origin are necessary to ensure that preferential trade actually benefits its targeted countries, overly restrictive rules may inhibit meaningful access and lead to under-utilisation of preferential access schemes. By contrast, liberal rules of origin may not benefit the targeted countries as much as intended, and the associated preferential access can invert the tariff structure and create problems for national manufacturers. Moreover, liberal rules of origin do not necessarily confer competitiveness. Inherent competitive factors explain why certain beneficiary countries of preferential arrangements are more likely to gain the most. Both distance between trading partners, which entails long transit periods for shipments, and the size of the cluster of expertise in beneficiary countries seem to matter. Finally, the identity of foreign investors also appears to influence the patterns of input procurement.

The recent modifications to the Canadian GSP regime offer interesting lessons. In 2003, Canada granted duty-free and quota-free entry to all textile and clothing imports originating from LDCs that meet the requirement that 25% of content originates from any LDCs, GSP beneficiaries or Canada. Four main issues are worth noting: *i)* the liberal rules of origin, with the right to group LDC or GSP beneficiaries, have allowed LDCs to drastically boost their clothing exports to Canada within a very short period of time; *ii)* this improved access has enabled many LDCs to expand their exports, although the gains were concentrated in two beneficiary countries, Bangladesh and Cambodia; *iii)* large trade gains also accrued to the largest developing countries, such as China and India, which shipped textiles to LDCs that were subsequently assembled into clothing products and then exported to Canada; and *iv)* duty-free treatment of clothing products inverted the tariff structure and created problems for Canadian manufacturers who claimed unfair competition. Instead of backtracking on its liberal commitments, Canada announced a series of new tariff cuts in early 2004 to address the problems caused by inverted tariff protection and, simultaneously, launched a programme designed to improve production efficiency of Canadian suppliers. One important lesson to draw from the Canadian experience is that the implementation of liberal rules of origin requires a comprehensive approach to ensure that the domestic processing industry also benefits from the trade liberalisation programmes.

With the imminent elimination of the ATC, the small developing countries and LDCs are increasingly vocal about their post-ATC vulnerability and are demanding access to developed country markets on an improved preferential basis as a way to compete more effectively with China and India. Recognising that there is at present virtually no production of high-quality textiles in LDCs, preferential access arrangements in favour of LDCs must take into account that they have to use competitive textiles originating from third countries to compete on export markets. Under these circumstances, it seems inevitable that in providing LDCs with preferential access, there will be some collateral benefits for suppliers of high-quality textiles. In the post-ATC period, provisions on rules of origin will be at the forefront of the trade policy agenda as demands from vulnerable offshore centres become more insistent. The challenge for policy makers in developed countries is to draft rules of origin for their preferential arrangements that will mainly benefit LDCs and small developing countries, which are most vulnerable to competition from the large and integrated suppliers in China and India. In addition, improvements concerning rules of origin under preferential trade arrangements will increase the competitive pressures on the domestic textile industry of developed countries.

Adjustment in the clothing industry

The main drivers of adjustment in the clothing industry in the post-ATC period are related to: *i)* the importance of time factors as determinants of international competitiveness; and *ii)* the adjustment in trade protection and WTO safeguard measures.

Time factors as determinants of international competitiveness

The role now played by textile and clothing production in the industrialisation process of developing countries is far more differentiated than it was a generation ago. While low wages can still give developing countries a competitive edge in world markets, time factors now play a far more crucial role in determining international competitiveness. With the imminent end of quantitative restrictions, several low-wage countries that had excelled as offshore assembly centres owing to their quota allocations find themselves vulnerable because of the inherent cost disadvantage of their business model based on production fragmentation. Time factors can be an important trade barrier for intermediary inputs involved in an internationally fragmented production process. There are trade-offs between low-wage cost and time factors, since temporal proximity to large consumer markets provides a competitive edge in the highly competitive, time-sensitive and fashion-oriented clothing market.

Moreover, the emergence of more competitive and integrated suppliers in China is exerting considerable pressure on such vulnerable offshore centres to shift domestic capacity towards more advanced processes and to diversify their economic activities. The comparative advantage of developing countries in the assembly process, *i.e.* in low-wage sewing, does not necessarily translate into a comparative advantage in the management of the entire supply chain when all services-related dimensions are taken into consideration. Efficiency in managing the entire supply chain is required, including in design, fabric procurement, logistical skills in transport, quality control, property rights protection, export financing and clearing of trade formalities.

To move beyond the assembly of imported inputs and along the supply chain into more advanced activities, exporting countries need to shift their expertise from manufacturing to services-related activities, such as design, materials sourcing, quality control, logistics and retail distribution. To pursue these avenues, national suppliers need to place greater emphasis on education and training of services-related skills and to encourage the establishment of joint structures through which domestic suppliers can share market knowledge and offer more integrated solutions to prospective buyers.

Efficient port infrastructure, reliable and competitive modes of transport and efficient customs procedures are also extremely important for maintaining an edge in the highly competitive textile and clothing markets. Reliable transport infrastructure and efficient customs procedures complement each other to minimise transit time for shipments involved in international trade and can make geographically remote locations more internationally competitive. Even if long transit times can be overcome to some extent by preferential market access arrangements, long periods in transit can essentially eliminate from international competition the offshore centres that are either geographically remote from the buyer's markets or nearby but with poor transport infrastructure.

Adjustment in trade protection

As noted earlier, access to high-quality textiles is considered one of the most important determinants of competitiveness for clothing suppliers. Therefore, high tariffs on textile inputs undermine the efforts of clothing suppliers to shift their production mix to goods that require imported high-quality textiles. Policy makers are often confronted with a policy dilemma when deciding which segments of the supply chain should be exposed to greater competition from imports to favour the processing sectors and ultimately consumers. On the one hand, textile suppliers will argue that they need protection to reach critical mass and compete on more equal terms with foreign textile suppliers. On the other hand, clothing suppliers will argue that duty-free access for their inputs is needed if they are to compete with imported clothing products. Various duty-remission programmes can help to reduce the impact of high tariffs on textile inputs, particularly when there is no domestic production of specific textile components. Each country thus needs to assess its competitive strengths and weaknesses along the supply chain, and to balance its tariffs so that tariff protection granted to fibres and textiles does not prevent the emergence of competitive suppliers in the high value-added segments of the supply chain.

India's potential

In India, the textile and clothing industries are based on a system of decentralised production, referred to as "reservation of garment manufacture for small-scale industry (SSI)" which provides certain economic advantages to small-scale labour-intensive firms, with high tariff protection throughout the supply chain, from natural and man-made fibres to textile and clothing products. Policy analysts have argued that the SSI framework has discouraged entrepreneurs from investing in optimal scale production plants and has created strong vested interests that are opposed to reforms. They have also argued that India faces formidable domestic hurdles if it is to meet international quality standards and thus is ill prepared to take advantage of the opportunities created by the elimination of quantitative restrictions. Mindful of all this, the Indian government has recently reduced import duties and is seeking to rationalise the imposition of the value-added tax across the textile and clothing supply chain. India's valuable assets for success in the post-ATC period include the domestic availability of several natural fibres, clusters of expertise in man-made fibres, low wages in manufacturing sectors, an increasingly affluent and educated middle class and a large domestic market. To unleash India's great potential, reforms are needed to remove domestic obstacles to growth and to inject a strong dose of import competition to encourage the modernisation of its production capacity. The case of India underscores the need for all vulnerable countries to assess and address their domestic competitive weaknesses if they want to pursue an export-led strategy in textiles and clothing.

WTO safeguard measures

The post-ATC situation has generated considerable anxiety about the emergence of more competitive suppliers in China. The potential disruption of markets in importing countries is also recognised in the WTO Protocol on the accession of China. The Protocol contains a transitional product-specific safeguard mechanism (Article 16) that enables

WTO members to restrict imports originating in China when such imports cause or threaten to cause market disruption to domestic producers of textile and clothing products. This transitional safeguard provision is valid for a period of 12 years after China's accession (or by December 2013). The WTO Report of the Working Party on the Accession of China (paragraph 242) also contains a textile safeguard provision that enables WTO members to restrict imports from China when they believe that imports of textile and clothing products of Chinese origin are, owing to market disruption, threatening to impede the orderly development of trade in these products. China's textile safeguard provision is valid until the end of December 2008. Otherwise, WTO members can apply temporary protection to products and sectors that are seriously injured by import competition. The implementation of this general safeguard measure is subject to a number of procedural provisions, including the determination of serious injury, consultations with affected trading partners and, potentially, the payment of offsetting compensation to aggrieved partners. Under the WTO Anti-dumping Agreement, members also can take action against dumping and may impose extra import duty on the particular product from the particular country in order to remove the dumping margin and hence the injury to the domestic industry in the importing country.

Whether or not WTO members will frequently invoke the WTO transitional safeguard provision, China's textile safeguard provision, the general safeguard provision or anti-dumping measures in the post-ATC period remains an open question. The United States invoked China's textile safeguard provision in December 2003 and, following consultations with China, restrained Chinese imports of knit fabrics, dressing gowns and brassieres for a period of 12 months. According to the US International Trade Commission ITC),[10] the WTO transitional safeguard provision creates an element of uncertainty regarding the capacity of Chinese exporters to access foreign markets, and the risk involved in sourcing from a single country will encourage buyers to diversify their sourcing networks among other low-cost alternatives to China. This diversification of imports will be influenced by competitive cost factors in other supplying countries which are themselves affected by market access opportunities offered under regional and preferential trade arrangements.

The potential in emerging economies

The demand for clothing products in developed countries is influenced by underlying changes in demography, disposable income and a growing tendency towards more relaxed and leisure wear, brand-name products and fashion wear. However, consumers in developed countries are spending a declining share of their disposable income on textile and clothing products. With the maturing of markets in developed countries, the opportunities for fastest growth in consumption are likely to be in the emerging and newly industrialised economies (NIEs). This underscores the importance of market access to developing countries in general and large emerging economies in particular.

For the overwhelming majority of developed and developing countries, average applied tariff protection on textiles and clothing remains high compared to average tariffs imposed on manufactured products.[11] In developed countries, there are considerable differences in the level of tariffs applied on textiles and clothing and in the recurrence of tariff peaks. In developing and least developed countries, there are similar imbalances. It is worth noting that in 2002 the tariffs imposed on textiles and clothing in China were roughly equivalent to the average tariffs applied by OECD countries and were thus considerably lower than in some OECD countries, such as Mexico, which is a large net exporter of clothing products. In the WTO, all of China's tariffs are bound, and most bound rates at the end of the implementation period will be much lower than the tariffs applied in 2002. This means that China is effectively reducing its tariff protection over the period. In other developing and least developed countries, high tariff protection remains the norm. Given their concerns about competition from China, they are, for the time being, reluctant to commit to tariff reductions in the ongoing multilateral trade negotiations. Therefore, the prospects of improving south-south trade in textiles and clothing are not promising. In terms of expanding north-south trade, the export interests of developed countries may be better served by seeking improved access to the retail distribution systems of developing countries.

Adjustment in retail distribution

The drivers of adjustment in retail distribution in the post-ATC period are related to: *i)* the leadership role played by large retail groups and brand-name marketers; *ii)* the importance of private codes of conduct and market knowledge; and *iii)* access to retail distribution in emerging economies.

Leadership role of large retail groups and brand-name marketers

Retail distribution is increasingly dominated by large retail organisations in the main consuming countries, where the trend is towards greater product specialisation, brand-name products and market segmentation. The large retail groups and brand-name marketers are also expanding their successful distribution models worldwide. These large retail groups collect market information about the latest trends in styles and tastes, and their integration of this information gives them considerable leverage in dealing with suppliers. Nevertheless, offshore suppliers can benefit from working in close co-operation with large retail groups and brand-name marketers as they learn to: *i)* manufacture quality products; *ii)* apply the buyer's codes of conduct; and *iii)* deliver products in a timely fashion. The development of business relationships between national clusters of expertise and the large retail groups and brand-name marketers plays an instrumental role in facilitating the qualitative transformation of the supply chain by facilitating backward and forward linkages in the local economy. For exporting countries seeking to develop their export-led strategies, nurturing contacts between domestic clusters and the large retail groups and brand-name marketers is a must.

Codes of conduct and market knowledge

Retail groups and brand-name marketers invest handsomely in building distinctive corporate images and in maintaining recognition of brand names. Through fear of tarnishing their reputation or losing the market knowledge that underpins their capacity to sell at premium prices, they are very careful to select suppliers that will protect their market knowledge and will not let their names be associated with exploitative working conditions. Hence, foreign suppliers that guarantee to protect market knowledge and implement the buyer's code of conduct have a competitive edge over other attractive business proposals that do not provide the same level of guarantee, even if they offer lower prices. In this respect, strong enforcement of intellectual property laws and private codes of conduct are considered assets for countries that aspire to maintain an export-led strategy in the upper market segment of clothing products. It also means that non-cost factors are becoming increasingly important in the supply chain, because buying decisions are not based exclusively on price competitiveness, particularly for brand-name and eco-labelled products.

Retail distribution in emerging economies

The large retail groups and brand-name marketers in textiles and clothing are expanding their distribution networks and pursuing business opportunities in countries with attractive growth prospects. In most developed countries, the establishment of retail distribution services is not hindered by restrictions on foreign ownership or obstacles to the right of establishment. Although the large retail groups and brand-name marketers are predominantly headquartered in developed countries and owned by developed countries' interests, some leading manufacturers in Hong Kong (China) have launched their brand names and are entering retail distribution. This strategic move requires services-related expertise in design, marketing, retailing, financing and the gathering of market intelligence on foreign markets. It also requires foreign direct investment (FDI) flows originating from Hong Kong (China) or from other emerging economies that are pursuing similar diversification strategies. In the absence of restrictions on FDI or limitations on access to retail distribution in developed countries, it is only a matter of time before retail distribution chains owned and controlled by Asian interests operate in developed countries and compete head to head with established large or small retail distributors.

In developing countries, access to retail distribution systems is less predictable. In China, as of December 2004, foreign retailing services will have the right to set up distribution networks without geographical and quantitative restrictions through wholly owned foreign enterprises, thereby offering considerable retailing opportunities in this large consumer market. Anecdotal sources estimate that the size of the Chinese affluent middle class is around 80-100 million people, or roughly equivalent to the combined populations of France and the United Kingdom. In India, another country with significant potential, foreign FDI in retailing is not allowed, and India has so far made no commitments under the General Agreement on Trade in Services (GATS) in respect of retail distribution services. Although the commercial presence of some large groups is currently increasing in India, these operations mainly facilitate the sourcing of Indian products for export. In the context of the Doha Development Agenda, countries have an opportunity to improve access for wholly owned foreign distribution services to developing countries that still maintain obstacles to FDI and/or restrict the right to distribute foreign-made goods.

Policy challenges

Trade policy measures have had a major impact on production, trade and investment decisions in the past. Their influence will lessen in the near future with the elimination of the quantitative restrictions that are probably the most restrictive of all trade instruments. As noted throughout this chapter, tariff reductions, preferential access under GSP regimes or regional trade arrangements and access to foreign retail distribution systems will remain on the policy agenda of trade policy makers in the post-ATC environment. To facilitate the process of sound structural adjustment in textile and clothing, governments can play a supporting role by establishing a coherent policy and regulatory framework that complements the competition-enhancing trade policy framework. Labour adjustment policies, technology and innovation policies, and other policy and regulatory dimensions, referred to as business facilitation, can play a complementary role in this process of structural adjustment. The salient points of these policy dimensions are summarised below.

Trade-related labour adjustment policies

It is difficult to isolate the causes of worker displacement. Technological change, productivity gains, increased import competition and shifts in production can all contribute to job losses. The difficulty has led many policy analysts to oppose targeted labour market adjustment policies and programmes for special groups of workers, *e.g.* workers who lose their jobs owing to increased imports, and instead propose broad labour adjustment programmes for all displaced workers. This issue is likely to remain prominent in the foreseeable future with the intensification of international relations among countries.

Available evidence on the impact of globalisation and international trade on labour adjustment suggests that workers who lose their jobs as a result of increased imports or shifts in production do not appear to be different from other dislocated workers. Similarly, their adjustment process does not seem to differ significantly. Trade-related dislocations may suggest the need for labour market adjustment policies and programmes but not necessarily a special response. An analysis of the characteristics of displaced workers from the textile and clothing industries shows that they tend to have a low level of education and low skill levels (thus earn low wages), and are predominantly women and minorities (including minority women). These characteristics make it more difficult for such workers to adjust to changes in the labour market.

In place of the debate over special *versus* general labour market adjustment policies and programmes, more effort needs to be directed towards determining which interventions are more effective. Most developed countries are attempting to improve the co-ordination of their unemployment benefits and employment services.

In most developed countries, unemployment insurance programmes are designed to assist all unemployed workers, regardless of industry, worker demographics or cause of displacement. The most significant exception to this general framework is the targeted Trade Adjustment Assistance (TAA) programme in the United States which provides assistance to workers displaced because of competition from imports and shifts in production. In most other developed countries, more comprehensive and generous labour market adjustment programmes tend to lessen the need for special programmes for workers from a specific industry or whose job loss can be traced to a specific cause.

There has been increasing reliance on training as part of the toolbox of labour market adjustment programmes. Many workers exiting traditional low-wage manufacturing industries lack basic language and mathematics skills, and this prevents them from acquiring the skills needed for the new jobs being created. The shift in the structure of the labour market in developed countries has also resulted in a gap between the skills workers needed in previous jobs and those required by future jobs. Governments are employing various subsidies and tax incentives to encourage training and skill enhancement.

The main goal of any labour adjustment programme should be re-employment: either by returning to one's previous job or finding a new job as soon as possible and with minimal disruption in earnings. With that objective in mind, countries have implemented various programmes to train workers and provide job search assistance. The recent introduction of "wage insurance" in Germany and the United States encourages workers to return to work as soon as possible. Wage insurance is designed for workers whose new wage is lower than their previous wage. By subsidising some portion of the difference between the new and previous wages, it is hoped that workers will be encouraged to take a new job sooner. It is also hoped that new employers will provide the worker with on-the-job training, which has proven to be more effective and cheaper than government-financed classroom training. These programmes also aim at minimising the economic and social impact of plant closings on communities. At the outset, the overall labour adjustment policy challenge is to devise ways to meet social goals in a cost-efficient and least trade-distorting manner.

Technology and innovation policies   *Product differentiation*

Different countries have different historical backgrounds in terms of their industrial development and thus differ with respect to optimal policy support for industries such as textiles and clothing. Some general lessons are learned from the examination of experiences with technology and innovation in many developed countries.

There seems to be no fundamental lack of invention and innovation. Hence, it does not seem appropriate for governments to launch large-scale basic research projects on textile and clothing technologies beyond the horizontal industrial research schemes based on public-private co-funding mechanisms. Although the textile and clothing industries can be considered mature, they use technological innovations that are largely generated in other industries, above all in chemicals and machinery. These suppliers of technology are well able to provide product and process innovations for textiles and clothing without financial support from public research programmes. While governments may stimulate collaborative innovation processes in the areas of dissemination and technology transfer, such approaches should not distort market-oriented innovation programmes.

Technology transfer between suppliers and users plays a pivotal role in the performance of textile and clothing suppliers. It is therefore appropriate for countries to seek to encourage technology transfer. However, to achieve faster productivity and welfare gains, the process of technology transfer could be strengthened by exploiting more efficiently the opportunities offered by modern information and communication technologies for the dissemination of advanced technological knowledge. Complementary public funding would be needed to give innovators financial incentives to pass proprietary technological knowledge to imitating firms.

Many small and medium-sized enterprises (SMEs) often face substantial difficulties for marketing their products, because they lack a widely recognised reputation for high product quality. Governments could support their marketing activities by promoting certification agencies and common brand names. At present, government activities in this area mainly concentrate on sponsoring fairs and exhibitions.

Governments should keep in mind that, in the long run, innovative capacities basically depend on the availability of suitable human capital. Therefore, a sound education and qualification system seems much more important for sustainable technical progress than public innovation programmes. This applies not only to textiles and clothing, but to any industry.

Business facilitation agenda

In the post-ATC period, there will be neither quantitative restrictions nor MFA-related guaranteed market access to mask the vulnerability of textile and clothing suppliers whose international competitiveness is hampered by inefficient domestic regulatory regimes, obsolete infrastructure in essential business services, cumbersome customs procedures and other distorted market structures. All these dimensions are influenced by the policy and regulatory framework set up by governments. From a trade policy perspective, efficiency in the areas of transport, telecommunications and electricity infrastructure and in customs services is an important determinant of a country's ability to integrate fully the world economy. Achieving greater synergy among the various policy and regulatory areas that affect the competitive position of national firms is, in essence, the purpose of a business facilitation agenda.

Foster a dynamic macroeconomic environment

Above all, the role of government is to pursue a sound and stable macroeconomic environment able to sustain non-inflationary economic growth. There is strong evidence that real economic growth and, in turn, net employment creation are stimulated in an environment of low inflation. The pursuit of sound macroeconomic policies fosters market adjustment to changes in the competitive environment and facilitates the redeployment of affected resources to other productive sectors. The pursuit of a business facilitation agenda complements other government actions at the macroeconomic and microeconomic levels, *i.e.* in trade, labour adjustment and innovation, and brings benefits that go well beyond the textile and clothing industries.

Minimise transit time for shipments

Reliability of transport infrastructure and efficiency in customs procedures complement each other to minimise transit periods for shipments involved in international trade and can make geographically remote locations more internationally competitive. Recognising that they have different geographical positions relative to large consumer regions and different transport options, countries need to assess the logistical costs involved in export markets with a view to: *i)* setting up an efficiency-enhancing environment in port infrastructure; *ii)* strengthening competition conditions in and between transport modes; *iii)* setting up a competition-enhancing environment in various port services; *iv)* addressing the terrorist risks in transport without losing sight of the benefits of frictionless transport systems; and *v)* better integrating the enforcement of national laws and regulations, *e.g.* customs procedures, taxation, sanitary and environment protection, with other service providers in ports.

Modernise customs procedures

In matters concerning the facilitation of international trade, textile and clothing traders are poised to benefit from streamlined border requirements with the dismantling of MFA export permits and related controls in formerly constrained exporting and importing countries. However, the internationally fragmented supply chain remains vulnerable to cumbersome and outdated customs procedures in countries that are less advanced in the implementation of modern customs systems. Export-led strategies suffer when shipments are held up in customs warehouses owing to inefficiencies in customs procedures, especially in countries that rely on imported inputs for a significant share of their production. In dealing with the added emphasis on security and safety, governments should not lose sight of the benefits of smoothly functioning transport and customs clearance systems.

Ensure reliable telecommunications and electricity infrastructures

Reliable and up-to-date telecommunications and electricity infrastructures give textile and clothing suppliers a competitive edge. Trade flows in differentiated products, such as textiles and clothing, are found to be sensitive to international variations in communication costs. Outdated regulatory frameworks in electricity and telecommunications services act as taxes on textile and clothing suppliers and, more importantly, undermine the capacity of national suppliers to focus production on the higher value-added segments of the supply chain that depend critically on reliable infrastructure to ensure quick market response. In the post-ATC period, the international competitiveness of textile and clothing suppliers will be enhanced in countries that maintain a competitive environment and spur investment in innovative telecommunications equipment, electricity generation and distribution systems.

Nurture SME-related entrepreneurship

It is important to nurture SME-related entrepreneurship, but when excessive fiscal advantages and labour law exemptions are offered to small-scale operations, there is a danger of creating distorting incentives to invest in sub-optimal productive capacity. Recent work by the OECD in the context of the Bologna Charter on SME Policies has found that education and training are the single most effective means of achieving the objective of fostering entrepreneurship in societies.

Notes

1. The WTO ATC superseded the Multi-Fibre Arrangement (MFA) regime of quantitative trade restrictions when it entered into force in January 1995 and provided the multilateral trade framework applicable for trade in textiles and clothing for all WTO members. The ATC provides for the elimination by 31 December 2004 of all forms of quantitative restrictions applied to trade in textile and clothing products, including those that originated under the MFA regime. The ATC phases itself out of existence at the end of 2004.

2. For more details about textile and clothing machinery trade by country, see Figure 4.3 in Chapter 4.

3. For more details about infrastructure, see the section on business facilitation in Chapter 5.

4. For more details about long-term productivity gains, see Figures 4.4a and 4.4b in Chapter 4.

5. WTO, Trade Policy Review of the United States, 2001, Geneva.

6. For more details about OPP-related logistics cost by country, see Table 2.10 in Chapter 2 and Table 5.2 in Chapter 5.

7. For more details, see Box 2.2 in Chapter 2.

8. For more details about the utilisation rates of preferential arrangements, see Tables 2.12 and 2.13 in Chapter 2.

9. For more details about the GSP regimes, see Box 2.1 in Chapter 2.

10. US International Trade Commission (2004), Textiles and Apparel: Assessments of the Competitiveness of Certain Foreign Suppliers to the U.S. Market, Investigation No. 332-448, Washington, DC, February.

11. For tariff information by country, see Tables 2.8 and 2.9 in Chapter 2.

Chapter 2

Market Developments and Trade Policies

This chapter reviews recent market developments in production, consumption and trade in textiles and clothing and assesses the trade policy framework in the post-ATC trading environment. It examines: the pattern of the international fragmentation of the supply chain; the role of large retail groups in production decisions; the productivity gap between producing countries; and the emergence of China as a leading producing country with an integrated supply chain. It assesses remaining sources of trade protection and the impact of regional and preferential trade arrangements. Countries that aspire to maintain an export-led strategy in textiles and clothing need to expand their manufacturing expertise to reach the higher value-added segments of the supply chain by upgrading their domestic skills in design, material sourcing, quality control, logistics and retail distribution.

Introduction

The scheduled elimination of quantitative restrictions under the WTO Agreement on Textiles and Clothing (ATC) at the end of December 2004 is taking place in an increasingly globalised world economy, where production and marketing activities depend on business decisions that respond to competitive opportunities around the world.[1] Trade policy measures have had major impacts on production and investment decisions in textiles and clothing and on trade flows. In particular, the trade quotas imposed on a bilateral country basis under the Multi-Fibre Arrangement (MFA) have contributed to the international fragmentation of the supply chain by accelerating the diversification of supply. This process has worked to the disadvantage of the more efficient and quota-constrained suppliers, many of which subcontracted clothing assembly to low–wage third countries. The MFA also benefited less competitive suppliers. In addition, the elimination of quantitative restrictions is challenging the global sourcing channels formed over decades of trade restrictions and will entail considerable adjustment for stakeholders, especially clothing assemblers in remote, low-wage countries. There is also considerable anxiety in the world textile and clothing community that the emergence of more competitive suppliers in China may give that country a disproportionate share of the economic benefits arising from the phasing out of quantitative restrictions.

In the 1980s, world trade in clothing exceeded world trade in textiles and since then has expanded at twice the annual growth rate of textiles: 6% *versus* 3% between 1990 and 2001. Several textile and clothing products were among the 20 most trade-dynamic products during the period 1980–98 (UNCTAD, 2002).[2] In 2002, world trade in textiles and clothing reached USD 152 billion and USD 200 billion, respectively, or 2.4% and 3.2%, respectively, of world merchandise exports (WTO, 2003, Tables IV.56 and IV.64).

It is anticipated that, with the scheduled elimination of the quantitative restrictions that have regulated international trade in these products for over four decades, world trade in textiles and clothing will remain dynamic in the foreseeable future. The deadline for quota elimination at the end of December 2004 coincides with the initial deadline of the Doha Development Agenda (DDA) when changes to existing WTO rules (or new WTO disciplines to be agreed) will also have an impact on international trade in these sectors. The multilateral trade negotiations in the textile and clothing industries are carried out under the negotiating group on market access whose mandate aims, *inter alia*, to reduce or eliminate, as appropriate, import tariffs and non-tariff-barriers. In these negotiations, WTO members have an opportunity to address remaining trade obstacles and other distorting measures that still constrain production and trade opportunities.

Trade liberalisation heightens pressures on firms to adapt their production mix to meet ever-changing consumer requirements in terms of design, quality and price, while putting in place efficient production methods that minimise production costs. Liberal trade regimes are an important component of this environment despite the fact that opening markets to international competition often leads to structural changes and imposes temporary hardships on certain segments of the economy. Governments can facilitate this structural adjustment in several ways.

In the post–ATC period, governments need to devise a coherent textile and clothing policy framework that strengthens the capacity of domestic producers to deal with rapid change and growing competition, and to capture more effectively trade opportunities that arise owing to improved market access. This process involves dismantling trade-distorting measures, improving the business environment for essential business services, supporting the emergence of qualified pools of expertise and the adaptability of the workforce, and negotiating improved market access for textile and clothing products and retail distribution systems. Liberal trade and investment policies play a key role in this process by restraining price pressure on imported inputs that cannot be secured from domestic suppliers, and by facilitating the emergence of competitive firms able to compete on domestic and international markets.

This chapter first presents recent key trends in production, consumption and trade in textiles and clothing and sets the background for the following discussion. In particular, it examines the pattern of international fragmentation of the supply chain, the role of large retail groups in production decisions, the productivity gap between producing countries and the emergence of China as a predominant producer with integrated suppliers. Then, in a discussion of trade policy challenges in the post-ATC period, the remaining sources of trade protection are identified and the trade impact of regional and preferential trade arrangements in these sectors is reviewed. A brief conclusion follows.

Key trends in production, consumption and trade

The interdependence of the textile and clothing industries is asymmetric. Whereas the clothing industry relies entirely on the textile industry to satisfy its textile needs, less than half of total textile production is used in clothing applications. Non-clothing textile applications are loosely defined as "technical textiles" and their growing importance is discussed in Chapter 4.[3] With the largest share of textile demand accounted for by non-clothing textile applications, growth in textile consumption is largely influenced by overall economic conditions and to a certain extent by consumption trends in clothing markets. It is estimated that technical textiles are growing at roughly twice the rate of textiles for clothing applications, where growth rates amounted to about 2% in recent years.

In developed countries, demand for clothing products has been influenced by underlying changes in demography, lifestyle and disposable income and a growing tendency towards more relaxed and leisure wear, brand-name products and fashion wear. Customers are now accustomed to easy access to a wide selection of seasonal products; this trend is expected to continue in the future. However, OECD consumers have been spending a decreasing share of their disposable income on textile and clothing products. A Eurostat report (2002) indicates that between 1970 and 1997 the share of textiles and clothing in total household expenditure in the European Union fell from 9.3% to 6.4%. A similar downward consumption trend is also apparent in the United States, where the share of clothing products in the Consumer Price Index (CPI) fell from 10.6% to 5.5% between 1963 and 1995 (Abernathy *et al.*, 1999).

In the large and diverse group of developing countries, income disparities remain significant, with the least developed countries (LDCs) lagging well behind the emerging and newly developed economies. In the latter, fast economic growth is linked to social mobility and a shift in consumption towards higher quality and branded products and away from traditional wear. With more than three-quarters of the world population living in non-OECD countries, large production and trading opportunities will materialise as their income levels increase. However, in the foreseeable future, the fastest consumption growth opportunities in textile and clothing products are likely to be concentrated in the emerging and newly developed economies.

Textile production is a capital–intensive process

The textile industry is composed of two main operations: *i)* the preparation of yarn, which involves spinning; and *ii)* textile preparation, which involves weaving, knitting and finishing. Technological innovations have greatly increased the speed of textile operations and have resulted in huge productivity gains.[4] In response to competitive pressures and technological progress, textile enterprises have seen a shift in production towards faster growth products, the specialisation of operations, the development of diversified inter-firms networks, lower levels of employment, the closure of uncompetitive plants and new work organisation which has involved the shift of production capacity to low-wage countries. Employment losses and production shifts by production segment are shown in Table 2.1 for the United States for the period 1970–2002 and for the European Union for the period 1996–2000. Between 1970 and 2000, the adjustment process in the textile industry has resulted in the net loss of 2.7 million jobs in five OECD countries, *e.g.* France (-337 000), Germany (-333 000), Japan (-997 000), the United Kingdom (-486 000) and the United States (-585 000), and a further loss of 1.4 million jobs in the clothing industry of these five countries.[5]

Reflecting faster growth in US demand for textiles for industrial and house furnishings applications, *i.e.* non–clothing applications of textiles or technical textiles, the shares of textile employment involved in the production of carpets and rugs and miscellaneous fabricated textile products, such as draperies, bed sheets, towels, bags and automotive trimmings, increased significantly (Table 2.1). The shares of employment in textile finishing and broad woven synthetic fabrics remained relatively stable. In the European Union, most losses of employment appear to have occurred in the preparation and spinning of textile fibres and knitted and crocheted articles.

Concurrently, textile firms have invested in new equipment that has boosted labour productivity. Table 2.2 shows capital expenditures and labour productivity indicators by production segment for the United States in 1997 and the European Union in 2000. In both regions, labour productivity and capital expenditure per employee are higher in textile manufacturing than in apparel manufacturing. Owing to data differences in respect of year, currency and classification system, it is difficult to compare productivity levels of the two regions. However, Annex Tables 2.A1.1 and 2.A1.2 compare various productivity indicators for 34 countries, and indicate that value added per employee is higher in the United States than in EU member states for both textile and clothing manufacturing.

Table 2.1. Textile and clothing employment in the United States and in the European Union, by production segment, 1970 and 2002

United States	Employment (thousands)		Change in employment	Segment as % of sector employment	
	1970	2002	2002/1970	1970	2002
Total textile employment	1 136.8	619.8	-517.0		
Textile mill products	974.8	431.8	-543.0	85.7%	69.7%
Broad woven fabric mills. cotton	212.1	49.5	-162.6	18.7%	8.0%
Broad woven fabric mills. synthetics	100.1	45.9	-54.2	8.8%	7.4%
Broad woven fabric mills. wool	36.6	5.3	-31.3	3.2%	0.9%
Narrow fabric mills	29.6	16.2	-13.4	2.6%	2.6%
Knitting mills	254.1	89.1	-165.0	22.4%	14.4%
Textile finishing. except wool	83.8	50.1	-33.7	7.4%	8.1%
Carpets and rugs	57.4	62.9	5.5	5.0%	10.1%
Yarn and thread mills	130.9	65.1	-65.8	11.5%	10.5%
Miscellaneous textile goods	70.3	47.7	-22.6	6.2%	7.7%
Miscellaneous fabricated textile products	162	188	26.0	14.3%	30.3%
Curtains and draperies	32[1]	16.6	-15.4	2.8%	2.7%
House furnishings, nec	47[1]	46.9	-0.1	4.1%	7.6%
Automotive and apparel trimmings	31.3[1]	57.3	26.0	2.8%	9.2%
Total clothing employment	1 108.4	322	-786.4		
Men's and boys' suits and coats	119	15.2	-103.8	10.7%	4.7%
Men's and boys' furnishings	374.9	105.7	-269.2	33.8%	32.8%
Women's and misses' outerwear	424.3	150.3	-274.0	38.3%	46.7%
Women's and children's undergarments	116.7	13.7	-103.0	10.5%	4.3%
Girls' and children's outerwear	73.5	9.6	-63.9	6.6%	3.0%
Fur goods. and misc. apparel and accessories	65.5[1]	27.5	-38.0	5.6%	8.5%
European Union	1996	2000	2000/1996	1996	2000
Total textile employment	1 166.0	1 110.1	-55.9		
Preparation and spinning of textile fibres	150.9	128.6	-22.3	12.9%	11.6%
Textile weaving	178.5	176.0	-2.6	15.3%	15.9%
Finishing of textiles	114.6	112.6	-2.0	9.8%	10.1%
Made-up articles, except apparel	128.7	126.6	-2.1	11.0%	11.4%
Other textiles	177.2	176.4	-0.8	15.2%	15.9%
Knitted and crocheted fabrics	48.0	50.5	2.5	4.1%	4.5%
Knitted and crocheted articles	188.9	142.3	-46.5	16.2%	12.8%
Total clothing employment	1 136.6	1 025.0	-111.5		
Leather clothes	13.4	10.4	-3.0	1.2%	1.0%
Other wearing apparel and accessories	959.3	803.6	-155.7	84.4%	78.4%
Dressing and dyeing of fur	14.7	13.6	-1.0	1.3%	1.3%

1. 1972 instead of 1970. Due to confidentiality rules, NACE 3-digit categories are aggregated in one or several categories in some EU member states.

Source: U.S. Bureau of Labor Statistics, National Employment, Hours, and Earnings Data: classified under the Standard Industrial Classification (SIC). EU data: Eurostat, Euratex calculations, classified under the General Industrial Classification of Economic Activities within the European Communities (NACE).

Detailed capital expenditures by production segment, shown in Table 2.2, give an indication of the capital intensity of the different production segments. The most capital-intensive textile segments are "other textiles", which includes carpets, rugs, rope, cordage and netting, in the European Union and the finishing and coating segment in the United States. Textile finishing operations are one of the most important operational steps for product differentiation, and specific applications are often copyrighted, thereby giving innovative firms a competitive edge.

Table 2.2. Productivity and capital intensity in textile and apparel manufacturing in the United States and the European Union

		Employment	Labour productivity	Capital expenditures	Capital expenditures
			(per employee)		(per employee)
United States, 1997	NAICS		(USD)	(USD thousands)	(USD)
Textile mills	313	391 899	60 467	2 691 704	6 868
Fibre, yarn and thread mills	3131	82 291	51 065	537 037	6 526
Fabric mills	3132	217 354	57 963	1 491 377	6 862
Finishing and coating	3133	92 254	74 754	663 290	7 190
Textile product mills	314	235 441	57 820	718 728	3 053
Furnishing (carpet and curtain)	3141	126 041	68 140	356 404	2 828
Other text. product mills	3149	109 400	45 929	362 324	3 312
Apparel manufacturing	315	710 796	47 524	941 178	1 324
Apparel knitting mills	3151	99 901	46 351	238 122	2 384
Cut and sew apparel mills	3152	558 328	48 001	629 588	1 128
Accessories and others	3159	52 567	44 697	73 468	1 398
European Union, 2000	NACE		EUR	EUR (1 000)	EUR
Manufacture of textiles	17	1 110 105	31 742	4 694 000	4 228
Spinning of textile fibres	171	128 588	36 603	710 800	5 528
Textile weaving	172	175 965	40 360	924 700	5 255
Finishing of textiles	173	112 569	38 041	659 900	5 862
Made-up articles, excl. apparel	174	126 631	36 996	548 700	4 333
Other textiles	175	176 395	47 121	1 094 600	6 205
Knitted and crocheted fabrics	176	50 476	32 934	298 900	5 922
Knitted and crocheted articles	177	142 349	31 015	532 200	3 739
Apparel manufacturing	18	1 025 032	21 896	1 892 600	1 846
Leather clothes	181	10 424	26 257	14 800	1 420
Other wearing apparel and acc.	182	803 583	26 984	1 635 200	2 035
Dressing and dyeing of fur	183	13 637	22 615	22 300	1 635

Note: Due to confidentiality rules, NACE 3-digit categories are aggregated in one or several categories in some EU member states.

Sources: US data: U.S. Census Bureau, 1997 Economic Census, June 2001, classified under the North American Industry Classification System (NAICS).; EU data, Eurostat, Euratex calculations, classified under the General Industrial Classification of Economic Activities within the European Communities (NACE).

Although EU and US firms face the same global environment, they have adopted slightly different industrial structures, as illustrated by the higher average number of employees per establishment in the United States than in the European Union, with 49.8 and 14.4 employees, respectively, per textile enterprise; and 41.8 and 9.5 employees, respectively per clothing enterprise (Table 2.3). It appears that US firms have adjusted by relying more heavily on consolidation, whereas EU firms have relied on developing diversified inter-firm networks to obtain production flexibility. However, these patterns do not predict how adjustment will occur during the post–ATC period.

Table 2.3. Employment by size of establishments in the United States and the European Union

	Establishments	Employees	Establishments	Employees	Establishments	Employees
United States	Textile mills		Textile product mills		Apparel mfg.	
1997	313 (NAICS)		314 (NAICS)		315 NAICS)	
1 to 4	1 305	2 686	3 519		5 202	
5 to 9	681		1 412	9 392	2 694	18 056
10 to 19	572	7 859	1 068		2 739	
20 to 49	620	19 413	975		3 194	100 217
50 to 99	450	32 348	421	29 713	1 495	
100 to 249	625		316		1 123	174 613
250 to 499	296	102 966	118	41 744	370	127 722
500 to 999	114	75 682	57	38 143	141	93 037
1 000 to 2499	29	37 933	12	15 133	28	37 155
2 500 or more	2		1		3	8 170
Total	4 694	391 899	7 899	235 441	16 989	710 796
Average		83.5		29.8		41.8
Average all textiles				49.8		
European Union	Textile mills				Apparel mfg.	
2000	17 (NACE)				18 (NACE)	
1 to 9	48 262	139 322			84 738	214 091
10 to 49	15 079	279 149			18 765	362 005
50 to 249	6 103	345 457			2 942	247 208
250 or more	3 082	280 667			1 162	196 434
Total	72 575	1 044 756			107 663	1 022 304
Average		14.4				9.5

Note: Due to confidentiality rules, NACE 3-digit categories are aggregated in one or several categories in some EU member states.

Sources: US data: U.S. Census Bureau, 1997 Economic Census, June 2001; EU data, Eurostat, Euratex calculations.

Different types of fibres, which can be mixed together to produce a wide range of textures and finishes, are used in the manufacture of textiles. Stengg (2001) estimates that in 1998 man–made fibres accounted for 72% of total industrial applications in the European Union; cotton accounted for 22%; wool for 5%; and the remaining share for flax and silk. However, cotton has become the main fibre in the manufacture of clothing products. A report by the American Apparel Manufacturers Association (1998) indicates that between 1980 and 1996 the share of cotton in apparel increased from 35% to 53%, while man-made fibres declined from 62% to 45%. The remaining 2% was accounted for by wool fibre. In the post-ATC period, continuing emphasis on the development of new materials for non-clothing textile applications will likely increase the share of man-made fibres in total demand.

Currently, textile production for clothing applications accounts for about one-third of total textile production, and faster growth rates are achieved for industrial and house furnishing applications. It is anticipated that the textile industry will continue to be challenged by product proliferation, particularly for industrial applications, and by the need to respond faster to rapidly changing market conditions without compromising quality. Over time, the textile industry has become a capital-intensive industry in which product differentiation, supported by R&D on material applications, and up-to-date equipment play crucial roles in defining the competitiveness of firms. This underscores the importance for governments to cultivate an innovation culture with a view to encouraging firms to invest in updated equipment and innovative processes. Chapter 4 examines the organisation of innovation systems in several OECD countries.

With the imminent elimination of quantitative restrictions, suppliers and investors are already anticipating quota-free market conditions and are investing in countries offering the best potential. In 2003, TCM imports into China reached USD 5 billion, an increase of over 200% from 1999 (see Figure 4.3 in Chapter 4). There is little doubt that China's textile and clothing enterprise clusters and expertise will become stronger. The textile industry in OECD countries will face intensified competition from the non-OECD countries that are upgrading their production capacity to meet higher production standards. The way in which the industry will innovate and adopt new technology will play a crucial role in defining the relative competitiveness of textile firms in the foreseeable future.

Clothing assembly is a labour–intensive process

The clothing industry is characterised by a highly labour-intensive assembly process, low barriers to entry (and exit) and therefore typically a large number of small and medium–sized enterprises (SMEs) that concentrate production on just a few product categories. Clothing production involves three main operations, pre-assembly, assembly and post-assembly, each of which with its own capital/labour ratio. The pre-assembly stage includes designing, grading and marking of patterns and cutting of textiles into individual components. It has been revolutionised with the application of computer–aided design (CAD) systems. The assembly stage is highly labour-intensive and involves complicated manipulation of soft and limp materials that are sewn into three-dimensional products (see Chapter 4, Annex 4.A2, for recent developments in the clothing production process).

Technological progress in telecommunications and transport networks has made it easier for clothing manufacturers to fragment production segments internationally and to perform the assembly stage in low-cost countries. However, this involves added costs owing to the transport of intermediary inputs, longer inventory holding and added managerial time involved in the co-ordination of an internationally fragmented supply chain. Clearly, these added costs must not exceed the cost advantages of offshore assembly. Time and distance act as important trade barriers for intermediary inputs involved in an internationally fragmented production process. However, efficient freight infrastructure and regular maritime services can make geographically distant locations competitive from a shipping standpoint (ITC, 2004).[6] The time factor is an important driver of investment and production decisions for the highly competitive, time-sensitive and fashion–oriented clothing market. Thus, there are tradeoffs between low wages and temporal proximity to large consumer markets (measured in the turnaround time during which orders must be filled and delivered). Chapter 5 looks at logistical dimensions of the international movement of textile and clothing products in the context of a business facilitation agenda.

The ability to switch the assembly process quickly to adapt to different designs, changing fashions and short production runs may be, on the one hand, a major obstacle to the development of automated assembly processes; on the other hand, it can give lean suppliers specialised in the fashion-oriented segments a competitive edge. Therefore, the location of assembly processes in low–wage countries is an advantage for standardised products in which the production cycle typically requires one year for completion. Its stages are: definition of specifications, selection of textiles, negotiations with potential assemblers, final selection of the assembler, shipment of inputs, assembly, shipment of clothing products, preparation for retail and display on retailers' shelves. For fashion-oriented segments, the cost and proximity advantages derived from quick responses and delivery on a just-in-time basis are sometimes sufficient to offset high wages and thus make business models that locate production in, or in close proximity to, consuming regions viable.

The post–ATC period will offer neither quantitative restrictions nor MFA-related guaranteed market access to mask the vulnerability of national suppliers whose international competitiveness is hampered by obsolete transport infrastructure, irregular transport services and various inefficient domestic regulatory regimes. With the elimination of quantitative restrictions, many exporting countries will lose the MFA–related economic rents that were linked to bilateral trade quotas and will have to address their competitive vulnerability if they aspire to maintain an export–led development strategy in textiles and clothing. The elimination of quantitative restrictions is challenging the global sourcing channels formed over decades of trade restrictions and entails considerable adjustments for all stakeholders. Adjusting to this new environment may require a shift in production methods and product mix, product specialisation in the higher value-added segments of the supply chain or possible diversification into other sectors.

Moving along the supply chain

The assembly of imported textiles into clothing is a simple form of industrial activity and is the starting point for an export-oriented strategy in low-income countries, typically in association with export-processing zones and outward processing programmes (OPP) that provide immediate access both to high-quality inputs and to foreign distribution networks. As technical and organisational skills develop, buyers in consuming countries will ask foreign manufacturers to supply finished products according to the buyers' specifications, typically buyers' brand-name products. This is known as full-package production. Transition from assembly of imported inputs to full–package production takes time, and foreign manufacturers have to demonstrate their entrepreneurial capacity to co-ordinate the entire supply chain, which encompasses a wide range of service–related skills, such as managerial know-how, designing, fabric procurement, property rights protection, export financing and handling of trade formalities. Full–package status gives foreign suppliers substantial autonomy and learning potential for industrial upgrading and provides an edge for export-oriented development (Gereffi, 2002).

The transition from the simple assembly of imported components to full–package production is far from automatic. Access to high-quality textiles is essential for moving upscale in the value chain. However, many small economies are hampered in this respect by various domestic obstacles: they lack backward linkages to national textile capacity;

they do not have an established tradition of clothing manufacturing; or they lack close proximity and/or easy transport to large consumer countries (Mortimore, 2002). Moreover, in some developing countries they may be hampered by excessive tariff protection on intermediary inputs, leading to inverted tariff escalation and distorted market structures.[7] To move beyond the assembly stage to more advanced activities, small economies need to shift their industrial cluster of expertise from manufacturing to design, material sourcing, quality control and logistics. National suppliers need to establish joint structures for sharing market knowledge and to offer more integrated solutions. Working towards closer co-ordination of national suppliers will make it possible to deal more efficiently with large buying groups and to face competition from other integrated suppliers. Hong Kong (China) and Singapore are small economies that have moved up the value chain by nurturing this shift in the industrial clustering of expertise and by providing a liberal trading environment to support private initiatives in these directions.

Chart 2.1 gives a schematic representation of the split between the buyers and suppliers of the main production segments in the supply chain under simple outward processing transactions and more advanced full-package transactions. In the case of simple outward processing transactions, only the sewing is done in the assembly country and all other activities are performed in the buyer's country. Considering that the input textiles usually represent about half of the total manufacturing cost of clothing products, the assembly of imported inputs does not generate much wealth for the country of final assembly, typically offshore centres. Under full–package transactions, the activities performed in the supplier country are diverse and create more backward and forward linkages to the local economy. Backward linkages are more important in countries where quality textiles are readily available from domestic sources, here referred to as integrated suppliers. Integrated suppliers can meet shorter delivery requirements because of the time saved in procuring the necessary inputs, and this confers a competitive cost advantage. The competitiveness of Chinese suppliers relies to a large extent on their ability to obtain high-quality textiles from domestic sources at attractive prices. China's low wages and its vibrant business climate complement these sourcing advantages and make Chinese suppliers highly cost-competitive on export markets.

Chart 2.1. Schematic representation of production-sharing possibilities

Buyer and supplier	Textiles		Clothing				Post-assembly		
	Yarn spinning	Weaving, knitting, finishing	Design	Grading, nesting and marking	Cutting	Sewing	Distribution	Marketing	Retail
OPP offshore suppliers									
Lead buyer									
Assembler									
Small non-integrated suppliers									
Lead buyer									
Full-package									
Integrated suppliers									
Lead buyer									
Full-package									

After full–package production, a further step is the co-ordination of the entire supply chain through triangular manufacturing. The lead supplier plays a role similar to that of an orchestra conductor by suggesting the design, procuring the textiles and overseeing the manufacturing process and the international movement of inputs and final products to the countries of final consumption. The supplier must have the necessary skills in design, transport logistics and quality control and broad knowledge in the areas of fabric and equipment procurement. In fulfilling buyers' orders, foreign manufacturers shift parts or all of the orders to subcontractors located in third low-cost countries with an appropriate MFA quota allocation in the buyer's markets. Entrepreneurs in Hong Kong (China) have mastered the triangular manufacturing model by developing a network of subcontractors located throughout the Asia region.

In the post–ATC period, triangular operations will remain attractive as a business model, but the selection of subcontractors will be made on grounds of business and efficiency rather than on the availability of an export quota allocation in the buyer's markets. In the new environment, the geographical reach of triangular operations is likely to be reduced in order to minimise the time involved in completing the entire fabrication process. Through triangular manufacturing, lead suppliers can concentrate activities in the highest value–added segments of the supply chain and develop their own brand-name products and ultimately begin selling them in their retail chains. Some of the leading clothing manufacturers in Hong Kong (China) have already launched brand-name products and entered retail business (Ramaswamy and Gereffi, 2000). In Hong Kong (China), where wages are too high to perform some manufacturing activities, future success depends on its promotion as fashion and regional procurement hubs, taking advantage of its international networks and supply chain co-ordination.

These developments suggest that the comparative advantage of low–income developing countries with an assembly process based on relatively low wages does not necessarily translate into a comparative advantage for the management of the entire supply chain when all services-related dimensions are taken into consideration. Efficiency in managing the entire supply chain is required, including for design, fabric procurement, logistical skills in transport, quality control, property rights protection, export financing and clearing of trade formalities. As quantitative restrictions are gradually phased out, several low-cost countries that excelled as offshore assembly centres because of their MFA quota allocations are gradually being exposed to the inherent vulnerability of production fragmentation. Countries that aspire to maintain an export-led strategy in textiles and clothing need to shift their industrial expertise from manufacturing to the higher value-added segments of the supply chain by upgrading their domestic skills in design, material sourcing, quality control, logistics and retail distribution. This process can be facilitated by encouraging national suppliers to share market knowledge and expertise with a view to offering more integrated solutions to prospective buyers.

Leadership role of large retail groups and brand-name marketers

The post–assembly stage involves packaging, inventory controls, marketing and retailing. Significant changes have taken place at the retailing stage with the blurring of the traditional boundaries between retailers, brand-name marketers and manufacturers. Retailers are increasingly involved in global sourcing through a wide variety of organisational channels, such as vertical integration, subcontracting and licensing arrangements for brand-name products. They may choose among various sourcing approaches – simple subcontracting of the assembly stage, full-package or triangular manufacturing – depending on their retail strategy. The retailer's decisions are influenced by the turnaround time during which the order must be filled and delivered, the quality of the clothing (staple or fashion) and the MFA quota availability for the type of product. This last factor will be irrelevant as of 2005.

The retail stage itself is increasingly dominated by large and lean organisations in the main consuming countries, which are moving towards greater product specialisation, brand-name products and market segmentation. The five largest US retailers accounted for 68% of all apparel sales in publicly held retail outlets in 1995 (Gereffi, 1999). Since then, the Wal-Mart, Carrefour and brand-name groups have expanded their market penetration in developed countries and have broadened their presence in emerging countries as well. Traditionally, clothing suppliers sold to a distribution network which was mainly composed of small- and medium-sized retailers. In this way, suppliers collected market information about the latest trends in styles and tastes. The integration of information is now carried out by the largest retailers who rely on electronic point-of-sales information; this gives them more leverage for dealing with manufacturers (Abernathy *et al.,* 1999). The shift from traditional retailing to the large and lean retail groups enables these groups to exert considerable pressure on suppliers and to capture a large share of any sources of cost savings or economic rents available throughout the supply chain. Moreover, considering that the largest value-added segments of the supply chain are in the distribution, marketing and retailing functions, a large share of wealth creation in the supply chain remains within the large retailers and brand-name marketers which are still predominantly based in developed countries.

Retail groups and brand-name marketers invest handsomely in building their corporate image and in maintaining brand-name recognition. Because they wish to avoid tarnishing their reputation or losing the market knowledge that underpins their capacity to sell at premium prices, they are careful to select suppliers that will protect their market knowledge and do not allow their names to be associated with exploitative working conditions. Hence, foreign suppliers that guarantee to protect market knowledge and implement the buyer's code of conduct have a competitive edge over other attractive business proposals that do not provide the same guarantees even if they offer lower prices. In this respect, strong enforcement of intellectual property laws and private codes of conduct are considered assets for countries that aspire to maintain an export-led strategy in the upper market segment of clothing products.

Large consumer groups and international civil society organisations active in the globalisation debate exert their own pressure on retailers and suppliers to advance their consumer and social agendas. As a result of ever closer scrutiny, several large retail groups are integrating social requirements in their private codes of conduct and, in turn, are imposing more stringent standards on their suppliers. This means that non–cost factors are increasingly important in the supply chain and that buying decisions are not based exclusively on price competitiveness, particularly for brand-name and eco-labelled products.

The development of Internet retailing has raised hopes for a new low-cost distribution system capable of capturing a large share of retail business and facilitating business-to-business (B2B) contacts. The Internet has largely succeeded in reducing costs in B2B transactions, but it faces considerable consumer resistance as a retail distribution system for clothing products. Much of the resistance is due to the fact that, for the present, Internet retailing is ill-suited to retailing clothing. Customers like to try on, touch and feel the texture and see the fit of clothes.

Research on the development of three-dimensional scanning technologies, clothing simulation software and integration process software is raising prospects for fully integrating retail functions into the supply chain, with individualised specifications electronically transferred to suppliers. In properly equipped retail outlets, customers would be scanned and could then view their body images dressed in the designs and materials of their choice. Moreover, with a personalised card containing individual body specifications, customers could order fashion products directly from Internet retailing sites. Such a fully integrated retail system raises the prospect of shorter delivery cycles, of a reduction of errors in specifications, of more efficient production and of better competitive conditions at the retail level. However, the current state–of–the-art computer–aided design (CAD) systems have difficulties in simulating accurately how all types of cloth drape a body (see Chapter 4).

Increasing weight of developing countries in the world economy

The globalisation of industrial activities that has been facilitated by economic and trade reforms is offering developing countries improved market opportunities and is encouraging an international fragmentation of manufacturing production on the basis of factor endowments. This is reflected in the steady increase in developing countries' share in world manufacturing, from 15.4% in 1985 to 24.3% in 2001 (Table 2.4). Not all developing countries and regions have participated to the same extent in this expansion. China has achieved impressive growth by more than tripling its world share during the period 1985–2001. Conversely, the share of industrial countries in total value added has declined, although the United States and Canada have succeeded in gaining additional market shares since 1995. Interestingly, 1995 corresponds to the second year of the implementation of NAFTA, of which Mexico is a member.

The increasing weight of developing countries in the world economy is also evident in the textile sector and in the aggregate sector composed of clothing, leather and footwear (CLF). Unfortunately, since the UN data do not cover China for this sectoral breakdown, the shares of developing countries in these sectors are under–reported. A further data problem is the lack of a breakdown for the clothing sector alone, without leather and footwear. Despite these shortcomings, the data show a continuing shift in the world distribution of production in favour of developing countries, with larger gains in textiles than in the CLF sector (Table 2.4).

Between 1985 and 2001, worldwide distribution of textile value added has also shifted considerably within developed countries. The declining competitiveness of Japanese textile manufacturers has led to a gradual shift of capacity to neighbouring countries and a loss of 7 percentage points in world textile share. Eastern European and the former USSR countries underwent a profound adjustment following the collapse of their centrally planned economic model, with a resulting loss of 11.4 percentage points in world share. Their adjustment process is beginning to bear results, as reflected in their increasing share in world production of clothing products since 1995 and a marked acceleration in 2001. The European Union and United States/Canada region pursued regional integration arrangements in the 1990s while simultaneously implementing MFA quotas and OPPs requiring regionally produced textiles. All these factors paved the way for each region to gain at a minimum 5 percentage points in world textile share up to 2000. However, the United States/Canada share dropped significantly in 2001 in the context of slower economic growth.

Table 2.4. Distribution of world value added, selected sectors

Percentages

	1985	1990	1995	2000	2001
All manufacturing sectors					
Developing countries	15.4	16.9	21.4	24.0	24.3
China	2.1	2.7	5.3	7.0	7.4
Industrialised countries	84.5	83.1	78.7	76.0	75.7
European Union	32.3	31.4	31.0	29.0	28.7
United States/Canada	23.9	23.4	25.2	26.1	26.3
Japan	15.4	16.8	15.8	14.0	13.8
Eastern European and former USSR	9.5	8.3	3.5	3.8	3.9
Textiles[1]					
Developing countries	23.0	25.1	29.9	32.5	33.0
Industrialised countries	77.0	74.9	70.1	67.5	67.0
European Union	27.4	27.7	32.3	32.6	32.7
United States/Canada	14.0	14.6	19.7	19.0	17.3
Japan	15.2	13.2	10.7	8.6	8.2
Eastern European and former USSR	18.0	17.2	4.9	5.0	6.6
Clothing, leather, footwear[1]					
Developing countries	22.7	24.7	25.0	27.8	27.8
Industrialised countries	77.3	75.3	75.0	72.2	72.2
European Union	33.9	31.2	33.5	30.8	31.5
United States/Canada	17.1	17.6	21.0	22.0	20.7
Japan	10.2	10.2	11.8	9.1	8.3
Eastern European and former USSR	13.6	13.7	5.6	7.1	8.6

Note: At constant 1990 prices.

1. Excludes China but not Hong Kong (China) or Chinese Taipei.

Source: International Yearbook of Industrial Statistics 2003, UN Industrial Development Organisation.

Developing countries are diversifying their production base

The relative importance of textiles and clothing in total manufacturing activities is diminishing with the diversification of production capacity and in line with the gradual redistribution of world capacity in textile and clothing in developing countries (Table 2.5). Their shares of total manufacturing value added in the textile and CLF industries fell to 5.4% and 3.2%, respectively, during the 1985–2001 period. The shares of industrial countries in total manufacturing value added for the textile and CLF industries fell even more dramatically to 2.0% and 1.5%, respectively. However, these aggregate numbers mask considerable disparity at the country level, and several developing countries have reached very high levels of export dependency on clothing exports (see Annex Table 2.A1.5).

The data shortcomings noted earlier complicate the assessment of production trends in textile and clothing industries. However, other UN data that report separate data for textiles and clothing (rather than in combination with leather and footwear) offer insights into the productivity and profitability levels achieved in many countries (see Annex Tables 2.A1.1 and 2.A1.2).[8]

Table 2.5. Shares of manufacturing value added in selected regions

Percentages

	1985	1990	1995	2000	2001
Textiles					
Developing countries	8.2	7.6	6.4	5.5	5.4
Industrialised countries	4.2	3.7	2.8	2.0	2.0
European Union	4.0	3.5	3.3	2.7	2.6
United States/Canada	2.8	2.6	2.5	1.4	1.3
Japan	4.2	3.0	2.2	1.6	1.6
Eastern European and former USSR	8.5	8.7	4.4	3.3	4.0
Clothing, leather, footwear					
Developing countries	6.3	5.4	3.9	3.2	3.2
Industrialised countries	3.3	2.7	2.2	1.5	1.5
European Union	3.8	2.9	2.5	1.7	1.7
United States/Canada	2.7	2.3	2.0	1.1	1.1
Japan	2.2	1.7	1.8	1.2	1.1
Eastern European and former USSR	5.0	5.1	3.7	3.3	3.7

Note: At constant 1990 prices. Excludes China but not Hong Kong (China) or Chinese Taipei.

Source: International YearGbook of Industrial Statistics 2003, UN Industrial Development Organisation.

Shrinking productivity gap

There are wide discrepancies in labour productivity in textile and clothing industries between developed and developing countries, as measured by value added per employee (Annex Tables 2.A1.1 and 2.A1.2). In the textile sector, the average value added of an OECD-area worker was about USD 36 700 in the late 1990s. In the listed non–OECD countries, the average value added per employee was USD 15 000 but there are considerable variations at the country level. For example, in Bangladesh and the Russian Federation, value added per worker was as low as USD 1 100 in the late 1990s. As a result, labour productivity levels in textile operations in Bangladesh, the Russian Federation, Vietnam, India, Sri Lanka and Egypt were at least ten times below those at that time in Germany, Korea, Japan, Finland or the United States.

Not surprisingly, labour productivity is lower for clothing than for textile operations in all reported countries except Chile, Egypt, India and Vietnam, and labour productivity levels are much higher in OECD countries than in non-OECD economies. Nine OECD countries have higher labour productivity than Hong Kong (China), the best performer among non-OECD economies. The Czech Republic and the Slovak Republic have the lowest productivity levels among OECD countries, slightly below that of Egypt. Labour productivity gaps in developing economies are significant. Hong Kong (China), the economy most heavily engaged in triangular manufacturing, has the highest level, while countries specialised in the assembly of imported inputs for re-export, *i.e.* Bangladesh, Vietnam, Sri Lanka, Indonesia, India and Morocco, have the lowest.

There are many reasons for the productivity gap between developed and developing countries, and they include both external and internal factors. As an external factor, decades of MFA-related quotas have prevented the textile industry from migrating to developing countries as fast as the clothing industry. With the imminent elimination of the ATC, there will be no major obstacles to the development of stronger clusters of textile expertise in the most competitive developing countries. The recent surge of imports of up-to-date textile and clothing equipment in China attests to this migration and foreshadows higher productivity levels and improved domestic availability of the high-quality textiles that are required for export markets. With the elimination of quotas and a world environment conducive to technology transfer through machinery imports and globalised knowledge networks, the efficient operation of modern equipment in developing countries is expected to shrink the productivity gap that has differentiated developed and developing countries.

Domestic obstacles also hamper the implementation of production-enhancing techniques. An inefficient regulatory framework and obsolete domestic infrastructure in essential business services, *e.g.* port infrastructure, transport modes, telecommunications, electricity and customs, act as a tax on textile and clothing suppliers and undermine their efforts to invest in productivity-enhancing equipment. These issues are examined in Chapter 5.

Moreover, many developing countries do not produce textiles of the quality required for export markets domestically and so must import them. Access to such textiles may be hampered by excessive tariff protection, inefficient customs clearance procedures and incentives that protect low-scale textile production that provides employment to a large pool of low-skilled workers. This situation is best illustrated by India, where high tariff protection is coupled with domestic policies that are designed to protect low-scale textile and clothing firms. This has resulted in a fragmented production capacity of sub-optimal scale and clothing that is of unsuitable quality for export markets. The employment displacement effects of trade liberalisation measures in textiles and clothing are a matter of concern for all countries, both developed and developing. The linkages between international trade and labour adjustment in the textile and clothing industries are discussed in Chapter 3.

In the post-ATC period, it will be crucial for countries wishing to remain active on export markets to reduce their productivity gaps by addressing domestic obstacles to growth, setting up an efficiency–enhancing policy environment and facilitating private initiatives to invest in modern equipment and production processes.

China: a threat and an opportunity

In the last two decades, China has sustained impressive economic growth and has become the world's largest exporter of clothing products and the second largest exporter of textiles. In the coming years, China's competitive position is expected to strengthen as it reaps the benefits of domestic reforms carried out pursuant to its recent accession to the WTO. Sustained flows of imports of modern TCM (see Figure 4.3 in Chapter 4) are improving China's capacity to produce high-quality textiles and strengthening its expertise. This will directly benefit domestic clothing suppliers who will have rapid access to high-quality textiles at competitive prices and can, in turn, meet short turnaround delivery requirements. Referring to the competitive factors underpinning the

Chinese textile and clothing industries, an ITC report (2004) underscores that China is expected to become the "supplier of choice" for most US importers because of its ability to make almost any type of textile and clothing product at any quality level at a competitive price.

The WTO Protocol on China's accession and its schedules contain specific provisions that require China to establish a legally based trading regime that is compatible with WTO principles and obligations, including a uniform trading regime, transparency of laws and regulations, non-discrimination and judicial review. Under its tariff commitments, China is committed to reduce its average tariff rate on textile and clothing articles by 33.7%, from an average applied rate of 17.1% in 2002 to 11.3% when all reduction commitments are implemented (OECD, 2002b). Moreover, all of China's tariffs are bound against increases in the WTO and most of its bound rates at the end of the implementation period are much lower than the tariffs applied in 2002, which means that China is effectively reducing its tariff protection over the period.[9]

Similarly, under its WTO services commitments, China has agreed to permit foreign suppliers to set up retailing services through wholly owned foreign enterprises by 11 December 2004. Upon China's accession to the WTO, foreign suppliers obtained the right to distribute, without limitations, goods that they produce in China. If these regulations are effectively enforced by that date, foreign retailing groups' retail distribution strategies in China will no longer be subject to geographical and quantitative restrictions. This will give them considerable retailing opportunities in this large consumer market. Anecdotal sources estimate that the size of the Chinese affluent middle class is around 80-100 million people, or roughly equivalent to the combined populations of France and the United Kingdom.

The WTO Protocol on the accession of China also contains a transitional product-specific safeguard mechanism that enables WTO members to restrict imports originating from China when the latter cause or threaten to cause market disruption to domestic producers of textile and clothing products (Article 16). This transitional safeguard provision is valid for a period of 12 years after China's accession (to December 2013). This provision recognises the potential market disruption in importing countries that would result from export surges from China. The WTO Report of the Working Party on the Accession of China (paragraph 242) also contains a textile safeguard provision that enables WTO members to restrict imports from China when they believe that imports of textile and clothing products of Chinese origin threaten to impede the orderly development of trade in these products owing to market disruption. The textile safeguard provision is valid until the end of December 2008. The United States has invoked this provision and, following consultations with China, has restrained Chinese imports for knit textiles, dressing gowns and brassieres for a period of 12 months. The post-ATC period creates considerable anxiety among the worldwide textile and clothing community about the emergence of more competitive suppliers in China that may capture a high (if not a disproportionate) share of the economic benefits arising from the phasing out of quantitative restrictions. What the post-ATC period may offer to China and countries competing with it may be illustrated by what happened to the import composition of Japan, a country that did not apply MFA restrictions. Between 1990 and 2002, the share of Japanese clothing imports originating from China soared from 31% to 79%.

Whether or not WTO members will frequently invoke the WTO transitional safeguard provision or China's textile safeguard provision remains an open question. However, based on the large consultation with US suppliers and retailers undertaken by the US

International Trade Commission (ITC, 2004), it is anticipated that the WTO transitional safeguard provision will bring an element of uncertainty to the capacity of Chinese suppliers to access foreign markets. Hence, the ITC argues that the ability of Chinese suppliers to expand export shipments in the post-ATC period will be tempered by the use by the United States and other WTO members of the transitional product-specific safeguard mechanism contained in China' WTO Protocol of accession. Furthermore, the ITC argues that US importers will address this risk of sourcing from a single country by diversifying their sourcing networks among other low-cost country alternatives. This diversification of imports will be influenced by competitive cost factors in other supplying countries which are themselves influenced by market access opportunities offered under regional and preferential trade arrangements. This underscores the importance of the preferential market access provided by developed countries to the least developed countries, some of which are highly dependent on clothing exports for their prosperity, *e.g.* Bangladesh and Cambodia (see Annex Table 2.A1.5).

It is not the first time that the world has witnessed the emergence of new competitive players in textiles and clothing. In the mid-nineteenth century, much anxiety resulted from innovative production techniques developed in the United Kingdom, and, immediately after World War II, there was much concern over the then low–wage countries of Japan and Korea. Both the industrial revolution and the expansion of the Japanese and Korean economies have led to considerable adjustment in the textile and clothing industries and, simultaneously, have stimulated world growth and offered broader trade opportunities. Spurred by China's strong growth prospects and the implementation of domestic reforms, increased market opportunities have already arisen and are expected to continue to appear in future for industrial and consumer products originating from both developed and developing countries. Driven by sustained high economic growth, China's total imports now exceed its exports. China's trade deficit reached USD 8.4 billion in the first quarter of 2004, fuelled by the country's growing need for raw materials and equipment.

In addition, in the past experience of the United Kingdom, Japan and Korea, high growth was accompanied by an increase in production and infrastructure bottlenecks, rising domestic wages and appreciating domestic currencies which chipped away at their competitiveness and provided more competitive producers with trade opportunities. Throughout 2003, power blackout measures were imposed to limit Chinese consumption of electricity and forced manufacturing plants to halve production temporarily. Power shortages are exacerbated by bottlenecks in the transport infrastructure which delay the distribution of imported coal and oil. The emergence of infrastructure bottlenecks raises questions about how reliably Chinese suppliers can meet tight delivery requirements in the just–in–time manufacturing sectors (see Box 5.2 in Chapter 5).

The analogy between the post-war situation of both Japan and Korea with the present situation in China should take into account China's huge untapped reservoir of low-skilled and low-wage labour, which is of a very different magnitude than that of Japan and Korea. It means that even if the Chinese currency appreciates relative to other currencies, Chinese suppliers would be able to partly offset the effects of a stronger currency on their competitiveness by reducing domestic wages without incurring undue labour shortages. Nevertheless, there are pressures on Chinese authorities to break the fixed parity with the US dollar and to let the yuan appreciate. So far, the authorities have resisted, but the presence of large accumulated foreign reserves (exceeding USD 435 billion in March 2004) is raising questions among currency market operators about the sustainability of the CNY/USD fixed parity.

With about one of every two textile employees working for China's state-owned enterprises (SOEs) (Table 2.6), trading partners have sought commitments that the trading transactions of China's SOEs would comply with WTO principles and agreements.[10] In the clothing industry, private firms' share of total clothing employment reached almost 90% in 2001, reflecting the relative ease of entry in this industry. Despite China's SOE commitments in the WTO, several competing suppliers argue that China's SOEs are not yet operating on a commercial basis so that they have unfair competitive advantages in both domestic and export markets. On the basis of Chinese statistics (Table 2.6), more than 40% of textile SOEs operated at a loss in 2001 and the average loss represented 2.2% of SOEs' output. The privatisation of China's large textile firms represents a politically sensitive task for the Chinese authorities who are likely to consider carefully the job displacement consequences of any privatisation programme. Moreover, the employment paradigm for Chinese authorities must be placed within its overall context of integrating into the urban regions the inflows of millions of job seekers who want better conditions than those in the rural regions where they originate.

Table 2.6. State–owned enterprises in China, 2001

	SOE employment as % of total employment	SOEs as % of total enterprises	SOE output as % of total output	SOEs operating at loss as % of total SOE	SOE losses as % of total SOE output
Textile industry	49.4	21.3	35.7	41.1	2.2
Natural fibres	48.4	21.1	31.1	40.7	2.4
Preparation of fibres	53.2	22.9	36.6	40.6	2.4
Finishing of textiles	29.2	16.2	16.7	46.0	3.2
Made-up cotton articles	29.1	20.8	18.4	35.4	1.8
Knitting textile	11.9	9.8	5.7	46.2	3.7
Synthetic fibres	58.2	22.7	51.4	43.8	1.8
Clothing industry	10.6	8.2	6.7	35.6	3.7
Knitwear	21.0	14.4	13.0	41.2	3.9
Garments and others	8.4	6.7	5.2	32.6	3.6
Equipment manufacturing	48.6	29.6	32.8	39.0	1.8

Source: OECD calculations based on CNTIC (2001/2002), *Report on China Textile Industry Development.*

In the more immediate future, export-oriented countries fear heightened competitive pressures from Chinese textile and clothing suppliers, despite the emergence of bottlenecks in essential energy and transport services. However, China's stellar economic performance, combined with its market opening measures, foreshadows improved trade opportunities in textile and clothing industries, for both natural and man-made fibres, related manufacturing equipment, and improved retail and marketing opportunities by the end of 2004. In the post-ATC period, Chinese suppliers will continue to exert considerable pressure on less competitive supplying countries to adjust domestic capacity towards more advanced processes and to diversify their economic activities. These market pressures call for domestic policies to facilitate structural adjustment and economic diversification through an emphasis on higher value-added production segments of the supply chain and diversification in other sectors and services.

Geographical patterns of trade shaped by trade measures

The composition of the world's largest textile and clothing exporters changed considerably over the 1990-2002 period (Table 2.7). Export shares of textiles declined the most in the European Union, Japan, Switzerland and Hong Kong (China), and increased the most in China, the United States and India. The most dramatic changes occurred in China, which became the world's second largest exporter, and in both Japan and Switzerland, whose world shares of textiles dropped by 1.6 percentage points. Nevertheless, Japan remained a very active player in the supply chain through the global sourcing operations of its large retail groups and as a major supplier of sewing machines.

On the import side, the European Union and the United States were the largest importing areas. Import shares grew particularly in the United States, China, Mexico and some eastern European and Mediterranean countries (Annex Table 2.A1.3). Textile exports from the European Union and the United States under outward processing programmes weighed heavily on clothing production decisions, which in turn created significant geographical patterns of trade in textiles and clothing. These programmes and their impacts are assessed below.

The reconfiguration of world clothing exports (also shown in Annex Table 2.A1.4) is marked by the emergence of China as the world's largest exporting country, ahead of the European Union (extra-regional exports). China's gains came mainly at the expense of middle- and high-income neighbouring countries that reduced production capacity or reconverted in the context of triangular manufacturing by transferring parts of their production to low-wage countries. Three economies, Hong Kong (China), Chinese Taipei and to a lesser extent Korea, are involved in triangular manufacturing and remain key world players in the supply chain, although their shares in direct exports of clothing indicate a considerable lessening of importance. New low-wage clothing suppliers with spare MFA quota allocations also emerged in East and South Asia, as well as in neighbouring countries to the European Union and the United States, which took advantage of preferential access in the form of free trade agreements or outward processing programmes.

Table 2.7. Leading exporters of textiles and clothing, 1990–2002

Exporters	2002	2002/1990	Exporters	2002	2002/1990
Textiles	Percentage share	Percentage point changes in world share	Clothing	Percentage share	Percentage point changes in world share
EU15	34.2	-14.5	EU15	25.1	-12.6
Extra-EU	*15.2*	*0.7*	*Extra-EU*	*8.3*	*-2.2*
China	13.5	6.6	China	20.6	11.6
Hong Kong, China	0.6	-1.5	Hong Kong, China	4.1	-4.4
United States	7.0	2.2	Turkey	4.0	0.9
Korea	7.0	1.2	Mexico	3.9	3.3
Chinese Taipei	6.3	0.4	United States	3.0	0.6
Japan	4.0	-1.6	India	2.8	0.5
India	3.7	1.6	Bangladesh	2.1	1.5
Pakistan	3.1	0.5	Indonesia	2.0	0.4
Turkey	2.8	1.4	Korea	1.8	-5.4
Indonesia	1.9	0.7	Thailand	1.7	-0.9
Mexico	1.5	0.8	Romania	1.6	1.3
Canada	1.4	0.7	Dominican Republic	1.4	0.7
Thailand	1.3	0.4	Tunisia	1.3	0.3
Switzerland	0.9	-1.6	Philippines	1.3	-0.3

Note: Data for India and Dominican Republic refer to 2001 instead of 2002.

Source: WTO, *International Trade Statistics 2003.*

Throughout the period, MFA quotas and trade preferences played a prominent role in the reconfiguration of trade flows. As a result, Mexico increased its world export share by almost eight-fold between 1990 and 2002 (see Annex Table 2.A1.4) and became the second largest supplier to the United States, behind China. Turkey also increased its world share during the period and is now the second largest supplier to the European Union. Romania and the Dominican Republic, which were virtually absent from export markets in the 1980s, had by 2002 joined the group of the 15 largest clothing exporters by taking advantage of preferential arrangements with the European Union and the United States, respectively.

In spite of the trade restrictiveness of quantitative restrictions, the OECD-area share of imports of clothing products originating from developing countries jumped from 40% to 65% between 1980 and 2000 (Annex Table 2.A1.9) and from 20% to 30% for textile imports (Annex Table 2.A1.8). The impact of MFA–driven triangular manufacturing, various free trade agreements and outward processing programmes on OECD imports is visible in the variations of import shares of individual suppliers. They broadly parallel the changes in world export shares discussed above. During the last 20 years, the destination of OECD-area exports of textiles has followed two opposite trends. The share of those moving within the OECD region increased during the 1980s and reached 80% in 1990. This share then gradually declined to 70% in 2001 (Annex Table 2.A1.6).

Three distinct geographical trade patterns have emerged. The Asia-Pacific region centres on key supply chain players, *i.e.* Hong Kong (China), Chinese Taipei, Korea and Japan, and involves a network of subcontracted suppliers located in China and other low-income East Asian countries. In Europe, the European Union has emerged as the region's supply chain manager with the Central and Eastern European and Mediterranean countries as the outward processors at the periphery. Finally, in North America, the United States is the supply chain manager and peripheral outward processors are found in Mexico and the Caribbean region.

Each exporting country has pursued its export interests on the basis of its own combination of factor endowments, cultural affinities, geographical proximity to large markets and preferential access networks. As an illustration, Annex Table 2.A1.5 shows the evolution of clothing export earnings for 33 countries for the period 1990–2002, and the evolution of the share of clothing in the country's total exports. It also identifies the countries that benefit from duty-free access to the European Union and the United States and qualifying countries under outward processing programmes in the European Union, the United States and Australia. The countries that have realised the largest proportional increase in their shares of clothing exports in total exports are listed in declining order. Jordan appears to have made the largest proportional gain by increasing its share in total exports by a factor of 12.9 during the period 1990-2002. Honduras's share increased about five-fold during the same period.

Among the 18 countries that have increased their shares of clothing in total exports, all except three – Sri Lanka, Indonesia and Macau (China) – have enjoyed preferential access under outward processing programmes or free trade arrangements to the markets of the European Union, the United States or Australia. Ten of those 18 countries now have export shares exceeding 30% of their total exports. Such a high level of export dependency on a single sector is not healthy, and many of these countries will be particularly vulnerable in the post–ATC as global sourcing channels reconfigure on the basis of cost competitiveness rather than the quota allocations of the MFA period.

Trade policy measures

Trade policy measures have had a major impact on production decisions in textiles and clothing and on trade flows. MFA restrictions have contributed to the international fragmentation of the supply chain by accelerating the diversification of supply to the benefit of less competitive producers when quota-constrained suppliers subcontract clothing assembly processes in third low–cost countries. The scheduled elimination of quantitative restrictions at the end of December 2004 is challenging the global sourcing channels established during the MFA period and represents a systemic change in trade policies. In the meantime, stakeholders are reassessing their global sourcing channels not only on the basis of price competitiveness but increasingly on the dynamics of inter-firm networks that are able to react quickly and meet the stringent specifications of large retail groups in terms of production quality and social requirements.

The deadline for quota elimination coincides with a key stage of negotiations under the Doha Development Agenda, as changes to existing WTO rules or new WTO disciplines to be agreed will also have an impact on international trade in textiles and clothing. During these negotiations, WTO members have an opportunity to deal with remaining sources of trade protection and trade-distorting measures with a view to establishing a framework of multilateral disciplines that effectively improves competitive conditions in all economies and offers improved market opportunities.

Several decades of trade liberalisation in other industrial sectors have benefited the world economy. Similar economic benefits will be achieved by tackling remaining trade restrictions affecting trade in textiles and clothing. Annex A reviews the economic literature on the impact of trade liberalisation reforms in these sectors and shows considerable variation in the expected annual welfare gains, ranging from USD 6.5 billion to USD 324 billion, or 0.02% to 1.49% of world GDP. In what follows, the remaining sources of trade protection and trade-distorting measures in OECD countries and non-OECD economies are examined. The roles that regional trade agreements and other preferential trade arrangements are likely to play in the post–ATC period are also reviewed.

High bound tariffs are one side of the coin

Following the full implementation of the Uruguay Round commitments, bound rates in textile and clothing are high in both developed and developing countries and remain an important impediment to achieving greater production efficiency and the realisation of welfare gains (Annex Table 2.A1.10). Bound tariffs for textiles and clothing average 9% in the Quad (versus 4.4% for all industrial products), (WTO, 2002b, pp. 4 and 5) 12% in developed countries as a whole and 29% in developing and transition economies (WTO, 2001, p. 29). When tariff levels are distinguished for textiles, clothing and manufactured products, as shown in Table 2.8 for 38 countries, tariffs are systematically higher on textiles than on manufactured products, and tariffs on clothing are higher than those on textiles. Annex Table 2.A1.10 shows a further breakdown of bound tariffs for five stages of the supply chain, beginning with raw agricultural products, vegetable fibres, man-made filament yarns, textiles and finally clothing products. While there are no identical tariff structures among countries, those with the lowest tariffs exhibit escalating tariffs; uniform tariff structures are found in countries applying the highest tariff levels.

Both escalating and uniform tariff structures have advantages and disadvantages. The advantage of a uniform tariff structure is that it makes the tariff regime more transparent and relatively easy to administer. Its disadvantage is that the costs of tariffs imposed on inputs are increased by manufacturer margins and domestic taxes that are ultimately borne by consumers. Tariffs on inputs act as taxes on domestic production and hinder the competitiveness of domestic production that relies on imported inputs. The opposite can be argued in instances of escalating tariffs. However, the assessment of tariff structures can only be meaningful when all tariff reduction schemes are taken into account. The impact of bound MFN tariffs is moderated by various tariff reduction measures, including the use of applied tariffs at lower levels than bound duties, preferential trade agreements and various forms of tariff relief programmes.

High bound and applied tariffs almost everywhere

Applied tariffs in 1996 by stages of production are notably lower than bound tariffs for several countries, many of which are OECD countries, such as Korea, Mexico, Australia, Turkey, Iceland and Switzerland (Annex Table 2.A1.11). Lower applied rates often reflect unilateral tariff reduction programmes implemented to stimulate domestic competition and to speed integration efforts in the world economy. However, they are less predictable as they can be ratcheted up to bound levels whenever domestic suppliers consider competition conditions to be unbearable.[11] Despite unilateral liberalisation efforts, average applied tariffs on textiles and clothing remain high compared to average tariffs imposed on manufactured products for the overwhelming majority of countries (Table 2.8).

Table 2.8. Simple average tariffs, selected countries

Percentages

Region	Country	Manufactures	Textiles	Clothing
OECD countries		6.2	9.4	16.1
	Australia	5.4	9.9	20.7
	Canada	4.9	10.7	18.4
	European Union	4.4	7.9	11.4
	Japan	2.9	6.5	11.0
	Korea	8.0	9.4	12.4
	Mexico	17.3	20.5	34.4
	New Zealand	3.1	2.4	13.7
	Turkey	5.9	8.6	11.8
	United States	4.0	9.1	11.4
Developing countries		13.5	18.1	23.0
Asia				
	China	9.6	9.7	16.1
	Hong Kong, China	0.0	0.0	0.0
	Indonesia	9.0	12.6	18.1
	Malaysia	9.9	16.7	19.6
	Philippines	7.4	10.7	19.2
	Singapore	0.0	0.0	0.0
	Chinese Taipei	6.4	8.3	13.1
	Thailand	16.1	18.7	39.7
South Asia				
	Bangladesh	22.1	30.2	..
	India	34.1	39.0	40.0
	Sri Lanka	8.0	3.4	11.0
Latin America				
	Argentina	16.1	20.1	22.9
	Bolivia	9.6	10	10.0
	Brazil	16.8	20	22.9
	Chile	9.0	9.0	9.0
	Colombia	12.1	18.0	19.9
	Costa Rica	4.8	8.3	13.8
	Dominican Republic	14.6	20.5	30.6
	El Salvador	6.9	17.0	23.9
	Jamaica	5.6	3.2	19.4
	Paraguay	13.7	19.5	22.4
	Peru	13.3	17.0	19.3
	Uruguay	14.7	20.1	22.9
	Venezuela	12.3	18.0	19.9
Africa				
	Algeria	24.1	35.3	44.5
	Egypt	22.3	42.0	39.7
	Morocco	28.2	38.2	49.6
	Tunisia	28.7	38.0	42.6
	Sub-Saharan Africa	16.8	21.8	34.5

Note: Tariff rates for the most recent year for which data are available; Manufactures are SITC 5-8 less 68; textiles (65); and clothing (84).

Source: UNCTAD (2002), World Integrated Trade Solution Database.

Tariff escalation and tariff peaks

Another difference between bound and applied rates is that the uniform structure of tariffs has practically vanished for applied rates, except for countries that have adopted duty–free access comprehensively, such as Hong Kong (China) and Singapore. At one extreme, steep tariff escalation affords a high degree of effective protection and can effectively shield domestic products from foreign competition. At the other extreme, inverted escalation or de-escalation, with higher tariffs on inputs than on finished products, hinders the competitiveness of finished products that rely on imported inputs. The trade-offs vary for each country depending on its factor endowments, production specialisation on fibres, textiles or clothing and degree of competitiveness.

Significant tariff escalation and thus high effective protection are revealed by the incidence of notable tariff peaks for textiles and clothing, as shown in Table 2.9. The tariffs used in the UNCTAD/WTO study were the final most–favoured nation (MFN) rates resulting from the Uruguay Round, or the most recent rates under applicable Generalised System of Preferences (GSP), or suspended MFN rates, whichever is lower.

Peak tariffs can be defined in various ways, such as three times the average tariffs on industrial products or above a fixed threshold rate. The UNCTAD/WTO study uses a 12% threshold rate, which is slightly below the 13.2% rate obtained by applying the three times rule for the Quad countries, *i.e.* 4.4% multiplied by three. Problems with tariff peaks are partly related to the fact that they are masked in measurements of average tariffs for an entire sector or for production segments and thus are not very transparent. They are also harder to administer and prone to incorrect customs declarations and discretionary interpretations in customs administrations where integrity concerns prevail.

Among Quad countries and four other large trading countries, the highest incidence of tariff peaks in the textile and clothing industries occurs in three developing countries where peak tariffs are concentrated in the 20-29% range. There are no incidences of tariff peaks in Korea and very few in the European Union and Japan. In Canada and the United States, there is a large incidence in the 12-19% tariff range and, for both countries, tariff peaks in textiles and clothing account for more than 50% of their total peak tariffs.

Table 2.9. Distribution of tariff peaks in textiles and clothing

		Post-Uruguay Round MFN rates[1]				Number of peaks	Share in total peaks
		12-19%	20-29%	30-99%	>=100%		
Korea	Textiles					0	0.0%
	Clothing					0	0.0%
EU	Textiles	3				3	0.2%
	Clothing					0	0.0%
Japan	Textiles	5			6	11	1.2%
	Clothing					0	0.0%
Canada	Textiles	177	7			184	31.9%
	Clothing	120	5			125	21.7%
United States	Textiles	184	25	1		210	23.0%
	Clothing	170	69	8		247	27.1%
Malaysia	Textiles	12	395	140		547	18.6%
	Clothing		235	3		238	8.1%
Brazil	Textiles	542	81			623	11.4%
	Clothing		238			238	4.5%
China (MFN 1998)	Textiles	181	219	292		692	16.1%
	Clothing		24	259		283	6.7%

1. Post-Uruguay Round MFN rates or most recent GSP rates or suspended MFN rates, whichever is lower.

Source: UNCTAD/WTO (2000).

Tariff relief measures

Many countries have general provisions in their respective customs tariff laws that grant duty-free or reduced rates for machinery, raw materials or inputs, so as to encourage downward processing. Tariff escalation is the result of this practice. In Australia, for example, textiles are imported at duty-free or low rates under various bylaws, including the Tariff Concession Orders. The Australian Industry Commission estimated that over 60% of all textile imports entered duty-free under these bylaws in 1995-96 (WTO, TPRM of Australia, June 1998, p. 67). In Canada, with the implementation of NAFTA, duty drawback and remission programmes conditional on domestic production levels and sourcing requirements were terminated in 1997, but six remission orders not related to performance were introduced in mid–1997 and are due to expire on 31 December 2004.[12] In India, duty–free imports of textile machinery are subject to an export obligation of six times the import value, to be realised over a fixed period of time (WTO, TPRM of India, March 1998, p. 58). Information about national duty-remission programmes applicable to textiles and clothing is sparse and obtaining updated information can be a time-consuming task. Further examples may not necessarily add much to the argument that such programmes exist and moderate the impact of high bound and applied tariffs.

Tariff liberalisation produces large consumer benefits

New Zealand commenced a significant unilateral tariff reduction programme in several sectors in 1988 and reaps large consumer benefits as a result. Tariffs on clothing dropped from a range of 40–65% in 1988 to 19% in 1999, and tariffs on textiles dropped from 40% to 12.5% during the same period. The NZ Institute of Economic Research estimates that the typical New Zealand household gained NZD 1 140 in 1998 as a result of the tariff cuts on cars, household appliances, shoes and clothing (NZ Institute of Economic Research (1999), pp. 4-5).

In Sweden, MFA restrictions were lifted in 1991 in the context of a deregulation package. However, slightly more stringent restrictions were re-introduced in January 1995 when Sweden acceded to the European Union. During the interim period, import competition strengthened significantly and clothing prices fell by an estimated 8% to 10%.[13] The composition of imports changed dramatically following the elimination of MFA restrictions but did not change significantly after their re-introduction in 1995. The EU's share of clothing imports dropped from 65% to 45% between 1990 and 1994, and inched up to 46% in 1996. China was the main beneficiary of the liberalisation process, with a gain of 16 percentage points in total Swedish clothing imports, followed by India with a 2.5 percentage point gain and a minimal gain for Bangladesh. Shortly thereafter, China's share fell to 16.3% of total Swedish imports and India's share receded to 3.1%. Portugal lost the most, with its import share falling by half from 16.8% in 1990 to 8.4% in 1996. The less dramatic trade impact following the re-introduction of MFA restrictions is partly explained by the generally weak macroeconomic environment of the mid-1990s. Swedish clothing buyers had likely developed new business relations with Asian and East Asian suppliers during the interim period which contributed to maintaining more stringent competitive conditions in the Swedish market after 1995. As noted earlier, Annex A provides a comprehensive review of the economic literature on the welfare gains associated with trade liberalisation reforms in textiles and clothing.

Preferential trade arrangements are another

Parallel to the phasing out of MFA restrictions, a complex web of preferential trade arrangements has developed. Some 250 regional trade agreements (RTAs) had been notified to the GATT/WTO as of June 2002, of which 129 notified since 1995, and only five WTO members were not party to a RTA at that time, *i.e.* China, Hong Kong (China), Japan, Macau (China) and Mongolia (WTO, 2002b). RTAs are primarily free trade agreements (FTAs) and customs union agreements that provide for tariff- and quota-free trade among beneficiary countries. In 2002, it was estimated that 43% of world trade was covered under RTAs, a percentage that will reach 55% by 2005 if all announced RTAs are effectively implemented (OECD, 2002a). Moreover, there are additional preferential arrangements of direct relevance to textiles and clothing, such as the Generalised System of Preferences for developing countries and outward processing programmes in which textile products are temporarily exported to low-wage countries for final assembly and are subsequently re-imported as clothing articles under preferential treatment. Examples of preferential trade arrangements offered by several economies are presented in Box 2.1.

Box 2.1. Preferential trade arrangements

The following examples of preferential arrangements concluded by the European Union, Japan and the United States give an indication of their diverging scope and of the large number of trading partners that are beneficiary countries under the various arrangements.

The EU has gradually built a pan-European free trade area covering 31 countries that provides duty-free access for all manufactured products and since 2002 duty- and quota-free trade of textiles and clothing, along with cumulative rules of origin.14 Since March 2001, 49 least developed countries (LDCs) have gained duty- and quota-free access to the EU textile and clothing markets under the programme Everything But Arms (EBA). Under the EU GSP programme, GSP benefits for textiles and clothing are generally limited to a 20% margin of the MFN rates.

Japan now has one free trade agreement with Singapore; another with Mexico will enter into force in January 2005 and negotiations are proceeding with Korea. Under the Japanese GSP regime, industrial goods, including textiles and clothing, originating from developing countries are generally reduced to half the applicable MFN rates and are admitted duty-free from LDCs. Japan has no country-specific outward processing programme; it has a general MFN provision to exclude the value of its goods sent abroad for further processing from the customs value of the returning products.

In the Western Hemisphere, NAFTA entered into force in 1994 and was instrumental in spearheading Mexico to its position as the world's fourth largest clothing exporter in 2001. Also in 1994, a process to integrate 34 economies into the Free Trade Area of the Americas (FTAA) was launched, the negotiations to be completed by 2005. The FTAA could supersede the complex web of sub-regional free trade agreements concluded in the interim. Since May 2000, the United States under the African Growth Opportunity Act (AGOA) provides growth opportunities for eligible Sub-Saharan Africa countries (38 in early 2003). Under the Caribbean Basin Trade Partnership Act (CBTPA), the United States provides opportunities for growth of duty- and quota-free clothing imports made from US textiles for 14 eligible countries. Under the Andean Trade Promotion and Drug Eradication Act (ATPDEA), similar benefits are provided to Colombia, Peru, Bolivia and Ecuador.

Although both the AGOA and CBTPA provide beneficiary countries improved trade opportunities in many sectors, their textile and clothing provisions are structured in such a manner that they are similar to OPPs. However, the use of third-country fabric is temporarily permitted for LDCs that are beneficiaries under AGOA until the end of September 2004.

Since January 2003, Canada provides duty-free access under all tariff items for imports from LDCs, except for outside of quota-tariff items for dairy, poultry and egg products. Canada also introduced multiple formula rules of origin for textile and clothing products originating from 48 LDCs that allows full cumulation of originating inputs from LDC or GSP beneficiary countries. Under the rules of origin, LDC imports must contain materials of LDC, GSP or Canadian origin that represent no less than 25% of the ex-factory price of the goods.

Australia also undertook commitments to offer duty-free and quota-free access to all exports originating from LDCs as of July 2003.

Depending on the scope and depth of the various RTAs and preferential arrangements, they provide improved access for beneficiary countries and accordingly influence production, trade and investment decisions. Each arrangement is associated with an economic rent that is not available to non-participants. The emergence of regional patterns of trade in textiles and clothing is partly attributable to these networks of preferential arrangements. Under NAFTA, Mexico became the second largest supplier to the United States; Turkey became the second largest supplier to the European Union under their customs union; and beneficiary countries under the Caribbean Basin Initiative increased their share of total US imports from 11.9% to 33.2% between 1990 and 2001 (OTEXA, 2001).

The scheduled elimination of bilateral quotas, examined below, will reduce the attractiveness of OPPs and, conversely, increase the relative attractiveness of other arrangements, such as RTAs and GSP regimes. The magnitude of economic benefits accruing under these arrangements varies greatly because of their differences in scope and the regimes of rules of origin that confer preferential access.

Reduced attractiveness of outward processing programmes

Outward processing transactions involve the temporary export of textiles or pre-cut textiles to low-wage countries for final assembly and re-import under preferential provisions, usually with customs tariffs imposed only on the value added of foreign processing and partial or total exemption from MFA quotas. Preferential access is often conditional upon the use of textiles made in the OPP-initiator country. Recently, the tendency has been to offer duty-free entry for OPP transactions (see Box 2.1).

For low-wage countries, the assembly of imported textiles into clothing is a simple form of industrial activity, and an OPP will often act as a booster for their export-oriented strategies by giving them immediate access to high–quality inputs and to foreign distribution networks. By being involved in an OPP, suppliers gain knowledge about working with international standards and meeting quality requirements and may benefit from transfers of technology (Senior Nello, 2002). Offshore centres involved in an OPP can accumulate knowledge more rapidly and learn how to manage the supply chain more efficiently.

For developed countries, outward processing transactions strengthen the competitive position of domestic suppliers by enabling them to transfer the labour–intensive sewing activities to low-wage countries. However, domestic clothing suppliers are constrained in their procurement when they are required to use domestic textiles. This may not be the most appropriate or the least-cost approach. It also provides domestic textile suppliers with a protected market, thereby blocking foreign competition from a significant share of the domestic textile market. In 1995, outward processing trade accounted for 15% of the EU's external trade in textiles and 70% of transactions originated from Central and Eastern European countries. In the United States, OPP imports increased from less than USD 6 billion in 1994 to 20 billion in 1999, and represented 24% of total clothing imports (WTO, Trade Policy Review of the United States, 2001).

Many countries have developed similar programmes. For example, Japan has a general provision to exclude the value of Japanese goods sent abroad for further processing from the customs value of the re-imported products.[15] This provision is applied on an MFN basis without country restrictions. In Australia, the assembly stage of clothing manufacturing is subcontracted in China, the Philippines, Vietnam and Indonesia on the basis of outward processing transactions.

Under normal circumstances, without the distorting influence of MFA quotas set on a bilateral basis, outward processing transactions make economic sense if the cost savings associated with low-wage assembly and tariff reductions exceed the inherent additional costs of production fragmentation, namely: two-way shipments, longer and larger inventory, and the added co–ordination needed to manage the fragmented supply chain. Moreover, outward processing transactions would occur in the offshore centres whose total logistical and transport costs are lowest. Comparing the total logistical and transport costs of offshore centres would indicate which centre is best positioned to engage in OPP transactions. Furthermore, comparison of the OPP–related costs with the logistical and transport costs for competing imports from an integrated supplier, *i.e.* one whose supply chain is not internationally fragmented, would indicate whether outward processing transactions are economically attractive relative to non-OPP transactions. Table 2.10 shows cost comparisons for several offshore suppliers involved in US outward processing transactions and compares the OPP-related costs with non-OPP transactions originating from China subject to the regular MFN duty rate.

Table 2.10. Cost competitiveness under outward processing programmes

Percentage of import values

Country of origin	Transit in days [1]			Time, freight and duty costs				Advantage
	Outbound from United States	Inbound for United States	Transit days	Time factor 0.5%/day	Freight cost	Customs duty	Total cost	Relative to China
CBTPA countries								
Dominican Republic								
Two-way shipments [2]	5	5	10	5.0%	3.4%	0.0%	8.4%	15.7%
MFN shipment		5	5	2.5%	1.7%	12.3%	16.5%	7.6%
Colombia								
Two-way shipments [2]	9	10	19	9.5%	3.4%	0.0%	12.9%	11.2%
MFN shipment		10	10	5.0%	1.7%	12.3%	19.0%	5.1%
AGOA recipients								
South Africa								
Two-way shipments [2]	34	25	59	29.5%	10.0%	0.0%	39.5%	-15.4%
MFN shipment		25	25	12.5%	5.0%	12.3%	29.8%	-5.7%
Kenya								
Two-way shipments [2]	62	61	123	61.5%	9.8%	0.0%	71.3%	-47.2%
One-way shipment [3]	n.a.	61	61	30.5%	4.9%	0.0%	35.4%	-11.3%
MFN shipment		61	61	30.5%	4.9%	12.3%	47.7%	-23.6%
Non-OPP recipient								
China								
MFN shipment		12	12	6.0%	5.8%	12.3%	24.1%	-

1. The outbound and inbound periods are average seaborne shipping and customs clearance periods calculated by ShipGuide.com. For Mexico and Canada, the transit periods are OECD estimates for rail shipments and customs clearance.

2. The average US customs duty on clothing imports was 12.3% MFN in 2002. Under various OPP-type programmes, the United States grants duty-free entry on imports of clothing articles assembled abroad from components produced in the United States.

3. Until the end of September 2004, duty-free entry is granted on clothing imports originating from AGOA's LDCs which are assembled from third country textiles. The reported transit period is underestimated since no time period is factored in for the importation of textiles from third countries.

Source: USAID (2003) for the transit data based on ShipGuide.com; OECD calculation of freight costs based on data from the US Department of Commerce, Bureau of the Census; and Hummels (2000) for the time factor per day.

The OPP–related cost is the sum of: *i)* the transit cost measured at the rate of 0.5% of import values for each transit day, which is the daily transit cost estimated by Hummels (2000); *ii)* the freight cost incurred over the relevant transport routes; and *iii)* the relevant customs duties.[16] The last column of Table 2.10 indicates the net cost advantage or disadvantage of the respective countries relative to competing imports from China subject to the regular MFN duty rate. It shows that OPP transactions provide a net cost advantage of 15.7% for the Dominican Republic and 11.2% for Colombia and a net cost disadvantage of –15.4% for South Africa and –47.2% for Kenya. For geographically remote suppliers, such as South Africa and Kenya, two-way outward processing transactions are the least competitive transactions of all trade possibilities.

With distance and time acting as trade barriers, outward processing transactions involving the final assembly of clothing articles from imported textiles in low-wage offshore centres remain economically attractive only if the margin of preferential duty exceeds the difference between the OPP-related cost and the logistical cost incurred for competitive suppliers. In other words, outward processing transactions are only attractive for offshore centres that are in close proximity to OPP-initiator countries. Proximity is a function of both geography and efficiency of transport infrastructure.

In the post–ATC period, the inherent vulnerability of production fragmentation in remote offshore centres will be exposed, and these centres will face the difficult task of competing with the most efficient and integrated suppliers. OPP recipients that have gradually developed their expertise are conscious of their vulnerability and are requesting improved trade opportunities to assist them in competing with the most competitive suppliers. Most requests concern the negotiation of comprehensive RTAs with developed countries and/or improved access through more liberal rules of origin under GSP programmes. These are discussed below.

Trade opportunities under regional trade arrangements

Turkey and Mexico have benefited from a customs union with the European Union and a free trade agreement under NAFTA, respectively. These arrangements have required deep integration commitments by Turkey and Mexico and given their suppliers improved opportunities to move along the supply chain by focusing on higher value-added production segments. For Mexico, NAFTA prompted a qualitative transformation with the emergence of new production facilities in higher value-added activities in textile finishing and in pre–assembly and post-assembly activities (see Box 2.2). Moreover, Mexico's close proximity to the United States with road and rail access (see Chapter 5) made it relatively easy and inexpensive to move manufacturing goods back and forth between the two countries. In spite of NAFTA, the competitiveness of Mexican textiles and clothing was recently eroded when improved trade opportunities were offered by the United States under the Trade Development Act and by competitive Asian suppliers. As a result, Mexican TCM imports fell back to pre-NAFTA levels in 2002, reflecting the prospective lesser competitiveness of Mexican suppliers (Table 2.11).

Turkey's customs union with the European Union entered into force in 1996, paving the way for improved opportunities for further integrating the Turkish textile and clothing markets into the larger European markets. Between 1995 and 1998, TCM imports in Turkey almost doubled compared to the previous four-year period, and even exceeded machinery imports by China in three consecutive years (1996-98) (Table 2.11). The enlarged competitive environment has allowed Turkey to build on its expertise and entrepreneurial skills. Between 1999 and 2001, Turkey's macroeconomic situation and high inflation rates have had a dampening effect on the overall economy and in particular in the textile and clothing industries, as reflected in lower levels of machinery imports.

Box 2.2. A new world blue jeans capital emerged in Mexico with NAFTA

Gereffi *et al.* (2002) have made an in-depth analysis of the North American apparel industry after NAFTA and argued that NAFTA has dramatically increased the export dynamism of the Mexican clothing industry and promoted the consolidation of clothing export production centres. To illustrate this transformation, they concentrated their analysis on the Torreón region, which has been called "The New Blue Jeans Capital of the World". Between 1993 and 1998, Torreón's blue jeans production jumped from 500 000 pairs a week to 4 million pairs.

Several factors contributed to this dynamism. Although not located in the immediate US border region, where most maquiladoras are found, the Torreón region is about a four-hour drive to the US border and has a tradition of cotton textile production that began in the late nineteenth century. During the period of import substitution that characterised the Mexican economy from the 1940s through the 1970s, the domestic jeans market was dominated by Torreón's suppliers, and several had developed their own brands, *e.g.* Jesus and Medalla Gacela. To survive through evolving economic circumstances, Torreón's suppliers underwent a significant transformation by moving from producers for the domestic market to maquiladora subcontractors for US manufacturers, and later to full-package exporters with considerable backward and forward linkages to the local economy. This transformation was influenced by four major factors: i) the devaluations of the peso; ii) the implementation of NAFTA; iii) the presence of new lead buyers, especially large retailers and brand marketers; and iv) the dynamism of the regional cluster of expertise.

The peso crises of 1982, 1985 and 1988 brought hyperinflation and forced jeans producers to redirect sales to export markets. Although the quality of their products was not up to international standards, they survived by assembling imported textiles as maquiladora subcontractors for US manufacturers (under 807/9802 production-sharing programmes or OPP). In the process, their skills in designing, cutting, finishing and marketing remained idle as their activities concentrated on sewing. However, the increased dependency on US manufacturers enabled Mexican suppliers to manufacture quality products and to deliver them in a timely fashion. Then, almost one year after the entry into force of NAFTA, the peso crisis of December 1994 resulted in a devalued peso and further enhanced the attractiveness of Mexican production.

Under NAFTA, the trade rules changed, which meant that all activities of the supply chain, not only sewing, could be performed in Mexico. Because of the significant production cost differential between the United States and Mexico, a large number of US clothing firms relocated to Mexico, resulting in the loss of 302 600 jobs in the United States and the creation of 294 800 jobs in Mexico between 1995 and 2000. New activities in the production of jeans destined for exports were quickly performed in Mexico, including cutting, finishing and even distribution.

The wider trade opportunities under NAFTA also attracted US retailers and brand marketers who require low-cost full-package suppliers to complement the activities that they themselves carry out, *i.e.* design, distribution and marketing. These new lead buyers introduced new aspects that have transformed the patterns of production. First, they required large volumes, which has encouraged Mexican firms to expand capacity. Second, Mexican suppliers were asked to produce higher value products. Finally, they did not want their names associated with alleged exploitative and unsafe working conditions. As a result, they have imposed their codes of conduct on full-package suppliers and prompted improved working conditions among Torreón suppliers.

Finally, prior to NAFTA, the Torreón region had developed diversified expertise, and regional suppliers had demonstrated flexibility in adapting during difficult periods. Hence, a cluster of diversified expertise was in place to manage the relationships between the Torreón cluster and lead buyers. While attracting the right kind of lead retailers, brand marketers and manufacturers to the Torreón regions was the prerequisite to move away from maquiladora production towards a full-package model, the dynamism of local entrepreneurship played a key role in reaping the opportunities that NAFTA created.

As employment by the Torreón apparel suppliers rose from 12 000 to 65 000 between 1993 and 1998, higher wages and labour shortages have encouraged some manufacturers to move their assembly operations to rural communities in the southern part of Mexico with few alternative sources of employment. While NAFTA has promoted the consolidation of regional clusters of textile and clothing expertise in Mexico, it also brought the maquiladora production model to rural and southern Mexico.

Table 2.11. Textile and clothing machinery imports, 1994–2002

USD millions

	Turkey	Mexico	China	World
2002	1 361	414	2 693	17 671
2001	594	508	2 051	17 948
2000	869	835	1 444	19 242
1999	498	782	958	17 399
1998	1 226	791	906	20 163
1997	1 823	778	1 645	22 888
1996	2 240	522	2 042	23 335
1995	1 503	349	2 146	24 240
1994	586	506	1 887	21 514

Source: UNCTAD.

The Turkish bilateral trade surplus in textiles and clothing with the European Union reached USD 13.6 billion in 2002, up from USD 9.1 billion in 1995, the year prior to the customs union. In terms of the composition of this trade surplus, Turkey maintains a small trade surplus in textile products and a huge surplus in clothing products. Despite the removal of quotas on several products by the European Union in January 2001, as scheduled under the ATC, the resulting intensification of competition from China and other suppliers did not seem to displace Turkish exports to the European Union. On the contrary, Turkish clothing exports increased by 17.4% between 2000 and 2002, and its trade surplus increased from USD 10.7 billion to USD 13.6 billion during the period. In 2002, Turkey machinery imports nearly doubled compared to 2001, reflecting improved macroeconomic conditions and most likely improved confidence about the prospects of Turkish textile and clothing industries.

Although comprehensive RTAs create production and trade opportunities, as attested in the cases of Mexico and Turkey, certain domestic factors have played an instrumental role in taking advantage of these opportunities. Among these factors are: the ability to attract the right kind of lead retailers, brand marketers and manufacturers; a pre–existing cluster of expertise; a vibrant entrepreneurship environment; and geographical proximity to minimise the transit time of shipments. A comprehensive RTA is necessary but on its own insufficient to promote trade flows and a qualitative transformation in production. As shown in Table 2.13, Israel has a long-established FTA with the United States but Israeli imports represented less than 1% of total US imports in 2003 or slightly more than imports originating from Egypt which has no bilateral FTA. In the post–ATC period, comprehensive RTAs can provide a useful policy framework to underpin the development of an integrated supply chain and to facilitate economic diversification strategies, but they do not necessarily imply competitiveness. Trade access is one important factor but others are equally if not more important. As discussed below, the regimes of rules of origin vary significantly among preferential arrangements and hence the magnitude of benefits accruing to the beneficiary countries.

Stringent rules of origin for textile and clothing products

Rules of origin (ROOs) are a necessary part of free trade agreements in order to preserve preferential treatment for member countries. They are a way to avoid the problem of trade deflection, *i.e.* of imports entering the region through the member country whose import tariff is the lowest. Specific rules of origin are often applied for sensitive products, such as textile and clothing, thus making it more difficult for suppliers to achieve the specified regional content. This creates an incentive for manufacturers to source inputs from regional suppliers and may act as a trade barrier. By limiting the sourcing of inputs from regional partners, ROOs may encourage vertical integration of the production chain that may not be competitive outside the regional market. A further problem with specific rules of origin is that the determination of regional content for yarns, textiles and final products requiring multiple components can be so burdensome and costly for suppliers that they prefer not to use the preferential arrangements. They also entail complex tasks for customs officials who are required to verify the relevant documentation. The cost of the formalities for determining the origin of products is estimated to amount to about 3% of the value of imports (UNCTAD, 2003). Within the OECD area, there are two major regimes of rules of origin applicable to textiles and clothing: the EU pan-European system and the yarn-forward rules of NAFTA.

The EU pan–European system of diagonal cumulation of origin applies virtually uniform rules of origin protocols for member countries to some 50 FTAs. Annex II to the Rules of Origin Protocol contains, for each tariff heading, a harmonised list of processing to be carried out on non-originating materials for the manufactured product to be granted originating status. The basic rules are those of the change in tariff heading at the 4-digit level of the Harmonised System (HS) of tariff classification, but for textiles and clothing these rules are replaced by specific technical requirements to qualify for preferential access. Brenton and Manchin (2002) note that 86% of textile product headings and 95% of clothing headings provide for specific technical requirements to confer regional origin. To confer origin for clothing products, the EU rules require not only that the sewing of textiles takes place in the qualifying region but also that the fabric itself is produced there.

Through the provisions of cumulation of origin implemented in 1997, distinct RTAs were merged into a pan-European network, including those between the EU and the European Free Trade Association (EFTA), the EU and Central and Eastern European countries, and the EFTA and Central and Eastern European countries. In contrast to the previously applied bilateral cumulation, diagonal cumulation implies that producers can use imports from any country in the zone to produce an originating product. For example, a producer in Switzerland is now able to use Polish inputs to produce goods for export to Germany. Prior to the pan–European network, the segmented regimes of rules of origin seriously impeded Swiss exports of textiles to the European Union as booming outward processing trade between the European Union and Central and Eastern Europe required EU–originating textiles (Nell, 1998). Despite the longstanding FTA between the European Union and Switzerland (initiated in 1972 and renewed in 1994) under the EU–EFTA FTA, outward processing transactions then only allowed temporary export of EU-originating goods and thus disqualified Swiss textiles. Diagonal cumulation has solved the problem. The Swiss example shows that diagonal cumulation expands the possibilities of outsourcing inputs and promotes the vertical integration of the production chains in a larger number of countries.

However, non-use of the pan-European provisions by many clothing suppliers in Poland, Hungary, Bulgaria and Romania led Brenton and Manchin (2002) to conclude that the costs of proving origin under the pan-European regime exceeded the tariff and administrative costs of export transactions under OPPs. Despite duty- and quota-free access for these countries since 1997, 35% of EU clothing imports from Poland, 40% from Hungary, 34% from Romania and 45% from Bulgaria were still carried out under dutiable OPPs in 2000.[17] In 1999, OPP clothing imports still accounted for more than a quarter of total EU clothing imports (Stengg, 2001).[18] These examples show that there are financial costs associated with the use of specific rules of origin to confer origin under FTAs so that exporters may elect not to take advantage of preferential access.

The European Union applies essentially the same technical requirements under its GSP regime for determining the origin of textile and clothing imports originating from GSP recipients. Under the EU GSP scheme, the cumulation of origin is permitted for four distinct regions of preference–receiving countries, namely: the Association of Southeast Asian Nations (ASEAN); the Central American Common Market; the Andean Group; and the South Asian Association for Regional Cooperation (SAARC). The trade data shown in Table 2.12 reveal two salient features of the EU GSP scheme. The first is that all textile and clothing imports are eligible for duty-free and quota-free imports, unlike the GSP schemes in the United States and Canada, although Canada expanded its GSP eligibility scheme to all textile and clothing imports from LDCs in 2003. The second is the low but increasing utilisation rate of actual imports receiving preferential rates to eligible imports, which reached 54% in 2002. The Japanese GSP scheme resembles the EU scheme with a 100% eligibility rate for textile and clothing imports and roughly similar utilisation rates (53%). Although there was no change in the rules of origin requirement under EBA, the increase of almost 10 percentage points in the utilisation rate in 2002 (54%) is explained by the rise in clothing exports originating from Bangladesh and Cambodia that met the requirement (UNCTAD, 2003). It is thought that Cambodian and Bangladeshi suppliers are adjusting their procurement and production mix in anticipation of the 2005 ATC deadline. By learning to work with EU inputs, they will be better positioned in 2005 to take advantage of the margin of preferences that the EU GSP scheme offers. This will help them to compete with the more efficient and integrated suppliers in China and India.

Table 2.12. LDC utilisation rates of GSP schemes in textiles and clothing, 2001

	Textile and clothing imports	Dutiable imports	Preferential imports	Eligibility rate	Utilisation rate
Canada	91.4	85.8	2.5	3.8%	2.9%
European Union	3 259	3 187	1 447	100%	45.4%
EU-EBA, 2002	3 648	3 424	1 847	100%	54.0%
Japan	54.5	47.5	25.2	100%	53.1%
United States	3 575	3 567	13.9	0.5%	0.4%

Note: USD million and percentage.

Source: UNCTAD (2003), various tables.

NAFTA's general rules of origin define the required transformation primarily in terms of prescribed changes in the tariff classification, except for certain goods, such as textiles and clothing, which are subject to additional content requirements. The basic rules of origin are known as yarn–forward, which requires that, to qualify for duty-free status, textiles and clothing must be produced from yarn made in a NAFTA country; one category of cotton fabric is subject to stricter rules, known as fibre-forward. These rules are supplemented by additional rules depending on the products, and derogations are provided for some non-NAFTA yarns and textiles, *i.e.* the special tariff preference-level provisions (TPLs).

Under various US preferential trade arrangements, specific content requirements must be met to confer origin and give preferential access. Under CBTPA, duty-free treatment is granted to clothing articles assembled from textiles made and cut in the United States and textiles manufactured from US yarns. This duty-free treatment is subject to annual volume caps and a few exceptions allow the use of third-country materials. Under AGOA, the general rule requires the use of US materials but the use of regional materials is permitted for hybrid apparel and sweaters knit to shape from cashmere. Moreover, AGOA's LDC beneficiaries are allowed to use third-country textiles under a special provision that expires at the end of September 2004. The United States also offers developing countries and LDCs GSP treatment for eligible goods, but the list of eligible textile and clothing products is narrow which explains that less than 1% of total textile and clothing from these countries qualifies for GSP preferential access (Tables 2.12 and 2.13).

Table 2.13. US textile and clothing imports under preferential trade arrangements, 2003

Regions and countries	Total imports (millions)	Preferential imports						Non-preferential imports	
		FTA duty-free	TPLs duty-free	9802	TDA 2000	GSP	% of total	MFN dutiable	% of total
Free trade agreements									
NAFTA	11 058.3	9 450.3	841.5	260.7			95.4%	506.6	4.6%
Mexico	7 940.8	7 259.3	67.0	260.7			95.5%	353.9	4.5%
Canada	3 118.3	2 191.0	774.5				95.1%	152.7	4.9%
United States-Israel	621.4	483.9					77.9%	137.5	22.1%
Preferential arrangements									
CBTPA	9 676.3			1 064.2	6 247.8		75.6%	2 364.3	24.4%
Honduras	2 507.3			172.8	1 951.9		84.7%	382.6	15.3%
Dominican Republic	2 128.4			221.8	1 720.2		91.2%	186.4	8.8%
Guatemala	1 773.4			195.1	597.0		44.7%	981.3	55.3%
El Salvador	1 758.0			293.5	1 105.6		79.6%	358.9	20.4%
Costa Rica	593.9			113.1	411.7		88.4%	69.1	11.6%
Nicaragua	483.9			8.8	149.2		32.7%	325.9	67.3%
ATPDEA	1 107.4			69.2	756.5		74.6%	281.7	25.4%
Colombia	538.9			67.6	261.5		61.1%	209.8	38.9%
Peru	516.1			0.0	452.6		87.7%	63.5	12.3%
AGOA	1 527.3			0.4	1 197.1		78.4%	329.8	21.6%
Mauritius	269.1			0.1	135.0		50.2%	134.0	49.8%
South Africa	253.4			0.0	126.6		50.0%	126.8	50.0%
Madagascar	196.3			0.0	186.3		94.9%	10.0	5.1%
Kenya	188.0			0.0	176.2		93.7%	11.8	6.3%
Swaziland	140.6			0.2	126.8		90.3%	13.6	9.7%
CBTPA+ATPDEA +AGOA	12 311.0			1 133.8	8 201.4		75.8%	2 975.8	24.2%
Generalised System of Preference									
Developing countries	34 072					249	0.7%	33 823	99.3%
Brazil	459					8	1.7%	451	98.3%
Egypt	558					0	0.0%	558	100.0%
India	3 556					91	2.6%	3 465	97.4%
Indonesia	2 334					10	0.4%	2 324	99.6%
Pakistan	2 201					19	0.9%	2 182	99.1%
Philippines	1 948					10	0.5%	1 938	99.5%
Thailand	2 062					41	2.0%	2 021	98.0%
Poland	66					0	0.0%	66	100.0%
Least developed countries	4 190					21	0.5%	4 169	99.5%
Bangladesh	1 868					18	1.0%	1 850	99.0%

Notes: TDA 2000 is the Trade Development Act of 2000; 9802 refers to imports under tariff heading for production-sharing programmes that provides for preferential duty rates for articles assembled abroad from components produced in the United States; TPLs refers to textile and clothing imports from Canada and Mexico that enter under special tariff preference-level provisions that permit the use of non–NAFTA materials. Total US imports of textiles and apparel reached USD 77.4 billion in 2003.

Source: US Department of Commerce, Bureau of the Census. For GSP data, US ITC, Trade Dataweb.

Recipient countries under CBTPA, AGOA and ATPDEA are more or less restricted in their procurement to exclusive use of US-made yarns and textiles in the context of production-sharing programmes in which the sewing activity is performed abroad, *i.e.* outward processing transactions. By contrast, under NAFTA, Mexican and Canadian suppliers have broader procurement choices in that they can use NAFTA–origin yarns and textiles to qualify for duty-free access and thus can perform basically all activities in the supply chain domestically. Thus, the textile and clothing trade opportunities under NAFTA are much broader than those offered under OPP-related preferential arrangements. Therefore, the extension of NAFTA to any OPP recipient countries would provide them with opportunities to move up the value-added chain and to diversify their manufacturing activities.

UNCTAD (2003) and Brenton and Manchin (2002) have argued that the main explanation for the low utilisation rate was the inability of preference-receiving countries to fully exploit the available preferences when these are subject to strict origin requirements and related administrative requirements. The review of the utilisation rate of actual imports receiving preferential rates to eligible imports under US preferential arrangements suggests, however, that other factors contribute to the difficulties that traders encounter for taking advantage of the preferential access. Table 2.13 shows considerable variations in the degree to which beneficiary countries of various US arrangements actually benefit from them.

Canadian and Mexican suppliers who secured duty-free entry for more than 95% of their exports have the highest utilisation rates. Almost a quarter of Canadian exports and 8.4% of Mexican exports qualified for duty-free entry under special tariff preference–level provisions which permit the use of non-NAFTA materials under certain conditions. For Mexico, a small and declining share of exports (3.3%) was still carried out under outward processing transactions in 2003.[19] The high utilisation rate under NAFTA reflects to some extent the built-in flexibility in the rules of origin requirements that permit the use of NATFA-origin materials and the conditional use of non–NAFTA materials. Other contributing factors include: the geographical proximity of the US market which enables short turnaround; the increasing market integration of the three economies with an increasingly integrated transport infrastructure and customs border partnerships; and a high rate of cross-ownership of firms.

By contrast, the United States–Israel FTA has a lower utilisation rate (77.9%) in spite of quite liberal rules of origin. These are based on substantial transformation provisions with 35% value-added content requirements, which are considered easier to meet than NAFTA yarn-forward provisions. However, the distance from Israel to the United States and the smaller clusters of Israeli textile and clothing expertise may lend themselves to fewer inter-firm relationships between the two countries and fewer trade transactions that satisfy the content requirements. As noted earlier, US imports from Egypt were slightly below imports from Israel in 2003, but there is no comprehensive FTA between Egypt and the United States. The attractiveness of Egypt stems in part from the quality of its cotton fibres and its related production expertise.

Under AGOA, three countries, *i.e.* Madagascar, Kenya and Swaziland, achieved high utilisation rates exceeding 90% in 2003, as they took advantage of the special LDC provision that permits use of third-country textiles. By contrast, the other AGOA countries, *i.e.* South Africa and Mauritius, have considerably lower utilisation rates (50%). Differences in utilisation rates are indicative of what is likely to happen to AGOA's LDCs as of October 2004 when they are no longer able to use this special provision. Nevertheless, as of January 2005, there will be no more bilateral quotas that would justify OPP transactions that are uneconomical owing to long transit periods (see Table 2.10). In the post-ATC period, the assembly of imported textiles in remote offshore centres will be a very vulnerable business model that will find it difficult to compete with integrated and competitive suppliers.

Under the CBTPA, utilisation rates by participating countries vary significantly, with a high rate for the Dominican Republic (91.2%) and low rates for Guatemala (44.7%) and Nicaragua (32.7%). Geographical proximity and efficient transport infrastructure make it easier for Dominican Republic suppliers to engage in two–way outward processing transactions and hence to achieve content requirements that qualify for preferential access. For Nicaragua and Guatemala, an ownership structure with predominantly Asian investors largely explains their low utilisation rates. Essentially, Asian investors selected these countries as offshore centres that rely on imported textiles originating primarily from Asia to assemble clothing articles that are destined for the US market. These investment projects were not exclusively intended to qualify under CBTPA and large shares of output are subject to MFN duties when entering the United States. In the post–ATC period, the transport infrastructure of the CBTPA beneficiaries will play a key role in maintaining the attractiveness of their OPP business models.

Canada significantly expanded product eligibility under its GSP system in favour of LDCs in 2003 and, in particular, granted duty-free entry to all textile and clothing imports that meet the 25% content requirement originating from any LDCs, GSP beneficiaries or Canada, thus basically excluding textiles from developed countries. The new rules of origin allow for full cumulation of originating inputs among LDC and GSP beneficiary countries. The measure provided a real boost to LDC clothing exports in 2003, which jumped from USD 110 million to USD 298 million, and captured 42.5% of the incremental total clothing imports for that year.[20] Two countries, Bangladesh and Cambodia, were the main beneficiaries. Together, they expanded their exports by USD 171 million (or 38.7% of total incremental clothing imports). The other main LDC beneficiaries were, in declining order: Lesotho, Haiti, Maldives, Laos, Nepal, Madagascar, Malawi, Sierra Leone and Swaziland. Altogether, the LDCs' share of total Canadian clothing imports more than doubled in 2003 from 3.1% to 7.5%. While the new rules of origin have undoubtedly benefited LDCs, China nevertheless captured 38.4% of incremental total imports in 2003, which is slightly less than the combined benefits that accrued to LDCs.

The strong responsiveness of LDC exports to Canadian trade opportunities is partly attributable to the inherent dynamism of the global textile and clothing industries in which production schedules can be quickly adapted to respond to new demand. It also partly reflects the export-constraining effect of MFA quotas, with growth of imports of non–constrained products and constrained products from countries with spare or unfilled quotas, mainly LDCs. There is also a size effect involved, in the sense that the Canadian market is relatively small compared to the US and EU markets, so that production runs for products destined for other markets can be easily increased and the incremental production exported to Canada. In the post-ATC period, LDCs will encounter stiffer competition from the most competitive suppliers and, as a result, they may be unable to benefit to the same extent as in 2003 when quotas still constrained the most competitive suppliers.

In the domestic market, the Canadian initiative has raised some controversy among national clothing manufacturers who claimed unfair competition from duty-free imports;

they had to pay import duties on some of their input requirements (the problem of inverted escalation of tariffs or de-escalation). Moreover, domestic manufacturers claimed that the new rules of origin are too loose because the largest developing countries (China and India) reaped huge benefits by shipping textiles to LDCs which subsequently assembled clothing products and exported them duty-free to Canada. In response to these concerns and to a number of closures of domestic plants, Canada announced a series of tariff cuts in early 2004 to address the problems caused by inverted tariff protection and simultaneously launched a programme designed to improve production efficiency among Canadian suppliers.

The above overview of rules of origin applied under various preferential trade arrangements shows considerable disparities among the various regimes and the utilisation rates of the various arrangements. While rules of origin are necessary to ensure that preferential trade actually benefits the targeted countries, overly restrictive or cumbersome rules may not provide meaningful access and result in an under-utilisation of preferential access schemes. By contrast, liberal rules of origin may not benefit the targeted group of countries as much as intended, and the associated preferential access can invert the structure of tariffs with negative consequences for national manufacturers. Moreover, liberal rules of origin do not necessarily confer competitiveness. Inherent competitive factors explain which beneficiaries of preferential arrangements are likely to gain the most. The distance between remote trading partners, which entails long transit periods for shipments, and the size of the cluster of expertise in beneficiary countries seem to matter. Finally, the identity of foreign investors also appears to influence the patterns of input procurement.

With the imminent elimination of the ATC, LDCs are increasingly vocal about their post-ATC vulnerability and are formulating demands to access developed country markets on an improved preferential basis to help them compete more effectively with the prime contenders, *i.e.* China and India. Recognising that there is at present virtually no production of high-quality textiles in LDCs, any preferential access arrangements granted to LDCs must take into account that they have to use competitive textiles originating from third countries to compete on export markets. As a result, it seems inevitable that in providing preferential access to LDCs, there will be some collateral benefits for suppliers of high-quality textiles. In the post-ATC period, rules of origin provisions will be at the forefront of the trade policy agenda as demands from vulnerable offshore centres will become more insistent.

Trade-distorting measures

There are concerns about the trade-distorting effect of numerous measures imposed at the borders and anti-competitive practices. Considerable concern is being voiced about counterfeiting and piracy in fashion products which is estimated to deprive owners and legitimate licensed holders of significant business opportunities and lost revenues. Another area of concern relates to the impact of production and export assistance to cotton production in several countries. Under the Uruguay Round Agreement on Agriculture, WTO members have agreed to discipline production assistance in agricultural products and have undertaken reduction commitments in respect of their total aggregate measure of support (AMS). They have also undertaken to notify to the WTO detailed information on production assistance entering the calculation of their total AMS. On the basis of the latest WTO notifications, the following support levels were notified for cotton production. For 1999 (the most recent year for which AMS data are available), the cotton-specific AMS payments amounted to USD 2 353 million in the United States,

EUR 623.7 million in the European Union and USD 55.4 million in Brazil.[21] India, Pakistan and Turkey, the third, fourth and fifth largest world producers of cotton, respectively, reported no cotton-specific AMS in 1999. The alleged trade-distorting impact of the US subsidies was the subject of a formal complaint by Brazil to the WTO in September 2002, and the trade dispute was dealt with under the dispute settlement procedure. Brazil argued that the US subsidies are not in conformity with the peace clause negotiated under the Uruguay Round Agreement on Agriculture that protects countries' commodity-specific domestic and export subsidies. This clause provides that countries' commodity-specific and domestic export subsidies cannot be challenged as long as they do not exceed their 1992 levels. The WTO dispute settlement report was released in September 2004.

Other non-tariff measures concern the imposition of specific levies, costly labelling and certification requirements, export restrictions on raw materials and semi–finished products, and export licences.[22] Within the context of the DDA, WTO members have the opportunity to level the playing field by dealing with these trade-distorting measures.

Conclusion

Trade policy measures have had a major impact on production decisions relating to textiles and clothing and on trade flows. MFA restrictions have contributed to the international fragmentation of the supply chain by accelerating the diversification of supply. This process has worked to the disadvantage of the more efficient and quota-constrained suppliers, many of which subcontracted clothing assembly to low-cost third countries. The arrangement also benefited less competitive suppliers. The scheduled elimination of quantitative restrictions is challenging the global sourcing channels established during the MFA period and represents a systemic change in trade policies. Stakeholders are now reassessing their global sourcing channels not only on the basis of price competitiveness but increasingly on that of the dynamics of inter-firm networks able to react quickly and meet the stringent specifications of large retail groups in terms of production quality and social requirements.

In the post-ATC period, the textile industry in OECD countries is likely to face intensified competition from the non–OECD economies that are investing in up-to-date equipment and upgrading quality and capacity to meet higher production standards. The textile industry will continue to be challenged by product proliferation, particularly for industrial applications, and by the need to respond much faster to rapidly changing market conditions without compromising quality. The way in which the industry innovates and adopts new technology will play a crucial role in defining the relative competitiveness of textile firms. Moreover, the continuing emphasis on the development of new materials in the non-clothing textile applications will likely increase the share of man-made fibres in total fibre demand.

With the imminent end to quantitative restrictions, several low-cost countries that had excelled as offshore assembly centres because of their quota allocations must now address the inherent vulnerability of production fragmentation. Time factors also act as important trade barriers for intermediary inputs involved in an internationally fragmented production process. There are tradeoffs between low-wage cost and time factors, since temporal proximity to large consumer markets provides a competitive edge in the highly competitive, time–sensitive and fashion-oriented clothing market. Moreover, the emergence of more competitive and integrated suppliers in China exerts considerable pressure on vulnerable offshore centres to adjust domestic capacity towards more advanced processes and to diversify their economic activities.

To move along the supply chain beyond assembly of imported inputs to more advanced activities, vulnerable offshore centres need to shift their cluster of expertise from manufacturing to services–related functions, such as design, material sourcing, quality control and logistics. To pursue these avenues, national suppliers need to establish joint structures through which they can share market knowledge and offer more integrated solutions to prospective buyers.

Retail distribution is increasingly dominated by large and lean retail organisations in the main consuming countries, which are moving towards greater product specialisation, brand-name products and market segmentation. The large retail groups and brand marketers are expanding their successful distribution models worldwide. With their sheer market size, large retail groups collect market information about the latest trends in styles and tastes and their integration of this information gives them considerable leverage in dealing with suppliers. Nevertheless, offshore suppliers can benefit from working in close co-operation with large retail groups and brand marketers and learn to: *i)* manufacture quality products; *ii)* apply the buyer's codes of conduct; and *iii)* deliver products in a timely fashion. The development of business relationships between national clusters of expertise and the large retail groups and brand marketers plays an instrumental role in facilitating the qualitative transformation of the supply chain with backward and forward linkages for the local economy.

For suppliers with experience in the services-related functions of the supply chain, the remaining stages in the value chain are the development of their brand-name products, the establishment of their retail distribution networks and their promotion as design and fashion hubs. This requires the development of services-related expertise in designing, marketing, retailing, financing and gathering of market intelligence in foreign markets. This will require foreign investment flows originating from emerging economies to sustain this strategic move.

In the post–ATC period, when quota considerations will no longer influence production and trade decisions, remote offshore centres will be faced with the difficult task of competing on the basis of quality, reliability and cost efficiency. With distance and time acting as trade barriers, preferential programmes designed to encourage the final assembly of clothing articles from imported textiles in low-wage offshore centres will only remain attractive if the margin of preferential duty exceeds inefficiency costs. In these new circumstances, outward processing programmes will provide cost advantages only to these offshore assembly centres that are nearest to the OPP-initiator countries. For geographically remote centres and nearby offshore centres with poor transport infrastructure, outward processing transactions will not offer cost advantages over non– OPP transactions originating from competing suppliers. Offshore assembly centres are conscious of their vulnerability and are seeking improved market access to developed countries' markets to help them to compete with the efficient and integrated suppliers.

Under NAFTA, Mexico has been able to promote the consolidation of its regional clusters of textile and clothing expertise and to move along the supply chain from the simple assembly of imported components and create backward and forward linkages to the local economy. Turkey has also built on its expertise and entrepreneurial skills to increase its bilateral trade surplus in textiles and clothing with the European Union in the context of their customs union. While the experience of Mexico and Turkey may serve as role models for offshore centres that aspire to maintain an export–led strategy in future, the analysis underscores the importance of a number of contributing factors that can maximise the trade opportunities created by regional trade arrangements. They include: the ability to attract the right kind of lead retailers, brand marketers and manufacturers; the pre-existence of a cluster of relevant expertise; a vibrant entrepreneurship environment; and geographical proximity so as to minimise transit time.

In the post–ATC period, rules of origin provisions that confer preferential access under FTAs and GSP programmes are likely to be at the forefront of the trade policy agenda, as vulnerable offshore centres make more insistent demands for improved access to developed countries' markets to help them to compete more effectively with the prime contenders, *i.e.* China and India. While rules of origin are necessary to ensure that preferential trade actually benefits the targeted countries, overly cumbersome rules lead to under-utilisation of preferential access schemes; conversely, liberal rules of origin do not benefit the targeted countries as much as intended and can invert the structure of tariffs, with negative consequences for the domestic processing industry. In respect of requests by LDCs, developed countries may need to consider that LDCs currently have virtually no domestic sources of high-quality textiles and, to compete on export markets, they need the most competitive textiles. It therefore seems inevitable that in providing preferential access to LDCs, some collateral benefits will accrue to the suppliers of high-quality textiles. It also means that any improvement in the rules of origin under preferential trade arrangements will increase the competitive pressure on the domestic textile industry of developed countries.

The quota-free period ahead presents all textile and clothing suppliers with the challenge to adapt their production mix to meet ever–changing consumer requirements in terms of design, quality and prices while setting up efficient and competitive production processes. The brunt of the adjustment pressures falls on the suppliers themselves, which are better placed to evaluate how to organise production methods, procure high-quality inputs and shift the production mix on the basis of evolving market signals. For governments, the structural adjustment challenges rest on devising a coherent textile and clothing policy framework that strengthens the capacity of domestic producers to deal with rapid change and growing competition and to capture more effectively the trade opportunities created by improved market access. This process involves: dismantling trade-distorting measures; improving the regulatory environment and infrastructure in essential business services; supporting the emergence of qualified pools of expertise and the adaptability of the workforce; enhancing the business environment for SMEs; negotiating improved market access for textile and clothing products; and eliminating the obstacles to the establishment of retail distribution systems in developing countries.

The deadline for quota elimination coincides with a key stage of negotiations under the Doha Development Agenda that may lead to changes in existing WTO rules or introduce new WTO disciplines, which will also have an impact on international trade in the textiles and clothing. During these negotiations, WTO members have an opportunity to deal with remaining trade protection and trade-distorting measures with a view to establishing a framework of multilateral disciplines that provides for both improved competitive conditions and enhanced market access opportunities across the globe.

Annex 2.A1. Tables

Annex Table 2.A1.1. Selected characteristics of textile branches, selected years and countries

	Latest year	Value added per employee	Wages and salaries per employee	Costs of input material and utilities	Costs of labour	Operating surplus
		Current USD (thousands)		Percent of output		
OECD countries (average)		**36.7**	**16.6**	**68.1%**	**17.2%**	**20.9%**
Australia	1997	36.1	21.8	66.8%	20.1%	13.1%
Belgium	1999	49.9	23.1	70.5%	13.6%	15.8%
Canada	1999	42.2	18.7	54.6%	20.2%	25.2%
Czech Republic	1998	6.1	3.1	69.9%	15.4%	14.7%
Finland	1999	48.2	23.2	57.0%	20.7%	22.3%
France	1999	39.0	21.9	71.1%	16.2%	12.7%
Germany	1999	42.4	26.8	65.7%	21.7%	12.6%
Italy	1998	45.0	18.0	70.9%	11.7%	17.4%
Japan	2000	57.9	15.7	57.0%	11.7%	31.3%
Korea	1999	42.7	11.0	55.6%	11.4%	32.9%
Norway	1999	40.4	25.7	61.3%	24.6%	14.1%
Mexico	1999	13.5	4.4	60.0%	13.0%	27.0%
Portugal	1998	15.1	6.8	69.7%	13.7%	16.7%
Slovak Republic	1998	4.2	2.4	68.5%	18.0%	13.5%
Spain	2000	25.3	13.3	68.7%	16.4%	14.9%
Turkey	1997	19.1	5.4	65.5%	9.7%	24.8%
United States	1999	60.0	24.4	57.1%	17.4%	25.4%
Non–OECD countries (average)		**15.0**	**5.6**	**72.6%**	**14.2%**	**25.0%**
Bangladesh	1997	1.1	0.5	66.7%	15.0%	18.3%
Cameroon	1999	35.4	5.1	35.6%	9.3%	55.1%
Chile	1998	19.4	7.5	70.5%	11.4%	18.1%
Colombia	2000	16.4	3.7	54.0%	10.4%	35.6%
Egypt	1998	3.4	1.7	67.5%	16.0%	16.5%
El Salvador	1998	8.9	2.9	56.7%	13.9%	29.4%
Hong Kong, China	2000	33.1	18.0	72.0%	15.3%	12.8%
India	1999	2.8	1.0	81.2%	6.9%	11.9%
Indonesia	1999	4.2	0.7	68.7%	4.9%	26.4%
Jordan	1997	7.8	2.5	68.5%	10.0%	21.6%
Malaysia	1999	14.0	4.0	67.6%	9.2%	23.2%
Mauritius	1998	9.0	2.9	63.8%	11.7%	24.5%
Morocco	1998	6.4	3.0	65.5%	16.3%	18.2%
Russian Federation	1998	1.1	0.7	64.5%	24.2%	11.3%
Singapore	2000	34.2	16.2	68.3%	15.0%	16.7%
Sri Lanka	1999	2.9	0.6	54.5%	10.3%	35.2%
Tunisia	2000	21.1	8.2	65.5%	13.4%	21.0%
Uruguay	1999	17.6	9.4	66.5%	17.9%	15.6%
Vietnam	2000	1.6	0.7	76.6%	10.6%	12.8%

Source: International Yearbook of Industrial Statistics 2003, UN Industrial Development Organisation.

Annex Table 2.A1.2. Selected characteristics of clothing branches, selected years and countries

	Latest year	Value added per employee	Wages and salaries per employee	Costs of input material and utilities	Costs of labour	Operating surplus
		Current USD (thousands)		Percent of output		
OECD countries		**27.71**	**13.67**	**66.7%**	**19.4%**	**20.6%**
Belgium	1999	40.9	22.4	77.3%	12.4%	10.3%
Canada	1999	30.5	15.1	53.1%	23.1%	23.8%
Czech Republic	1998	4.5	2.6	59.7%	23.7%	16.7%
Finland	1999	32.1	19.5	65.9%	20.7%	13.4%
France	1999	33.6	20.2	71.0%	17.4%	11.6%
Germany	1999	39.6	25.3	73.5%	16.9%	9.5%
Italy	1998	32.4	14.0	71.4%	12.4%	16.2%
Japan	2000	36.9	10.8	47.1%	15.5%	37.4%
Korea	1999	23.8	9.1	50.8%	18.8%	30.4%
Norway	1999	30.5	22.4	61.1%	28.6%	10.3%
Mexico	1999	9.3	3.2	60.3%	13.8%	26.0%
Portugal	1998	10.0	5.4	67.4%	17.7%	14.9%
Slovak Republic	1998	3.9	2.3	55.6%	25.7%	18.7%
Spain	2000	17.3	9.8	68.1%	18.2%	13.7%
Turkey	1997	15.6	4.1	67.3%	8.6%	24.2%
United States	1999	54.8	18.9	51.0%	16.9%	32.1%
Non–OECD countries		**8.5**	**3.8**	**64.5%**	**16.7%**	**24.7%**
Bangladesh	1997	0.9	0.4	75.4%	9.7%	15.0%
Cameroon	1999	2.6	0.9	50.7%	17.0%	32.3%
Chile	1997	25.2	7.9	51.3%	15.3%	33.4%
Colombia	1999	8.2	2.4	53.4%	13.5%	33.0%
Egypt	1998	4.8	1.1	56.4%	9.9%	33.7%
El Salvador	1998	5.1	2.5	30.7%	33.5%	35.7%
Hong Kong, China	1999	27.6	14.8	71.1%	15.5%	13.4%
India	1999	2.9	0.7	75.7%	6.4%	17.9%
Indonesia	1999	2.5	0.6	63.4%	8.5%	28.1%
Jordan	1997	4.7	1.8	58.4%	16.0%	25.6%
Malaysia	1999	6.4	3.1	66.1%	16.5%	17.4%
Mauritius	1997	5.0	2.6	64.2%	19.0%	16.8%
Morocco	1998	4.0	2.5	55.9%	27.9%	16.2%
Singapore	2000	17.6	11.0	75.6%	15.3%	9.1%
Sri Lanka	1999	2.3	0.7	54.1%	14.2%	31.8%
Tunisia	2000	6.6	3.3	71.4%	14.1%	14.6%
Uruguay	1997	8.0	3.4	62.2%	15.8%	22.0%
Vietnam	2000	1.8	0.7	60.2%	16.5%	23.2%

Source: International Yearbook of Industrial Statistics 2003, UN Industrial Development Organisation.

Annex Table 2.A1.3. Leading exporters and importers of textiles, 1980-2002

Percentage share in world exports and values in USD billions

	1990	2001	2002	2002/1990	% change 2002	Value 2002
World value	104.33	146.98	152.15	Change in world share	3.5%	**USD billions**
Percent of world merchandise exports	3.1%	2.5%	2.4%			
Exporters						
EU15	48.7%	35.1%	34.2%	-14.5%	0.9%	52.05
Extra-EU	*14.5%*	*15.1%*	*15.2%*	*0.7%*	*4.3%*	*23.12*
China	6.9%	11.4%	13.5%	6.6%	22.2%	20.56
Hong Kong, China	2.1%	0.7%	0.6%	-1.5%	-7.0%	0.98
Re-exports					*2.1%*	*11.40*
United States	4.8%	7.1%	7.0%	2.2%	2.0%	10.70
Korea	5.8%	7.4%	7.0%	1.2%	-3.2%	10.59
Chinese Taipei	5.9%	6.7%	6.3%	0.4%	-3.8%	9.53
Japan	5.6%	4.2%	4.0%	-1.6%	-2.7%	6.03
India	2.1%	3.9%	3.7%	1.6%	-10.4%	5.38
Pakistan	2.6%	3.1%	3.1%	0.5%	5.9%	4.79
Turkey	1.4%	2.7%	2.8%	1.4%	7.6%	4.24
Indonesia	1.2%	2.2%	1.9%	0.7%	-9.6%	2.90
Mexico	0.7%	1.4%	1.5%	0.8%	5.8%	2.21
Canada	0.7%	1.5%	1.4%	0.7%	0.9%	2.18
Thailand	0.9%	1.3%	1.3%	0.4%	2.2%	1.93
Switzerland	2.5%	1.0%	0.9%	-1.6%	-1.6%	1.42
Importers						
EU15	46.7%	31.7%	30.4%	-16.3%	-0.8%	46.21
Extra-EU	*13.2%*	*11.7%*	*11.3%*	*-1.9%*	*0.5%*	*17.27*
United States	6.2%	10.5%	10.6%	4.4%	10.2%	17.00
China	4.9%	8.6%	8.1%	3.2%	3.9%	13.06
Hong Kong, China					-1.3%	12.02
Retained imports	*3.8%*	*0.7%*	*0.4%*	*-3.4%*	*-38.7%*	*0.62*
Mexico	0.9%	4.1%	4.0%	3.1%	5.7%	6.37
Japan	3.8%	3.2%	2.8%	-1.0%	-4.6%	4.54
Canada	2.2%	2.6%	2.4%	0.2%	-0.1%	3.81
Korea	1.8%	2.1%	2.0%	0.2%	3.3%	3.17
Turkey	0.5%	1.3%	1.8%	1.3%	47.8%	2.84
Poland	0.2%	1.8%	1.7%	1.5%	4.4%	2.73
Romania	0.1%	1.4%	1.5%	1.4%	17.8%	2.37
United Arab Emirates	0.9%	1.2%	1.2%	-	-7.1%	1.69
Thailand	0.8%	1.0%	0.9%	0.1%	-2.5%	1.50
Russian Federation	-	1.0%	1.0%	-	3.3%	1.48
Australia	1.3%	0.9%	0.9%	-0.4%	13.1%	1.47
Morocco	0.3%	1.0%	0.9%	0.6%	-0.6%	1.39
Sri Lanka	0.4%	0.9%	0.9%	0.5%	0.1%	1.36
Bangladesh	0.4%	1.0%	0.8%	0.4%	-22.2%	1.16

Notes: Data for India and United Arab Emirates refer to 2001 instead of 2002 and 2000 instead of 2001.

Total exports exclude Hong Kong (China) re-exports. Data for the Russian Federation and United Arab Emirates include estimates. Imports for Australia and Canada are valued on an fob basis. Data for China, Mexico and Morocco include shipments through processing zones.

Source: WTO, *International Trade Statistics 2003*.

Annex Table 2.A1.4. Leading exporters and importers of clothing, 1980–2002

Percentage share in world exports and values in USD billions

	1990	2001	2002	2002/1990	% change 2002	Value 2002 USD billions
World value	108.13	193.69	200.85	Change in world share	3.7%	
Percent of world merchandise exports	3.2%	3.3%	3.2%			
Exporters						
EU15	37.7%	24.9%	25.1%	-12.6%	4.4%	50.45
Extra-EU	*10.5%*	*8.1%*	*8.3%*	*-2.2%*	*5.6%*	*16.59*
China	8.9%	18.9%	20.6%	11.6%	12.7%	41.30
Hong Kong, China	8.6%	4.8%	4.1%	-4.4%	-10.3%	8.31
Re-exports						*14.04*
Turkey	3.1%	3.4%	4.0%	0.9%	21.0%	8.06
Mexico	0.5%	4.1%	3.9%	3.3%	-3.2%	7.75
United States	2.4%	3.6%	3.0%	0.6%	-14.0%	6.03
India	2.3%	2.8%	2.8%	0.5%	-11.2%	5.48
Bangladesh	0.6%	2.2%	2.1%	1.5%	-3.0%	4.13
Indonesia	1.5%	2.3%	2.0%	0.4%	-12.9%	3.95
Korea	7.3%	2.2%	1.8%	-5.4%	-14.2%	3.69
Thailand	2.6%	1.8%	1.7%	-0.9%	-5.8%	3.37
Romania	0.3%	1.4%	1.6%	1.3%	16.9%	3.25
Dominican Republic	0.7%	1.5%	1.4%	0.7%	-5.8%	2.71
Tunisia	1.0%	1.3%	1.3%	0.3%	3.3%	2.69
Philippines	1.6%	1.2%	1.3%	-0.3%	9.5%	2.61
Chinese Taipei	3.7%	1.3%	1.1%	-2.6%	-11.6%	2.20
Importers						
EU15	52.6%	41.8%	42.3%	-10.3%	5.0%	84.88
Extra-EU	*26.2%*	*24.9%*	*25.4%*	*-0.8%*	*5.7%*	*51.02*
United States	24.0%	34.3%	31.7%	7.7%	0.5%	66.73
Japan	7.8%	9.9%	8.4%	0.6%	-8.3%	17.60
Hong Kong, China						15.64
Retained imports	*0.7%*	*1.0%*	*0.8%*	*0.1%*	*-16.3%*	*1.60*
Mexico	0.5%	2.0%	1.9%	1.4%	5.7%	4.06
Canada	2.1%	2.0%	1.9%	-0.2%	2.1%	4.01
Russian Federation	-	1.6%	1.8%		27.4%	3.86
Switzerland	3.1%	1.7%	1.6%	-1.4%	6.8%	3.45
Korea	0.1%	0.8%	1.0%	0.9%	33.0%	2.17
Australia	0.6%	0.8%	0.9%	0.2%	11.0%	1.82
Singapore	*0.3%*	*0.2%*	*0.3%*	*0.0%*	17.7%	*0.54*
United Arab Emirates	0.5%	0.7%	0.8%	0.3%	9.0%	1.55
Norway	1.1%	0.6%	0.6%	-0.4%	10.3%	1.36
China	0.0%	0.7%	0.6%	0.6%	6.4%	1.36
Saudi Arabia	0.7%	0.4%	0.4%	-0.3%	5.9%	0.86
Chinese Taipei	0.3%	0.5%	0.4%	0.1%	-10.5%	0.83

Notes: Share in economy's total merchandise exports refers to latest year available.

For Egypt: the United States provides duty-free treatment for textiles and clothing made in qualifying industrial zones since March 1998. CBERA: Caribbean Basin Economic and Recovery Act; AGOA: African Growth Opportunity Act. CU96: Customs Union, 1996; EBA01: Everything but Arms, March 2001. CO-OP: Co-operation Agreement to be replaced by Euro-Mediterranean Agreements.

Data for Cambodia and the Dominican Republic include estimates. Data for China, Costa Rica, Dominican Republic, El Salvador, Malaysia, Mexico, Morocco and Philippines include exports from processing zones.

Source: WTO, *International Trade Statistics 2002 and 2003*.

Annex Table 2.A1.5. Clothing exports in selected economies, 1980–2002

	Value USD millions				Share in economy's total merchandise exports (%)		Free trade agreements (FTA)		Outward processing programmes (OPP)		
	1990	1995	2001	2002	1990	2002	United States	EU	United States	EU	Australia
Largest Increase in export shares 1990-2002											
Jordan	11	29	296	...	1.0%	12.9%	2001	CO-OP			
Honduras	64	299	505	475	7.7%	37.4%			CBERA		
Mexico	587	2 731	8 011	7 751	1.4%	4.8%	1994	FTA00			
Romania	363	1 360	2 780	3 251	7.3%	23.4%		FTA94	OPP 99	OPP	
Canada	328	1 016	1 943	1 988	0.3%	0.8%	1989				
Costa Rica	54	50	376	397	3.7%	7.6%			CBERA		
El Salvador	184	700	1 725	1 841	31.6%	61.5%			CBERA		
Morocco	722	797	2 342	2 413	16.9%	30.4%		CO-OP		OPP	
Bangladesh	643	1 969	4 261	4 131	38.5%	67.8%		EBA01			
Cambodia	...	...	1 125	...	...	81.7%		EBA01			
Bulgaria	...	236	880	1 066	...	18.6%		FTA94		OPP	
Sri Lanka	638	1 758	2 441	2 326	33.4%	49.5%					
Dominican Republic	782	1 721	2 712	...	36.0%	50.9%			CBERA		
Pakistan	1 014	1 611	2 136	2 228	18.1%	22.5%			OPP 02		
Tunisia	1 126	2 322	2 601	2 688	31.9%	39.5%		CO-OP		OPP	
Indonesia	1 646	3 376	4 531	3 945	6.4%	6.9%					OPP
Macau, China	1 111	1 377	1 663	1 648	65.3%	70.0%					
Mauritius	619	808	860	949	51.9%	54.1%		EBA01	AGOA		
Declining export shares 1990-2002											
Philippines	1 733	2 420	2 384	2 611	21.4%	7.2%					OPP
China	9 669	24 049	36 650	41 302	15.6%	12.7%					OPP
EU15 (extra)	11 338	14 939	15 719	16 592	2.1%	1.8%					
India	2 530	4 110	5 483	...	14.1%	12.4%					
Turkey	3 331	6 119	6 661	8 057	25.7%	23.3%		CU96			
Declining export values 1995-2002											
Thailand	2 817	5 008	3 575	3 369	12.2%	4.9%					
Korea	7 879	4 957	4 306	3 694	12.1%	2.3%					
Hong Kong, China	9 266	9 540	9 263	8 306	31.9%	45.5%					
Chinese Taipei	3 987	3 251	2 484	2 197	5.9%	1.6%					
United States	2 565	6 651	7 012	6 032	0.7%	0.9%					
Poland	384	2 304	1 949	1 915	2.7%	4.7%		FTA94		OPP	
Malaysia	1 315	2 266	2 071	1 963	4.5%	2.1%					
Israel	482	663	602	549	4.0%	1.9%	1985				
Jamaica	83	287	116	...	7.2%	9.5%			CBERA		
Egypt	144	253	239	...	4.2%	5.8%	1998				

Notes: Share in economy's total merchandise exports refers to latest year available.

For Egypt: The United States provides duty-free treatment for textiles and clothing made in qualifying industrial zones since March 1998. CBERA: Caribbean Basin Economic and Recovery Act; AGOA: African Growth Opportunity Act. CU96: Customs Union, 1996; EBA01: Everything but Arms, March 2001. CO-OP: Co-operation Agreement to be replaced by Euro-Mediterranean Agreements.

Data for Cambodia and the Dominican Republic include estimates. Data for China, Costa Rica, Dominican Republic, El Salvador, Malaysia, Mexico, Morocco and Philippines include exports from processing zones.

Source: WTO, *International Trade Statistics,* 2002 and 2003.

Annex Table 2.A1.6. OECD textile exports by destination, 1980–2001

OECD exports	OECD-24						OECD-29		
Textiles	1980	1985	1990	1995	2000	2001	1995	2000	2001
Total exports USD millions	38 886	35 525	66 773	75 300	72 546	71 243	98 268	96 888	93 344
OECD (% of total exports)	73.4%	75.5%	80.0%	74.4%	72.1%	70.5%	68.8%	67.9%	67.2%
EU15	57.6%	55.5%	61.3%	51.0%	42.2%	41.7%	47.0%	39.5%	39.8%
Greece	0.9%	1.2%	1.6%	1.1%	0.9%	0.9%	1.0%	0.8%	0.7%
Portugal	0.6%	0.8%	2.2%	2.2%	2.0%	2.0%	1.8%	1.7%	1.7%
Turkey	0.2%	0.3%	0.6%	1.1%	1.4%	1.3%	1.0%	1.4%	1.2%
Four eastern European	1.4%	1.1%	1.5%	4.6%	5.4%	5.7%	4.2%	4.7%	5.1%
NAFTA	6.0%	10.0%	7.9%	9.9%	17.7%	16.6%	9.5%	17.3%	16.2%
United States	3.2%	6.7%	4.5%	5.3%	7.7%	7.5%	5.8%	9.4%	8.8%
Mexico	0.5%	0.5%	0.9%	1.4%	5.5%	5.0%	1.2%	4.4%	4.0%
Japan	1.4%	1.6%	2.5%	2.1%	1.3%	1.3%	2.3%	1.5%	1.4%
Korea	0.8%	1.2%	1.5%	1.8%	1.3%	1.2%	1.4%	1.1%	1.0%
Australia + New Zealand	2.0%	2.2%	1.3%	1.2%	0.9%	0.8%	1.1%	0.9%	0.8%
Non-OECD	26.2%	24.3%	19.1%	24.4%	26.4%	28.0%	29.8%	30.8%	31.6%
Hong Kong, China	2.4%	3.0%	2.6%	3.0%	2.8%	2.7%	5.2%	3.7%	3.3%
China	1.1%	1.5%	0.9%	3.1%	4.2%	4.2%	3.8%	5.4%	5.4%
Chinese Taipei	0.5%	0.8%	1.0%	1.1%	0.8%	0.6%	1.1%	0.8%	0.6%
Asia-6	1.7%	1.6%	1.7%	2.2%	1.9%	1.6%	3.0%	2.8%	2.5%
India	0.1%	0.2%	0.1%	0.2%	0.2%	0.3%	0.2%	0.3%	0.4%
Bangladesh	0.0%	0.0%	0.0%	0.0%	0.1%	0.1%	0.3%	0.3%	0.3%
Pakistan	0.2%	0.2%	0.1%	0.1%	0.1%	0.1%	0.1%	0.1%	0.1%
Vietnam	0.0%	0.0%	0.0%	0.2%	0.4%	0.4%	0.5%	0.7%	0.7%
Africa	6.1%	4.0%	4.1%	4.4%	4.5%	4.9%	4.0%	3.9%	4.4%
Morocco	0.4%	0.5%	1.1%	1.4%	1.6%	1.7%	1.2%	1.3%	1.4%
Tunisia	0.6%	0.6%	1.0%	1.5%	1.7%	1.9%	1.3%	1.4%	1.6%
Non-OECD eastern Europe	0.4%	0.5%	0.4%	2.2%	3.1%	3.6%	1.8%	2.5%	3.0%
Russian Federation	0.0%	0.0%	0.2%	0.6%	0.5%	0.7%	0.7%	0.6%	0.8%
Non-OECD America	2.8%	1.9%	1.4%	2.3%	2.8%	3.6%	3.1%	3.6%	4.1%
MERCOSUR	0.6%	0.2%	0.3%	0.7%	0.7%	0.5%	1.0%	0.9%	0.7%
Rest of the world	9.2%	9.1%	4.1%	1.6%	1.1%	1.1%	2.6%	2.4%	2.5%

Note: OECD-29 = all present OECD members except the Slovak Republic.

OECD-24 = OECD 29 except Mexico, Czech Republic, Hungary, Poland and Korea.

Asia-6 = Brunei, Indonesia, Malaysia, Philippines, Singapore and Thailand.

Non-OECD eastern Europe = Albania, Bulgaria, Romania and Slovenia.

Textile products defined in SITC Revision 2, category 65.

Source: OECD International Trade Statistics.

Annex Table 2.A1.7. OECD clothing exports by destination, 1980–2001

OECD exports	OECD-24						OECD-29		
Clothing	1980	1985	1990	1995	2000	2001	1995	2000	2001
Total exports USD millions	19 615	20 415	47 683	60 460	61 606	60 970	74 772	82 983	81 547
OECD (% of total exports)	87.7%	89.2%	91.0%	84.6%	81.7%	82.3%	86.4%	85.1%	85.4%
EU15	70.5%	64.5%	70.3%	60.3%	55.3%	55.9%	57.6%	50.4%	51.6%
Greece	0.3%	0.4%	0.9%	0.9%	1.1%	1.1%	0.8%	0.9%	0.9%
Portugal	0.1%	0.2%	0.8%	1.4%	1.7%	1.9%	1.1%	1.3%	1.4%
Turkey	0.0%	0.0%	0.1%	0.1%	0.4%	0.3%	0.1%	0.3%	0.3%
Four eastern European	0.4%	0.3%	0.7%	2.2%	1.8%	2.0%	1.9%	1.5%	1.7%
NAFTA	5.5%	13.1%	7.9%	9.7%	15.4%	14.9%	14.2%	24.8%	23.7%
United States	3.8%	11.0%	5.7%	6.0%	9.6%	9.6%	11.0%	20.1%	19.4%
Mexico	0.9%	0.8%	0.9%	2.4%	4.2%	3.6%	1.9%	3.2%	2.8%
Japan	1.9%	1.6%	4.0%	5.1%	3.1%	3.1%	6.6%	3.6%	3.4%
Korea	0.0%	0.1%	0.2%	0.8%	0.5%	0.7%	0.6%	0.4%	0.5%
Australia + New Zealand	0.4%	0.4%	0.4%	0.6%	0.5%	0.4%	0.5%	0.4%	0.4%
Non-OECD	12.2%	10.8%	9.0%	15.3%	18.1%	17.4%	13.4%	14.7%	14.3%
Hong Kong, China	0.6%	0.8%	1.1%	1.6%	1.1%	1.3%	1.4%	0.9%	1.0%
China	0.0%	0.0%	0.1%	0.2%	0.2%	0.2%	0.2%	0.3%	0.4%
Chinese Taipei	0.0%	0.0%	0.3%	0.6%	0.5%	0.5%	0.6%	0.4%	0.4%
Asia-6	0.2%	0.3%	0.4%	0.5%	0.3%	0.3%	0.5%	0.3%	0.3%
India	0.0%	0.0%	0.0%	0.0%	0.0%	0.0%	0.0%	0.0%	0.0%
Bangladesh	0.0%	0.0%	0.0%	0.0%	0.0%	0.0%	0.0%	0.0%	0.0%
Pakistan	0.0%	0.0%	0.0%	0.0%	0.0%	0.0%	0.0%	0.0%	0.0%
Vietnam	0.0%	0.0%	0.0%	0.0%	0.0%	0.0%	0.0%	0.0%	0.0%
Africa	3.1%	1.4%	1.1%	1.5%	1.8%	1.7%	1.3%	1.4%	1.4%
Morocco	0.0%	0.1%	0.2%	0.3%	0.6%	0.6%	0.2%	0.4%	0.4%
Tunisia	0.4%	0.2%	0.4%	0.6%	0.6%	0.7%	0.5%	0.5%	0.5%
Non-OECD eastern Europe	0.2%	0.1%	0.2%	0.8%	1.5%	1.8%	0.7%	1.2%	1.4%
Russian Federation	0.0%	0.0%	0.0%	1.5%	1.4%	1.8%	1.4%	1.2%	1.4%
Non-OECD America	2.8%	2.1%	2.5%	5.2%	7.6%	5.8%	4.3%	6.1%	4.7%
MERCOSUR	0.5%	0.0%	0.1%	0.2%	0.2%	0.2%	0.2%	0.2%	0.2%
Rest of the world	4.2%	5.7%	2.8%	2.2%	2.2%	2.4%	1.9%	1.8%	2.0%

Note: OECD-29 = all present OECD members except the Slovak Republic.

OECD-24 = OECD 29 except Mexico, the Czech Republic, Hungary, Poland and Korea.

Asia-6 = Brunei, Indonesia, Malaysia, Philippines, Singapore and Thailand.

Non-OECD eastern Europe = Albania, Bulgaria, Romania and Slovenia.

Clothing products defined in SITC Revision 2, category 84.

Source: OECD International Trade Statistics.

Annex Table 2.A1.8. OECD textile imports by origin, 1980–2001

OECD imports	OECD-24						OECD-29		
Textiles	1980	1985	1990	1995	2000	2001	1995	2000	2001
Total imports USD millions	35 835	34 618	69 482	76 014	73 476	70 247	89 792	91 391	87 543
OECD (% of total exports)	80.3%	78.4%	79.3%	73.2%	69.3%	68.9%	72.8%	70.7%	70.7%
EU15	60.9%	58.9%	61.9%	52.8%	44.4%	44.1%	51.6%	42.9%	43.0%
Greece	1.2%	1.2%	0.7%	0.5%	0.4%	0.4%	0.4%	0.4%	0.4%
Portugal	1.5%	1.9%	1.8%	1.9%	1.8%	1.9%	1.6%	1.6%	1.6%
Turkey	0.8%	1.3%	1.7%	2.0%	3.2%	3.5%	1.8%	2.8%	3.1%
Four eastern European	0.7%	0.4%	0.5%	1.9%	2.6%	3.0%	1.9%	2.5%	2.8%
NAFTA	7.9%	5.8%	5.9%	8.1%	11.2%	10.9%	9.2%	15.0%	14.6%
United States	6.9%	4.7%	4.5%	5.3%	6.1%	5.7%	6.8%	10.8%	10.3%
Mexico	0.3%	0.3%	0.6%	1.2%	2.3%	2.3%	1.0%	1.9%	1.9%
Japan	3.1%	4.6%	2.6%	2.0%	1.9%	1.7%	2.5%	2.1%	1.9%
Korea	2.5%	3.0%	2.8%	3.1%	3.7%	3.4%	2.8%	3.4%	3.2%
Australia + New Zealand	0.4%	0.6%	0.4%	0.6%	0.5%	0.6%	0.6%	0.5%	0.5%
Non-OECD	19.5%	21.5%	20.5%	26.1%	30.1%	30.9%	26.4%	28.8%	29.1%
Hong Kong, China	1.4%	1.4%	0.9%	0.6%	0.7%	0.7%	0.5%	0.6%	0.6%
China	3.0%	4.6%	4.2%	6.7%	8.7%	9.3%	7.3%	8.4%	8.9%
Chinese Taipei	1.4%	2.4%	2.3%	2.3%	2.6%	2.3%	2.6%	2.6%	2.3%
Asia-6	1.3%	1.7%	2.2%	3.5%	3.6%	3.5%	3.5%	3.6%	3.4%
India	2.6%	2.1%	2.2%	3.6%	4.6%	4.7%	3.5%	4.3%	4.3%
Bangladesh	0.6%	0.5%	0.3%	0.3%	0.3%	0.4%	0.3%	0.3%	0.3%
Pakistan	1.3%	1.7%	2.3%	2.9%	3.1%	3.3%	2.9%	2.9%	3.0%
Vietnam	0.0%	0.0%	0.0%	0.1%	0.2%	0.2%	0.1%	0.2%	0.2%
Africa	1.5%	1.5%	1.3%	1.4%	1.3%	1.4%	1.4%	1.1%	1.2%
Morocco	0.3%	0.2%	0.2%	0.2%	0.1%	0.2%	0.2%	0.1%	0.1%
Tunisia	0.2%	0.1%	0.1%	0.2%	0.2%	0.2%	0.2%	0.2%	0.2%
Non-OECD eastern Europe	0.3%	0.3%	0.2%	0.6%	0.6%	0.7%	0.6%	0.5%	0.7%
Russian Federation	0.0%	0.0%	0.0%	0.3%	0.2%	0.2%	0.3%	0.2%	0.2%
Non-OECD America	2.3%	2.7%	1.8%	1.2%	1.0%	1.0%	1.1%	1.1%	1.0%
MERCOSUR	1.7%	2.0%	1.2%	0.8%	0.6%	0.6%	0.7%	0.5%	0.6%
Rest of the world	1.5%	0.1%	1.2%	1.5%	2.3%	2.1%	1.4%	2.1%	1.9%

Note: OECD-29 = all present OECD members except the Slovak Republic.

OECD-24 = OECD 29 except Mexico, the Czech Republic, Hungary, Poland and Korea.

Asia-6 = Brunei, Indonesia, Malaysia, Philippines, Singapore and Thailand.

Non-OECD eastern Europe = Albania, Bulgaria, Romania and Slovenia.

Textile products defined in SITC Revision 2, category 65.

Source: OECD International Trade Statistics.

Annex Table 2.A1.9. OECD clothing imports by origin, 1980-2001

OECD imports	OECD-24						OECD-29		
Clothing	1980	1985	1990	1995	2000	2001	1995	2000	2001
Total imports USD millions	34 676	42 152	100 735	135 541	164 701	165 699	143 892	176 043	177 826
OECD (% of total exports)	61.7%	53.8%	52.3%	40.7%	35.0%	34.4%	42.6%	36.8%	36.2%
EU15	45.7%	36.6%	36.3%	24.7%	17.6%	17.6%	42.6%	36.8%	36.2%
Greece	2.9%	1.8%	2.0%	1.1%	0.5%	0.6%	25.8%	18.4%	18.5%
Portugal	1.9%	2.5%	3.7%	2.6%	1.5%	1.5%	1.0%	0.5%	0.6%
Turkey	0.3%	1.7%	3.6%	4.0%	3.9%	4.1%	2.5%	1.5%	1.5%
Four eastern European	1.8%	1.0%	1.4%	3.1%	2.4%	2.5%	3.1%	2.4%	2.5%
NAFTA	3.4%	1.9%	2.2%	4.7%	7.6%	7.0%	5.7%	8.9%	8.2%
United States	2.2%	0.7%	1.2%	1.7%	1.0%	0.8%	2.9%	2.6%	2.4%
Mexico	0.8%	0.7%	0.7%	2.2%	5.4%	5.0%	2.1%	5.1%	4.7%
Japan	1.1%	1.5%	0.4%	0.2%	0.2%	0.2%	0.2%	0.2%	0.2%
Korea	8.1%	10.2%	7.8%	3.4%	2.8%	2.5%	3.2%	2.7%	2.3%
Australia + New Zealand	0.1%	0.1%	0.2%	0.2%	0.2%	0.2%	0.2%	0.2%	0.2%
Non-OECD	38.2%	46.1%	47.6%	59.2%	65.0%	65.6%	57.3%	63.1%	63.7%
Hong Kong, China	13.5%	14.4%	9.2%	6.9%	5.9%	5.4%	6.6%	5.7%	5.2%
China	2.7%	5.1%	9.8%	17.9%	20.5%	20.9%	17.4%	20.0%	20.5%
Chinese Taipei	6.1%	8.0%	3.9%	2.3%	1.8%	1.6%	2.2%	1.7%	1.5%
Asia-6	3.6%	5.2%	7.2%	8.2%	8.2%	8.0%	7.9%	7.9%	7.7%
India	2.0%	1.9%	2.6%	3.4%	3.0%	3.0%	3.3%	2.9%	2.9%
Bangladesh	0.0%	0.4%	0.8%	1.9%	2.8%	2.9%	1.8%	2.7%	2.8%
Pakistan	0.2%	0.5%	0.9%	1.2%	1.2%	1.2%	1.1%	1.1%	1.2%
Vietnam	0.0%	0.0%	0.0%	0.6%	0.9%	0.8%	0.6%	0.9%	0.8%
Africa	2.0%	2.1%	3.7%	4.5%	4.3%	4.7%	4.5%	4.3%	4.7%
Morocco	0.4%	0.6%	1.4%	1.6%	1.4%	1.5%	1.6%	1.4%	1.5%
Tunisia	1.1%	0.8%	1.3%	1.5%	1.4%	1.6%	1.7%	1.5%	1.7%
Non-OECD eastern Europe	1.2%	1.1%	0.6%	1.8%	2.4%	2.9%	1.7%	2.3%	2.8%
Russian Federation	0.0%	0.0%	0.0%	0.2%	0.3%	0.3%	0.2%	0.3%	0.3%
Non-OECD America	1.7%	2.4%	2.9%	5.0%	6.7%	6.6%	4.7%	6.4%	6.3%
MERCOSUR	0.7%	0.7%	0.5%	0.2%	0.1%	0.1%	0.2%	0.1%	0.1%
Rest of the world	3.1%	2.9%	2.7%	2.1%	4.2%	4.1%	1.8%	3.8%	3.7%

Note: OECD-29 = all present OECD members except the Slovak Republic.

OECD-24 = OECD 29 except Mexico, Czech Republic, Hungary, Poland and Korea.

Asian-6 = Brunei, Indonesia, Malaysia, Philippines, Singapore and Thailand.

Non-OECD eastern Europe = Albania, Bulgaria, Romania and Slovenia.

Clothing products defined in SITC Revision 2, category 84.

Source: OECD International Trade Statistics.

Annex Table 2.A1.10. Bound tariffs in textiles and clothing, post-Uruguay Round

Percentages

Country	Raw agricultural products		Vegetable fibres		Man-made filaments yarn		Products made of fabric		Clothing	
HS number	HS 50.04-.07		HS 51-53		HS 54-55		HS 56-60 + 63		HS 61-62	
Bound rate	Average	Maximum	Average	Maximum	Average	Maximum	Average	Maximum	Average	Maximum
European Union	0.00	0.00	5.10	8.00	6.29	8.00	7.91	12.00	11.51	12.00
Japan	0.00	0.00	4.24	12.53	6.27	8.10	5.65	14.20	9.23	13.40
Switzerland	0.00	0.00	2.91	10.80	4.57	15.10	4.79	20.00	5.96	15.90
Norway	0.53	0.70	6.12	12.00	7.35	13.10	7.69	13.70	11.06	13.70
Slovak Republic	0.38	0.70	4.96	10.80	5.64	17.00	8.08	31.50	9.04	16.40
Czech Republic	0.38	0.70	4.96	10.80	5.64	17.00	8.12	31.50	9.04	16.40
Iceland	0.00	0.00	1.18	11.50	3.31	6.50	14.22	28.00	20.51	21.00
Canada	0.00	0.00	8.13	14.00	10.89	14.00	13.12	18.00	17.46	18.00
United States	0.61	2.43	5.98	15.22	10.01	17.78	5.70	18.80	10.72	26.40
Hungary	3.75	6.00	5.89	10.00	6.11	17.41	8.17	44.00	11.35	13.00
Poland	2.50	5.00	10.33	38.00	8.55	12.00	14.10	26.30	18.00	18.00
Malaysia	5.00	5.00	13.23	30.00	18.02	30.00	23.74	40.00	20.87	31.00
Philippines	10.00	10.00	21.91	30.00	24.57	30.00	30.90	50.00	30.00	30.00
Korea	27.53	51.00	12.08	30.00	13.24	30.00	21.42	30.00	28.31	35.00
Australia	0.45	0.94	12.68	42.75	16.80	40.31	15.23	52.79	39.20	89.30
Argentina	35.00	35.00	35.00	35.00	35.00	35.00	35.00	35.00	35.00	35.00
Mexico	20.00	20.00	34.54	50.00	35.00	35.00	34.93	40.00	35.13	50.00
Venezuela	40.00	40.00	35.46	40.00	35.00	35.00	32.13	35.00	35.00	35.00
Brazil	35.00	35.00	35.34	55.00	35.00	35.00	34.78	35.00	35.00	35.00
Indonesia	40.00	40.00	39.94	40.00	40.00	40.00	40.00	40.00	40.00	40.00
New Zealand	0.00	0.00	3.19	30.00	6.48	20.00	19.11	42.50	43.94	313.50
Colombia	70.00	70.00	38.91	99.00	34.61	35.00	36.60	40.00	40.00	40.00
Romania	18.50	60.00	39.90	270.00	34.89	35.00	27.15	35.00	20.43	35.00
Tunisia	62.00	62.00	60.21	62.00	49.85	60.00	51.82	60.00	60.00	60.00
Thailand	63.25	226.00	23.89	30.00	30.00	30.00	30.05	35.00	30.60	100.00
Turkey	18.48	19.50	51.36	150.00	88.34	150.00	68.46	200.00	99.22	100.00
India	100.00	100.00	89.17	160.00	75.20	100.00	83.25	100.00	100.00	100.00

Note: Post-Uruguay Round bound tariff rates; only tariffs with *ad valorem* equivalents are included.

Source: CD-ROM Tariffs and Trade, OECD Query and Simulation Package, OECD Trade Directorate 2003.

Annex Table 2.A1.11. Applied tariffs in textile and clothing products, 1996

Percentages

HS numbers	Raw agricultural products HS 50.04-.07		Vegetable fibres HS 51-53		Man-made filaments yarn HS 54-55		Products made of fabric HS 56-60 + 63		Clothing HS 61-62	
Applied rate	Average	Maximum	Average	Maximum	Average	Maximum	Average	Maximum	Average	Maximum
Iceland	0.00	0.00	0.00	0.00	0.00	0.00	3.98	10.00	14.59	15.00
Korea	3.50	8.00	6.91	8.00	7.93	8.00	8.00	8.00	8.00	8.00
European Union	0.80	2.50	6.43	14.30	8.83	10.10	9.36	21.10	12.59	13.40
Japan	1.56	6.25	5.81	16.00	7.82	10.85	6.96	17.90	12.29	14.50
Turkey	3.75	6.00	8.09	17.00	10.33	11.00	11.68	15.00	13.85	14.00
Slovakia	1.58	2.90	5.43	11.50	6.17	18.80	8.71	33.60	9.59	17.20
Czech Republic	1.58	2.90	5.43	11.50	6.17	18.80	8.75	33.60	9.59	17.20
Hungary	5.08	8.90	11.26	15.00	9.26	15.00	12.12	20.00	10.14	20.00
Norway	0.45	0.60	8.82	18.40	11.12	21.00	11.29	22.70	16.96	22.70
United States	1.13	4.50	7.94	20.45	13.05	18.85	9.05	22.40	13.80	29.66
Canada	0.00	0.00	10.50	19.00	14.33	19.00	17.05	23.60	22.67	24.50
Switzerland	0.00	0.00	3.92	28.80	6.10	27.10	6.71	52.72	8.74	28.62
Brazil	4.00	4.00	14.48	18.00	16.44	18.00	18.20	20.00	20.04	30.00
Argentina	4.00	4.00	14.66	18.00	16.65	21.00	18.12	20.00	21.45	28.00
Malaysia	0.00	0.00	10.45	30.00	13.53	20.00	19.48	30.00	19.96	30.00
Colombia	7.50	10.00	16.36	20.00	17.40	25.00	18.46	20.00	20.00	20.00
Poland	6.70	11.70	13.07	20.00	10.88	17.70	19.91	30.00	26.60	26.60
Australia	0.00	0.00	11.84	24.00	15.70	25.00	13.59	37.00	32.60	37.00
Mexico	10.00	10.00	13.76	15.00	14.11	15.00	20.72	35.00	35.00	35.00
Indonesia	5.00	5.00	15.48	27.50	17.60	25.00	21.49	30.00	28.22	30.00
Romania	5.00	5.00	16.08	25.00	20.59	25.00	26.21	40.00	30.00	30.00
New Zealand	0.00	0.00	1.06	21.00	3.21	14.00	10.92	26.25	39.60	219.35
Thailand	7.50	10.00	20.55	42.50	25.66	30.00	34.63	45.00	44.71	100.00
India	1.25	5.00	91.82	160.00	97.68	175.00	97.07	100.00	100.00	100.00

Note: Applied tariff rates in 1996; only tariffs with *ad valorem* equivalents are included.

Source: CD-ROM Tariffs and Trade, OECD Query and Simulation Package, OECD Trade Directorate 2003.

Notes

1. The WTO ATC superseded the Multi-Fibre Arrangement regime of quantitative trade restrictions when it entered into force in January 1995 and provided the multilateral trade framework applicable for trade in textiles and clothing for all WTO members. The ATC provides for the elimination by 31 December 2004 of all forms of quantitative restrictions applied to trade in textile and clothing products, including those that originated under the MFA regime. The ATC phases itself out of existence at the end of 2004. For the purpose of qualifying the period when no more quantitative restrictions will be applied to trade in textile and clothing products, the term "the post-ATC period" is used throughout this publication.

2. According to UNCTAD (2002, pp. 54-58), the 20 most dynamic products have grown at an average annual rate of 12.9%, compared to an average annual growth rate of 8% for merchandise exports. Among these are four textile and clothing products: silk (SITC 261) with an average annual growth rate of 13.2%; knitted undergarments (846) at 13.1%; textile undergarments (844) at 11.9%; and knitted textiles (655) at 11.7%.

3. The technical textiles are materials and products manufactured primarily for their technical performance and functional properties rather than their aesthetic or decorative characteristics. They embrace a wide range of materials, processes and applications and share overlapping interests with other materials, such as chemicals, plastics, fibreglass and various composite materials. Technical textiles are used in many industries, including furniture, automotive, health and hygiene, transport, construction and environment.

4. Technology and recent trends in the production process are analysed in greater detail in Chapter 4.

5. See Table 3.1 in Chapter 3 on labour adjustment policies.

6. Hummels (2000) has estimated that each day saved in shipping time is equivalent to a reduction of 0.5% in import tariffs. Limão and Venables (2001) have investigated the dependence of transport costs on geography and infrastructure and estimated that a 10 percentage point increase in transport costs typically reduces trade volumes by approximately 20%. Radelet and Sachs (1998) have also compared transport costs for 97 developing countries and estimated that the costs of freight and insurance for landlocked developing countries was on average 50% higher than for coastal economies.

7. In India, the industry is based on a system of decentralised production, referred to as "reservation of garment manufacture for small-scale industry", which provides a series of economic advantages to small-scale labour-intensive firms. Verma (2002) argues that these domestic measures create deep distortions so that Indian clothing can neither attain optimal economies of scale nor produce clothing products that meet international standards of quality. In the same vein, Kathuria and Bhardwaj (1998) argue that India faces formidable domestic hurdles if it is to meet international standards and competition. These include: the reservation system for the small-scale sector, restrictive labour laws, limitations on foreign ownership of the garment industry, inefficient transport and customs clearance systems and a policy bias against synthetic fibres.

8.   Annex Tables 2.A1.1 and 2.A1.2 show for the textile and the clothing sectors, respectively, value added per employee, annual wages and salaries per employee, breakdown of total cost among the costs of input material and of labour, and the operating surplus for over 30 countries.

9.   China's simple average applied tariff rate for all goods was 12.1% in 2002, and it is committed to reduce its average bound rate to a level of 9.8% when all tariff reductions are implemented, by 2010 at the latest (OECD, 2002b).

10.   On the import purchasing procedures of SOEs, China undertook to refrain from taking any measures to influence the quantity, the value or the origin of goods purchased or sold by SOEs. On export transactions, China is required to provide full information on the pricing mechanism of its SOEs. Moreover, it undertook to phase out within three years after its accession limitations on the right to trade products subject to designated trading rights, which include certain wool products covered under HS 51 and certain acrylic filament yarns covered under HS 54 and 55 categories.

11.   An added complexity in dealing with bound and applied tariffs is that some developing countries consolidate their tariff regime incompletely, *e.g.* they do not bind all their tariff lines, therefore there are no upward limits on increasing their tariffs. Such situations make tariff regimes unpredictable.

12.   These remission orders cover imports of children's blouses and shirts; women's and girls' knitted blouses and shirts; women's and girls' blouses and shirts; saris; women's and girls' ensembles; babies' snowsuits, coats and jackets; and rainwear. WTO, TPRM of Canada, November 1998, p. 93.

13.   "The Taste of Free Trade – the Forbidden Fruit – in Textiles and Clothing is Sweet", a report on the Swedish deregulation of quotas and a view on EU textile trade policy under ATC to the ITCB meeting in San Salvador, June 1997.

14.   The 31 pan-European members include the EU15, ten central and eastern European countries (Bulgaria, the Czech Republic, Estonia, Hungary, Latvia, Lithuania, Poland, Romania, Slovenia and the Slovak Republic) and Cyprus, Malta, Turkey, Iceland, Norway and Switzerland. The pan-European regime of cumulative rules of origin allows parts and components produced in any country member to be treated as domestic components.

15.   Under Article 45 of the Cabinet Order for Enforcement of the Temporary Tariff Measures Law, the reduction of the customs value is equal to the value of exported Japanese goods multiplied by 1.06.

16.   Chapter 5 discusses the logistical dimensions of the international movement of textile and clothing products. Table 5.2 compares the logistical and dutiable cost of textile and clothing shipments for a large number of countries.

17.   Brenton and Manchin further illustrate their argument about the costs of compliance to rules of origin by noting that the EU and Turkey have a customs union and implement a common external tariff that does not require rules of origin and that, as a result, OPP transactions are negligible.

18.   The estimate is drawn from a report prepared in 2000 by l'Observatoire Européen du Textile et de l'Habillement (OETH).

19.   During the initial NAFTA implementation period, bilateral trade tariffs between Mexico and the United States have maintained the attractiveness of OPP transactions that provided for duty-free entry. As bilateral tariffs were gradually eliminated over a seven-year period for textile and clothing products, the attractiveness of OPPs waned. However, OPPs are still used for transactions involving third-country textiles that were

cut in the United States and then assembled in Mexico before re-export to the United States. With the improvement in the availability of high-quality textiles from domestic sources that qualify for NAFTA origin, Mexican suppliers have fewer commercial reasons to pursue OPP transactions.

20.   Trade Data Online, www.strategic.ic.gc.ca. Measured in Canadian dollars, Canadian clothing imports grew by a mere 0.5%. Preliminary import data for the first two months of 2004 indicate continuing strong growth of imports from LDCs.

21.   The WTO notifications are, respectively: G/AG/N/USA/43; G/AG/N/EEC/38; and G/AG/N/BRA/18.

22.   For a comprehensive list of non-tariff measures applied to exports, readers should consult the WTO document TN/MA/W/25 and its addendum. These documents provide a compilation of submissions by WTO members of non-tariff measures affecting their exports that they wish to have addressed during the Doha negotiations.

References

Abernathy, F., J. Dunlop, J. Hammond and D. Weil (1999), *A Stitch in Time, Lean Retailing and the Transformation of Manufacturing – Lessons from the Apparel and Textile Industries*, New York, Oxford, Oxford University Press.

American Apparel Manufacturers Association (1998), *Focus: An Economic Profile of the Apparel Industry*, Arlington, VA.

Brenton, P. and M. Manchin (2002), "Making EU Trade Agreements Work, The Role of Rules of Origin", Centre for European Policy Studies, CEPS Working Document No. 183, March.

Eurostat (2002), *European Business Facts and Figures, data 1990–2000, Theme 4 Industry, Trade and Services, 2002 Edition*, European Commission.

Gereffi, Gary (1999), "International Trade and Industrial Upgrading in the Apparel Commodity Chain", *Journal of International Economics*, 48: 37–70.

Gereffi, Gary (2002), "The International Competitiveness of Asian Economies in the Apparel Commodity Chain", Asian Development Bank, Economics and Research Department, ERD Working Paper series No. 5, February.

Gereffi, G., D. Spener and J. Bair (eds.) (2002), *Free Trade and Uneven Development, The North American Apparel Industry after NAFTA*, Temple University Press, Philadelphia.

Hummels, D. (2000), "Time as a Trade Barrier", Purdue University, October, Hummelsd@purdue.edu.

ITC (US International Trade Commission) (2004), "Textiles and Apparels: Assessments of the Competitiveness of Certain Foreign Suppliers to the U.S. Market", Investigation No. 332–448, Washington, DC, February.

Kathuria, S. and A. Bhardwaj (1998), "Export Quotas and Policy Constraints in the Indian Textile and Garment Industries", Policy Research Working Paper, No. WPS 2012, The World Bank, New Delhi Office.

Limão, N. and A.J. Venables (2001), "Infrastructure, Geographical Disadvantage, Transport Costs and Trade", *The World Bank Economic Review*, Vol. 15, No. 3, p. 451-479.

Mortimore, D. (2002), "When Does Apparel Become a Peril? On the Nature of Industrialization in the Caribbean Basin", in G. Gereffi, D. Spener and J. Bair (eds.) (2002), *Free Trade and Uneven Development, The North American Apparel Industry after NAFTA*, Temple University Press, Philadelphia.

Nell, P. (1998), "EFTA and the EU/Eastern Europe Regime for Outward Processing of Textiles: Major Integration through Paneuropean Cumulation", *Aussenwirtschaft*, 53, 2: 289–309.

NZ Institute of Economic Research (1999), "Consumer Benefits from Import Liberalisation: A New Zealand Case Study", report prepared for the Ministry of Foreign Affairs and Trade, Wellington, June.

OECD (2002a), "Regional Trade Agreements and the Multilateral Trading System", TD/TC(2002)8/FINAL, Paris.

OECD (2002b), "China's Tariff Regime", CCNM/TD(2002)9/FINAL, Paris.

OTEXA (The Office of Textiles and Apparel) (2001), TQ data of December 2001.

Radelet, S. and J. Sachs (1998), "Shipping Costs, Manufactured Exports and Economic Growth", mimeo, Harvard Institute for International Development, Cambridge.

Ramaswamy, K. and G. Gereffi (2000), "India's Apparel Exports: The Challenge of Global Markets", *The Developing Economies*, Volume 38, 2: 186–210.

Senior Nello, S. (2002), "Progress in Preparing for EU Enlargement: The Tensions between Economic and Political Integration", *International Political Science Review*, Vol. 23, No. 3, July..

Stengg, W. (2001), "The Textile and Clothing industry in the EU: A Survey", Enterprise Papers No. 2, June.

UNCTAD (2002), *Trade and Development Report 2002*, United Nations, Geneva.

UNCTAD (2003), *Trade Preferences for LDCs: An Early Assessment of Benefits and Possible Improvements*, United Nations, Geneva.

UNCTAD/WTO (2000), *The Post-Uruguay Round Tariff Environment for Developing Country Exports: Tariff Peaks and Tariff Escalation*, United Nations, Geneva.

Verma, S. (2002), "Export Competitiveness of Indian Textile and Garment Industry, Indian Council for Research on International Economic Relations", Working Paper No. 94, New Delhi.

WTO (2001), *Overview of Development in the international Trading Environment, Annual Reports by the Director-General*, Geneva.

WTO (2002a), *International Trade Statistics 2002*, Geneva.

WTO (2002b), *Overview of Development in the International Trading Environment, Annual Report by the Director–General,* Geneva.

WTO (2003), *International Trade Statistics 2003*, Geneva.

Chapter 3

Trade-Related Labour Adjustment Policies

Although trade liberalisation yields economy-wide benefits, the opening of markets to international competition puts pressure on labour markets and results in both temporary and permanent hardships for displaced workers. This chapter outlines the main characteristics of displaced workers in the textile and clothing industries in OECD countries and analyses recent developments and policy reforms in labour adjustment programmes. The analysis underscores the difficulty of isolating the causes of worker displacement and suggests the need for broad labour adjustment programmes, regardless of the causes of worker displacement. It notes the increasing reliance on training as part of the toolbox of labour market adjustment programmes and the advent of wage insurance programmes.

Introduction

During the last decade, OECD countries have gradually liberalised trade in the textile and clothing industries in accordance with their international commitments. Although liberalisation yields economy-wide benefits, the opening of markets to international competition puts pressure on labour markets and can result in both temporary and permanent hardships for workers displaced in the process. The prospective elimination of the quantitative restrictions covered under the WTO Agreement on Textiles and Clothing (ATC) has already led to major adjustment, challenging the global sourcing channels that were formed over decades of trade restrictions.[1] As a result, there is considerable anxiety among textile and clothing workers about the future of their jobs.

Although trade policy will continue to affect economic outcomes in these sectors, mainly through relatively high import tariffs and preferential trade arrangements, the labour policy challenge is likely to become more prominent in the post-ATC period. How and what kinds of labour adjustment programmes for displaced workers would allow governments to play their role in redistribution and thus contribute to social cohesion? Most OECD countries have already established programmes to deal with displaced workers' needs. In non–OECD countries, displaced workers tend to rely on less sophisticated social safety networks, with family solidarity often the main source of assistance. Due to difficulty in gathering detailed information on non–OECD countries, this chapter focuses on policies and programmes in certain OECD countries.

The chapter is structured as follows. First, it examines the linkages between international trade and labour adjustment. It stresses the difficulty of disentangling import competition from other causes of job displacement and emphasises the role of public policy in providing assistance to displaced workers. It then turns to the main characteristics of displaced workers in the textile and clothing industries in OECD countries, before describing and analysing recent developments and policy reforms in labour adjustment programmes in some OECD countries. Finally, some concluding remarks are offered. Annex 3.A2 describes the main characteristics of unemployment insurance programmes in France, Germany, Japan, the United Kingdom and the United States.

International trade and labour adjustment

Although liberalisation yields economy-wide benefits, the opening of markets to international competition puts pressure on labour markets which can result in both temporary and permanent hardships for displaced workers. Moreover, these negative consequences tend to be highly concentrated by industry, by location and by worker demographics. Accordingly, the gains from trade tend to be unevenly distributed throughout the economy, resulting in both winners and losers.

Adverse labour effects

Workers can be adversely affected in varying degrees by increased import competition, falling export sales and shifts in production. Workers employed by the domestic import-competing industry are considered front-line or "primary" workers. Workers who produce inputs for the domestic competing industry are considered "secondary" workers. Tertiary workers are those who provide goods and services to primary and secondary workers and their families but not directly to the industries for which they work. For example, in the case of clothing imports, workers who produce men's pants are considered primary workers. Workers who produce zippers are considered secondary workers, and those employed by restaurants and retail stores in the community where the clothing and zipper producers are located are considered tertiary workers.

In the above example, primary workers are most likely to face job loss as a result of increased import competition. Depending on the state of the economy, it may take some time for those workers to find new jobs. Furthermore, if they finally find a new job, the salary may be less than what they earned before being laid off. Secondary workers may experience similar losses, although the probability of layoff may be less than that for primary workers, especially if they have a diversified set of buyers and/or production lines. Likewise, tertiary workers may experience losses, but to a lesser degree than primary and secondary workers.

Beyond the hardships for workers employed by the firm, plant closures due to severe competition from abroad are likely to have serious implications for the entire community. If a community's economy is highly dependent on a certain firm or industry, as well as the inputs necessary for its production, the adjustment burden will also be felt by local workers in retail sales and other services. In addition, the loss of a large plant can erode a community's tax base, thereby leaving no one untouched by the closure.

In larger communities and during times of economic prosperity, the adjustment burden – although present – may be less pronounced. In this case, the negative consequences of the closure of a single plant may be concentrated on the primary workers and not affect the broader community. In any case, some workers may lose their jobs and have to go without a salary for several weeks or months while trying to find new jobs. In addition, depending on their skills and experience, they may have to accept jobs at lower salaries. The mere threat of moving production facilities overseas is often used as a means of keeping wages low and reducing workers' health insurance and pension benefits.

Table 3.1. Net job losses in textiles and clothing between 1970 and 2000

	Textiles	Clothing	Total loss	Total loss (%)	Employment levels, 2000
France	-337000	-238 000	-575 000	72.9%	241 000
Germany	-333 000	-262 000	-595 000	67.6%	285 000
Japan	-997 000	-140 000	-1 137 000	66.4%	576 000
United Kingdom	-486 000	-248 000	-724 000	73.7%	258 000
United States	-585 000	-531 000	-1 116 000	49.0%	1 161 000
Total	-2 738 000	-1 419 000	-4 147 000	62.2%	2 521 000

Source: Extracted from Annex Table 3.A1.1.

Table 3.1 shows that textile and clothing employment in France, Germany, Japan, the United Kingdom and the United States fell by more than 4 million between 1970 and 2000. The *net* number of job losses masks the actual *gross* job losses and gains during this period (see the following section on creative destruction). The largest drop in terms of employment level and share of textile and clothing employment occurred in Japan and in the United Kingdom, respectively. Job losses occurred in each of the three decades covered but with less intensity during the first half of the 1990s for all countries (Annex Table 3.A1.1). Although Japan did not apply quantitative restrictions, its percentage of employment losses is marginally lower than that of Germany and slightly lower than those of France and the United Kingdom, three countries that applied MFA restrictions to smooth out the adjustment.

A longer historical analysis provides a better appreciation of textile and clothing employment in Japan. It should be recalled that the Short-term Arrangement regarding International Trade in Textiles (STA) and the Long-term Arrangement regarding International Trade in Cotton Textiles (LTA) came into force in 1961 and 1962, respectively, to protect the most advanced countries from the then low-cost production from Japan, Hong Kong (China) and other developing countries. Internal factors, such as wage pressure from competing industrial activities in Japan and the appreciation of the yen, steadily eroded the competitiveness of Japanese textile and clothing firms (the same is also true for Hong Kong, China). The rise and fall of the Japanese textile and clothing industries illustrates the importance of macroeconomic factors, *e.g.* exchange rates and aggregate labour supply and demand conditions as determining factors for sectoral activities.

The broader picture

Changes in textile and clothing employment over the last 30 years have not occurred in a vacuum. In many economies, the decline in textile and clothing employment occurred against the backdrop of broader employment declines throughout the manufacturing sector and intensified globalisation of industrial activities. For example, total non-farm employment in the United States increased by more than 55 million between 1974 and 2000, which is equivalent to a 70.9% increase in employment (Table 3.2).[2] During this period, employment in manufacturing and mining fell by almost 2 million, and employment in service-related industries, such as transport, wholesale and retail trade, finance, insurance, real estate, construction, government and services, increased by 57 million.

Table 3.2. Changes in US employment by sectors, 1974-2000

	Employment change 1974 to 2000	
	Thousands	%
Total manufacturing (see Table 3.3)	-1 604	-8.0%
Mining	-154	-22.1%
Transport	2 306	48.8%
Wholesale trade	2 500	56.2%
Finance, insurance and real estate	3 428	82.6%
Construction	4 633	11.5%
Government	6 532	46.1%
Retail trade	10 798	86.1%
Services	27 016	20.1%
Total	55 455	70.9%

Source: US Department of Labor.

Developments in employment in the manufacturing sector were also considerable over the period, with 14 of the 20 manufacturing industries experiencing declines in total employment of more than 2.5 million jobs (Table 3.3). These job losses were somewhat offset by an increase in employment of approximately 1 million workers in the remaining six manufacturing industries. Almost half of the manufacturing job losses were concentrated in textiles and clothing. In fact, the two largest employment declines occurred in the textile and clothing industries.

Table 3.3. Changes in US employment in manufacturing industries, 1974 to 2000

	Employment change, 1974 to 2000	
	Thousands	%
Clothing	-729	-53.5%
Textiles	-434.5	-45.0%
Primary metal industries	-390.4	-30.3%
Paper	-239.9	-26.8%
Leather	-200.9	-74.1%
Industrial machinery	-109.2	-4.9%
Stone, clay and glass	-94.4	-14.0%
Fabricated metal products	-93.2	-5.7%
Petroleum	-70	-35.5%
Miscellaneous mfg. industries	-69.7	-15.4%
Tobacco	-42.8	-55.5%
Instruments	-40.2	-4.5%
Chemicals	-26.5	-2.5%
Food	-21.7	-1.3%
Transport equipment	8.8	0.5%
Electronic equipment	59.8	3.6%
Furniture	69.6	14.2%
Lumber and wood	103.8	14.3%
Rubber	273	37.0%
Printing and publishing	436.2	39.3%

Source: US Department of Labor.

These data suggest that, at least in the United States, the decline in textile and clothing employment coincided with a decline, or at least a slowdown, in overall manufacturing employment. Other OECD countries also experienced a similar shift out of manufacturing and into services-related industries, resulting in considerable changes in labour demand and supply over the last three decades.

Creative destruction and jobs in textiles and clothing

While the evidence points to considerable net job losses in advanced countries, import competition has also brought new dynamism, resulting in the creation of new jobs in the same sectors with different specialisations. In many ways the textile and clothing industries have reinvented themselves through the adoption of improved textile technologies and new organisational structures in the clothing industry. In Italy, for example, textile employment increased by 20 000 between 1995 and 2000 (Annex Table 3.A1.1). In Japan, Korea and the United States, job losses were accompanied by shifts in production towards faster growth segments such as industrial and house furnishing applications in the United States, the finishing of textiles in Korea and made-up textile articles in Japan (Annex Table 3.A1.2).

Levinsohn and Petropoulos (2001) discuss the process of creative destruction in the textile and clothing industries. They document a substantial level of entry in US textile and clothing industries and a high job creation rate from the early 1970s to the mid–1990s. They find that many jobs disappeared but new and higher paying jobs replaced some of those lost. They concluded that, in spite of strong import competition, these industries are good examples of creative destruction in which surviving firms emerge stronger while less productive plants exit.

In comparing the behaviour of US firms that are globally engaged and those that are not, Lewis and Richardson (2001) reveal that the productivity of plants with investment links to foreign plants is typically higher than that of plants without such linkages. Similarly, a typical assembly–line worker in a plant that exports or outsources abroad earns more than an otherwise comparable assembly–line worker in a plant that does neither. They also find that the global commitment through imports of inputs, capital goods inputs, and finished products induces significant productivity gains that more than offset the losses of the workers and firms that are displaced by imports. Against the background of these rewards, their policy suggestion is to encourage the global integration of firms and to minimise the burden on firms that do not make that choice.

The many causes of job loss

The effects of international trade and globalisation on labour markets have been the focus of considerable debate and analytical research. Kletzer (2001a) has made one of the most interesting and in-depth analyses of the labour adjustment induced by import competition and globalisation. Her work shows that import-competing workers have reasons to be anxious about the prospect of losing their jobs, because those who lose their jobs experience large and persistent earning losses. However, she also found that earning losses are experienced by all displaced manufacturing workers, irrespective of the causes of the job loss, *i.e.* import competition and/or technological change. While she agrees that there is a need for political recognition of trade-related adjustment problems, her research supports the need for broad labour adjustment programmes for all displaced workers irrespective of the causes of job displacement.

In the same vein, Field and Graham (1997) studied the re–employment experiences of displaced workers in the textile and clothing industries to determine both if the unemployment experience was significantly different for these and other sectors, and to relate these findings to possible adjustment costs resulting from trade liberalisation initiatives by the United States. They conclude that textile and clothing workers displaced due to mass layoffs or large plant closures do not represent a special case, different from that of workers who lose their jobs under similar circumstances in other industries. Although they find that displaced textile and clothing workers who find new jobs in different sectors experienced a somewhat longer period of unemployment than displaced workers in other sectors, they tended to find jobs in higher-wage sectors. They also argue that although the case might be made for policies to alleviate the hardships of older workers in the textile and clothing industries, "industry-specific protection from imports does not appear to be an effective way to assist classes of laid-off workers who might experience extraordinary difficulty due to lay-off" (Field and Graham, 1997, p. 156).

In a review of the empirical literature on the effects of international trade on the US labour market, Blancflower (2000) concludes that globalisation "did not appear to be the main, or even one of the major, causes of the labour market changes that occurred in the USA or elsewhere since the 1970s" (p. 54). Other influential factors included skill-biased technological change, immigration, declining unionisation, declining real minimum wages and reductions in the supply of college-educated workers. Although noting the dramatic changes in labour markets that occurred during the previous decades, Blancflower stresses technology as an important factor in explaining the shift in demand away from less skilled jobs.

Labour adjustment as a public policy issue

Unlike capital, the free movement of labour is confronted with significant barriers. At the international level, most countries have restrictions on immigration, while within an economy, labour mobility is restricted more by natural factors than by laws. There are significant financial, economic, social and psychological costs associated with the movement of labour.

There are three rationales for government action on labour market adjustment. The first is economic: labour market policies and programmes may enable a more efficient allocation of resources. In the area of international trade, devoting some resources to easing the adjustment burden may help facilitate further trade liberalisation, which may result in significant gains for the entire economy. The second is political: politicians tend to avoid policies, like trade liberalisation, that may harm employment. One way to make such policy decisions more palatable to politicians is for them to make a commitment to assist workers and communities that are adversely affected by the policy. The third is equity: there are costs and benefits to most government policies, including trade policy. For example, trade liberalisation may help some people and hurt others. In these cases, there is an argument that those who benefit from a specific policy should be asked to assist those who are hurt by that policy.

The absence of policies and programmes designed to respond to trade-related dislocations may result in the imposition of broader measures to protect an industry from increased import competition. The costs to the economy associated with these measures will most likely be greater than the cost of providing assistance to workers who might otherwise lose their jobs. Annex A presents a review of quantitative studies of the welfare gains from complete trade liberalisation in textiles and clothing and shows the estimated annual global benefits ranging from USD 6.5 billion to USD 324 billion. Moreover, the trade policy community has recently begun paying closer attention to the social and economic consequences of international trade. Policy makers from all countries, whether they have a constitutional democracy or parliamentary system, are being asked to think about the labour market adjustment issues related to trade liberalisation.

Developed countries are not alone in attempting to face the new realities associated with trade policy. Policy makers from developing countries are increasingly asked to consider the domestic consequences of trade liberalisation. The emergence of China as a major exporter has made this a very real concern. Countries in which low wages have played an important role in their export strategy are now learning that they can be out-competed on price (see Chapters 2 and 5). Most of these countries do not have a sophisticated social welfare system, and furthermore, many have very restrictive labour laws that make it extremely difficult to fire workers.

It is becoming clear that all countries, regardless of their level of development, must begin to address the social and economic consequences of trade liberalisation. In recent years, there has been a tendency for policy makers to call for international co-operation to address challenges that are common to many countries. Examples include AIDS, poverty and environmental issues. By contrast, responding to the pressures associated with trade liberalisation, despite the fact that countries around the world face these pressures, continues to be seen primarily as a national responsibility. For example, although workers in many developing countries will benefit from the removal of quantitative restrictions, the responsibility of assisting adversely affected workers and communities falls more directly on the formerly protected economies, *i.e.* the United States, the European Union and Canada, and those developing countries that have built an export–led strategy based on MFA quota allocations. There is considerable anxiety in the world textile and clothing community about the emergence of more competitive and integrated suppliers, particularly in China, that may capture a disproportional share of the economic benefits arising from the phasing out of the ATC.

Against the background of closer international integration, the systemic shift towards services-related activities and the phasing out of quantitative restrictions, the main policy challenge is to secure the benefits from liberalised trade and investment while, simultaneously, minimising the resulting adjustment burdens on adversely affected workers and communities. To achieve this goal, governments must transfer some of the benefits of trade and investment enjoyed by the vast majority of people to help offset some of the costs incurred by those adversely affected by import competition. The main goal of any labour adjustment programme should be re-employment, either a return to one's previous job or the finding of a new one, as soon as possible, with minimal disruption in earnings. Such programmes should also aim at minimising the economic and social impact of plant closures on communities. Therefore, the overall policy challenge is to devise ways to meet the social goals in a cost-efficient and least trade-distorting manner.

Characteristics of displaced workers

As mentioned above (see Table 3.1), a change in net employment is only one aspect of the labour adjustment story. Net figures do not provide any insight into the actual number of job losses and gains. The issue of *net versus gross* changes in employment gets to the heart of the burdens associated with labour market adjustment. Many workers do not (and, some may argue, cannot) move freely from job to job, owing to skill requirements, location, family responsibilities and wage and benefit differentials. In some cases, the labour market is in fact segmented. Thus, the mere existence of a job opportunity does not erase the adjustment burden.

In order to fully appreciate the burdens of labour market adjustment, it is important to develop a deeper understanding of the individual workers who are forced to adjust to changes in the labour market. This requires detailed labour data. Until recently, the United States was the only country that surveyed displaced workers in order to gain insight into the adjustment process.[3] In addition to providing more information about displaced workers by age, sex, marital status, and education, these data also enable a deeper understanding of the adjustment burden facing workers. The data include information on the industry from which the worker was separated, his/her pre-separation wage, tenure and length of unemployment. Workers are surveyed over time to gain information on the adjustment process, *i.e.* if the worker is re-employed and if he/she has experienced any income loss. The availability of these surveys has facilitated the analysis of labour adjustment developments in the United States.

Kletzer (2001a) undertook a very ambitious study of displaced workers, which includes an in-depth analysis of the adjustment process and the costs of adjustment for displaced workers. Box 3.1 presents a summary of her major findings.

Box 3.1. Job loss from imports: measuring the costs

Like manufacturing workers displaced for other reasons, import-competing displaced workers are older, less formally educated, and more tenured than displaced non-manufacturing workers. Generally, these are not the characteristics of workers who succeed in training programmes.

For many workers, import-competing job loss is very costly, owing to difficulties in finding new employment at a level of pay similar to the old job. Two-thirds of re-employed workers earn less on their new job than they did on their previous job, and one-quarter experience earnings losses in excess of 30%. The average earnings loss is more modest, but still sizeable at 13%. The distribution of earnings losses is very similar to that found for all workers displaced from manufacturing jobs for other reasons.

Import competition is associated with low re-employment rates because workers vulnerable to rising imports experience difficulty in gaining re–employment owing to their individual characteristics. The characteristics that limit the re-employment of import-competing displaced workers are: low educational attainment, advancing age, high tenure, minority status and marital status. Workers with high tenure and/or low skill levels may encounter serious skill-related adjustment problems, as well as having rusty job search skills.

For most workers, the costs of job loss occur as re-employment earnings losses. Less formally educated workers experience the greatest difficulty in maintaining earnings. More generally, re-employment earnings losses rise with age, fall with education, and rise with job tenure. Workers whose earning losses rise appear to need the most help.

Re-employment in manufacturing minimises the earnings losses (on average). An advantageous outcome for production workers with manufacturing-specific skills is to stay employed in manufacturing. Earnings losses are reduced by re-employment in the old industry. Re-employment in services is associated with the largest earnings losses. There may be little retraining associated with these moves.

Source: Kletzer (2001a).

More recently, Kletzer carried out additional calculations focusing on displaced workers in the textile and clothing industries for the period 1993-2001. These data are presented in Tables 3.4 to 3.7. Data are presented for displaced workers previously employed in clothing, in textiles, in other import-sensitive industries and in all other manufacturing industries.[4]

Table 3.4 presents the basic demographic characteristics of displaced workers and shows that those from the clothing and textile industries represent only 11% of all surveyed displaced workers. Although there does not appear to be any discernable difference in age between the four groups, there is a higher prevalence of women and minorities in the textile and clothing industries. This finding can play an important role in the adjustment process, since in many families women tend to be second wage earners and are thus less likely to relocate in order to take a new job.

Table 3.4. Demographic characteristics of displaced workers

	Share	Age	Female	Minority	Married
Clothing	8%	39.47	75%	46%	56%
Textiles	3%	38.36	54%	35%	69%
Other import–sensitive	34%	39.61	36%	24%	63%
Other manufacturing	55%	39.11	31%	21%	61%

Source: Kletzer, unpublished calculations.

Table 3.5 shows that displaced workers from the textile and clothing industries are twice as likely as other displaced workers to have less than a high school education, and they are far less likely to have attended college. This finding supports the widely held perception that textile and clothing workers are low-skilled.

Table 3.5. Education characteristics of displaced workers

	Less than high school	High school graduate	Some college	College or more
Clothing	34%	40%	21%	6%
Textiles	23%	40%	30%	7%
Other import–sensitive	11%	37%	30%	23%
Other manufacturing	14%	38%	30%	18%

Source: Kletzer, unpublished calculations.

Table 3.6 provides insight into the jobs from which workers were separated. It appears that all four groups of displaced workers were separated from full-time (FT) jobs. Textile workers tend to have the longest average job tenure (approximately ten years), almost twice as long as workers displaced from the clothing industry. In fact, of the four groups, displaced workers from the clothing industry experienced the shortest average job tenure. On the other hand, approximately 80% of the workers displaced from the clothing industry were employed for more than ten years. This is considerably higher than for other displaced manufacturing workers. Data in the last two columns complement earlier findings concerning the level of education. According to these data, there is a higher probability that displaced workers from the clothing and textile industries will be operators and a lower probability that they will have a craft. Both of these findings support the conclusion that the textile and clothing industries tend to require low-skill work.

Table 3.6. Tenure characteristics of displaced workers

	Displaced from full-time job	Job tenure (years)	Tenure less than 10 years	Craft	Operator
Clothing	94%	5.59	19%	8%	76%
Textiles	97%	9.64	36%	11%	63%
Other import-sensitive	97%	7.33	28%	21%	35%
Other manufacturing	95%	6.96	26%	17%	42%

Source: Kletzer, unpublished calculations.

Table 3.7 provides some insight into workers' pre-separation earnings. Displaced textile and clothing workers earned significantly less than other displaced manufacturing workers. It is particularly interesting that the mean earnings for displaced textile and clothing workers are much lower than mean and median earnings for displaced workers from other import-sensitive industries. Approximately one-quarter of displaced clothing workers had earnings of less than USD 200 a week. This is considerably higher than the per cent of textile workers (9%) and the per cent of all other displaced workers (5%) earning less than USD 200 a week. This suggests that, in addition to being primarily low-skill industries, textile and clothing also tend to pay low wages.

Table 3.7. Earnings and replacement rates of displaced workers

	Mean earnings (USD)	Median earnings (USD)	Earnings less than USD 200/week	Earnings greater than USD 800/week	Wage replacement rate
Clothing	247.31	201.58	26%	3%	56%
Textiles	346.37	283.09	9%	4%	63%
Other import-sensitive	529.96	420.44	5%	22%	69%
Other manufacturing	471.37	383.89	5%	18%	69%

Source: Kletzer, unpublished calculations.

Overall, the preceding tables suggest that displaced workers from the textile and clothing industries tend to have a low level of education, low skills (and thus earn low wages), and are predominantly women and minorities (including minority women). All of these characteristics make it more difficult for them to adjust to changes in the labour market. Therefore, it is not surprising that the probability of re–employment within the two–year survey period is significantly lower for workers displaced from the clothing industry and somewhat lower for workers displaced from the textile industry than for workers displaced from other manufacturing industries.

Labour market adjustment policies

This section sets out a framework for analysing labour market adjustment policies and programmes in the developed countries. The framework may also assist policy makers in developing countries, as they consider options for responding to labour market adjustment burdens. Labour adjustment policies are only one part of a country's overall set of policies designed to respond to each country's unique economic and social conditions. They tend to fall into three major categories: *i)* preventive and reactive; *ii)* direct and indirect; and *iii)* targeted and general.

Classification of labour adjustment policies

In the first category, *preventive* measures are put in place primarily to *avoid* dislocations. They typically take the form of protecting an industry and its workers from foreign competition or some other economic development. *Reactive* measures are put in place in *response* to dislocations. They usually take the form of assisting workers during their period of unemployment and may include unemployment insurance, job search assistance and training.

Specific measures within these two major types of policies can also be qualified in terms of their effects. *Direct* measures aim at addressing workers' immediate needs. They are sometimes referred to as "active" labour market policies. Examples of direct labour market programmes for unemployed workers include financial assistance during the period of unemployment, job search assistance and training. *Indirect* measures have an indirect effect on such workers, in particular, and on the labour market, more generally. For example, raising a customs tariff on a particular product or group of products will likely have an indirect effect on the workers who produce those goods. In this case, the increased tariff may assist an industry facing foreign competition and prevent, or at least postpone, worker displacement from the industry.

The third major classification deals with the scope and reach of the labour market programmes and policies. *Targeted* measures tend to be highly focused on assisting either one or a limited group of industries and its workers. A government subsidy to a particular industry is an example of a targeted measure. *General* measures are designed to assist all industries and/or workers without discrimination or preference. Table 3.8 shows some examples of direct and indirect, targeted and general labour market policies and programmes.

Table 3.8. Classification of labour market adjustment policies

Measures	Direct	Indirect
General	Unemployment insurance, training and job search assistance for all displaced workers.	Macroeconomic, exchange rate and tax policies; across-the-board trade policy measures, *e.g.* an import surcharge.
Targeted	Special assistance for a particular group of workers, *e.g.* workers who lose their jobs owing to increased import competition.	Industry subsidies and preferential tax treatment, tariffs, quotas and other industry–specific trade policy measures.

Direct adjustment programmes have traditionally focused on providing financial assistance to unemployed workers through unemployment insurance. Over the last few years, there has been a shift in emphasis towards re–employment services, like training and job search assistance. Recent reforms in Germany, Japan and the United States have gone beyond job search assistance to include re-employment incentives, such as wage subsidies.

Direct programmes in most countries also tend to be general in nature and designed to assist all unemployed workers, regardless of worker demographics, industry of origin or cause of dislocation. The US Trade Adjustment Assistance (TAA) programme is an example of a targeted and direct programme. Under TAA, additional assistance beyond the traditional unemployment insurance system is offered to workers adversely affected by increased import competition and shifts in production.

Figure 3.1. Main phases in labour market adjustment policies and programmes

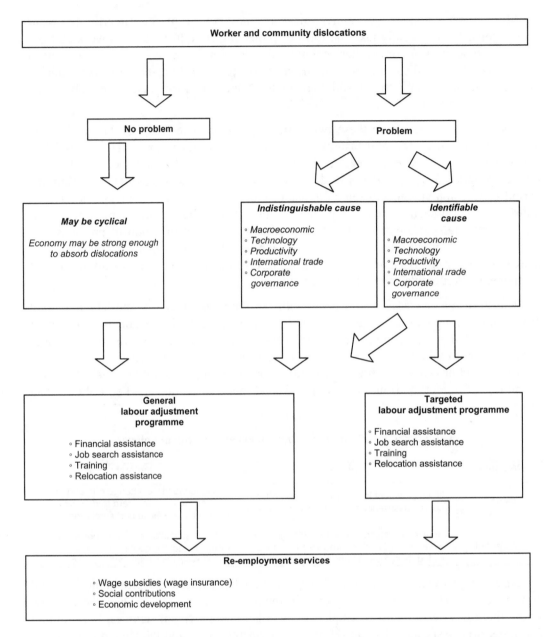

Macroeconomic policies – monetary and fiscal policies – although not specifically and exclusively designed to affect labour markets, can have a significant impact. They are therefore classified as general and indirect labour adjustment policies. One example would be the macroeconomic policies implemented in the United States during most of the 1990s, which resulted in a significant expansion in total employment. The rise in job creation reduced some of the adjustment burden that some workers experienced as a result of losing their jobs.

Exchange rate policies may also be seen as an example of general economic policies that have an indirect effect on labour market adjustment. The strong appreciation of the US dollar against the major trading currencies during the first part of the 1980s intensified competition for the US tradable-goods sector, resulting in a loss of export markets overseas and a significant increase in imports. This burden has more recently shifted to Japan and somewhat to Europe, as the values of the yen and the euro have appreciated against the US dollar.

Since it is difficult to trace the direct impact of macroeconomic and exchange rate policies on labour markets, these policies tend to be ignored in discussions of labour market adjustment policies and programmes. In addition, it is difficult to fine tune these policies. Yet, the macroeconomic environment is extremely important in determining the extent of the adjustment burden and the speed with which workers can find new jobs. For example, job search assistance is helped by an economy that is creating large numbers of jobs.

The most traditional examples of direct and preventive policies are industry subsidies, tax incentives and various kinds of trade policy measures. These measures tend to target a particular industry or group of industries, but they can also be designed to affect an entire economy. A schematic representation of labour market adjustment policies and programmes is shown in Figure 3.1.

Unemployment insurance

Unemployment insurance is the most common form of labour market adjustment programme throughout the world. Instituted in the early part of the twentieth century, unemployment insurance programmes have become a central element of the social safety net in most developed countries and more recently in some developing countries. As a general rule, unemployment insurance programmes provide some financial assistance to workers during their period of unemployment. The programmes tend to be financed through payroll taxes paid by employers and employees. For the most part, unemployment insurance programmes provide assistance to workers who involuntarily lose their jobs without cause. In rare cases, such as Japan, workers who voluntarily leave their jobs may also be eligible for assistance.[5]

Table 3.9 presents recent unemployment rates for France, Germany, Japan, the United Kingdom and the United States. Japan has traditionally experienced low unemployment rates, although that has been changing in recent years, with rates more than doubling during the 1990s. Among these countries, France has experienced the highest unemployment rates and the United States the most stable unemployment rates.

Table 3.9. Standardised unemployment rates

	1990	1995	2000
France	8.6%	11.4%	9.3%
Germany[1]	4.8%	8.2%	7.9%
Japan	2.1%	3.1%	4.7%
United Kingdom	6.9%	8.5%	5.4%
United States	5.6%	5.6%	4.0%
Total OECD	n.a.	7.4%	6.3%

1. For 1990 the unemployment rate is only for the former West Germany.

Source: OECD Employment Outlook 2002.

Information on the unemployment insurance programmes in five OECD countries is presented in Tables 3.10 and 3.11. More detailed information about the assistance programmes provided in each of these countries can be found in Annex 3.A2. There is wide variance among unemployment insurance programmes in these countries. Major differences occur in the amount and duration of financial assistance paid to unemployed workers. This reflects an ongoing debate over the potential disincentives of providing financial assistance to unemployed workers.

Some people argue that unemployment insurance should operate like any other type of insurance programme – workers pay a premium to insure themselves against the possibility of losing their job. When that occurs, the argument goes, workers would be entitled to compensation. This position is balanced against those who argue that providing financial assistance to unemployed workers may serve as a disincentive for finding a new job. This group argues that generous assistance to unemployed workers prolongs the duration of unemployment, thereby causing a moral hazard.

Table 3.10. Unemployment insurance provisions

	Replacement rate[1]	Minimum payment USD	Maximum payment USD	Duration (months)
France[2]	75%	8 214	60 184	60
Germany[2]	60%		30 890	12
Japan	80%		20 209	10
United Kingdom	Flat rate		4 084	6
United States	50%	4 524	15 600	6

1. The replacement rate is the percentage of the previous wage received by workers; the relevant exchange rates are mentioned in Annex 3.A2.

2. Country provides additional assistance once unemployment insurance is exhausted.

Source: *OECD Employment Outlook 2002.*

Programmes in each of the five countries covered fall along the spectrum of this debate. Following recent reforms, the United Kingdom provides the lowest amount of financial assistance to its unemployed workers. The US programme is next. Both the United Kingdom and the United States provide initial financial assistance for only six months, the shortest duration among the five countries analysed.[6] France, Germany and Japan provide more financial assistance for longer periods of time. The Japanese unemployment insurance programme is the closest to a true "insurance" programme, in that all unemployed workers are eligible for assistance, whether their separation is voluntary or not. The French programme appears to be the most generous.

Table 3.11. Brief summary of unemployment insurance programmes in five countries

	Qualifying period	Duration of benefits	Replacement rate	"Fallback" programmes	Comments
France	5 alternative ways to qualify for different benefit durations, depending on work history in the previous 3 years	4 months to 33 months, depending on employment history and age	57% to 75% of previous earnings (no maximum); benefit rate falls after an initial jobless period.		
Germany	12 months in the last 3 years	156-832 days, depending on age and employment history	67% of previous net wage (60% for workers without children)	57% of previous net wage (50% without children) Means-tested; unlimited duration	12-week waiting period for quitters
Japan	26 weeks of work in past year	90-360 days; increases with age, years worked and full-time status	50% to 80%, depending on age and rate of pay, to a maximum	Universal welfare, unlimited duration	Some restrictions on quitters
United Kingdom	2 years continuous employment	6 months	Flat rate cash benefits (GBP 48.25 in 1996) per week.	Means-tested unemployment assistance, based on household income; unlimited duration	Unemployment assistance is more generous than unemployment insurance, especially if no other earners in the household; can include full rent and property tax subsidies
United States	26 weeks of work in past year	26 weeks (plus 13 weeks extended benefits in cases of high unemployment)	50% to 70% maximum Average replacement rate 30% to 40%	Means-tested welfare benefits available to single parents only Lifetime limit of 5 years	Very low take-up rate; quitters are disqualified; benefits are taxed as income

Source: Author's summary based on available information.

Training programmes

Next to unemployment insurance, training is probably the second most prevalent aspect of direct or active labour market adjustment programmes in OECD countries. In countries like Germany, providing training to unemployed workers is part of a comprehensive policy of training and vocational programmes. Other countries employ a mix of private and public training schemes.

Training programmes fall into two broad categories: providing basic skills in language and maths to those with low educational attainment; and providing specific job-related skills. Deficiencies in basic skills are particularly common among workers in traditional low-skill manufacturing jobs, for example in the textile and clothing industries, where many workers have less than a high school education. The lack of basic skills places an added burden on an already arduous adjustment process when such workers face the need to find a new job.

In recent years, there have been efforts to engage the private sector more in the provision of specific job-related skills training. In Germany, tax credits are used to encourage firms to hire and train new workers. In the United States in recent years, there has been a shift from government-provided training to government-financed privately provided training. Workers are given what amounts to vouchers, which they can use to finance approved training.

Analysis of training programmes is severely limited by the lack of data concerning who is trained, for what, at what cost, and how useful the training is in helping the worker find a new job. In spite of the lack of useful empirical research on the effectiveness of various training schemes, there is evidence that on-the-job training tends to be more efficient than classroom training. Accordingly, government-sponsored training programmes have moved more in that direction in recent years.

Table 3.12 compares expenditures on training and unemployment insurance in the five countries. France and Germany spend the most on training and unemployment insurance. This is due to a combination of ambitious training programmes, generous assistance and relatively higher unemployment rates than in the other countries. In relative terms, the cost of the rather generous assistance in the Japanese programme is offset in part by the lower incidence of unemployment. The United States appears to spend the least on assisting its unemployed workers. A similar pattern exists regarding expenditures on training. France and Germany spend the most, while the low percentage for Japan is primarily due to its low unemployment rate. The United Kingdom and the United States spend relatively less on training their unemployed workers than the other countries.

It is interesting to note the gap in expenditures on training between France and Germany at one extreme and Japan, the United Kingdom and the United States at the other. Training programmes in France and Germany do not appear to be a substitute for unemployment compensation but a complement. There is also no evidence that training reduces the adjustment period and thus the need for more unemployment compensation. In fact, it some cases, training may actually prolong the adjustment process, but may also prevent workers from experiencing long-term income losses as a result of their job loss.

Table 3.12. Expenditure on training and unemployment compensation, 2000

	Training	Unemployment compensation
	(% of GDP)	(% of GDP)
France	0.22%	1.38%
Germany	0.34%	1.89%
Japan	0.03%	0.55%
United Kingdom	0.04%	0.56%
United States	0.04%	0.30%

Source: OECD Employment Outlook 2002.

Trade adjustment assistance

As mentioned above, unemployment insurance programmes in most OECD countries are designed to assist all unemployed workers, regardless of industry, worker demographics or cause of dislocation. The most significant exception to this general framework is the US TAA programme. By comparison, more generous labour market adjustment programmes in most other OECD countries somehow lessen the need for special programmes for workers from a specific industry or whose job loss can be traced to a specific cause, *i.e.* import competition. The absence of targeted trade-related labour programmes in other OECD countries may also be a reflection of the inherent difficulty of isolating worker dislocations due to trade from other causes, *e.g.* technological change, productivity gains and shifts in labour demand and supply.

The US Trade Expansion Act of 1962, which provided President Kennedy with the authority to enter into GATT negotiations, established the TAA. Initially, the programme was designed to provide extended financial assistance, beyond the traditional 26 weeks of unemployment insurance, to workers who lose their jobs owing to an increase in imports. Very few workers received assistance during the programme's first 12 years, largely because of rigid eligibility criteria. In 1974, Congress eased the eligibility criteria and expanded the assistance to include training.[7] Since 1975, over 3 million American workers have been certified as eligible for assistance under TAA, and approximately 1.9 million have received assistance.

Between 1975 and 1999, workers from the steel, auto, textile and clothing industries comprised a large majority of TAA participants (Figure 3.2). According to more recent data, between January 2002 and July 2003 a little more than 23% of the petitions, representing close to 28% of eligible workers, were from the textile and clothing industries (Annex Table 3.A2.13).

Figure 3.2. TAA participants by industry, 1975 to 1999

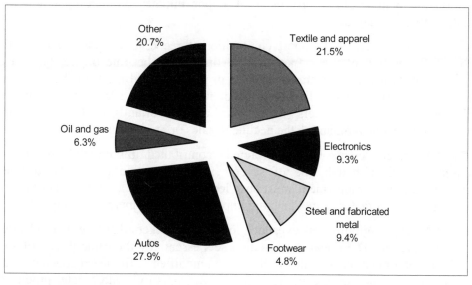

Source: US General Accounting Office (2001).

Under the programme, workers who enrol in training can currently receive up to 78 weeks of financial assistance, beyond the standard 26 weeks of unemployment insurance. In addition, they can receive job search and relocation assistance. The financial assistance is considered an entitlement, and Congress must appropriate sufficient funds to provide payments to all eligible workers. Training is a *capped* entitlement, and Congress fixes the total amount of funds appropriated for training, but every eligible participant is entitled to enrol in some government-sponsored training.[8] TAA also provides funds for job search and relocation assistance, although not many workers request this assistance.

With the approval of NAFTA in 1993, Congress established a separate programme for workers who lose their jobs in industries that face increased imports from and/or relocate production to Canada or Mexico. Assistance provided to workers under the NAFTA–TAA programme was almost identical to that provided under the general TAA programme, but there were some differences in coverage. In addition to covering workers who lost their jobs from import-competing industries, NAFTA–TAA provided assistance to workers who lost their jobs owing to shifts in production to Canada or Mexico. In addition, some secondary workers, who lost jobs because they worked for suppliers or downstream producers for firms that faced increased import competition from Canada or Mexico, received assistance. Annex Table 3.A2.15 shows the characteristics of workers who received assistance under TAA and NAFTA–TAA in 1999 and 2000.

In August 2002, President George W. Bush signed the Trade Act of 2002, which granted him the authority to enter into multilateral and bilateral trade negotiations. The Act also included the most extensive reform and expansion of the Trade Adjustment Assistance programme since it was established (Box 3.2). The new TAA provisions must now be fully enacted and the necessary funds appropriated to enable the reformed programme to operate. With its broader scope, the TAA annual budget is estimated to triple over the next few years.

One of the key issues regarding TAA is the mechanism by which a worker's job loss can be traced to increased imports. The TAA Act sets out a rather sophisticated process for making this determination. A group of workers, or some organisation acting on behalf of a group of workers, *e.g.* a firm or union, may petition the US Department of Labor. Based on the petition, the Department of Labor initiates an investigation into the circumstances of the lay-offs.

In the case of increased import competition, three criteria apply: *i)* a significant number or proportion of the workers in the firms have become or are threatened to become totally or partially separated; *ii)* sales or production of the firms have decreased absolutely; and *iii)* imports of like products or those that are directly competitive with articles produced by the workers' firms contributed importantly to the total or partial separation or threat thereof, and to the decline in sales or production.

The US judicial courts have interpreted "contributed importantly" to mean that increased imports, although one of several factors contributing to the decline in production, sales and employment, must be at least as important as all the other factors. In other words, another factor cannot be more important than the increase in imports.

In 2002, TAA eligibility was expanded to include workers that lose their jobs due to shifts in production. The relevant legislation sets essentially the same three criteria for making this determination, with the third criterion modified to fit the expanded definition: *iii)* a shift in production of like articles or directly competitive with articles produced by such workers' firm contributed importantly to the total or partial separation or threat thereof, and to the decline in sales or production. Since the programme was only expanded in 2002 to cover eligibility under the shift in production criteria, the courts have not yet had an opportunity to interpret the legislation. It is fair to assume that none of these determinations will be clear-cut and easy to make. Workers have the right to appeal the Department of Labor's initial determination. They can also take their complaints to the US Court of International Trade.

Box 3.2. Some of the key TAA reforms of 2002

Secondary workers: TAA eligibility criteria were expanded to include workers who lose their jobs in plants producing parts that are inputs into import-competing final goods. Some of these workers were already covered under NAFTA–TAA. This provision could result in a doubling in the number of workers eligible for assistance.

Refundable tax credit for health insurance: Workers are eligible to receive an advance of 65% of a refundable tax credit to help offset the cost of maintaining health insurance for up to two years.

Shift in production: TAA eligibility criteria were expanded to include workers who lose their jobs owing to shifts in production to countries which have bilateral agreements with the United States or "where there has been or is likely to be an increase in imports...."

Wage insurance: Workers over 50 years old and earning less than USD 50 000 a year may be eligible to receive 50% of the difference between their old and new wage for up to two years, if the new wage is lower than the old wage.

NAFTA-TAA and TAA: NAFTA-TAA and TAA were harmonised and combined.

Training appropriation: Congress doubled the legislative cap on the training appropriation, from USD 110 million to USD 220 million a year. Congress also has to agree to the actual annual appropriation for training.

Extension of income maintenance by 26 weeks: Workers enrolled in training may be eligible to receive income maintenance for up to two years. This constitutes an increase 26 weeks from the previous limit.

Increased job search and relocation assistance: The assistance was updated for inflation.

TAA for farmers: A programme was established to provide assistance to farmers and fishermen when the international price of a commodity falls more than 20% below the previous five-year average.

Increased funds for TAA for firms: Congress raised the appropriation cap on this very small programme which provides loan guarantees to firms for the purpose of retooling and responding to international competition.

The inherent difficulties associated with determining the cause of a job loss, *i.e.* increased imports or a shift in production, will now be compounded by the inclusion of secondary workers. The 2002 law defines secondary workers as workers employed by supplier firms, downstream producers, and firms that provide contract services who are separated or threatened with separation if their separation is due to a loss of business with a firm where workers have been certified as eligible to apply for trade adjustment assistance.

Difficulties associated with identifying the cause of displacement, together with the issue of providing different unemployment and re–employment services based on that cause, have led many policy analysts to recommend implementation of broad labour adjustment programmes for all displaced workers regardless of the causes of displacement.[9] In an overview of the Globalisation Balance Sheet project undertaken by the Institute for International Economics, Richardson (2003) stresses the emerging consensus that policies should: "*i)* move away from specific industry- and job-based relief and towards worker empowerment; *ii)* move towards education and skill-building experience, including on-the-job training; and *iii)* move towards insurance programmes that preserve an individual's lifetime earnings potential" (Richardson, 2003, p. 12).

At the outset, it appears that the TAA is a reflection of the unique way of granting trade negotiating authority to the president in which political compromises are reached on many trade-related issues, including the means for offering some kind of compensation for workers adversely affected by trade. The ultimate priority for any labour market adjustment programme should be its effectiveness in assisting workers to find new jobs, as soon as possible, with the least amount of permanent income loss. Since the United States is the only country with a targeted programme devoted to workers adversely affected by trade, there is insufficient evidence to test the effectiveness of this approach.

Other labour adjustment measures

Labour market adjustment policies and programmes in most OECD countries are currently undergoing reform. The reform is motivated by three factors. First, many have been experiencing high unemployment rates that coincide with long periods of unemployment. Second, the high incidence of unemployment has raised the cost of maintaining generous unemployment insurance systems. Third, there is an ongoing debate over the effect of unemployment assistance on prolonging unemployment. It is argued that generous assistance serves as a disincentive to work, prolonging the period of unemployment and exacerbating a country's unemployment rate. Although there is limited empirical evidence to support the argument, it has gained attention in countries with high unemployment, like Germany and France.

In general, reforms of labour market adjustment programmes are proceeding on the basis of three principles. First, direct financial assistance has been reduced in an effort to address the disincentive argument – the weekly amount of financial assistance has been reduced in France, Germany and the United Kingdom. Second, there has been a shift in emphasis from unemployment compensation to re-employment assistance. Third, in providing re–employment assistance, efforts have been made to improve the management and co-ordination of services. There has been an effort to make unemployment assistance programmes more "customer friendly" in each of the five countries analysed. Job seekers work with re-employment counsellors, who assist them in identifying and obtaining new employment. In some cases, workers are required to actually sign a "contract" with the counsellors, formalising their job search plans.

In recent years, the policy focus concerning unemployment assistance in the United States has also shifted toward re-employment services. The idea of a "one-stop shop" for unemployment assistance – inspired by the German system – has been further developed and promoted by the United States. Japan has also established "Hello Work" centres, similar to the one-stop centres in the United States. On the other hand, the United States has not followed the other large OECD countries in reducing direct financial assistance. It periodically extends the provision of unemployment insurance during periods of prolonged high unemployment.

Probably the most creative innovation in unemployment assistance over the last few years is the introduction of "wage insurance". Both Germany and the United States (under TAA) have recently introduced a limited version. Under the US programme, workers who are over 50 years of age and who earned less than USD 50 000 at their previous job, may be eligible to receive half of the difference between their new and old wage, if their new wage is less than their previous wage. The programme is aimed at reducing one of the major barriers to re-employment. It is also hoped that workers will receive on-the-job training at their new job, as this tends to be more effective than government-financed classroom training.

Conclusion

Available analytical work on the impact of globalisation and international trade on labour adjustment suggests that workers who lose their jobs owing to increased imports or shifts in production do not appear to be different from other displaced workers. Similarly, their adjustment process does not appear to differ significantly. Trade-related displacement may suggest the need for labour market adjustment policies and programmes but not necessarily a special response.

It is increasingly difficult to isolate the causes of worker displacement. Technological change, productivity gains, increased import competition and shifts in production can all contribute to job losses. This difficulty has led many policy analysts to oppose targeted labour market adjustment policies and programmes for special groups of workers, *e.g.* workers who lose their jobs owing to increased imports or shifts in production, and instead put into place broad labour adjustment programmes for all displaced workers. This issue is likely to remain prominent in the foreseeable future with the intensification of international relations among countries and improved technological developments.

Instead of debating special *versus* general labour market adjustment policies and programmes, more effort needs to be made to determine which interventions are more effective. Most OECD countries are attempting to improve the co-ordination of their unemployment benefits and employment services. There has been an effort to make the process more "customer-friendly".

There is increasing reliance on training as part of the toolbox of labour market adjustment programmes. Many workers coming out of traditional low-wage manufacturing industries lack basic language and maths skills, which prevents them from acquiring the specific skills required in the new jobs being created. The shift in the structure of the labour market in the OECD countries has also resulted in gaps between the skills that workers needed in their old jobs and those demanded by their future jobs. Governments are employing various subsidies and tax incentives to encourage training and skills enhancement.

One creative innovation in recent years has been the advent of wage insurance. Although somewhat similar to existing wage subsidy programmes, wage insurance is designed for workers whose new wage is lower than their previous wage. By subsidising some portion of the difference between the two, it is hoped that workers will be encouraged to take a new job sooner. It is also hoped that new employers will provide the worker with on-the-job training, which has proven to be more effective and cheaper than government-financed classroom training. Germany and the United States have recently introduced limited programmes for older workers.

It is also important to see labour market adjustment policies and programmes in the context of a country's broader social safety net. The best example is the issue of health care in the United States. The United States is one of the few developed countries without universal health care. Since employers provide health insurance and pensions for many workers, when workers lose their jobs, they and their families also face losing their health insurance and pensions. One way to reduce the "special-ness" of TAA would be to provide the new health insurance tax credit to all unemployed workers, regardless of the cause of displacement.

With only a few months before the scheduled elimination of the ATC, there is considerable anxiety in the worldwide textile and clothing community about the emergence of more competitive and integrated suppliers, particularly in China, that may capture a disproportional share of the economic benefits arising from the phasing out of the ATC. In particular, several developing countries that have excelled as offshore assembly centres, owing in part to their MFA quota allocations, will be exposed in the post-ATC period to the inherent vulnerability of international production fragmentation. Developing countries are certainly not exempt from labour pressures due to changes in international trade and investment.

In some ways, developing countries are at a disadvantage, as many do not have well-developed social safety nets. On the other hand, the wealth of experience in the developed countries may provide developing countries, particularly the most advanced ones, with important lessons from which to develop their own labour market adjustment policies and programmes. International financial institutions may also help them overcome the resource constraints associated with developing a response to issues related to structural adjustment.

In stark contrast to the amount of resources being devoted to labour market adjustment measures, governments do not collect the data necessary to determine the effectiveness of such programmes. More information about the experience of displaced workers and the effectiveness of the various elements in labour market adjustment programmes could make an important contribution to the reform of existing programmes and the development of new ones. The technology exists for such data collection; governments need to see better data collection as a priority and commit sufficient resources to this effort.

Finally, it needs to be stressed that a sound and dynamic macroeconomic environment is the most important factor in addressing labour market pressures. The main objective is for workers to be employed in high-skill and high-wage jobs. All of the labour market adjustment policies and programmes discussed in this chapter are only effective if they result in workers finding new employment.

Annex 3.A1. Tables

Annex Table 3.A1.1. Job losses in textiles and clothing in six countries, 1970-2000

Thousands

	France			Germany			Japan		
	Textiles	Clothing	Total	Textiles	Clothing	Total	Textiles	Clothing	Total
1970	451	338	789	501	379	880	1 349	364	1 713
1975	364	304	668	357	288	645	1 093	467	1 560
1980	297	272	569	320	227	547	776	437	1 213
1985	n.a.	n.a.	n.a.	246	170	416	706	459	1 165
1990	150	143	293	229	143	372	634	488	1 122
1995	131	139	270	261	122	383	491	375	866
2000	114	100	214	168	117	285	352	224	576
1970-2000	-337	-238	-575	-333	-262	-595	-997	-140	−1 137
% change	-74.7%	-70.4%	-72.9%	-66.5%	-69.1%	-67.6%	-73.9%	-38.5%	-66.4%

	United Kingdom			United States			Italy		
	Textiles	Clothing	Total	Textiles	Clothing	Total	Textiles	Clothing	Total
1970	625	357	982	1 113	1 164	2 277			
1975	511	346	857	996	1 065	2 061			
1980	351	277	628	986	1 150	2 136			
1985	259	237	496	840	887	1 727			
1990	227	203	430	829	807	1 636			
1995	188	173	361	842	724	1 566	332	274	606
2000	149	109	258	528	633	1 161	352	206	558
1970-2000	-476	-248	-724	-585	-531	-1116	20[1]	-68[1]	-48[1]
% change	-76.2%	-69.5%	-73.7%	-52.6%	-45.6%	-49.0%			

1. 1995-2000.

Source: *United Nations Yearbook of Industrial Statistics*; Bureau of Labour Statistics, US Department of Labor; and Cline (1990).

Annex Table 3.A1.2. Employment in textiles and clothing, by production segment

		Employment (thousands)		Segment as % of total employment	
	China	2000	2001	2000	2001
	Textile industry	4 211.5	4 244.3		
	Natural fibres	3 782.7	3 808.6	89.7%	89.8%
	Preparation of textile fibres	3 057.8	3 081.9	72.6%	72.6%
	Finishing of textiles	379.8	379.2	8.9%	9.0%
	Made-up cotton articles and cordage	299.2	303.1	7.1%	7.1%
	Knitting textile industry, excluding knitwear	45.9	44.5	1.0%	1.1%
	Synthetic fibres	428.8	435.7	10.3%	10.2%
	Clothing industry	2 871.9	2 664.5		
	Knitwear	499.4	476.1	17.9%	17.4%
	Garment textile industry and others	2 372.5	2 188.3	82.1%	82.6%
	Equipment manufacturing industry	165.3	164.2		
NACE	**European Union**	1996	2000	1996	2000
17	**Total textile**	1 165.961	1 110.1		
171	Preparation and spinning of textile fibres	150.857	128.6	12.9%	11.6%
172	Textile weaving	178.526	176.0	15.3%	15.9%
173	Finishing of textiles	114.584	112.6	9.8%	10.1%
174	Made-up articles, except apparel	128.729	126.6	11.0%	11.4%
175	Other textiles	177.235	176.4	15.2%	15.9%
176	Knitted and crocheted fabrics	47.969	50.5	4.1%	4.5%
177	Knitted and crocheted articles	188.85	142.3	16.2%	12.8%
18	**Total clothing**	1 136.559	1 025.0		
181	Leather clothes	13.427	10.4	1.2%	1.0%
182	Other wearing apparel and accessories	959.303	803.6	84.4%	78.4%
183	Dressing and dyeing of fur	14.7	13.6	1.3%	1.3%
JSIC Rev. 10	**Japan**	1994	2000	1994	2000
1700	**Textiles**	517.7	352.4		
1710	Spinning, weaving and finishing of textiles	217.5	130.4	42.0%	37.0%
1711	Preparation of textile fibres; weaving of textiles	133.9	76.2	25.9%	21.6%
1712	Finishing of textiles	83.6	54.2	16.2%	15.4%
1720	Other textiles	139.1	114.5	26.9%	32.5%
1721	Made-up textile articles, except apparel	78.2	64.5	15.1%	18.3%
1722	Carpets and rugs	9.3	7.2	1.8%	2.1%
1723	Cordage, rope, twine and netting	10.3	8.5	2.0%	2.4%
1729	Other textiles, nec	41.2	34.3	8.0%	9.7%
1730	Knitted and crocheted fabrics and articles	161.1	107.4	31.1%	30.5%
1800	**Wearing apparel and fur**	407.0	223.7		
1810	Wearing apparel, except fur apparel	406.0	223.0	99.8%	99.7%
1820	Dressing and dyeing of fur; articles of fur	1.0	0.7	0.2%	0.3%
1900	**Leather and articles; footwear**	82.7	58.9		
1910	Leather and articles of leather	35.9	24.3	43.4%	41.3%
1911	Tanning and dressing of leather	11.1	8.4	13.5%	14.3%
1912	Luggage, handbags and the like, saddlery and harness	24.8	15.9	29.9%	27.0%
1920	Footwear	46.8	34.5	56.6%	58.7%

Annex Table 3.A1.2. Employment in textiles and clothing, by production segment (continued)

SIC	Korea	Employment (thousands)		Segment as % of total employment	
		1990	2000	1990	2000
1700	**Textiles**	355.2	232.2		
1710	Spinning, weaving and finishing of textiles	269.3	154.7	75.8%	66.6%
1711	Preparation of textile fibres; weaving of textiles	219.7	95.8	61.9%	41.3%
1712	Finishing of textiles	49.6	58.9	14.0%	25.4%
1720	Other textiles	46.1	46.2	13.0%	19.9%
1721	Made-up textile articles, except apparel	24.4	27.2	6.9%	11.7%
1722	Carpets and rugs	1.1	1.0	0.3%	0.5%
1723	Cordage, rope, twine and netting	7.5	4.9	2.1%	2.1%
1729	Other textiles, nec	13.2	13.1	3.7%	5.6%
1730	Knitted and crocheted fabrics and articles	39.8	31.3	11.2%	13.5%
1800	**Wearing apparel and fur**	240.4	152.5		
1810	Wearing apparel, except fur apparel	234.6	150.1	97.6%	98.4%
1820	Dressing and dyeing of fur; articles of fur	5.8	2.4	2.4%	1.6%
1900	**Leather and articles; footwear**	217.1	52.9		
1910	Leather and articles of leather	37.5	19.4	17.3%	36.7%
1911	Tanning and dressing of leather	20.2	10.3	9.3%	19.4%
1912	Luggage, handbags and the like, saddlery and harness	17.3	9.1	8.0%	17.2%
1920	Footwear	179.6	33.5	82.7%	63.3%

SIC	United States	1970	2002	1970	2002
22+239	**Total textile**	1 136.8	619.8		
22	Textile mill products	974.8	431.8	85.7%	69.7%
221	Broad woven fabric mills, cotton	212.1	49.5	18.7%	8.0%
222	Broad woven fabric mills, synthetics	100.1	45.9	8.8%	7.4%
223	Broad woven fabric mills, wool	36.6	5.3	3.2%	0.9%
224	Narrow fabric mills	29.6	16.2	2.6%	2.6%
225	Knitting mills	254.1	89.1	22.4%	14.4%
226	Textile finishing, except wool	83.8	50.1	7.4%	8.1%
227	Carpets and rugs	57.4	62.9	5.0%	10.1%
228	Yarn and thread mills	130.9	65.1	11.5%	10.5%
229	Miscellaneous textile goods	70.3	47.7	6.2%	7.7%
239	Miscellaneous fabricated textile products	162	188	14.3%	30.3%
2391	Curtains and draperies	32[1]	16.6	2.8%	2.7%
2392	House furnishings, nec	47[1]	46.9	4.1%	7.6%
2396	Automotive and apparel trimmings	31.3[1]	57.3	2.8%	9.2%
231-8	**Total clothing**	1 108.4	322		
231	Men's and boys' suits and coats	119	15.2	10.7%	4.7%
232	Men's and boys' furnishings	374.9	105.7	33.8%	32.8%
234	Women's and misses' outerwear	424.3	150.3	38.3%	46.7%
235	Women's and children's undergarments	116.7	13.7	10.5%	4.3%
236	Girls' and children's outerwear	73.5	9.6	6.6%	3.0%
238	Fur goods, and misc. apparel and accessories	65.5[1]	27.5	5.6%	8.5%

Note: Due to confidentiality rules, NACE 3-digit categories are aggregated into one or several categories in some EU member states.

1. 1972 instead of 1970.

Source: For Japan and Korea, OECD Structural Statistics for Industry and Services Database. For China, OECD calculations based on CNTIC (2001/02), Report on China Textile Industry Development. For the United States, US Bureau of Labor Statistics, National Employment, Hours, and Earnings Data. For the EU, EURATEX data.

Annex 3.A2. Country-specific systems

The French unemployment insurance system

The French unemployment insurance system is probably the most generous among the five countries. The programme consists of two parts: unemployment insurance, financed by employer and employee contributions, and a "solidarity scheme", financed by the state. Workers who involuntarily lose their jobs and have made contributions to the system are eligible to receive assistance under the programme. The level of assistance is based on the worker's previous earnings. Workers who exhaust their unemployment insurance, have difficulty finding employment or are near retirement, may be eligible for assistance under the solidarity scheme.

The French unemployment insurance system is unique, in that it is managed by a combination of private organisations, including numerous employers' associations and trade unions. At the national level, this organisation is called Unedic, and it is responsible for setting the overall policy for the programme. At the local level, the joint organisation is called Assedic, and it is responsible for administering the programme. Annex Table 3.A2.1 presents the basic elements of the unemployment insurance programme and the solidarity scheme.

Annex Table 3.A2.1. The French unemployment insurance and solidarity scheme

Group	Unemployment Insurance	Solidarity scheme
Management	The "social partners" through Unedic	The state
Assistance	Earnings-related assistance, for a limited period of time	Fixed amount of assistance for an unlimited period
Financing	Employer and employee contributions	State budget
Target population	Workers who have involuntarily lost their jobs	Workers who have exhausted unemployment insurance; hard to re-employ; and older workers
Administering agency	Assedic	Assedic

Source: Assedic (2003).

Currently, total contributions for unemployment insurance equal 6.4% of payroll, up to a maximum of 8.5 times the minimum wage, or USD 1 044.45 (unless otherwise noted, EUR 1=USD 1.10). The employer's share is 4% of payroll and the employee's share is 2.4% of payroll. Among the five countries surveyed, France is the only one in which the employer's contribution is larger than the employee's.

Workers applying for unemployment assistance, are asked to sign a "Return to Employment Aid Plan" (PARE), which commits them actively to seek re-employment. Companies with fewer than 1 000 employees must provide workers with a PARE as a form of advance notification of job termination. This allows workers to file for unemployment insurance and begin meeting with the employment service, even before their last day of work.

Once workers meet with representative from the National Agency for Employment (ANPE), they are asked to develop and sign a "Personal Action Plan" (PAP), which covers the type of jobs the worker is seeking as well as the worker's request for training. The local Assedic office monitors the worker's progress in achieving the goals set forth in the PAP. If the worker remains unemployed after six months, he or she may be asked to develop a new plan. If the worker remains unemployed after 12 months, the local Assedic may provide a subsidy to a prospective employer.

Workers who sign a PAP are eligible to receive: *i)* unemployment insurance for the entire duration of eligibility; *ii)* a mobility grant equal to travel expenses up to USD 2 086.70; *iii)* a training grant covering part of the costs for tuition, travel and accommodation during training; and *iv)* a special grant for those unemployed for more than 12 months. Workers can receive the special grant for up to three years, at a declining scale (40% of gross salary during the first year, 30% of gross salary during the second year and 20% of gross salary during the third).

The French unemployment insurance system also provides assistance to workers who leave their jobs in order to follow a spouse who moves for professional reasons. Another unique aspect of the French unemployment insurance programme is that workers under 50 years of age can continue to receive financial assistance for a maximum of 18 months *after* re-employment. This is designed to help workers who take temporary or part-time jobs while they continue to look for full-time employment or workers who have lost their major employment, although they maintain a secondary job. To be eligible, the worker's current salary can not be greater than 70% of his or her pre-layoff income.

Annex Tables 3.A2.2 to 3.A2.4 provide more details about the French unemployment insurance programme. Annex Table 3.A2.2 presents information on the amount of assistance workers receive and Table 3.A2.3 presents information on the duration of that assistance, while Annex Table 3.A2.4 provides information on re-employment benefits.

Annex Table 3.A2.2. Unemployment insurance assistance

Monthly gross earnings	Initial assistance	Social contribution USD
Less than USD 1 089.44	75% of salary	
Between USD 1 089.44 and USD 1 193.39	Minimum assistance 27.24 per day	
Between USD 1 193.39 and USD 1 970.30	40.4% of gross daily earnings plus USD 11.17 per day	3% of previous earnings (for pension)
Between USD 1 970.30 and USD 10 700.80	57.4% of gross daily earnings	11.25% of assistance, if above USD 33

Source: Assedic (2003).

Annex Table 3.A2.3. Duration of assistance

Duration of previous employment	Duration of assistance
6 months within the last 22 months	7 months
14 months within the last 24 months	23 months
Between the age of 50 and 57, over 27 months within the last 36 months	36 months
Above 57 years old, 27 months within the last 36 months and 100 quarters of contributions to retirement pension	42 months

Source: Assedic (2003).

Annex Table 3.A2.4. Re–employment benefits

Gross salary and other income	Amount of assistance while working	Example
During the first six months of new employment		
Level of monthly earnings equal to or less than half the guaranteed minimum wage *i.e.* USD 668.32	Full amount of assistance	Before taking a new job, assistance was USD 447.48 a month. Assuming the monthly salary from the new job equals USD 419.23, the worker will continue to receive the full amount of unemployment insurance, in addition to his/her new salary.
Level of monthly earnings is greater than half the guaranteed minimum wage *i.e.* greater than USD 668.32	40% of unemployment insurance assistance, in excess of USD 668.32	Before taking a new job, assistance was USD 447.48 a month. Assuming the monthly salary from the new job equals USD 838.48, the worker will receive USD 379.41 a month of unemployment insurance, in addition to his/her new salary.
During the following six months		
All levels of earnings	Unemployment assistance will be reduced by 40% of gross earnings.	Before taking a new job, assistance was USD 447.48 a month. Assuming the monthly salary from the new job equals USD 838.48, the worker will receive USD 112.09 a month of unemployment insurance, in addition to his/her new salary.

Source: Assedic (2003).

Annex Table 3.A2.5 presents data on the minimum amount of daily assistance under unemployment insurance, the solidarity scheme and early retirement programmes. The programmes are designed so that a worker can move through all three, if necessary. For example, an older worker who has difficulty finding a new job may initially receive unemployment insurance. If the worker has not found a new job by the end of the benefit period, he or she may be eligible to continue receiving assistance under the solidarity scheme. Workers may be eligible for an early retirement pension, if they are over 57 years of age and if they have made at least 100 quarterly contributions to the national pension fund.

Annex Table 3.A2.5. Minimum daily assistance

Programme	Minimum daily assistance
Unemployment insurance	
Minimum assistance	USD 27.24
Fixed amount	USD 11.17
Solidarity allowance	
Allowance for special categories of job seekers	USD 10.51
Specific solidarity allowance	USD 14.92
Increased allowance	USD 21.42
Retirement-equivalent assistance	USD 32.19
Early retirement	
Minimum amount	USD 29.58
Minimum gradual early retirement	USD 14.78

Source: Assedic (2003).

The German unemployment insurance system

The German unemployment insurance programme is one of the oldest in the world. Until recently, it was also one of the more generous. It is similar to others, in that it is financed through a payroll tax paid by employers and employees. The Federal Employment Office (*Bundesanstalt fur Arbeit*), an independent government agency, administers the programme. The German unemployment insurance system has recently been the focus of much attention as its reform is at the centre of Chancellor Schroeder's Agenda 2010. A commission established by Chancellor Schroeder and chaired by Peter Hartz, CEO of Volkswagen, developed most of the reform proposals.

Until recently the German unemployment insurance system consisted of three parts: *i)* unemployment money (*Arbeitslosengeld*), based on previous wages and financed exclusively through payroll taxes, provided assistance to workers for 12 to 32 months; *ii)* unemployment assistance (*Arbeitslosenhilfe*), was means-tested and financed exclusively though expenditures from the federal budget. Workers could receive unlimited unemployment assistance once they exhausted their unemployment money; and *iii)* social assistance (*Sozialhilfe*), based on family assets and financed exclusively through expenditures from state budgets, was available to workers who were not eligible for unemployment assistance.

Although there is limited direct empirical evidence of the relationship, many people have argued that the potential for significant government assistance for an almost unlimited period contributed to the high rate of long–term unemployment in Germany. Table 3.A2.6 provides a comparison of long-term unemployment rates in the five large OECD countries. Long-term unemployed as a share of total unemployed is in fact higher in Germany than in France, Japan, the United Kingdom and the United States. It is also substantially higher than the average for all OECD countries.

Annex Table 3.A2.6. Long-term unemployed as a share of total unemployed

	1990		1998		2001	
	>6 months	>1 year	>6 months	>1 year	>6 months	>1 year
France	55.5%	38.0%	64.3%	44.2%	57.2%	37.6%
Germany	64.7%[1]	46.8%[1]	69.6%	52.6%	67.6%[2]	51.5%[2]
Japan	39.0%	19.1%	39.3%	20.9%	46.2%	26.6%
United Kingdom	50.3%	34.4%	47.3%	32.7%	43.6%	27.7%
United States	10.0%	5.5%	14.1%	8.0%	11.8%	6.1%
Total OECD	44.6%	30.9%	48.6%	33.4%	41.8%	27.5%

1. Only covers West Germany.
2. Data for 2000.

Source: OECD Employment Outlook 2002.

Reducing the duration of unemployment assistance and tightening the eligibility requirements were among the major objectives of the Hartz Commission. The following is a list of the Commission's recommendations, as well as a comment on implementation. They are listed in order of their appearance in the Commission's report to the Chancellor.

1. Creation of job centres. Unemployment insurance offices, currently financed by the federal government, and social assistance offices, currently financed by the state governments would be combined. The federal government would fully finance the new combined office. Another recommendation was to organise the job centres by region, not according to political jurisdictions. The government did not adopt these recommendations.

2. Rapid response activities. Workers would be required to register for unemployment insurance as soon as they were notified of potential layoff. Workers could gain access to all job search tools, such as a national job openings database. Workers could also take time from work to search/interview for a new job. Workers would not receive income assistance until they were officially unemployed. The government adopted this proposal and it was implemented on 1 July 2003.

3. Accepting job offers (neue Zumutbarkeit). Under this proposal, all unemployed workers would have to accept new job offers, taking geographic mobility factors into account. If the first offer is refused, the worker's unemployment assistance could be stopped for four to 12 weeks. During this time, the workers could get social assistance if he/she met the eligibility criteria. After one year, workers must be willing to accept a job offer anywhere in Germany. Refusing a second job offer could result in forfeiting further unemployment assistance. In that event, a worker could continue to receive social assistance, if he or she was eligible. These proposals were adopted by the government and have already been implemented.

4. Education and training of young people. This recommendation deals with alternative means of financing training. One option calls for a new apprenticeship programme for young workers based on a credit system. Individuals would have an account, which they could use to finance their training. The government rejected these proposals, since training is not compulsory under the unemployment insurance system.

5.   Incentives for hiring older workers.

Wage insurance for older workers. Workers over 55 can be eligible for a government subsidy of 50% of the difference between the old and new wages for up to 12 months. As in the case of unemployment insurance payments, workers would receive a monthly transfer in the amount of the wage subsidy. The government has adopted this proposal. The wage insurance system has been implemented and a few workers are already receiving assistance.

Early retirement. The Commission proposed allowing workers over 55 to receive the full amount of unemployment assistance in a lump sum. In the end, the government did not adopt this proposal.

Develop incentives to hire older workers, e.g. reduce social contributions, allow more flexibility in application of labour laws, permit short-term contracts.

6.   Unemployment benefit reform.

Unemployment money. The Commission proposed to reduce the maximum length of assistance from 32 to 18 months for older workers. The level of assistance would be linked to the previous wage – 67% of previous wage if worker has children, 60% if not. The length of assistance would depend on age. Workers under 45 years old would be eligible for 12 months of assistance. Workers over 55 years old could receive assistance for up to 18 months.

Unemployment money is financed through a social contribution of 6.5% of wages, split equally between employees and employers, up to the first USD 5 610 per month.

Unemployment assistance. The Commission proposed harmonising unemployment assistance and social assistance. Workers would continue to be eligible for social assistance if they remained unemployed after their unemployment money expired, but the level of assistance would be set at the current level of social assistance. The commission also recommended tightening the means test for social assistance. Workers must be available for work, including temporary jobs, or training, and must accept new job offers, in order to continue receiving assistance.

7.   Incentives to employers for hiring and retaining workers. The Commission recommended proposals designed to reward companies – possibly by reducing social benefit contributions – and employers that hire unemployed workers and retain their existing workers. This proposal included some kind of experience rating for hiring. The government has not yet acted on these proposals.

8.   Temporary job placement agencies (PSA). Beginning January 2004, workers can enter into temporary contracts with job placement agencies (PSA). PSAs are responsible for paying wages and making social contributions for workers, regardless of whether they do or do not receive placement. If a temporary assignment turns into a permanent job offer, the hiring company takes on the responsibility of paying wages and social contributions directly. Workers must be willing to accept short-term contracts with PSAs. If a temporary job does not become permanent, a worker can re-enter the unemployment insurance system.

9.   "Ich AG". This proposal aims at encouraging self-employment. Self-employed workers would be eligible for government assistance, including lower taxes and simplified accounting requirements. Self-employed workers could also receive up to three years of unemployment assistance, if they do not generate income. Self-employed workers

cannot hire others, except for family members. The government adopted this proposal and it is being implemented.

10. Promotion of low-wage jobs. The Commission recommended developing preferences for low-wage jobs. Workers making less than USD 440 per month would not have to pay any social benefit contributions. Employers would be paid a lump sum payment of 25% of wages, which would include all taxes and social contributions. For wages between USD 440 and USD 880, workers would pay some social benefit contribution and the employer would pay the full 21% of wages. Above USD 880, workers and employers would pay full social benefit contributions and taxes. The government adopted this proposal.

11. Reorganisation of the Federal Employment Service. The Commission recommended reorganising the Federal Employment Service to be more like a private company than a government authority. Federal Employment Service workers would have contracts similar to private employees, not government workers. The government has not yet adopted this proposal.

12. Clusters and competence centres. The proposal was to combine economic development, regional planning and employment functions. The government rejected this proposal.

13. Tax incentives for hiring unemployed workers (capital for work). Firms hiring unemployed workers would be eligible to borrow up to USD 110 000 for each worker, at a reduced interest rate, from the Credit Anstalt. The government would subsidise the lower interest rate. The firm would only need to secure half the loan, and the federal government would guarantee the other half. The government adopted this proposal.

These steps are probably the most ambitious set of reforms undertaken by any country in recent years. The German unemployment insurance system, once considered one of the most generous programmes, is becoming more like programmes in most OECD countries.

One of the major criticisms of these reforms is that they will do little to reduce the high rate of German unemployment. The connection between the amount of unemployment assistance and the unemployment rate in Germany has primarily been based on anecdotal evidence. Critics also argue that the reform of the Federal Employment Office and the unemployment insurance system will do little to create additional jobs in Germany. There seems to be an assumption implicit in this reform effort that increasing the supply of workers actively seeking employment will somehow increase the demand for those workers.

Reforming the unemployment assistance programme alone does little to help create new jobs. The Chancellor's Agenda 2010 includes little direct assistance for economic development. More importantly, a large share of German employment remains under collective wage-setting agreements. Inflexible German wage-setting policies may make it difficult for the increase in labour supply to translate into lower wages, which in turn might encourage more job creation.

An important aspect of the reformed German unemployment insurance system is the interaction between the unemployed and Federal Employment Office counsellors. These counsellors are responsible for assisting workers in their job search. They are also responsible for enforcing the new rules that dictate that assistance can be terminated if a worker is not willing to accept a job, regardless of the wage offered or its location. The ultimate success of most of the recently implemented reforms lies with these counsellors.

The conventional wisdom is that Germany is the paragon of training. Based on the data presented in Table 3.12, Germany spends ten times more on training that Japan, the United Kingdom and the United States. It appears that most of that money is devoted to apprenticeship programmes and active worker training. Training is not considered an "entitlement" as part of the German unemployment assistance programme. Training funds are available on a "first come, first served" basis. If funds are available, unemployed workers can take one course per year. Courses tend to be short. Federal Employment Service counsellors are the primary "gate keepers" for training.

Health insurance is not an issue for the unemployed since German law requires that everyone have health insurance. Employers are responsible for paying health insurance premiums for their employees. The federal government subsidises health insurance premiums for unemployed workers. This serves as an incentive for unemployed workers to register with the Federal Employment Office.

In addition to providing unemployment assistance, the German system has several incentives for hiring new workers. Companies that hire unemployed workers are eligible for a reduction in the amount of social contributions they are required to make. In addition, companies may be eligible to receive up to four months of salary for a worker during his or her initial probation period.

The Japanese unemployment insurance system

Until recently, Japanese labour market adjustment policies could be characterised as predominately preventive. The measures were primarily subsidies to firms to prevent or postpone worker layoffs. Recent macroeconomic developments in Japan have increased pressures on firms, forcing the government to reduce its reliance on programmes that forestall adjustment and expand programmes that assist in the adjustment process.

The following is a list of various preventive Japanese labour market adjustment programmes: *i)* industry assistance; *ii)* employment adjustment subsidy (*koyo chosei joseikin*); *iii)* labour movement employment-stability subsidy (*rodo ido koyo antei joseikin*); *iv)* labour movement ability-development subsidy (*rodo ido noryoku kaihatsu joseikin*); and *v)* lifetime ability-development subsidy (*shogai noryoku kaihatsu kyuhukin*).

Like the other five large OECD countries, the primary reactive labour market adjustment programme in Japan is unemployment insurance, known as employment insurance (EI). As a rule, the Japanese unemployment insurance system covers all workers under the age of 65, except for those employed by the government and in the shipbuilding industry. To be eligible for assistance, EI contributions must be made on behalf of the worker, and the worker must be employed for at least six months during the year prior to job separation. Workers must register at a government-sponsored placement office in order to receive EI.

The Japanese unemployment insurance scheme covers any worker separated from his or her job, regardless of the reason for the separation. Workers who voluntarily leave their jobs can be eligible for EI assistance. In fact, one unofficial estimate suggests that currently only one-third of workers receiving assistance under EI were involuntarily laid off.

Until recently, EI assistance was set at between 60% and 80% of a worker's previous wage (50% to 80% of the previous wage for workers between the ages of 60 and 64), subject to a maximum amount. Workers receive payments for 90 to 360 days, depending on age, years of EI coverage and work status (full-time) (Annex Tables 3.A2.7-3.A2.9).

A combination of very liberal eligibility requirements, the amount of payment and the length of payments (Annex Table 3.A2.10) have made the Japanese system one of the most generous unemployment insurance schemes among OECD countries. It is true that the Japanese economy had a very tight labour market for much of the last 30 years. During the 1980s and the beginning of the 1990s, the Japanese unemployment rate remained between 1% and 2%. Few workers left their jobs voluntarily or involuntarily and few workers received assistance under the EI programme.

All of this has changed over the last decade. The Japanese unemployment rate has been increasing since 1993. The added demand on EI has almost completed depleted any reserves accumulated from previous years. The EI trust fund is currently facing a serious financial crisis. This has prompted the Japanese government to institute some reforms in the EI system.

Annex Table 3.A2.7. Level of assistance under the Japanese unemployment system

Age	Upper limit of daily wages	Upper limit of daily basic allowance
Up to 29	USD 108.83	USD 54.42
30 to 44	USD 120.92	USD 60.46
45 to 59	USD 133	USD 66.5
60 to 64	USD 128.83	USD 57.98

Note: USD 1.00 = JPY 110.

Source: Japanese Ministry of Health, Labour and Welfare (2003).

Annex Table 3.A2.8. Benefits for workers under 60 years of age

Amount of daily wage	Benefit rate
USD 17.67 to USD 34.83	80%
USD 34.83 to USD 101.08	50% to 80%
USD 101.08 to USD 133.00	50%

Source: Japanese Ministry of Health, Labour and Welfare (2003).

Table 3.A2.9. Duration of assistance for unemployed who lose their jobs as a result of bankruptcy or dismissal

Age	< 1 year	1 to 4 years	5 to 9 years	10 to 19 years	> 20 years
Under 30	90 days	90 days	120 days	180 days	Na
30 to 34	90 days	90 days	180 days	210 days	240 days
35 to 44	90 days	90 days	180 days	240 days	270 days
45 to 59	90 days	180 days	240 days	270 days	330 days
60 to 64	90 days	150 days	180 days	210 days	240 days

Source: Japanese Ministry of Health, Labour and Welfare (2003).

Annex Table 3.A2.10. Duration of assistance for unemployed

Age	< 1 year	1 to 4 years	5 to 9 years	10 to 19 years	> 20 years
For ordinary unemployed					
All ages	90 days	90 days	90 days	120 days	150 days
For workers hard to re–employ					
Less than 44 years old	150 days	300 days	300 days	300 days	300 days
45 to 64 years old	150 days	360 days	360 days	360 days	360 days

Source: Japanese Ministry of Health, Labour and Welfare (2003).

The UK unemployment insurance system

UK unemployment insurance has also recently undergone significant reform, making it considerably less generous than programmes in France, Germany, Japan and the United States. In contrast to some other countries, firms in the United Kingdom are required to notify workers well in advance of any potential layoff. Employers must also provide severance pay to qualified workers. Workers who qualify for redundancy rights are eligible to the following notice of potential job loss: i) a minimum of one week for each year of service, up to a maximum of 12 weeks; and ii) employers must provide severance pay based on length of service and previous weekly earnings (up to a maximum of USD 341.25 [GBP 1=USD 1.625]); for ages 18 to 21, half a week's pay for each year of service; for age 22 to 40, one week's pay for each year of service; and for ages 41 to 60, one and a half week's pay for each year of service. The maximum severance package is USD 10 237.50, approximately one-third annual average earnings.

The British Job Seekers Assistance (JSA) has two components: *i)* contribution-based unemployment insurance (UI); and *ii)* non–contribution, means-tested unemployment assistance (UA). Workers earning above USD 102.38 per week must make contributions to the UI system. In order to receive UI, workers must have been employed for two years prior to separation. In 1996, the duration of UI payments was reduced from 12 to six months. After exhausting UI assistance, workers can apply for the means-tested UA programme. Eligibility for UA is based on family income, not the worker's previous income. Workers with children may be eligible for additional assistance.

JSA is based on unemployment and is not related to the cause of displacement. There is no special assistance for workers whose job loss may be associated with changes in international trade. There are also no special provisions for workers from specific industries. One objective in recent reforms to JSA was to make assistance less attractive and encourage people to return to work sooner.

Annex Table 3.A2.11. Amount of unemployment insurance assistance

Age	Weekly amount
16 to 17	USD 53.46
18 to 24	USD 70.28
Above 25	USD 88.81

Note: GBP 1 = USD 1.625.

The US unemployment insurance system and TAA programme

The US unemployment insurance programme is mandated by the federal government and administered by the states. Although there are many similarities among the various state programmes, the United States has some 50 different unemployment insurance programmes. The Federal Unemployment Tax is 0.8% of the first USD 7 000 of gross payroll, split evenly between employers and employees. Contributions are experience-rated, *i.e.* some portion of the contribution is based on past experience with the unemployment insurance system.

The weekly benefit amount is based on some portion of an individual's wage, and is set by the states. Benefits vary widely by state. In 2000, the average benefit was approximately USD 200 per week. Minimum weekly benefits ranged from zero in New Jersey to USD 102 in Rhode Island. Maximum weekly benefits ranged from USD 133 in Puerto Rico to USD 646 in Massachusetts.

Data presented in Annex Table 3.A2.12 suggest that the average replacement rate has tended to be about 35% of average weekly wages over the last 30 years. Replacement rates vary not only across states, but also among individual recipients. Workers with higher previous wages tend to experience lower wage replacement rates, while the opposite is true for workers with lower incomes.

Annex Table 3.A2.12. Unemployment insurance assistance

	Unemployment insurance average weekly benefit		Recipiency rates[1]
	Nominal USD	Ratio to average weekly wage	
1970	USD 50.31	35.7%	43.0%
1975	USD 70.23	37.1%	49.2%
1980	USD 99.66	36.6%	43.3%
1985	USD 128.14	35.3%	30.8%
1990	USD 161.56	36.0%	35.2%
1995	USD 187.29	35.5%	34.0%

1. Percentage of unemployed receiving unemployment insurance.

Source: BLS, US Department of Labor, *ET Handbook Number 394*.

The duration for receiving unemployment insurance also varies by state. The minimum duration ranges from four weeks in Oregon to 26 weeks in 12 states. Federal law sets the maximum duration at 26 weeks, but the maximum duration is 30 weeks in Massachusetts and Washington. Extended benefits (EB), equal to 13 additional weeks of unemployment insurance, may be triggered when unemployment rates remains high over a period of time. In 1992, the US Congress established an optional trigger for an additional seven weeks, but very few states have adopted it.

The initial 26 weeks of unemployment insurance is fully financed by employer and employee contributions to the UI Trust Fund. Half of the additional 26 weeks of extended benefits is funded as a direct expenditure of the federal government. The other half is financed out of the UI Trust Fund. Extended benefit levels are identical to those under the initial 26 weeks of unemployment insurance. Annex Tables 3.A2.13 to 3.A2.15 provide more detailed information about TAA and NAFTA–TAA participants.

Annex Table 3.A2.13. TAA and NAFTA–TAA, 2002 to July 2003

	Number of certifications		Employees covered by certifications	
	Unit	%	Unit	%
All industries	3 606	100%	376 428	100%
Clothing	563	15.6%	69 150	18.4%
Textiles	281	7.8%	35 436	9.4%
Textiles and clothing	844	23.4%	104 586	27.8%

Source: US General Accounting Office (2001).

Annex Table 3.A2.14. TAA services by participant

	1995	1996	1997	1998	1999	2000	Total
Total workers certified	118 837	166 310	165 898	153 804	227 650	145 112	977 611
Basic allowance							
Recipients	25 641	32 856	3 4158	26 241	36 910	32 368	18 8174
Average USD	4 270.5	3 889.7	4 332.81	4 542.51	4 310.48	5 564.14	4 483.62
Additional allowance USD							
Recipients	5 856	7 132	15 215	7 736	8 166	10 010	54 115
Average USD	7 103.83	6 113.29	3 522.84	6 489.14	62 08.67	7 472.53	5 811.7
Training							
Recipients	28 645	32 971	26 865	25 235	32 120	24 106	16 9942
Average USD	2 126.03	2 077.58	3 104.41	3 166.24	3 029.27	4 322.58	2 908.05
Job search assistance USD							
Recipients	927	752	520	289	314	359	3161
Average USD	323.62	398.94	384.62	346.02	318.47	278.55	347.99
Job relocation assistance USD							
Recipients	1 678	940	875	473	771	731	5 468
Average USD	1 668.65	1 914.89	1 942.86	1 691.33	1 297.02	1 504.79	1 682.52
Total services (USD millions)	215.1	242	286.9	250.2	308.2	360.3	1 662.7

Source: US General Accounting Office (2001).

Annex Table 3.A2.15. Profile of TAA and NAFTA-TAA participants, 1999 and 2000

	TAA and NAFTA–TAA participants	Total US workforce
Male	36%	53%
Female	64%	47%
Average age	43	n.a.
Limited English proficiency	12%	n.a.
Average pre–lay off wage	USD 12.13/hour (at separation)	USD 13.36/hour (production worker)
Average new wage	USD 10.31	n.a.
Median job tenure	7 years (at separation)	3.5 years
Education		
Less than high school	25%	10%
High school graduate	55%	32%
Some post high school	17%	28%
College graduate	4%	30%

Source: US General Accounting Office (2001).

Notes

1. The WTO ATC superseded the Multi-Fibre Arrangement (MFA) regime of quantitative trade restrictions when it entered into force in January 1995 and provided the multilateral trade framework applicable for trade in textiles and clothing for all WTO members. The ATC provides for the elimination by 31 December 2004 of all forms of quantitative restrictions applied to trade in textile and clothing products, including those that originated under the MFA regime. The ATC phases itself out of existence at the end of 2004. For the purpose of qualifying the period when quantitative restrictions will no longer be applied to trade in textile and clothing products, the term "the post-ATC period" is used throughout this publication.

2. The United States is taken in an example given the availability of data over a sufficiently long period of time.

3. The future of the Bureau of Labor Statistics (BLS) is currently in doubt. By contrast, in light of the significant reforms of its labour market assistance programmes, Germany is beginning an ambitious effort to survey its displaced workers.

4. For an explanation of import-sensitive industries, see Kletzer (2001a).

5. One Japanese official unofficially estimated that only one-third of those currently receiving unemployment insurance were separated from their jobs involuntarily.

6. The United States has a programme of extended assistance in times of high unemployment. Workers who exhaust their unemployment insurance in the United Kingdom may be eligible for assistance under the country's welfare programme.

7. The eligibility criteria were liberalised, so that imports had to "contribute importantly" to job loss. In other words, the increase in imports had to be only one of several contributing factors to the job loss.

8. By contrast, the Workforce Investment Act (WIA) – the programme that provides assistance to dislocated workers regardless of cause – is not an entitlement. Workers only receive training if there are adequate funds available. Most states exhaust training funds under WIA well before the end of the year, thereby denying workers the possibility to enrol in training. In addition, states can deny training, if it is determined that a worker can find a job that pays a subsistence wage.

9. See, in particular, Richardson (2003), Kletzer (2001a), Field and Graham (1997) and Blancflower (2000).

References

Assedic (2003), "Unemployment Insurance: A Scheme for Social Protection within the Dynamics of Employment, Notice DAJ 266", July.

Blancflower, D.G. (2000), "Globalization and the Labor Market", paper commissioned by the Trade Deficit Review Commission, Washington, September.

Blien, U., U. Walwei and H. Werner (2002), "Labour Market Policy in Germany", Institute for Employment Research of the Federal Employment Service, Germany.

China National Textile Industry Council (CNTIC) (2002), "Report on China Textile Industry Development 2001/2002", www.cnfi.com.en.

Cline, W. (1990), *The Future of World Trade in Textiles and Apparel*, Revised Edition, Washington: Institute for International Economics.

Field, A.J. and E.M. Graham (1997), "Is there a Special Case for Import Protection for the Textile and Apparel Sectors Based on labour Adjustment?", *The World Economy* 20, No. 2, pp. 137-157.

Higuchi, T. (1997), "Trends in Japanese Labour Markets", in Mari Sako and Hiroki Sato (eds.), *Japanese Labour and Management in Transition*, Routledge, London.

Higuchi, T. (2003), "Rising Unemployment Rate and Reform of Employment Insurance in Japan", World Bank project, The World Bank, Washington, DC.

International Labour Organisation (2000), "Labour Practices in the Footwear, Leather, Textile and Clothing Industries", report for the discussion at the Tripartite Meeting on Labour Practices in the Footwear, Leather, Textiles and Clothing Industries, Geneva.

Japanese Ministry of Health, Labour and Welfare (2003), "Employment Insurance System of Japan", Employment Insurance Division, Employment Security Bureau, memo, 28 August.

Keller, B. (2003), "The Hartz Commission's Recommendations and Beyond – An Intermediary Assessment", paper presented at the expert meeting, "Towards a New labour Market Order in Germany," 30-31 January.

Kletzer, L.G. (2001a), "Job Loss from Imports: Measuring the Costs", Institute for International Economics, Washington, DC, September.

Kletzer, L.G. (2001b), "A Prescription to Relieve Worker Anxiety", Policy Brief 01-2, Institute for International Economics, Washington, DC, February, www.iie.com/publications/pb/pb01-2.htm.

Kletzer, L.G. (forthcoming), *Workers at Risk: Job Loss from Apparel, Textiles, Footwear and Furniture, 1979 to 2001*, Institute for International Economics, Washington, DC.

Levinsohn, J. and W. Petropoulos (2001), "Creative Destruction or Just Plain Destruction? The U.S. Textile and Apparel Industries since 1972", National Bureau of Economic Research, Working Paper 8348, June, www.nber.org/papers/w8348.

Lewis, H. and D. Richardson (2001), "Why Global Commitment Really Matters!", Institute for International Economics, Washington, DC, October.

OECD (2002a), *OECD Employment Outlook 2002*, Paris.

OECD (2002b), *Benefits and Wages, OECD Indicators*, Paris.

Richardson, D. (2003), "Some Measurable Costs and Benefits of Economic Globalisation for Americans", presentation at a conference, Responding to Globalisation: Societies, Groups, and Individuals, University of Colorado, Boulder, April.

Seike, A. and H.W. Tan (1994), "Labour Fixity and Labour Market Adjustments in Japan and the United States", in H.W. Tan and H. Shimada (eds.), *Troubled Industries in the United States and Japan*, St. Martin's Press.

Sekiguchi, S. (1994), "An Overview of Adjustment Assistance Policies in Japan", in H.W. Tan and H. Shimada (eds.), *Troubled Industries in the United States and Japan*, St. Martin's Press.

Tan, H.W. (1994), "Troubled Industries in the United States", in Hong W. Tan and Haruo Shimada (eds.), *Troubled Industries in the United States and Japan*, St. Martin's Press.

US General Accounting Office (2001), "Trade Adjustment Assistance: Improvements Necessary, but Programmes Cannot Solve Communities' Long-term Problems", GAO-01-988T, Washington, DC.

Walwei, U. (2002), "Labour Market Effects of Employment Protection", Institute for Employment Research of the Federal Employment Service, Germany.

Chapter 4

Technology and Innovation

This chapter focuses on recent world trends in applied technology in the textile and clothing industries and reviews innovation and technology diffusion approaches in OECD countries, including production and trade of TCM. It summarises recent technological changes in the transformation stages of textiles into final clothing products, outlining productivity gaps between the various production stages and highlighting opportunities for fragmenting the supply chain on the basis of comparative advantages. It examines various policy approaches taken by OECD countries to promote innovation and innovative clusters in the textile and clothing industries and notes best practices. The role now played by textile and clothing production in the industrialisation process of developing countries is far more differentiated than it was a generation ago. While low wages can still give developing countries a competitive edge in world markets, quick turnaround times now play a far more crucial role in determining international competitiveness in these fashion-oriented and time-sensitive markets.

Introduction

This chapter focuses on recent trends in applied technology in the textile and clothing industries and reviews innovation and technology diffusion approaches in OECD countries. First, it offers a global perspective on production and trade of textile and clothing machinery (TCM). Then, it summarises recent technological changes in the transformation stages of fabrics into final clothing products, outlining productivity gaps between the various production stages and highlighting opportunities for fragmenting the supply chain on the basis of comparative advantages. Next, it examines various policy approaches taken by OECD countries to promote innovation and innovative clusters in the textile and clothing industries and outlines best practices in innovation policies. Some concluding remarks follow. Annex 4.A2 provides details on the main production stages involved in the fabrication of clothing products.

Technology and trade in the textile and clothing industries

In recent decades, the textile and clothing industries have been subject both to normal growth patterns, with all their consequences, but also to deviations from the normally agreed trade rules in most OECD countries. This led to the introduction of numerous non-tariff barriers, in addition to above-average tariff rates, including the Multi-Fibre Arrangement (MFA). The MFA quantitative restrictions are due to be eliminated by the end of 2004.[1]

At least until the 1980s, exports of textiles grew faster than exports of clothing. Then, exports of textile and clothing products expanded roughly in line with the growth in total world trade (Figure 4.1). Towards the mid-1990s, however, textile exports levelled off as production shifted closer to locations where clothing was produced or as new textile-producing plants were established in countries that produced clothing. This is particularly the case in China, where the expansion of the textile and clothing industries is driven by accession to the WTO and by the prospect of quota-free exports at the end of 2004. However, despite these developments, exports of textile and clothing machinery are not expanding (Figure 4.2). In fact, exports of TCM have declined, with the major exception of exports to China (Figure 4.3). Imports of TCM in China reached USD 5 billion in 2003, an increase of over 200% compared to 1999. This may well lead to the establishment of very strong textile and clothing clusters of enterprises and expertise.

Over the centuries and across countries, the textile and clothing industries have has served as a motor of industrialisation or as a key driver of exports (Deane, 1965, pp. 84–88). First came the invention and the production of commercially viable TCM and then adequate access to imports of such machinery. In the past, a symbiotic relationship often existed between efficient and creative TCM production and competitive textile and clothing industries and helped to ensure the international competitiveness of the textile and clothing products produced and exported. In recent times, this relationship has faded, if not disappeared.

Figure 4.1. World exports, 1965–2002

USD billions

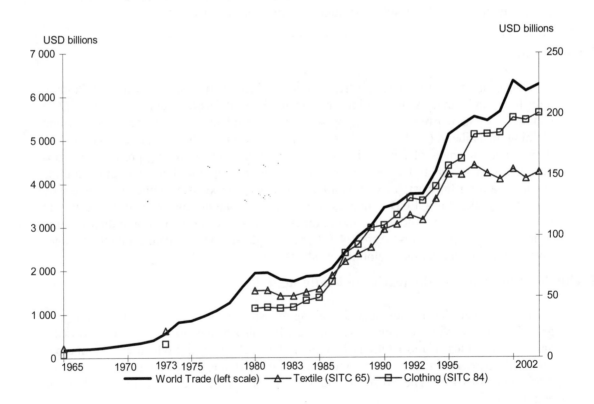

Source: *WTO Annual Report*, various issues.

Figure 4.2. Total merchandise exports (left scale), exports of textile and clothing products and textile and clothing machinery, 1992–2002

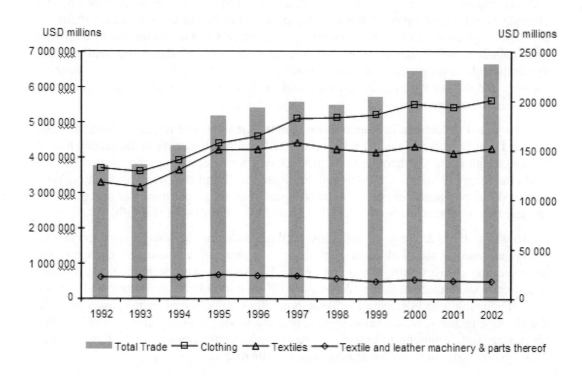

Source: Own calculations based on UNCTAD tabulations.

Figure 4.3. Textile and clothing machinery exports to major regions/countries

USD millions

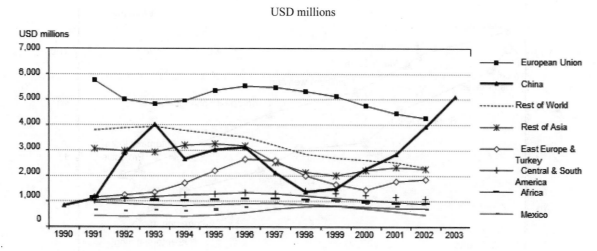

Source: WTO Annual Report and own calculations based on UNCTAD and Chinese customs data. Data for China for the entire year 2003 are estimated on the basis of the first ten months.

A case in point is Germany's sewing machine industry, which competed very well in international markets as long as it could draw on feedback from a viable clothing industry. However, once it was no longer possible to test machine prototypes nearby at a clothing producing company, German sewing machines began to lose market share.[2] A productive symbiosis still exists in Germany with respect to the production of industrial grade needles, which represent on average roughly 60% of the world market. The symbiotic relationship involves needle manufacturers, the steel industry, the clothing industry and the sewing machine industry and likely requires less direct interaction than in the case of sewing machines.

The initial inventions in England, *i.e.* spinning jennies and mules, helped maintain England's early leadership in the textile industry from the eighteenth to the second half of the nineteenth century, when the more productive US ring-spinning innovations took the lead (Sandberg, 1970, pp. 120–140) and dominated well into the twentieth century. With similar developments taking place in the weaving of cloth, labour input per unit of output in these two processes has been reduced dramatically (Figures 4.4a and 4.4b).

However, these are only the steps involved in producing the intermediary inputs that are largely used in the production of clothing. The story of technological change in the latter industry evolves more slowly. As Figure 4.4a shows, many technological advances had already taken place in the textile industry by the mid-nineteenth century, and – in the case of spinning – had decreased working hours for a kilogram of yarn by over 90%. In the clothing industry, which basically involves the sewing process, commercially viable ideas were just beginning to emerge in the mid-nineteenth century. Until then, various ideas on both sides of the Atlantic never reached the market.

Figure 4.4a. Working hours per unit output in spinning and weaving from 1750

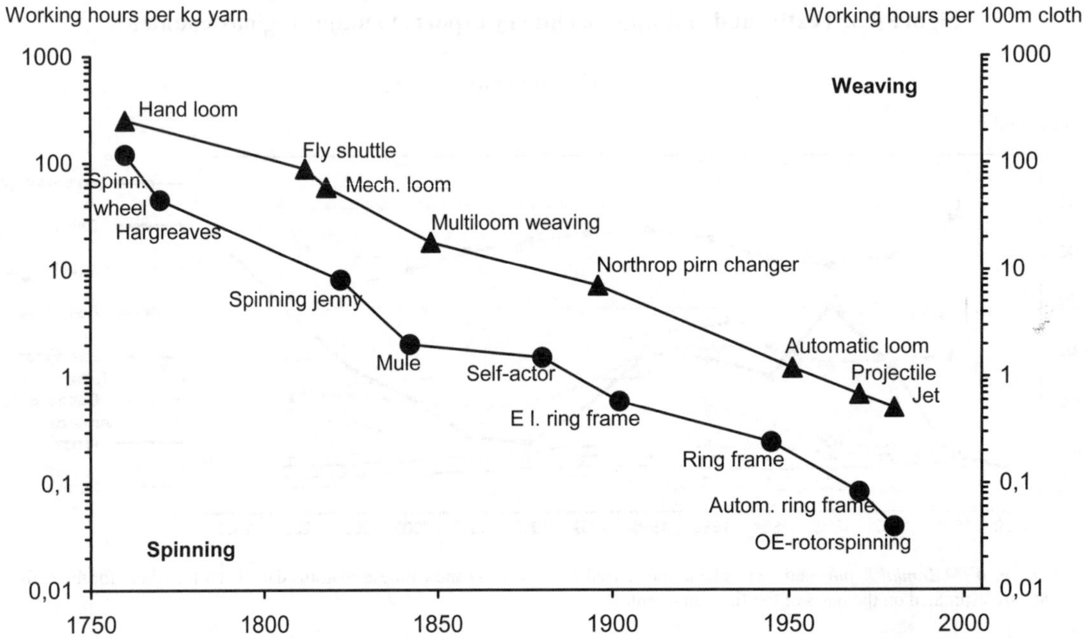

Figure 4.4b. Working hours per unit output in spinning and weaving from 1925

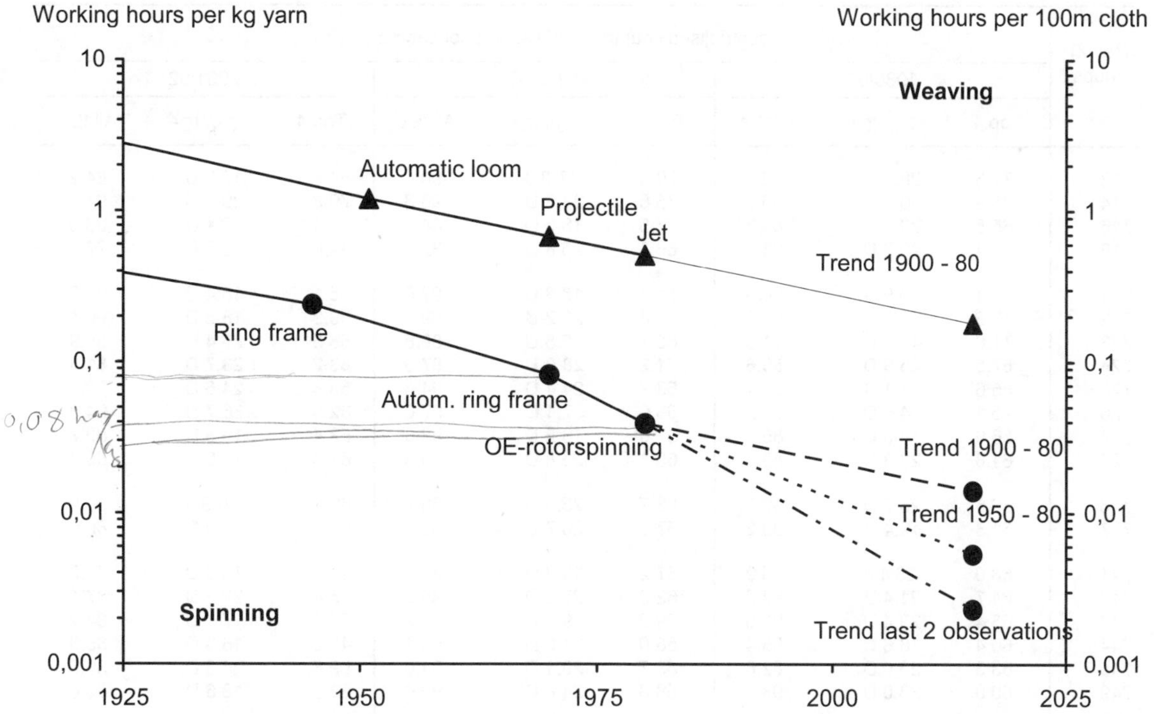

Working hours per kg yarn

Working hours per 100m cloth

Weaving

Automatic loom

Projectile

Jet

Trend 1900 - 80

Ring frame

Autom. ring frame

OE-rotorspinning

Trend 1900 - 80

Trend 1950 - 80

Spinning

Trend last 2 observations

Source: Adapted from Hartman (1993, p. 66); own calculations.

The first successful patent for a machine that used thread from two different sources was granted in the United States to Elias Howe in 1846.[3] However, it was Isaac Singer who commercialised the process in the early 1850s (although he was later found guilty of infringing upon Howe's patent), redesigned the needle position to up and down movements and installed a foot treadle instead of a hand crank. By the early twentieth century, electrically powered sewing machines were in widespread use. Since then, major technical advances in the clothing industry (with wide-scale replacement of labour inputs by capital equipment) have not occurred.

In the production process, current sewing techniques do not basically differ from those that prevailed following the integration of the sewing machine into the production process during the course of the last century. The production process continues to be labour-intensive, and in almost no other major industry are labour inputs coupled with such small amounts of physical capital equipment.[4] The basic reason is the nature of the production process itself, where two-dimensional materials, *i.e.* cloth that is rather soft and limp in nature, are subjected to a series of individual labour-intensive handling/assembly steps, culminating in the formation of a product which then fits/drapes a three-dimensional human body. While some steps in the upstream end of the clothes manufacturing process, *e.g.* computer-aided design (CAD), or some specific items have been adapted to more capital-intensive methods, *e.g.* jeans, the process as a whole remains fragmented.

Table 4.1. Concentration in world machinery and transport equipment exports, 1981–2002

SITC (Rev.2) groups	Industrialised countries' (IC) export concentration (%)[1]								
	1980/81			1989/90			2001/02		
	Top 4	Top IC[2]	All ICs	Top 4	Top IC[2]	All ICs	Top 4	Top IC[2]	All ICs
713	71.6	28.2 U	92.7	59.0	17.8 J	90.1	54.9	17.9 U	84.2
714	78.9	36.3 U	96.7	75.6	33.9 U	96.3	70.8	29.7 U	94.4
716	65.5	20.5 U	86.2	57.5	18.3 D	84.2	39.1	12.1 D	68.5
718	50.4	20.3 D	86.6	66.1	25.8 D	82.5	44.8	16.3 D	77.7
721	61.1	27.9 U	90.9	54.1	18.8 U	92.0	55.1	18.4 D	90.2
722	75.8	33.9 U	92.0	71.8	23.2 D	89.5	59.9	18.8 D	90.4
723	71.6	42.8 U	91.3	60.7	25.5 U	89.8	58.5	26.4 U	85.9
724	**67.5**	**25.9 D**	**86.6**	**71.2**	**28.0 D**	**87.9**	**63.2**	**23.7 D**	**81.5**
725	55.6	25.1 D	96.1	53.7	24.4 D	94.3	53.8	24.6 D	93.5
726	75.1	34.5 D	97.2	68.0	37.1 D	97.0	62.5	36.7 D	94.8
727	56.6	18.5 U	85.5	57.0	18.2 D	92.6	53.4	19.8 D	89.7
728	61.8	23.3 D	89.2	65.1	23.8 D	89.5	62.4	17.9 D	88.4
736	66.6	26.7 D	90.3	63.7	25.3 D	88.7	63.1	20.9 J	86.9
737	61.8	19.4 U	88.2	57.9	20.7 D	92.0	54.1	17.0 D	86.6
741	68.0	23.1 J	95.9	57.2	16.2 U	91.6	45.7	15.0 U	76.5
742	64.7	21.4 U	93.5	62.3	27.2 D	95.2	56.4	22.3 D	87.1
743	63.4	23.4 U	95.5	59.2	19.9 D	91.9	52.3	17.1 U	84.2
744	60.4	18.6 U	95.4	56.0	21.0 D	90.1	46.2	16.3 D	85.9
745	63.5	26.0 D	82.8	63.7	29.1 D	94.0	59.8	24.3 D	89.6
749	60.0	23.0 D	93.5	58.3	24.6 D	90.0	52.0	18.6 D	80.6
751	73.1	44.7 J	89.8	66.1	35.3 J	84.6	39.0	12.3 D	65.2
752	66.6	39.0 U	94.8	63.3	23.9 U	77.4	33.2	10.7 U	53.7
759	72.1	43.8 U	92.5	48.2	23.5 U	80.6	37.6	12.2 J	55.7
761	65.3	36.5 J	83.2	43.3	14.9 D	60.3	24.8	12.6 J	37.3
762	63.1	54.1 J	68.8	31.0	21.8 J	42.3	22.2	6.1 J	34.3
763	86.1	76.0 J	90.2	67.5	58.2 J	72.9	41.8	34.1 J	52.3
764	59.0	25.4 J	80.7	55.7	27.4 J	79.0	34.7	9.9 G	64.2
771	59.3	20.6 J	85.7	49.3	17.0 D	73.4	30.9	10.7 D	56.8
772	61.6	20.0 D	88.2	62.5	21.0 D	88.3	48.2	15.1 D	70.4
773	56.8	21.3 J	87.9	47.6	16.7 U	79.3	30.1	11.6 U	52.2
774	72.9	34.7 U	97.3	72.7	25.0 U	98.5	68.0	29.1 U	94.0
775	59.1	17.9 D	83.1	54.3	21.3 D	79.3	39.0	14.5 D	57.3
776	60.0	29.3 U	71.2	57.9	22.7 U	66.5	44.1	17.4 U	57.3
778	61.1	18.6 J	88.8	60.4	20.7 J	86.4	46.5	17.1 J	68.4
781	72.7	31.8 J	97.1	66.1	24.8 J	95.2	57.4	22.0 D	86.0
782	70.5	31.0 J	94.7	64.6	23.4 J	95.9	50.8	16.2 C	79.2
783	68.5	32.1 D	92.1	60.0	21.4 D	94.6	50.1	21.1 D	82.3
784	66.5	27.8 U	93.5	65.2	21.5 D	89.9	54.2	18.1 U	84.6
785	84.7	68.9 J	88.5	71.3	44.6 J	72.1	54.0	32.2 J	70.3
786	56.1	25.7 D	81.1	53.7	23.7 D	68.7	40.8	22.2 D	60.5
791	67.1	19.6 F	77.1	58.0	19.0 D	76.7	44.0	17.1 D	75.5
792	82.9	53.8 U	95.0	77.9	48.1 U	96.5	75.5	37.3 U	94.7
793	57.6	39.5 J	81.5	55.2	21.4 J	73.7	38.6	20.7 J	58.0

SITC 724 is machinery for the textile and clothing industries.

1. % share in total world exports of given group. In case of all ICs data refer to 1980/81 and 1989/90 and 2001/02.

2. Letters following shares designate the following countries: C = Canada; F = France; D = Germany; G = Great Britain (United Kingdom); J = Japan; U = United States.

Source: Own calculations based on UNCTAD (1992: Table 4.3A and 2002 4.2A) and unpublished UNCTAD sources, respective tables. See Annex Table 4A.1 for description of groups.

Table 4.2. Shares, changes in shares and yearly growth rates for SITC product groups, 1980–2002

SITC (Rev.2) groups	Share in total SITC 7 exports			Change in shares			Growth rates	
	1980/81	1989/90	2001/02	89/90-80/81	01/02-89/90	01/02-80/81	80/81 - 89/90	89/90-01/02
Total								
713	3.2	3.2	3.0	-0.0	-0.2	-0.2	8.3	6.4
714	1.6	2.1	2.4	0.5	0.2	0.8	11.0	8.1
716	1.5	1.1	1.3	-0.4	0.2	-0.2	6.8	8.5
718	0.4	0.3	0.2	-0.1	-0.1	-0.2	3.7	5.0
721	1.2	0.8	0.5	-0.4	-0.3	-0.7	3.4	2.7
722	1.4	0.6	0.3	-0.8	-0.2	-1.1	-1.5	2.5
723	3.4	1.6	1.2	-1.8	-0.4	-2.2	1.5	4.2
724	**2.1**	**1.8**	**0.8**	**-0.3**	**-1.0**	**-1.3**	**6.1**	**-0.5**
725	0.5	0.6	0.3	0.1	-0.3	-0.2	8.9	-0.4
726	0.7	1.0	0.6	0.3	-0.4	-0.1	10.1	1.8
727	0.5	0.5	0.2	-0.0	-0.2	-0.3	7.2	1.0
728	3.3	3.3	2.7	0.0	-0.6	-0.6	8.3	5.0
736	2.5	2.0	1.2	-0.5	-0.9	-1.3	5.8	1.9
737	0.7	0.6	0.4	-0.1	-0.2	-0.3	6.3	2.2
741	2.4	2.1	1.7	-0.3	-0.4	-0.7	7.2	5.0
742	1.2	1.1	0.9	-0.1	-0.2	-0.3	6.8	5.2
743	1.8	1.8	1.7	0.0	-0.1	-0.1	8.3	6.7
744	2.3	2.1	1.6	-0.2	-0.5	-0.7	6.5	4.3
745	1.7	1.5	1.0	-0.2	-0.4	-0.7	6.1	3.6
749	3.3	3.2	2.8	-0.1	-0.4	-0.5	7.9	5.8
751	1.3	0.9	0.4	-0.4	-0.5	-0.9	5.3	0.1
752	2.7	5.2	6.8	2.5	1.7	4.1	16.7	9.8
759	2.0	3.9	5.2	1.9	1.2	3.2	17.4	9.7
761	1.1	1.0	1.2	-0.1	0.2	0.1	11.1	8.9
762	1.2	0.5	0.5	-0.7	0.1	-0.7	6.7	8.2
763	1.4	1.1	1.1	-0.3	-0.0	-0.3	9.5	6.9
764	4.4	4.5	8.0	0.1	3.5	3.6	10.6	12.7
771	0.8	0.8	1.2	-0.0	0.4	0.4	11.0	11.2
772	2.8	3.1	3.4	0.3	0.3	0.6	9.8	7.9
773	1.2	1.1	1.5	-0.1	0.4	0.3	9.1	10.4
774	0.6	0.8	0.7	0.2	-0.1	0.1	10.9	6.0
775	1.8	1.6	1.6	-0.2	-0.0	-0.2	8.7	6.9
776	3.0	4.0	8.8	1.0	4.8	5.8	14.8	15.0
778	3.0	3.2	3.6	0.2	0.4	0.6	9.2	8.2
781	12.3	15.6	13.5	3.3	-2.0	1.2	10.0	5.7
782	4.8	3.5	2.4	-1.3	-1.1	-2.4	5.0	3.5
783	0.8	0.7	0.6	-0.1	-0.0	-0.2	6.5	6.4
784	7.0	7.3	6.2	0.3	-1.1	-0.8	8.7	5.5
785	1.3	0.7	0.8	-0.6	0.0	-0.5	5.6	7.7
786	0.8	0.5	0.5	-0.3	-0.0	-0.3	5.9	6.7
791	0.7	0.4	0.4	-0.3	0.0	-0.3	3.3	7.8
792	5.6	6.6	5.0	1.0	-1.6	-0.6	10.8	4.4
793	3.5	1.9	1.9	-1.6	0.0	-1.6	4.9	7.2

Source: Own calculations and sources noted in Table 4.1. See Annex Table 4.A1.1 for a description of product groups.

The labour intensity of production in the clothing manufacturing process has driven shifts in locations within countries but particularly between countries with differing relative endowments of labour and capital. While other products also incorporate inputs for which the degree of labour intensity has meant that they are assembled in locations that minimise labour costs, the major difference with the clothing manufacturing process is that the labour intensity of the entire production process means that not only parts of the process are shifted to other locations but the entire manufacturing process.

Given that the textile complex employed roughly 2 million workers in the European Union and about 1 million in the United States in early 2000, it is clearly important to be able to assess the potential impact of changes in technology that could help preserve these jobs, or as many as possible, in their current locations or at least in the same countries. Chapter 3 has looked at the characteristics of displaced workers in the textile and clothing industries and examined the linkages between international trade and labour adjustment and recent developments and reforms in labour adjustment programmes in some OECD countries.

What shapes the exports of the textile and clothing machinery industry? Table 4.1 gives an overview of the 43 industries that constitute the machinery and transport sector: textile and clothing machinery is classified under the 724 SITC group. It lists the shares of the top four exporters from OECD countries (column labelled "Top 4") in that given industry. It lists the share attributed to the largest exporting country (a letter designates the country). It also shows for a given year the share of all industrialised countries in total world exports of the given industry. It reveals that the TCM industry has remained one of the most concentrated industries over the 20-year period. The share of the top four exporting countries has only slipped slightly since 1981, and just three industries have higher shares, as opposed to 15 in 1981. In respect of the country with the highest share in TCM, *i.e.* Germany, its share fell slightly from 25.9% to 23.7% between 1981 and 2002. In 1981, 23 other industries had ratios above the TCM ratio of the country with the highest share. In 2002, only nine industries had higher ratios than the country with the highest share.

Insights into technology trends in the textile and clothing industries

Clothing applications of textiles

Without going into the specifics for all types of materials and for every operation, the production of textile and clothing products covers the following spectrum of activities:

- Basic inputs: Gins; Bailing equipment; Cards; Frames.

- Textile production:
    - Production of filaments, fibres and yarns: Filament- and fibre-producing equipment; Twisters/winders; Spinning frames; Doffing machines/devices; Winding and reeling machines.
    - Weaving preparation and machines; Creels, warping and beaming machines; Rapier, air/water jets, shuttle looms, circular looms.
    - Knitwear and hosiery production: Beam warping machines; Circular knitting machines; Printing machines; Flat knitting machines.
    - Washing, bleaching, drying, etc.: Washings machines; Yarn/fabric dyeing machines; Printing machines; Inspecting machines

- Clothing production: Designing; Pattern making; Grading; Nesting and marking; Cutting; Sewing; Inspecting; Pressing; Packaging.
- Post-clothing production: Inventory; Transport.

On the upstream end of the above list, progressing from raw materials to a finished woven or knitted garment involves perhaps the two most capital-intensive steps, namely spinning and weaving. Given the advances achieved over the last decades (see Figures 4.4a and 4.4b), prevailing production frontiers permit speed, quality and flexibility of a sort that was unheard of 50 years ago. While the level of physical capital intensity has made the textile sector one of the more capital-intensive of manufacturing sectors, the human capital intensity required to operate the new equipment has increased less, given the embodied-intelligence in the software included in such new equipment. Annex 4.A2 provides details of productivity changes that have occurred in the main production stages from fabric to a finished clothing product. It also provides some insight into the area of technical textiles, which are not discussed at length in this chapter (see below), as their production processes and uses differ widely from those that are used for clothing or home furnishings.

One parameter that cannot yet be changed significantly is fabric width. If it could be adapted to fit the design optimally for grading, nesting and marking, fabric utilisation would be greatly improved. This would yield particularly great returns for top-of-the-line garments, which currently have much lower fabric utilisation rates. Another parameter which requires attention is set by the cutting machines, as high-ply lays still present problems. Finally, while the quality of needles has improved to the extent that a 10% to 20% increase in productivity can be achieved in some cases vis-à-vis the situation some decades ago, the quality (strength) of threads creates constraints. There are no major technical problems in downstream sewing activities, with the exception of the inability to compress clothes to optimal weight/volume for shipping.

Although the number of persons employed for a given output in each of these stages in the production process differs depending on the type of product and the length of the production run, it is generally accepted that the assembly stage, *i.e.* sewing, accounts for up to 80% of total labour costs. However, when shares in value added are calculated, it is clear that wage/salary levels are higher in the upstream activities. It is thus hardly surprising that the major technological changes to date have occurred upstream from sewing. However, it would be incorrect to assume that higher relative labour costs were the sole factor in major technological breakthroughs in this area; there is also the simple fact that the technological constraints in sewing and other downstream activities are more binding.

In order to determine what technological trends mean for the location of the textile and clothing industries, it is instructive to move back to the post-World War II period in Europe. That was when Swiss and German firms began to dominate weaving technology and later spinning. Their experience gives a picture of how important changes in the production of inputs play a role in the global textile and clothing production processes (Box 4.1).

Box 4.1. The essence of globalisation in the textile machinery sector at the micro level

In the mid-1970s, Schlafhorst was a company producing numerous winders (accounting for about 50% of total sales), cotton drawing and ring-spinning frames as well as warping and hosiery machines. It had many production units in Germany, with roughly 4 000 employees, and had experienced a continual decline in sales throughout the decade. In the late 1970s, it introduced a technologically advanced spinning frame, the culmination of five years of research. It ran at faster speeds, produced finer yarn counts and was equipped with a full range of automatic devices. The labour–saving potential dovetailed perfectly with the restructuring of textile mills in developed countries which were under considerable competitive pressure from textile mills in developing countries.

At the same time, Schlafhorst decided to eliminate eight production lines and to focus production on spinning equipment and cone winders. With a view to offering a fully integrated spinning process, it acquired the ring-spinning firm Zinser and became the world leader in spinning equipment. In late 1980s, owing to economic difficulties, Schlafhorst was taken over by Saurer, a Swiss equipment firm specialised in embroidery, quilt stitching and twisting machines. After acquiring Schlafhorst, Saurer's world share in spinning frames approached 50%.

To secure an adequate share in the fast-growing China/Asia markets, Saurer decided to establish ties with Chinese textile machinery manufacturers. As a result, the Saurer group has noticeably expanded activities in China and other parts of Asia, and these ties now form a crucial part of the company's global activities. This underscores the importance of ensuring that technological advances are interfaced and tested with textile firms operating under real-world conditions. The consolidation process, combined with the establishment of ties to Chinese machinery manufacturers, has paved the way for spinning frames produced in Germany to be exported to new destinations. In 2002, more than 60% of German-made spinning frames were exported to non-OECD countries.

Technological advances over the past quarter century have in fact had a major impact on the location of the textile and clothing industries, but also on the structure of textile and clothing machinery industry. The newer technologies have led to a departure from traditional practices whereby textile companies maintained a large stock of machinery and components (Landis, 1970, p. 184). They now concentrate more on producing and selling textiles and clothing.[5]

The continuing concentration of TCM in OECD countries is a result of evolving, multifaceted technological demands which can be best met by drawing on state-of-the-art technical and scientific knowledge that is readily accessible in OECD countries, where an effective interface between textile and clothing manufacturers is available (see below).[6] In the textile industry particularly, technical progress has been less restrained than in the clothing industry by the physical properties of the intermediary inputs.[7] The interface has been strengthened by a demand for ever higher quality and by more rapid changes in fashions, which have required more effective production controls and a greater degree of flexibility. Hence, successful exporting of textile and clothing products by OECD countries has increasingly become a function of quality. The level of quality demanded is often attainable only by employing capital equipment from OECD countries, with its embodied technologies and other essential components.[8] This has applied to the upstream end of the textile manufacturing process, *e.g.* spinning, and, to a lesser degree, to the sewing process.[9]

Thus, while the TCM industry has tended to be concentrated in OECD countries, exports of textiles and clothing have advanced strongly in non-OECD countries. There are essentially two reasons. First, in the first half of the 1980s, they began to acquire the new generation of textile machines, thereby increasing their productive capacities and the quality of output. Second, stronger competition in export markets has meant that effective labour cost differentials played a greater role even in such highly capital-intensive production processes.[10] Consequently, in 2001, the share of clothing exports originating in non–OECD countries had increased by 20% to over 50% and the share of textile exports by over a third to represent more than 40% of total world textile exports.[11]

As non-OECD economies came to play a greater role in the clothing and textile industries, they accounted for an increasing share of TCM imports but not of TCM production. In all of the 3–digit categories in the seven series of the SITC classification system, the share of TCM exports destined for non-OECD countries increased the most over the 1980s, and by 1990 represented the largest share of all 43 major categories of machinery and transport equipment. Thus, producers of TCM, more than exporters of any other machinery, rapidly began to sell to new customers, often in new markets.

Accompanying this international shift in demand for capital equipment from OECD to non-OECD countries was a definite trend towards seeking new production locations, primarily in Asian countries. In the 1980s, this was evident in most of the machinery and transport equipment categories. However, at the end of the 1980s, exports to OECD countries still largely dominated in textile and clothing machinery (Table 4.1). In the course of the 1990s, the share of TCM exports to OECD countries dropped slightly as non-OECD countries increased production and exports of such machines. Nonetheless, the OECD area's share of exports of TCM did not drop nearly as much as that in most other machinery categories. While the three major European producers of machinery concentrated their shipments to the European continent, Japan had already begun to use its locational advantage to supply the fast-growing Asian markets.[12]

Table 4.3. Germany's employment in manufacturing industries, 1993-2001

	Employees (thousands)			Annual percentage change		
	1993	1997	2001	93-97	97-01	93-01
Manufacturing	8 035.2	6 494.6	6 641.1	-5.18	0.75	-2.35
Mechanical engineering	1 084.8	1 014.6	1 030.8	-1.66	0.53	-0.64
Textile/clothing machinery	51.3	44.9	36.1	-3.28	-7.05	-4.31
Textiles	193.6	143.3	129.8	-7.25	-3.25	-4.88
Clothing	153.2	92.1	67.3	-11.95	-9.93	-9.77
Employees by establishment						
Manufacturing	75.3	69.3	64	-2.05	-2.6	-2
Mechanical engineering	96.3	98.6	88	0.59	-3.73	-1.12
Textile/clothing machinery	162.3	144.8	118.6	-2.81	-6.43	-3.84
Textiles	61	43.6	40.7	-8.05	-2.26	-4.93
Clothing	34.7	39.4	35	3.23	-3.89	0.1

Source: Own calculations based on *Statistisches Bundesamt, Fachserie 4, Reihe 4.1.2*, various years.

Before moving to the innovation policies implemented in individual OECD countries, it is worthwhile focusing briefly on how the entire textile and clothing complex has adjusted to various parameter shifts over the past decades. Germany, as the leading exporter of TCM and having been a major exporter of textile and clothing products offers a useful example. As Table 4.3 shows, the large employment shifts out of the clothing industry were followed by shifts out of the textile industry and then to a lesser degree out of the TCM industry, while mechanical engineering as a whole maintained its share or exhibited fewer employment losses. In clothing manufacturing, both employment and number of establishments have dropped in equal proportion, leaving the number of employees per establishment unchanged. In the textile industry, the number of employees per establishment dropped significantly, implying productivity increases.

Non-clothing applications of textiles or technical textiles

What precisely are technical textiles?[13] That is, where does the range of textiles for clothing end and that of technical textiles begin? The Textile Institute in the United Kingdom adopted in 1994 the following definition: "technical textiles are those textile materials and products manufactured primarily for their technical and performance properties rather than their aesthetic or decorative characteristics". In essence, this suggests the basic Bauhaus philosophy that "Form follows Function". Yet, a hiking jacket may be made entirely of specially designed technical textile fibres (function) but still be meant to be fashionable (form), so that a clear distinction between a clothing product and a technical textile is not possible. The problem is complicated by the speed with which new differentiated products are being developed. It may be best to refer either to the application groups used at the major fairs organised by the Messe Frankfurt or to the products produced. The latter are defined in terms of the properties of the product, e.g. non-woven, technical fabrics, etc., while the former use the areas in which the products are used, such as: Agrotech, Bondtech, Buildtech, Geotech, Hometech, Medtech, Mobiltech, Packtech, etc.

It is estimated that technical textiles are growing at roughly twice the rate of textiles for the clothing industry, where growth rates have been about 2% a year in recent years. In areas such as ecological protective textiles, geotextiles or protective textiles the growth rate may be twice that of the traditional clothing sector or even more. Technical textiles now account more than half of total textile production. Their growing importance is reflected in the globalisation of activities to support such industries. Hence, one of the world's largest fair organisers, Messe Frankfurt, now carries out five fairs focused on technical textiles worldwide, i.e. in Frankfurt, Atlanta, Moscow, Sao Paulo and Shanghai, compared to just two fairs some 12 years ago (Frankfurt and Osaka).

The growing importance of non-woven products, which accounted for about 25% of technical textile production in 2000, can be clearly demonstrated by examining the participation of machinery manufacturers at the fairs of the International Textile Machinery Association (ITMA) in the 1991 and 2003 (ITMA fairs are held every four years). Whereas in 1991, it was difficult to locate technical textile machinery exhibitors, an entire hall was dedicated to such equipment in 2003. This development underlines that the application potential of technical textiles is rapidly expanding.

The textile industry's major shift towards technical textiles has so far been widely associated with industries in OECD countries. Whereas many non-OECD countries can or can almost copy the quality of thread/yarn and woven fabrics produced in OECD countries, the processes involved in technical textiles are, for the moment, well beyond what many non-OECD countries can achieve.

Will technical textiles continue to be produced in OECD countries? Or, as in the case of the textile and clothing industries, will production move to non-OECD countries? The processes involved have developed through the same type of intersectoral co-operation and research as occurred between the TCM industry and the textile and clothing industries. However, as the new processes become standardised and technology flows to non-OECD countries, where universities are already connected to global developments, these industries are likely to be established as well. Whenever major industries shift to or expand production in non-OECD countries, it is only a matter of time before inputs are produced there as well. Hence, the question is to what extent the production of technical textiles can be maintained in OECD countries. To answer this question, additional research is needed on the drivers of the technical textile industry. If the migration occurs, it could take place faster than before, since the textile industry failed to migrate as fast as the clothing industry owing to MFA-related quotas applied on textile and clothing products in OECD countries.

Innovation systems in OECD countries

Economic and innovative performance of textiles and clothing

Over two centuries ago, the textile and iron industries were the main drivers of the industrial revolution. The mechanical loom, the substitution of cotton for wool, and the steam engine as a device for converting heat into work emerged as the core elements of the cotton mill. This paved the way for the factory system, which expanded further when sewing machines were introduced in the mid-nineteenth century.

The role that textile and clothing production plays in the industrialisation process of developing countries is very different from what it was some 30 years ago when the MFA regime was instituted. The clothing industry, where time-tested technology is linked to low labour costs, still gives developing countries a competitive edge in world markets. Today, the situation is becoming more complicated, however, as time factors now play a far more crucial role in determining competitiveness (Hummels, 2001). In order to remain competitive, the more developed countries need to climb the technology ladder, through either product or process innovations.

Following the imposition of MFA quotas and the broader application of quotas that ensued, textile and clothing producers in OECD countries understood that they would be increasingly subjected to competitive pressures, stemming also from technological challenges in the rapidly expanding developing countries. Nevertheless, they were unable to prevent significant downsizing in these industries. On average, the employment share of textiles and clothing in total manufacturing declined by one-third over the past two decades (Table 4.4). There are no exceptions to this trend, as even relatively labour-rich countries, such as Greece, Mexico and Portugal, saw shrinking employment shares in textiles and clothing between 1980 and 2001.

Although there are considerable differences in technology and factor intensity between the textile and clothing industries,[14] their relative decline was similar for the OECD area as a whole. Employment shares have declined in textiles in all countries, and, while the shares of clothing increased in Greece, Italy and Portugal, they fell in the other countries. By and large, for textiles, the relative reduction in employment was greatest in the major textile and clothing producing countries; for clothing, it was greatest in countries where the shares of both textiles and clothing in total employment are quite low.

As more developing countries expanded exports of textile and clothing products over the last two decades, locations close to the European Union (e.g. eastern Europe) and the United States (e.g. Mexico and the Caribbean) proved to be very attractive for textile and clothing production. The speed of downward adjustment in textiles and clothing accelerated from the 1980s to the 1990s, demonstrating that structural change in these industries is far from complete and can be expected to continue.

Table 4.4. Share of textiles and clothing in total manufacturing employment in OECD countries

	Textiles and clothing			Textiles			Clothing		
	1980	1990	2001	1980	1990	2001	1980	1990	2001
Australia	8.6	8.3	6.3	3.5	3.4	2.9	5.1	4.9	3.4
Austria	11.7	9.1	5.3	6.0	4.8	3.2	5.7	4.3	2.1
Belgium	13.2	11.9	8.5	7.4	7.0	6.8	5.8	4.9	1.7
Canada	8.9	7.9	6.1	3.0	2.5	2.0	5.9	5.4	4.1
Denmark	7.1	5.6	2.9	3.1	2.8	1.8	4.0	2.8	1.1
Finland	11.3	6.8	3.6	4.2	2.5	1.7	7.1	4.3	1.9
France	11.0	8.5	5.4	4.9	3.9	2.9	6.1	4.6	2.5
Germany	7.6	5.2	2.8	4.3	3.0	1.8	3.3	2.2	1.0
Greece	30.5	28.8	22.1	17.8	14.5	6.6	12.7	14.3	15.5
Italy	17.3	16.5	14.6	11.7	7.9	8.0	5.6	8.6	6.6
Japan	15.4	12.4	7.6	7.2	4.5	2.7	8.2	7.9	4.9
Korea	30.9	22.0	14.7	19.5	11.8	7.7	11.4	10.2	7.0
Mexico	18.4	16.1	16.6	7.7	7.3	7.1	10.7	8.8	9.5
Netherlands	5.0	3.9	2.7	3.3	2.4	1.9	1.7	1.5	0.8
Norway	5.2	3.1	2.6	3.5	2.3	1.9	1.7	0.8	0.7
Poland	-	-	12.7	-	-	-	-	-	-
Portugal	31.1	31.2	28.0	18.4	15.3	11.5	12.7	15.9	16.5
Spain	13.4	11.8	9.7	6.9	5.1	4.3	6.5	6.7	5.4
Sweden	3.9	2.7	1.7	2.0	1.7	1.1	1.9	1.0	1.6
United Kingdom	10.9	9.9	8.8	5.2	4.6	4.1	5.7	4.3	4.7
United States	10.4	9.1	5.9	4.8	4.6	3.5	5.6	4.5	2.4
OECD average	13.6	11.5	8.8	7.2	5.6	4.2	6.4	5.9	4.6

Notes: Clothing includes leather. Instead of 2001, Belgium and Germany refer to 2000, Australia, Norway, Portugal and Sweden to 1999, Mexico and United Kingdom to 1997, and Korea to 1996. In 1980 and 1990, Germany only refers to West Germany.

Source: OECD, STAN database.

Structural adjustment pressures mainly result from changes in the international division of labour. Export and import shares in textiles and clothing are high, international investment activities are expanding and subcontracting (largely in the form of outward processing programmes) plays a dominant role (Matthes, 2002; Grömling and Matthes, 2003). In a global setting, countries' economic performance crucially depends on the ability of domestic producers to gain a competitive edge.

Revealed comparative advantage (RCA) is a well-established concept for measuring the sectoral performance of countries in the international division of labour. Balassa (1965) argued that a country's comparative advantage in a specific industry should be revealed by a positive balance in international trade, normalised by the country's total trade balance. To obtain an unbounded and symmetric measure, the formula originally proposed by Balassa was modified as follows (Klodt et Maurer, 1995):

$$RCA_i^j = \ln(x_i^j / m_i^j : \sum_i x_i^j / \sum_i m_i^j) \cdot 100 \cdot$$

where x and m denote exports and imports and i and j denote industries and countries. This index, which is limited to a range between plus and minus infinity, is positive for those industries in which country j has a revealed comparative advantage and negative for industries in which it has a revealed comparative disadvantage. Trade in textiles is covered by SITC categories 26 and 65 and trade in clothing SITC categories 84 (United Nations, 1986).

Of the 28 countries for which comprehensive trade data are available, 13 showed a comparative advantage in textiles and clothing in 2001, and 15 showed a comparative disadvantage (Table 4.5). With 15 positive and 13 negative RCA coefficients, the picture was quite similar in 1991. According to this concept, the most competitive countries in textiles and clothing are Belgium, Greece, Italy, Korea, Mexico, Portugal, Turkey, China, Hong Kong (China) and Chinese Taipei.

Comparative advantage looks different, however, when textiles and clothing are analysed separately. In 2001, only six countries had a positive RCA coefficient in both industries (Belgium, China, Italy, Korea, Chinese Taipei and Turkey) and nine countries had a negative coefficient in both industries (Canada, Finland, France, Ireland, Spain, Norway, Sweden, the United Kingdom and the United States). As a rule of thumb, positive RCA coefficients for textiles tend to dominate in relatively capital-rich countries, whereas positive coefficients for clothing are found in relatively labour-rich ones.

In addition to factor intensity, historical and cultural roots matter. Carpets from Belgium and fashions from Italy are cases in point. It is probably no accident that the famous case study used by Krugman (1991, pp. 59-61) to illustrate path dependencies in the "new economic geography" (bedspreads from Georgia) is taken from textiles and clothing.

The sign of the comparative position of most countries in textiles and clothing has not changed over time. There is a general deterioration, however, in the position of advanced countries and a corresponding improvement in that of China, Mexico and Chinese Taipei. The export opportunities of Mexico have been enlarged by the preferential access to US and Canadian markets granted under NAFTA. China's performance cannot be explained by its WTO accession, as it only acceded at the end of 2001. The situation is different in the Central and Eastern European countries which obtained access to EU markets after the signing of the Europe Agreements.[15] These countries may be interested in expanding exports to the EU in industries other than textiles and clothing, and it is likely that most will become net importers of textiles and clothing in the near future.[16]

Table 4.5. Revealed comparative advantages in textiles and clothing

	Textiles and clothing		Textiles		Clothing	
	1991	2001	1991	2001	1991	2001
Australia	75	27	77	79	-128	-123
Austria	5	-24	5	7	-3	-58
Belgium	29	33	52	44	-20	15
Canada	-100	-50	-109	-65	-106	-39
Czech Republic	61	15	44	-16	74	61
Denmark	6	-7	-38	-24	50	9
Finland	-47	-69	-67	-41	-22	-104
France	-9	-28	-26	-10	9	-46
Germany	-22	-27	2	9	-46	-64
Greece	62	22	-68	-33	200	60
Hungary	50	15	-91	-105	162	111
Ireland	-2	-63	-15	-19	11	-106
Italy	92	72	11	33	194	106
Japan	-39	-104	4	17	-208	-340
Korea	123	119	81	101	233	128
Mexico	-38	22	-49	-103	-74	114
Netherlands	-17	-19	-24	5	-5	-34
Norway	-171	-182	-118	-112	-232	-261
Poland	47	-5	-48	-123	146	146
Portugal	90	54	-50	-19	250	130
Spain	-45	-22	-48	-19	-68	-34
Sweden	-95	-67	-69	-36	-113	-93
Turkey	206	141	62	32	560	364
United Kingdom	-25	-72	-44	-43	-7	-99
United States	-74	-119	10	-172	-145	-189
China	110	133	-3	6	394	367
Hong Kong, China	42	36	-19	-9	96	69
Chinese Taipei	134	171	54	128	1 323	1 266

Note: For a definition of revealed comparative advantage, see text. Instead of 1991, Belgium, the Czech Republic and Korea refer to 1993, Poland and Hong Kong, China, to 1992. Chinese Taipei 2001 data refers to 1999.

Source: Own calculations based on OECD, International Trade by Commodity Statistics.

It has repeatedly been shown, both theoretically and empirically, that the competitive position of producers from advanced countries on world markets is closely related to the technology intensity of their products or production processes. However, technology intensity not only depends on appropriate business strategies of firms, but also on the technological potential of the respective industry. As compared to other manufacturing industries, this potential seems to be largely exploited in textiles and clothing. Consequently, the R&D intensity of the textile and clothing industries is quite low throughout the OECD area (Table 4.6). Today, the countries with the highest R&D intensity are Ireland (where R&D intensity in textiles and clothing is almost as high as in manufacturing on average), Finland, Japan, Belgium and Germany.

Table 4.6. R&D intensity of OECD countries, 1990–2000

	Textiles and clothing		Total manufacturing	
	1990	**2000**	**1990**	**2000**
Belgium	1.2	2.2	5.2	6.6
Canada	0.7	1.0	3.4	4.0
Denmark	0.4	0.9	4.2	5.9
Finland	1.1	2.4	4.7	8.8
France	0.4	0.9	7.0	7.0
Germany	1.5	2.0	6.7	7.4
Ireland	2.0	2.8	2.7	3.3
Italy	0.0	0.1	2.9	2.1
Japan	1.6	2.1	7.3	7.6
Korea	0.6	0.9	5.2	4.5
Netherlands	0.7	1.3	5.5	5.7
Norway	0.9	1.9	5.1	4.3
Spain	0.1	0.6	2.0	2.1
Sweden	1.5	1.1	8.7	12.3
United Kingdom	0.3	0.4	5.9	6.1
United States	0.6	0.5	8.5	8.3
OECD area	0.9	1.4	5.3	6.0

Notes: Intensity refers to direct R&D expenditures as a percentage of gross output. Textile and clothing includes leather. OECD average is an unweighted average. Ireland and Italy 1990 refer to 1991. Belgium 1990 refers to 1992. Germany and Korea 1990 refer to 1995. Canada and Norway 2000 refer to 1997. Ireland, Japan and Sweden 2000 refer to 1998. Denmark, France, Korea, Netherlands, Spain and United Kingdom 2000 refer to 1999.

Source: OECD, ANBERD database.

Nevertheless, research intensity in textiles and clothing has increased substantially in almost all OECD countries over the past decade. This is the case not only in absolute terms, but also relative to total manufacturing. With Ricardian trade theory in mind, where relative technology levels determine comparative advantage, one might expect that the countries with the highest relative increase in R&D intensity should exhibit the most pronounced improvement in their RCA indices. In order to check this hypothesis, an index was calculated which measures the change in R&D specialisation by the ratio of relative R&D intensity of textiles and clothing in 2000 divided by the corresponding relative R&D intensity in 1990 (calculated from Table 4.6). When the resulting coefficient exceeds unity, the respective country has increased its R&D specialisation in textiles and clothing over time. Change in comparative advantage was measured by the difference between the RCA coefficients of 2001 and 1991 (calculated from Table 4.5). Positive differences indicate improved international competitiveness and negative ones indicate deterioration.

According to these calculations, the most significant increase in R&D specialisation took place in Spain (Table 4.7). Spain has also substantially improved its trade performance in textiles and clothing as measured by the RCA concept. This observation supports the Ricardian trade model. On the other hand, Sweden was able to improve its trade performance even more, although the R&D intensity of textiles and clothing declined not only in relative, but even in absolute terms. France and Norway have increased their R&D specialisation, but lost ground in international competitiveness. All in all, there is no significant correlation between the increase in R&D and trade performance for the countries covered in Table 4.6. Therefore, it does not follow that more money for industrial R&D would more or less automatically lead to improved competitiveness on world markets.

The major reason for the weak relationship between technological specialisation and trade performance is the fact that most innovations in textiles and clothing are created in other industries. New materials are mainly developed in the chemical industry, and new processes are developed in the machinery industry. As shown above, these industries contribute substantially to improving the technological sophistication of textiles and clothing.

As a result, the technological competitiveness of producers of textiles and clothing largely depends on their ability to adopt new products and processes developed elsewhere. Therefore, technology transfer is the major source of innovative activities within these industries. The main features of these activities for major OECD countries are surveyed below.

Table 4.7. R&D specialisation and trade performance of textiles and clothing

	R&D specialisation	Change in comparative advantage
Belgium	1.44	4
Canada	1.21	50
Denmark	1.6	-13
Finland	1.17	-22
France	2.25	-17
Germany	1.21	-5
Ireland	1.15	-61
Japan	1.26	-65
Korea	1.73	-4
Netherlands	1.79	-2
Norway	2.5	-11
Spain	5.71	23
Sweden	0.52	28
United Kingdom	1.29	-47
United States	0.85	-45

Notes: The R&D specialisation is the ratio of percentage change in textile and clothing R&D intensity shares between 2000 and 1990 to same ratio for total manufacturing, *e.g.* for Belgium: [(2.2/1.2) / (6.6/5.2)] = 1.44. Change in comparative advantage is measures by the difference between the RCA coefficient of 2001 and 1991: for Belgium: 33-29 = 4.

Source: Own calculations based on Tables 4.5 and 4.6.

Innovation and technology diffusion approaches by country

The following survey of the most important institutions engaged in research on textiles and clothing in the OECD area focuses on countries in which these industries contribute substantially to total manufacturing output and employment (see Table 4.4). The major focus of these institutions is on innovation-oriented consulting and on technology transfer from chemicals and machinery. Furthermore, they often have close links to specialised university departments and focus on technology transfer from university research to innovative activities in the textile and clothing industries.

Innovation and technology diffusion approaches in OECD countries largely concentrate on support for such research institutions. By contrast to popular high-technology industries, such as microelectronics and aerospace, specific research and innovation programmes are rare and there are almost no specific government institutions or public budgets for the textile and clothing industries. Instead, innovation policy can be characterised as a hybrid system of private and public research institutions. Understanding the innovation system of this industry therefore requires an understanding of the network of private firms and semi-private research institutions. As textiles and clothing are mature and traditional industries, these networks often have deep historical roots.

As a further common denominator, the research institutions usually are geographically scattered and highly diversified in their innovative activities. Usually, there is no central co-ordination by the government, and most institutions define the aim and scope of their activities independently. In most countries, their work is supported by national employer organisations and certain supranational institutions.

Corporate and individual members from over 90 countries are represented by the Textile Institute (www.textileinstitute.org), which has its headquarters in Manchester (United Kingdom) and provides various technical and market-related information relating to textiles, clothing and footwear. However, it does not engage in research, and its information capacities are basically limited to library services.

EURATEX (www.euratex.org), a non-profit trade organisation dedicated to the promotion of the European textile and clothing industries, is the most important supranational institution at the European level. It is located in Brussels. Its members are national textile and clothing associations from 24 European countries, including seven associations from new EU member states, as well as from Turkey and Morocco. In the area of R&D, it concentrates on the provision of information about European R&D policies and funding opportunities, European research institutions and relevant research and technology developments, and on the co-ordination, promotion and support of European R&D projects. In addition, EURATEX supports the industry in defining commercial strategies, in developing an integrated environmental strategy and in defending intellectual property rights against counterfeiting and piracy. Bulletins, position papers and newsletters contain relevant information about market trends, new technologies and policy initiatives.

The second major European institution is TEXTRANET (www.textranet.org), which is located in Paris and was established by national textile research and technology organisations from the European Union and EFTA. It promotes co-operation among technical centres in various countries, especially in areas that require an intense exchange of information or significant funding for individual projects. It has set up data banks on textile technology and is promoting research projects on specific themes. The projects are carried out at national technical centres which are selected and co-ordinated by TEXTRANET. These activities mainly serve the needs of small and medium-sized enterprises that would be unable to afford such projects on their own. A further goal of TEXTRANET is to avoid duplication and scattering of research efforts by improving communication and co-ordination of national research and technology institutions.

In addition, there are a number of smaller European institutions with limited or no own R&D facilities. Examples are Eurocotton (Committee of the Cotton and Allied Textile Industries of the EU), Interlaine (Committee of the Wool Textile Industry in the EU), ECA (European Carpet Association) in Brussels and ETAP (European Association for Textile Polyolefins), all four in Brussels, Aertel (European Ribbon, Braid and Elastic Fabric Association) in Ghent, or EUROCORD (European Federation of Wire Rope Industries) in Paris.

Belgium

Centexbel (www.centexbel.be) is the major research institution of the Belgium textile industry. A private organisation with 120 staff members, it is engaged in developing and promoting technological innovation and providing information and training about technological trends and new applications. It has offices in Brussels, Zwijnaarde (near Ghent) and Herve. In yarn engineering, for instance, Centexbel concentrates on extrusion and thermomechanical processes, on crystal structure and thermostability characteristics, and on improving the quality and processability of synthetic yarns. Further topics include microbiology and hygiene, flax and carpet technology, and standardisation, certification, patents and testing. Technical information for the textile industry is also provided by Febeltex (www.febeltex.be), an employer organisation which represents about 500 textile companies.

Czech Republic

Based on the long tradition of Bohemian textiles, Inotex (www.inotex.cz) is both a producer of textiles, dyes and textile machinery and a provider of standardisation and technical assistance to the Czech textile industry. It was founded in 1992 as a successor to the Research Textile Finishing Institute. Since 1993, it also runs a scientific-technical park called the Centre of Textile Technology and Education.

France

The Institut Français Textile-Habillement (French Textile and Apparel Institute, www.ifth.org) carries out general interest missions and provides a variety of services for the French textile and clothing industries. It has 350 staff members working at 13 sites throughout the country. Research projects, financed both by private contracts and by public funds, are concerned with fibres, structures and composites, measurement and control systems, design and production processes, training tools and exchange of information. Among others, fire resistance, manufacturability, comfort of clothing, and microbiological properties are analysed. IFTH supports research projects of private firms through consulting, training and the publication of scientific and technical documents. Its services also include certification of products and companies, and participation in French and international standardisation commissions.

Technological consulting, promotion and training are provided by Espace Textile (www.espacetextile.com), set up by French textile companies, by the Fédération Française des Industries Diverses de l'Habillement (www.lamode=francaise.org), the Fédération Nationale de l'Habillement (www.federation-habillement.fr), the Federation de l'Ennoblissement Textile (www.textile.fr/fet), and the Fédération Française des Industries Lainière et Cotonnière (www.fedcoton-laine.com).

Research and innovation activities of the French textile and clothing industries benefit significantly from a number of public schools and universities. The most important ones are ENSAIT (Ecole Nationale Supérieure des Arts et Industries Textiles), ENSITM (Ecole Nationale Supérieure des Industries Textiles), ESIM (Ecole Supérieure des Industries et de la Mode), ESITE (Ecole Supérieure des Industries Textiles), ESIV (Ecole Supérieure des Industries du Vêtement), and ESTIT (Ecole Supérieure des Techniques Industrielles et des Textiles).

To a certain extent, innovative activities of the French textile and clothing industries are co-ordinated by its employer organisation, the Union of Textile Industries (www.textile.fr), which is otherwise mainly concerned with lobbying and training initiatives.

Germany

Research and innovation activities in German textiles and clothing are co-ordinated by the Forschungskuratorium Textil (Textile Research Council, www.textil-online.de/forschung). Members are the German employer organisation Gesamttextil (www.textil-online.de) and a number of technical and regional associations. Other members include the Deutsche Institute für Textil- und Faserforschung (German Institute for Textile and Fibre Research) at the University of Stuttgart (www.uni-stuttgart.de), the Textilforschungszentrum Aachen at the Technical University of Aachen (www.rwth-aachen.de), the Deutsches Textilforschungszentrum (German Textile Research Centre) at the University of Duisburg (www.dtnw.de), the Hohenheimer Institute (www.hohenstein.de), the Textilforschungsverbund Nord-Ost, which covers five research institutes in eastern Germany, and four smaller individual institutes in Krefeld, Bremen and Munster. One of these is the STFI (Sächsesches Textil Forschungs Institut, www.stfi.de) which is specialised in technical textiles, non-wovens, geotextiles, environmental applications and protective clothing.

The Deutsche Institute für Textil- und Faserforschung at the University of Stuttgart has been split up into three separate institutes which conduct research on chemical fibres, polymers and spinning (Institut für Chemiefasern, www.uni-stuttgart.de/icf), on weaving, spinning and texturing (Institut für Textil- und Verfahrenstechnik, www.itv-denkendorf.de), and on dyeing and composite materials (Institut für Textilchemie, www.uni-stuttgart.de/itc). These three institutes employ about 100 scientists and engineers and their research projects are typically carried out in co-operation with and co-financed by private firms.

The same applies to the three institutes of the Textilforschungszentrum Aachen, which are working on quality assessment of yarn, on weaving, on technical and medical textiles, on recycling and on new materials (Institut für Textiltechnik, www.ita.rwth-aachen.de), on carpets and carpet processing (Deutsches Teppich-Forschungsinstitut, www.tfi-online.de), and on chemical, physical and biological properties of wool and wool processing (Deutsches Wollforschungsinstitut, www.dwi.rwth-aachen.de).

The Deutsches Textilforschungszentrum at the University of Duisburg (www.dtnw.de) specialises in innovation in textile processing. Major German research institutes are at Hohenheim (www.hohenstein.de) and conduct public-private projects, mainly on product and design innovations in garments (Bekleidungsphysiologisches Institut), on testing and certifying textile materials (Forschungsinstitut Hohenstein), and on cleaning of textiles and apparel (Forschungsstelle Textilreinigung). All in all, the German innovation system is characterised by close links between specialised university institutes and private companies which co-operate on many co-financed projects.

Greece

In the decades leading up to its EU membership, Greece was a traditional location for outward processing trade with other European countries. Since this type of trade basically aims at circumventing tariff barriers, Greece only had limited research activities. Since its EU accession, outward processing trade is less attractive and Greece has had to rely upon its own technological base.

The major institution for providing scientific and technological services to private companies in textiles and clothing is the Clothing Textile and Fibre Technology Development Company (CLOTEFI, www.etakei.gr), which was founded in 1986. It is a non-profit organisation under the supervision of the Ministry of Development's General Secretariat for Research and Technology. CLOTEFI's activities include: product testing and quality control; troubleshooting relating to quality problems and technology implementation; pilot studies to simulate industrial processes at laboratory scale; and designing and implementing research projects on behalf of the European Commission or the Greek government.

Hungary

INNOVATEXT (www.innovatext.hn) is the central textile engineering and testing institute of Hungary. Founded in 1949, its services to private firms include laboratory tests and site inspections, assistance with the distribution of self-developed branded products, scientific and technical information, and special training courses. In addition, it provides services on quality control and standardisation, environmental protection and textile recycling. It participates in several international research projects commissioned by the EU.

Italy

The innovation landscape in Italy is marked by a number of regionally and sectorally specialised firms that provide research assistance to textile and clothing producers. An example is the Como Textile Company (www.textilecomo.com) which offers training and communication services and technical consulting to firms in the Como District. Another is Tecnotessile (www.tecnotex.it) which carries out R&D projects on the behalf of private firms, offers consultancy support for application for European and national R&D funds, and helps to meet the requirements of quality and environment standards. A similar institution for the Emilia Romagna region is ASTER (Agenzia per lo Sviluppo Tecnologico dell' Emilia Romagna; www.aster.it), although it does not specialise in textiles and clothing but offers assistance for innovation activities in a variety of industries. In the same region, CITER (Centro di Informazione Tessile dell'Emilia Romagna; www.citer.it) offers a variety of information services about technological and fashion trends in textiles and clothing.

CENTROCOT (Centre Tessile Cotoniero e Abbigliamento, www.centrocot.it) runs its own laboratories for material and product testing. They are open to any Italian textile and clothing producer. Its research activities concentrate on the promotion of joint research projects of small and medium-sized firms and academic institutions. In addition, Centrocot offers certification and quality control services.

The activities of these and many other smaller research institutions are linked to corresponding research departments at universities (for instance the Politecnico di Torino) and to the network of the Italian National Research Council (www.cnr.it), the major public organisation for the support of scientific and technological research in Italy.

Korea

In Korea, the main industry association is the Korea Federation of Textile Industries (KOFOTI) (www.kofoti.or.kr), founded in 1967. It aims at strengthening the competitiveness of the Korean textile industry as the industry's leading organisation. It organises trade fairs, engages in lobbying and public relations activities regarding government regulation and trade policy, runs a fashion information library, and offers information about national and international market trends.

Another major institution is the Korea Chemical Fibers Association (www.kcfa.or.kr) which represents 14 companies engaged in chemical fibre production. It represents the interests of member companies and provides various services in support of technological development, productivity improvement and product quality.

These two institutions do not carry out research projects. The most important Korean institutions that engage in research on textiles and clothing are KTDI (Korean Textile Development Institute, www.textile.or.kr) and KATRI (Korea Apparel Testing and Research Institute, www.katri.re.kr). Both are private non-profit organisations and run research laboratories and testing facilities. They give technological support to private firms and offer certification services. In addition, the Korean government has launched the "Milano Project", which aims at developing the Daegu region into a "worldwide textile and fashion mecca" by linking fashion, design and clothing industries with the local weaving and dyeing industry (www.milano.daegu.kr). The project, started in 1999, supports R&D in design and apparel and in yarn, dyeing, fabrication, textile machinery and synthetic fabrics. Total funding of KRW 680 billion (about USD 500 million) is covered by the central government (54%), private enterprises (28.5%) and local government (7.5%).

Portugal

In Portugal, the major institution for the support of research and innovation in textiles and clothing is CITEVE (Technological Centre for the Textile and Garment Industries of Portugal, www.citeve.pt). A non-profit company, it offers consulting and technological assistance to Portuguese companies. Its laboratories specialise in quality control, environmental certification and defect analysis. They are also able to provide services for laboratory equipment calibration and textile conditioning and storage. CITEVE is divided into nine technology transfer units that range from dyeing, printing and finishing to technical textiles to health and safety at work. A major area of technological activity is support to Portuguese firms in their application for research projects financed by the European Commission. Furthermore, CITEVE offers technical assistance in training and participates in public debate on industrial policy issues.

Spain

AITEX (Instituto Tecnológico Textil, www.aitex.es) is a private non-profit organisation for the promotion of innovation and technological development in the Spanish textile industry. It has its own laboratories and research staff and offers support to private firms in several technological areas such as improving the water resistance of fibres.

The major academic research institution for textiles and clothing is INTEXTER (Institute of Textile Research and Industrial Cooperation, www.ct.upc.es/intexter) at the Universidad Politécnica de Catalunya at Barcelona. It offers technical assistance, material analyses and tests, quality control and standardisation services, education and training, and runs its own research projects. These are carried out in nine different laboratories which specialise in the control of environmental contamination, the physiochemistry of dyeing, physical textile parametry, textile polymers, textile mechanical systems and processes, surfactants and detergency, textile chemistry technology, special and knitted fabrics, and environmental toxicology. Many of the individual research projects are commissioned by the European Commission under its BRITE/EURAM, ESPRIT or CRAFT programmes.

Turkey

Despite the high importance of clothing for the Turkish economy, there are few institutions for the promotion of research and innovation in this industry. Industry interests are mainly articulated by ITKIB (Istanbul Textile and Apparel Exporters' Association) (www.itkib.org.tr) which organises trade fairs, provides a data bank for the clothing sector and represents its member companies in dealing with the Turkish government and at international level. It also operates a quality control and research laboratory. Another representative institution is TCMA (Turkish Clothing Manufacturer's Association, www.tgsd.org). As a member of IAF (International Apparel Federation) and EURATEX, it represents the clothing industry, organises trade fairs and provides data. A major focus is to fully exploit the advantages of the customs union with the European Union.

The Turkish clothing industry would seem to have a significant potential for innovation and development. The main research and innovation institution is TUBITAK-TRC (Scientific and Technical Research Council of Turkey – Textiles Research Centre). It was founded in 2001 and conducts research activities in co-operation with the industry and related universities. The Department of Textile Engineering of the Aegean University (www.ege.edu.tr) carries out R&D activities and pilot projects. Textile engineering education is also offered in the Istanbul Technical University (www.tekstil.itu.edu.tr). Most recent research projects are carried out for SMEs. Turkey possesses a rich human capital base for the manufacturing of clothing, but national firms lack appropriate facilities for material testing and development. Likewise, they have only limited access to consulting services for improving market research and marketing strategies which might allow Turkish manufacturers to earn higher prices for their products on world markets.

United Kingdom

UK research and innovation activities in textiles and clothing are dominated by non-profit research companies established by private firms. The most important is the British Textile Technology Group (www.bttg.co.uk) at Manchester, which offers a variety of standardisation and testing services and is also engaged in the development of innovative materials and production technologies. Its research fields relate to fire protection, testing of technical textiles, new carpet and floor covering technologies, certification of equipment and products, and innovation in spinning and non–woven fabrics.

Furthermore, several British universities have strong expertise in textiles and clothing, above all the University of Manchester Institute of Science and Technology (www.umist.ac.uk). It offers research and technology translation and executive training and consultancy for private customers from the textile and clothing industries. In addition, collaborative research is promoted by a subsidiary of this university, UMIST Venture Ltd., which is dedicated to facilitating the start-up of new companies in any industry able to exploit commercially the results of academic research.

United States

Information about the US textile and clothing industries is collected and disseminated by OTEXA (Office of Textiles and Apparel, www.otexa.ita.doc.gov), which is part of the

Department of Commerce. Although not directly engaged in research and innovation, it informs about trends in international trade and trade policy which might help to design sustainable innovation strategies. Moreover, it administers the basic research projects of the National Textile Center and the Textile and Clothing Technology Center.

The National Textile Center (www.ntcresearch.org) is a research consortium of eight universities, which gets research funds from the US Congress. Its research projects are concerned with chemical systems (dyeing, finishing, waste reduction), fabrication of fibres, management systems (innovations in production, distribution and consumption applications), and materials science (natural and synthetic polymers and fibres).

Another university-related institute is Clemson Apparel Research (http://car.clemson.edu) at Clemson University, South Carolina. It is dedicated to the support of the sewing industry, but is also active in textiles and related materials research and applications. A further field of activity is manufacturing and supply chain optimisation. Its core facility is a model plant which produces military garments for the Department of Defense. Research activities concentrate on the development of supply chain execution software, mass customisation software and software for colour inventory management, cost-benefit analysis, and computer-aided design and production.

Similar research institutions are the School of Polymer, Textile and Fiber Engineering (www.tfe.gatech.edu) at the Georgia Institute of Technology, the Department of Textile Engineering (www.eng.auburn.edu/department/te) at Auburn University, and the School of Textiles and Materials Technology (www.philau.edu/schools/tmt) at Philadelphia University.

In addition, several other research institutions carry out projects for private firms and are linked to universities. An example is the Institute of Textile Technology (www.itt.edu) at the North Carolina State University. Its research services include a Textile Analysis and Troubleshooting Laboratory which provides chemical testing and defect analysis.

By contrast, the Textile and Clothing Technology Corporation (www.tc2.com) and the Textile Research Institute (www.triprinceton.org) are independent from universities. The former is a joint non-profit company of more than 200 textile and clothing producers throughout the United States and is mainly concerned with mass customisation technologies. The most prominent project in this area is related to 3–D body measurement, which assists retailers and customers in selecting the appropriate size of clothing. The latter is a joint non-profit company of about 30 corporate member firms and specialises in materials testing and the development of innovative fibres, films and porous materials.

Innovation and marketing activities of private firms are further supported by various trade organisations, such as the American Apparel and Footwear Association, the American Fiber Manufacturers Association and the National Cotton Council, although these institutions do not have research facilities.

Towards best practice in innovation policies

History also matters in industrial policy. Different countries have different backgrounds of industrial development and thus differ with respect to optimal policy support for specific industries, such as textiles and clothing. However, some general lessons can be drawn from cross-country experience.

First, there seems to be no fundamental lack of invention and innovation. It would not be appropriate for governments, therefore, to launch large-scale basic research projects on textile and clothing technologies beyond the horizontal industrial research schemes based on public-private co-funding mechanisms. Although the textile and clothing industries can be considered mature, they use technological innovations that are largely generated in other industries, above all in chemicals and machinery. These technology suppliers are well able to provide product and process innovations for textiles and clothing without financial support from public research programmes. While governments may stimulate collaborative innovation processes in the fields of dissemination and technology transfer, such approaches should not distort market-oriented innovation programmes.

Second, technology transfer between technology suppliers and technology users plays a pivotal role in the technological performance of textiles and clothing. It seems appropriate, therefore, that all countries surveyed above are concentrating their innovation policies in this area. Nevertheless, this approach should probably be strengthened, because the opportunities offered by modern information and communication technologies for the dissemination of advanced technological knowledge are not yet fully exploited. Such a policy would require complementary public funding to give innovators financial incentives for passing proprietary technological knowledge to other firms.

Third, many SMEs often face substantial difficulties in the marketing of their products, because they lack a widely recognised reputation for high product quality. Governments could support marketing activities by promoting certification agencies and common brand names. At present, government activities in this area mainly concentrate on sponsoring fairs and exhibitions.

Finally, governments should keep in mind that, in the long run, innovative capacities basically depend on the availability of suitable human capital. Therefore, a sound education and qualification system seems much more important for sustainable technical progress than public innovation programmes. This applies not only to textiles and clothing, but to any industry.

Conclusion

Applied technologies in the textile and clothing industries over the past decade, as in earlier periods, have assumed a differentiated path. While the textile industry can point to numerous improvements and innovations which should allow it to extend its secular productivity trend, the clothing industry can only point to various improvements in the fragmented process of sewing a garment. In fact, today's sewing techniques in the core production process do not differ much from those of a century ago, and a labour–intensive production process remains the norm. In hardly any other major industry are labour inputs coupled with such small amounts of physical capital. While the gap between productivity in weaving and spinning may be widening to the advantage of spinning, the mix of highly differing processes upstream and downstream from the actual sewing process makes it difficult to judge how great the overall changes in productivity will be. If the technology path in the textile industry can be viewed as a rather straight highway, that traced by the clothing industry is best pictured as a road heading up productivity peaks and then down into valleys of low productivity, with hardly an option to shift into a higher gear.

Perhaps the automobile industry and its computer-controlled, just-in-time, automated production process can serve as an example for the clothing industry. When the automobile industry was just beginning, Henry Ford saw the potential to turn a piecemeal production process into a production line. By radically changing the production parameters and introducing the production line, where myriads of pieces come together to form the final product, he opened up an era, which has now been again subjected to major shifts, with state-of-the-art production structures.[17] Could the textile and clothing industries undergo a similar shift?

It seems unlikely. There would seem to be little potential for massively shifting the productivity of the sewing process, although major developments in otherwise bonding pieces of cloth together to form clothes might emerge. While the efforts currently undertaken in the sewing process will eventually change productivity, over the medium run these results are bound to be more in the line of automating certain sewing operations, such as sleeve assembly, rather than the entire production line. And when automation of the entire production line is finally achieved, it will probably be used more for long production runs, involving large volumes of standardised articles, rather than short runs dictated by quickly changing fashions.

In matters concerning exports of the TCM industry over the last 20 years, the four main exporting countries, *i.e.* Germany, Italy, Japan and Switzerland, were quite successful in retaining their relatively large share of the sector's worldwide exports. However, in the 1990s, the TCM industry was the only machinery industry that experienced negative growth rates. This, combined with the very strong growth of TCM imports in China in recent years, foreshadows a major source of future textile and clothing exports, owing to stronger textile and clothing clusters, consisting of a larger number of enterprises and higher levels of expertise.

This chapter argues that the role now played by textile and clothing production in the industrialisation process of developing countries is far more differentiated than it was some 30 years ago. While low labour costs still give developing countries a competitive edge in world markets, time factors now play a far more crucial role in determining international competitiveness. Nonetheless, to remain competitive, developed countries are forced to climb the technology ladder, either through product or process innovations.

In most countries, intensified research efforts have not prevented a decline in the share of textiles and clothing in total manufacturing employment since the early 1980s. The share of textiles declined in all countries reviewed and the share of clothing declined everywhere except in Greece, Italy and Portugal. The trade data show that structural adjustment pressures in the OECD area do not result from a shrinking of world markets but largely from the rapid expansion of Chinese exports of textiles and clothing. As the integration of China into the world economy continues, OECD countries will have to face intensified competition on world markets and structural adjustment pressures within their domestic economies.

This chapter finds a weak relationship between technological specialisation and trade performance of OECD countries as measured by the difference between the revealed comparative advantage indices for 2001 and 1991. The major reason is that most innovations in textiles and clothing are created in other industries. New materials are mainly developed in the chemical industry, and new processes are developed in the machinery industry. As a result, the technological competitiveness of producers of textiles and clothing largely depends on their ability to adopt new products and processes developed elsewhere. Therefore, the major focus of innovative activities in these industries is on technology transfer.

In turning to developments across OECD countries, it was shown that innovative activities in textiles and clothing are broadly scattered across most of the countries surveyed. As a rule, central institutions do not co-ordinate individual research agendas, with Korea the only exception. It is difficult to assess whether this bottom-up type of organisation is advantageous or disadvantageous. It may result in parallel research and missed opportunities for synergies, but it may also promote institutional competition.

Despite the lack of central co-ordination, the opportunities for networking and information exchange via the Internet are increasingly exploited by research and innovation-oriented institutions. Most offer electronic information services and provide contacts to other institutions within and beyond national borders. In many countries, research collaboration between universities and private firms plays a dominant role. This form of public-private partnership is especially well established in the United States and Germany. In France, Italy and the United Kingdom, by contrast, joint research is mainly carried out through joint ventures established by private firms and backed by financial contributions from government. Again, it is difficult to assess which type of joint research is more beneficial. Each can be said to have its own historical roots and its own specific merits.

Among the research topics addressed by the institutions surveyed above, textiles clearly dominate. This obviously reflects different technological potentials and different expected marginal returns from R&D. The promotion of joint research and innovation activities in textiles and clothing is undoubtedly difficult for SMEs. Especially in textiles, a substantial part of R&D is carried out by large companies from the chemical industry, which do not have to rely on joint research. Any approach to promote public-private research institutions in textiles and clothing can be regarded to a large degree, therefore, as an approach to promote the business opportunities of SMEs. Turkey, for instance, might adopt this approach. If such a strategy was successfully implemented, Turkish manufacturers might well be able to earn higher prices for their products on world markets. Subsequently, if such a strategy proved successful, it might be instituted in other countries.

As industrial policies have to take into account specific path dependencies as well as indigenous industrial structures, it is hard to identify a one-size-fits-all policy approach for supporting innovation in textile and clothing industries. Nevertheless, this chapter draws four general lessons. First, there is no significant lack of inventions and innovations. Governments should therefore refrain from launching large-scale basic research programmes for textiles and clothing. Second, governments are right to emphasise technology transfer and the diffusion of innovations. This approach could be developed further by better exploiting the potential of modern information and communication technologies for the dissemination of technological knowledge. Third, reputation increasingly becomes a key factor of competitiveness. Governments could support the creation of reputation, especially among SMEs, by promoting quality certification and common brand names. Lastly, in the long run, the technological performance of industries basically depends upon the stock of human capital. Therefore, education and qualification policy should be regarded as the most important precondition of technological success, not only in the textile and clothing industries, but in all industries.

Annex 4.A1. Table

Annex Table 4A.1. Description of 3–digit SITC (Rev.2) categories in Section 7, Machinery and Transport Equipment 2000

Divisions/categories	Description
71	**Power Generating Machinery and Equipment**
713	Internal combustion piston engines, and parts
714	Engines and motors, non-electric
716	Rotating electric plant and parts
718	Other power generating machinery and parts
72	**Machinery Specialized for Particular Industries**
721	Agricultural machinery and parts
722	Tractors fitted or not with power take-offs
723	Civil engineering and contractors plant and parts
724	**Textile and Leather Machinery and Parts**
725	Paper and pulp mill machinery, machinery for manufacture of paper
726	Printing and bookbinding machinery, and parts
727	Food processing machines and parts
728	Machinery and equipment specialized for particular industries
73	**Metalworking Machinery**
736	Machine-tools for working metal or metal carbides, and parts
737	Metalworking machinery, and parts
74	**General Industrial Machinery and Equipment, N.E.S. and Parts, N.E.S.**
741	Heating and cooling equipment, and parts
742	Pumps for liquids, liquid elevators, and parts
743	Pumps, compressors, fans and blowers
744	Mechanical handling equipment, and parts
745	Other non-electrical machinery, tools, apparatus, and parts
749	Non-electric accessories of machinery
75	**Office Machines and Automatic Data Processing Equipment**
751	Office machines
752	Automatic data processing machines and units thereof
759	Parts of and accessories suitable for 751, 752
76	**Telecommunications and Sound Recording and Producing Apparatus/Equipment**
761	Television receivers
762	Radio-broadcast receivers
763	Gramophones, dictating and sound recorders
764	Telecommunications equipment, and parts
77	**Electrical Machinery, Apparatus and Appliances, N.E.S., and Parts thereof, N.E.S.**
771	Electric power machinery, and parts thereof
772	Electrical apparatus such as switches, relays, fuses and plugs
773	Equipment for distributing electricity
774	Electric and radiological apparatus, for medical purposes
775	Household type, electrical and non-electrical equipment
776	Thermionic, cold and photocathode valves, tubes, and parts
778	Electrical machinery and apparatus, n.e.s.
78	**Road Vehicles (Including Air-Cushion Vehicles)**
781	Passenger motor cars, for transport of passengers and goods
782	Motor vehicles for transport of goods materials
783	Road motor vehicles, n.e.s.
784	Parts and accessories of 722, 781, 782, 783
785	Motorcycles, motor scooters and invalid carriages
786	Trailers and other vehicles, not motorized
79	**Other Transport Equipment**
791	Railway vehicles and associated equipment
792	Aircraft and associated equipment, and parts
793	Ships, boats and floating structures

Source: United Nations (1975, pp. 65-83).

Annex 4.A2. The Clothing Production process

The production process, from the designing of a collection to the pressing and packaging of finished clothing products, encompasses a wide range of activities, each of which has a distinct composition of capital and labour. To better appreciate the production specificity of each stage and the technological progress made in recent years, this annex provides technical details about the main production stages involved in the fabrication of clothing products.

Designing

The current state-of-the-art CAD systems for this step of the production process have one major weakness: they have difficulty in simulating accurately how all types of cloth drape a body.

The designing of clothes can be a very human-capital intensive process, depending largely on the level of the fashion content. At one end of the spectrum, there is the designing of standard clothing items, where the fashion content is close to zero; in this case, the design share would amount to no more than a technical description of standardised inputs. At the other end, there is the *haute couture*, where creative, highly individual design activities can represent a sizeable portion of the final sales price. It is at this end of the spectrum that the use of computed-aided design (CAD) systems has greatly increased the productivity of individual designers. The ability to design on a full-colour screen with a light pen, and thus fewer limitations than with a piece of paper and coloured drawing tools, and also to incorporate a wide range of structuring and patterning options implies that the trial and error process before the "creation" is considered completed can be considerably shortened. The setting up of a fashion collection for a season is simplified; quick additions are easily accomplished by retouching/modifying in the computer system the fashion items that prove to be more popular.

Moreover, the on-screen, full-colour patterned "cloth" can be printed in a pre–selected width to ensure that the visual conception is replicated in two dimensions on a textile fabric. Likewise, colour and material input requirements can be sent on line to the producers of these intermediary inputs to have them checked in terms of technical feasibility as well as price, production and delivery specifications. Hence, almost the entire time-consuming and human-capital-intensive range of activities that precede the so-called pre-assembly process can be enormously simplified and accelerated through CAD.

The current state-of-the-art CAD systems for this step of the production process have one major weakness: they have difficulty simulating how all types of cloth drape a body. This problem is slowly being resolved for known materials. The basic reasons for this weakness can be found in inherent characteristics of clothes: they fit/drape individuals in a manner that depends on the kind of material, its thickness and patterning as well as the demands of fashion. Thus, while a snug-fitting, cotton t-shirt on a computer-generated individual can be assumed to present no problems for existing PC/micro–based systems, this is not yet the case for a long flowing gown, incorporating various types of materials, patterns and cuts. The snug-fitting t-shirt can be portrayed in the same manner as shoes: the mirror image of the side already designed in three dimensions can be used to create the opposite side. In essence, the final product when designing a shoe or a snug-fitting t–shirt is basically an extension of the outer surface of the computer-generated foot or torso. However, the further a piece of clothing is removed from the outer surface of a normed torso, the greater the number of parameters which have to be taken into consideration. In the case of the gown, this would require information on so many individual parameters that currently only a mainframe computer would have the capacity to handle the task. Given the price of such systems today, this would only seem to be economically viable for the largest companies. As computers become more powerful and faster, this constraint will only be eliminated to the extent that the various properties of the materials used can be correctly captured and portrayed.

Pattern making

The impact of technology in this area can be expected to be greater in the future, as the individual steps are more standardised. Small firms will be able to benefit by outsourcing their pattern-making requirements.

Pattern making in the clothing industry is the art of transforming a finished design for a three-dimensional piece of clothing into two-dimensional segments which, when reproduced, are capable of being assembled in a production process into any number of replicas of the original model. There are two basic constraints. First, and most obvious, the pattern must be able to replicate the original model (fashion constraint). Second, the pattern must be able to be structured in a manner which allows it to be adapted to a production process under certain time and cost constraints. To achieve these results, highly paid, skilled personnel use powerful computers and interactive software. Although the two steps are connected, a separate examination makes it easier to understand the technological implications of the pattern-making process.

Dissecting a designed clothing product into segments which, when reassembled, replicate the original design requires familiarity with the various attributes of cloth, when sewn or otherwise combined with the same or other types of cloth to wrap around, drape or otherwise fit a human body or part thereof in a certain manner. Beyond this, the structure of the material, the type of patterns printed on it and the other specifications of the design, *e.g.* type of pockets, number of fasteners, etc., all present demands which are currently best fulfilled by skilled individuals. In larger companies, a CAD system helps the skilled individuals to break down more efficiently – on a screen, using simple commands – a piece of clothing into manageable components. Although computers can assist automatically when applying standard procedures to certain parts of a piece of clothing, *e.g.* collars, cuffs and seams, when products are only slightly changed or when single-material products with simple lines, *e.g.* jeans, are to be produced, they have yet to assume tasks for which optical and sensorial attributes must also be taken into consideration.

Once a pattern has been created that fulfils the fashion constraint for a given piece of clothing, downstream production specifications must be defined. This means that each step needed to assemble the individual parts into the final product must be identified and the relevant production costs estimated. Since the lead time for new fashions is quite short, time constraints preclude any investment in new product-specific equipment. As the technical capabilities of a given equipment are known and since the sequence as well as the demands of certain steps are dictated either by the nature of the product and/or have evolved from past experience (and are thus available from computer databases), this task can be reduced to filling in the gaps with guesstimates if there is a computer-based production planning system. Here again only the larger companies have installed such systems.

The result of these calculations is a set of figures on the material, labour and capital costs of production, plus the time necessary to produce a given amount of output. This set of figures is also used to set up production schedules and map out material flows from incoming fabrics to outgoing packaged final products. The impact of technology in this area can be expected to increase in future as individual steps are more standardised. Small firms will be able to benefit by outsourcing their pattern-making requirements. However, given the similarity of production processes in clothing factories, there is obviously room for inter-firm production planning services, particularly if an overall strategy to improve the competitive position of the national industry is being pursued.

Grading

The once tedious and time-consuming process of grading is now the work of a computer software package.

Following the use of CAD systems in connection with most aspects of pattern making, they can be used in the pre-assembly process to add on the necessary fabric leeway for seams, hems and the like. Since grading (that is, the production of patterns of different sizes from an initial pattern to correspond to the entire spectrum of normed sizes) is a similar procedure, state-of-the-art CAD systems permit virtually instantaneous grading, be it for European/US or any other set of size specifications. The once tedious and time-consuming process of grading is now the work of a computer software package, which includes standard grading factors that can also be modified to fit individual firm or fashion parameters.

Nesting and marking

Today's state-of-the-art CAD systems perform the structuring of an entire marker on fabric of any size.

These are the final steps of the pre-assembly layout process before the fabric to be used is integrated. At this point, the graded patterns consisting of *n* pieces per size for *m* sizes which have to be arranged, *i.e.* nested, in such a manner on a master pattern sheet, *i.e.* on a marker, so that they cover as much of the fabric as possible. Whereas in the past, each piece of a pattern had to be hand-placed, nested and marked on a pattern sheet (marker), today's state-of-the-art CAD systems can structure an entire marker on fabric of any size. Such systems make it possible to utilise, depending on the type of fabric, over 90% of the fabric, with time savings of over 50% and a 5% reduction in wastage. Today, such jobs can be easily outsourced, including the necessary fabrics.

Since material costs represent a major share of the final product price and since fabric wastage has little reuse value, this aspect is quite important in improving the competitive edge. The prevailing computer systems assist the operator in moving around the individual pattern pieces, nesting them and creating multiples of given nesting structures across the width or length of the marker, provide tolerance checks as concerns the distance between the individual pieces vis-à-vis the cutting system specifications. Such checks ensure that costly mistakes are not made by trying to squeeze as many pattern segments as possible out of the fabric, thereby nesting them closer than cutting tolerances allow.

These systems cannot yet replace highly skilled workers who have developed over the years a feeling for how to nest and structure markers by software packages that can take $n \times m$ number of pattern pieces and optimise their nesting across and down a given marker. However, these jobs are being deskilled in the sense that they can almost be replaced by software. Soon perhaps, there will no longer be individuals who have mastered this trade. However, the power and speed of PCs/micros will have to be expanded and have a certain degree of human intelligence capabilities. Utilisation of fabric beyond perhaps 95% for normal products and 80% for high fashions will only be possible if individual pattern components become more congruent, the size of individual components increases, fabric dimensions are adjusted to specific nesting structures and, in particular, weaving/knitting techniques are developed that allow individual pattern components to be produced almost without wastage.

Cutting

Cutting still require skilled labour, particularly as the quality of the work performed provides the basis for producing the clothing items.

Beginning with the cutting process, the actual fabric enters the pre-assembly path. It is delivered on rolls of between 90 and 140 centimetres in width, which contain the length of fabric necessary to produce the required number of clothing items (the length of a production run for a given item is a function of fashion content and price). The fabric is carefully unrolled, inspected for flaws, cut into specified lengths as dictated by the marker (they rarely exceed 30 meters for practical purposes), and then precisely laid out and stacked in what is called a lay. On top of a lay for a given production run, where the number of fabric layers is mainly dictated by the type of cutting equipment and type of fabric, the marker printed by the CAD and computer-assisted methods (CAM) is placed or the marker information in the CAD/CAM system is interfaced directly with the cutting system.

All the above described steps still require skilled labour, particularly as the quality of the work performed provides the basis for producing the clothing items. Inroads have been made here in ensuring that the cutter does not damage the fabric and that the individual pieces being cut out of a deep-piled lay are completely identical. Since cutters are among the best-paid workers in a clothing factory, the automation and consequent deskilling of this step implies a considerable reduction in wage costs both directly and in terms of shortened training periods. At the same time, productivity increases and wastage is decreased considerably.

As important as the automation of the cutting process itself might be in terms of improving the competitive position of a larger company today, it stands alone when compared with the labour-intensive tasks on both sides of it. Particularly, the bundling and tagging of the individual pattern components from the lay for the sewing process is an area where much progress has been made by the introduction of CAM. However, the constraints are those mentioned earlier, namely the fact that the workers are dealing with limp pieces and not hard components (as in the automobile industry).

Sewing

Totally automated procedures have made only minor inroads in sewing. Among other things, productivity improvement can be attributed to better needles.

As mentioned at the outset, sewing is the core production process in the clothing industry. It is the area in which automated procedures have made only minor inroads. Given this and in order to be brief, it probably suffices to state that aside from certain parts of the sewing process or some materials or some specific items of clothing, all the ideas of the last two decades for totally automated sewing systems have led to little more than the conclusion that they will not happen in the near future.

Two basic approaches were taken to attempt to solve the difficulties involved: *i)* the Japanese chose an overall strategy with a view to developing an automated clothing factory; and *ii)* the United States and Europe chose a marginal approach either to automate initially a certain segment (the United States) or concentrate on particular problems (the European Union).

By far the most ambitious project is the Japanese Automated Sewing System which was officially initiated in 1982 by the Ministry of Economic and Trade and Industry (METI) and launched in January 1983 in the form of an Association of Technology Research of Automated Sewing System. The goal of this project was to create an automated clothing production system which could efficiently manufacture clothes even if produced in small lots to satisfy the variety of consumer tastes. The timeframe for the project foresaw a factory going on stream in 1989. Despite rather generous funding (figures differ, but probably USD 100 million will have been spent) and periodic optimistic statements, the vision of having textiles enter one side of a factory virtually void of workers and clothes coming out on the other side could not be realised as planned. It was primarily the insurmountable difficulties connected with the 3-D sewing technology, as well as the handling of fabrics, which put the project so far behind projected deadlines. Partial results could be seen at numerous IMBs (World Fair for Apparel Production Technology and Textile Processing), but the project has since disappeared from the headlines.

In the United States, with more than 21 000 establishments of which 70% employed fewer than 50 workers and 25% fewer than five, the thrust of the research on automating the clothing manufacturing process concentrated on one specific task, the benefits of which were expected to have implications for many facets of clothing production. Beginning in 1979, this project, which is organised under the Textile/Clothing Technology Corporation (TC²), set out to increase labour productivity after having established that US clothing manufacturers, given equal quality and service inputs, can compete with foreign imports on a price basis. With funding equally shared between the industry and the Department of Commerce, TC² was supported by a coalition of producers' organisations and unions. Research efforts were directed towards that part of the assembly operation which takes the most time (75%) and hence induces the most labour costs: handling. This decision seemed all the more justified given that 130 years of research had been invested in perfecting sewing techniques and that sewing speeds of 10 000 stitches per minute were already possible in the late 1980s.

The task chosen to research and automate was the sleeve of a man's suit. This sub-assembly step was selected because it embodied the full range of problems encountered in the assembly process, *i.e.* sewing inseams, folding cuffs, tacking vents and sewing outseams. It also placed strict demands on aligning the seams and adjusting sleeve sub-components so as to achieve a smooth mating at the shoulder end of the sleeve.

The fabric handling/transport problems were solved using foam-backed, parallel moving belts, which clamp the entire surface of the fabric. The fabric, held by the belts, was fed to a perpendicularly positioned sewing machine mounted on a plate which was designed to rotate around the needle position. The parallel and interlocking moving belts opened up immediately prior to the intended stitch position. With a series of other belts, the machine could move one ply of fabric with respect to the other. Following the successful computer-controlled transport and sewing of fabric with high-quality stitch results, the next step consisted of aligning the edges of the next seam.

This was accomplished by using a robot fitted with a vision system geared to recognise the free edges of the fabric to be joined. Once this was done, the pieces were fed through the sewing unit described above. Instead of carrying out the process step by step on different units, the entire system was built into one unit, with the clothing components moving back and forth between the vision system, robot and sewing machine.

Obviously the success of this project depended on its adaptability to other pre-cut clothing components. This meant that software had to be developed that would guide the equipment through the same steps that would be used by experienced sewing machine operators. The technology was put in the hands of the Singer Company, which received it from Draper Laboratory, the institution responsible for developing it for TC^2. It failed to achieve the necessary commercial viability.

In essence, the sewing process focuses, as it did a century ago, on the needle's ability to transport a thread flawlessly through pre-cut pieces of fabric so as to join them in a prescribed manner into the desired type of apparel. Unlike a century ago, the speed with which needles penetrate fabrics and the wide range of fabric strengths increase the ever-present danger of needles being snagged in the fabric (and damaging the fabric) when pieces are being rapidly repositioned and threads cut. Selecting the correct needle is obviously of paramount importance, as this helps avoid machine downtime and thus results in savings. Investment in producing better needles has led to an increase in productivity of roughly 10% to 20% over the last 20 years with respect to sewing jeans (based on interviews with needle producers).

Finally, the analogy to sewing pieces of fabric together to produce a garment can be found in turning yarn into garments. In the past, wool sweaters would have to be stitched together from knitted flatware. Now, a complete sweater (simple pattern) can be produced in 30 minutes, but would take two hours if done by a manual knitting machine. However owing to the high cost (roughly USD 7 per sweater and roughly a 300% cost differential with manual knitting machines), such machines will only be used for the higher end of the market.

Inspecting, pressing and packaging

Technological innovations have been important in the pressing process.

On the downstream side of the clothing production process, technological innovations have been important in the pressing process and to some extent for operations coupled with "repairing" rejects from the inspection process. Although the finishing process (as these three steps are called) is the more important the higher the value of the final product, it is the key interface between the production process and a company's reputation in the market. Money saved here will lead to lower quality output and will feed back via lower prices and hence lower profits. Obviously, there is a trade-off at this point between thoroughness and speed. However, if the production process functions correctly, the number of rejects will be small and there will be no bottleneck. An indication of an increase in rejects means that certain parts of the process are imperfect and should be corrected before additional time and materials are wasted.

Highly automated pressing units have been devised which ensure a high-quality finish. As expensive as these machines are (they use inflatable bags or flexible dummies over which the garments are placed), they are proving their worth not only by speeding up the process but also by being able to rectify certain types of garment defects. They have been initially installed in high-income countries and are used particularly for operations dealing with higher-quality apparel.

Throughout the production process from design to packaging

CAD systems interfaced with a modern telecommunications network have made it possible to delink human-capital-intensive activities from locations where purely labour-intensive production activities take place, without sacrificing the necessary information linkages. Already almost 20 years ago, there were trans-Pacific links between design studios on the west coast of the United States and manufacturing operations in Hong Kong, China. Inroads are now being made on the labour-intensive core of the clothing manufacturing process that still remains in OECD countries. It is highly probable that this process will continue and induce further migration of certain other services, as noted in the Economic Report of the President of February 2004. Other factors being equal, such migration will only be limited by the availability of adequate infrastructure in any location. It will increase further as telecommunication links become less expensive and the necessary software to deal with fashion issues comes on the market.

Aside from transport costs, which are always a factor in identifying least-cost production locations, be they within or between countries, access to qualitatively acceptable inputs can be a barrier restricting locational shifts, particularly between continents. Since the close and often longstanding links between the textile and clothing industries are considered by some to be especially important to ensure that demanding up-market customers can be satisfied, this type of barrier may prove to be less binding for the wide range of medium-priced products, as textile producers in the newly industrialised economies are approaching or already have reached production standards in OECD countries. Obviously the implications for textile producers in OECD countries cannot be overlooked. The role of adequate infrastructure in telecommunications and transport for competition are discussed in Chapter 5.

Notes

1.   Already in the mid-1800s in Germany, Prussia complained to the Zollverein about the South German cotton spinners and their continuing "assistance and their disregard for the interests of other industries and of consumers" (Henderson, 1959, p. 184).

2.   However, this was not the only reason for the disappearance of some German sewing machine manufacturers.

3.   While Howe introduced the lockstitch, it was James Gibbs who produced the first single-thread chain stitch (1857).

4.   In a study assessing the impact of industrialisation policies on trade performance (Spinanger, 1987), which examined the factor intensities of 28 industries in six economies (*i.e.* United States, Malaysia, Chinese Taipei, Singapore, Korea and the Philippines) over a ten-year period, the clothing industry was the only one that consistently had the lowest physical capital intensity (fixed assets/employee) and the lowest human capital intensity (wages/employee).

5.   A particularly relevant point is the preparation of textiles for the sewing process. Whereas this was previously carried out in house, the selection of the fabric, the cutting of patterns and bundling for assembly in the in-house sewing process can now be completely outsourced. This obviously reduces a clothing company's activities to its "core competence." It also helps SMEs to be competitive, as they no longer need to maintain underutilised expensive capital stock.

6.   The interface between the textile industry and the textile machine industry continues to play an important role, from which both parties profit. It is not only the synergy effect due to approaching problems from different angles; it is also the ability to test machines under true working conditions before they come on the market.

7.   Technological shifts, however, can shorten the replacement life cycle of equipment. "Twenty years ago, 15 years was considered to be the normal life of textile equipment. Today it is no more than ten years, and for some technologies, such as texturising, the useful life of the equipment can even be shorter." (Hartmann, 1993, p. 67).

8.   Countries like India and China produce considerable and increasing amounts of TCM, but most is likely used to produce for domestic markets or for other developing countries. However, given the crucial interface between the TCM industry and the textile and clothing industries, the inherently competitive textile and clothing industries offer a potential basis for competitive, exportable TCM if the other essential inputs are available. The question is: When will they become actual competitors for OECD countries?

9.   In a study dealing with the textile and clothing industries in Germany, companies interviewed often noted that when contracting for work to be done offshore, they stipulated which machines should be used to produce the required quality output. Some companies, particularly those with offshore processing operations carried out in eastern

Europe, even provide the necessary machines (on a lease or joint-venture basis). Whatever the arrangement, the machines come from OECD countries (Piatti and Spinanger, 1994). A study of Hong Kong (China)'s clothing industry showed a similar, albeit less direct, stipulation of machinery inputs. That is, companies setting up operations in other Asian countries tended to use the same equipment as in Hong Kong (China), and it usually came from OECD countries (Spinanger, 1994).

10. Thus, major textile companies in OECD countries began to outsource certain products from non-OECD countries. In Morocco and Tunisia, where numerous German, French and other EU companies have operations, mill operations can be carried out on 35% more days a year than in Germany, while wages are only 8% to 17% of German levels. Hence, companies outsource "greige away from Europe and into the lower-cost countries, like Tunisia, in order to focus efforts in Europe on finishing, where the real addition to value-added is". Interview with the president and CEO of Dominion Textiles, one of world's top 20 textile companies (*Textile Asia*, November 1992, p. 22).

11. Figures for the 25 largest exporters of textile and clothing products.

12. Japan's pattern of exports during the decade and across all categories is very different from that of the other three major suppliers: the latter's exports were largely destined to OECD countries, whereas Japan's overall shares of TCM exports to non-OECD countries averaged 60% and even exceeded 70% in 1991. The shares of the other three suppliers were usually 50% less even if somewhat more in the second half of the period. Over the period 1983-91, Japan's exports of TCM to Asian countries grew by 23%, while those to European countries grew by 13%.

13. The Chinese, some three millennia BC, were already using silk for industrial purposes, and the Romans are known to have used woven fabrics and meshes to "stabilise marshy ground for road building which are early examples of what would now be termed geo-textiles and geo-grids"(Byrne, 2000, p. 1).

14. The clothing industry can probably be considered the most labour-intensive and least human-capital-intensive (Spinanger, 1988); the textile industry in OECD countries is one of the most capital-intensive.

15. Even before these agreements, the European countries east of the EU had profited widely from offshore production legislation, which permitted EU countries to ship EU textiles to these countries to be turned into clothing products. They were then reshipped to the EU and duty was only applied on the value added produced outside the EU.

16. On the trade effects of the latest EU enlargement, see Klodt (2003). Based on the trade effects of the Europe Agreements and on a comparison to previous enlargement rounds, it is argued that new patterns of trade specialisation will not emerge in future, but are already established.

17. By 1914, just four years after starting the production line, the Ford company's 13 000 workers were producing 260 000 cars, while the rest of the industry employed 66 350 workers to make 286 000 cars.

References

Balassa, B. (1965), "Trade Liberalization and 'Revealed' Comparative Advantage", *The Manchester School of Economics and Social Studies*, Vol. 33, pp. 99-123.

Byrne, C. (2000), "Technical Textiles Market – An Overview", in A.R. Horrocks and S.C. Anand (eds.), *Handbook of Technical Textiles*, Cambridge, pp. 1-23.

Deane, P. (1965), *The First Industrial Revolution*, Cambridge University Press, Cambridge.

Grömling, J. and J. Matthes (2003), *Globalisierung und Strukturwandel in der Deutschen Textil – und Bekleidungsindustrie*, Deutscher Instituts-Verlag, Cologne.

Hartmann, U. (1993), "Trends in Textile Capacity", *Textile Asia* 24 (7). pp. 66-71.

Henderson, W.O. (1959), *The Zollverein*, Quadrangle Books, Chicago.

Hoffmann, K. and H.J. Rush (1988), *Microelectronics and Clothing, The Impact of Technical Change on a Global Industry*, Praeger, New York.

Hummels, D.(2001), "Time as A Trade Barrier", Purdue University.

Klodt, H. (2003), "Prospective Trade Effects of Eastern EU Enlargement", in R. Pethig and M. Rauscher (eds.), *Challenges to the World Economy, Festschrift for Horst Siebert*, Springer, Berlin.

Klodt, H. and R. Maurer (1995), "Determinants of the Capacity to Innovate: Is Germany Losing its Competitiveness in High-Tech Industries?", in H. Siebert (ed.), *Locational Competition in the World Economy*, Mohr Siebeck, Tübingen.

Krugman, P. (1991), *Geography and Trade*, MIT Press, Cambridge, MA.

Landis, D.S. (1970), *The Unbound Prometheus - Technological Change and Industrial Development in Western Europe from 1750 to the Present*, Cambridge University Press, Cambridge.

Matthes, J. (2002), Internationalisierungsstrategien im Deutschen Textil- und Bekleidungsgewerbe, *iw-trends* (4): 39–48.

Piatti, L. and D. Spinanger (1994), "Germany's Textile Complex under the MFA: Making it under Protection and Going International", Institute of World Economics, Kiel Working Paper, No. 651, September.

Sandberg, L.G. (1969), "American Rings and English Mules: the Role of Economic Rationality", *Quarterly Journal of Economics*, Vol. 83, No. 1. Also published in S.B. Saul (ed.) (1970), *Technological Change: The United States and Britain in the 19th Century*, Methuen and Co, Ltd., London.

Spinanger, D. (1988), "Does Trade Performance Say Anything about Efficient Industrialization Policies, Evidence from Pacific Rim Countries?", Kiel Working Paper 302.

Spinanger, D. (1994), "Profiting from Protection in an Open Economy – Hong Kong's Supply Response to EU's MFA Restrictions", Institute of World Economics, Kiel Working Papers, No. 653, September.

Textile Asia (1992), "Weathering the Storm", Interview between Kayser Sung (*Textile Asia* Publisher and Editor-in-Chief) and Charles H. Hantho (President and CEO of Dominion Textiles). November, pp. 17-24.

The Textile Institute (1994), *Textile Terms and Definitions*, Tenth Edition, Manchester.

UNCTAD (1992, 2002), *Handbook of International Trade and Development Statistics*, United Nations, New York.

United Nations (1975), *Monthly Bulletin of Statistics*, Geneva.

United Nations (1986), *Standard International Trade Classification. Revision 3*, Statistical Papers, Series 11 (34), New York.

World Trade Organisation (WTO) (various years), *WTO Annual Report*, Geneva.

Chapter 5

Business Facilitation

Exporting countries seeking to maintain an export-led development strategy in textiles and clothing have to address their competitive weaknesses due to: inefficient domestic regulatory regimes; obsolete infrastructure in essential business services; cumbersome customs procedures; and other distorted market structures. The chapter highlights the business environment in which trade in textiles and clothing takes place, underscoring the importance of a sound macroeconomic environment for facilitating the process of structural adjustment. It emphasises the importance of minimising the time involved in the international movement of textile and clothing products through more efficient transport infrastructure and customs procedures as well as the value of modern electricity and telecommunications infrastructure for the competitiveness of textile and clothing firms. Moreover, it stresses the importance of nurturing a culture of entrepreneurship to support these industries where small- and medium-sized enterprises predominate.

Introduction

In preparation for the market liberalisation initiated by the WTO Agreement on Textiles and Clothing (ATC), countries involved in the textile and clothing supply chain need to prioritise their policy agenda on the basis of an analysis of their competitive strengths and weaknesses.[1] The new competitive environment may be such that exporting countries have to consider changes in production methods: specialising in specific sub-segments of the supply chain, shifting production segments towards higher value-added articles and diversifying into other industrial activities. Although the prime responsibility for adjustment falls on firms themselves because they are better placed to evaluate how to react to evolving market signals, governments play a supporting role by establishing a coherent policy and regulatory framework that strengthens the capacity of the private sector to deal with the new competitive environment.

In the post-ATC period, there will be neither quantitative restrictions nor MFA-related guaranteed market access to mask the vulnerable situation of national suppliers whose international competitiveness is hampered by inefficient domestic regulatory regimes, obsolete infrastructure in essential business services, cumbersome customs procedures and other distorted market structures. Exporting countries will have to address their competitive vulnerability if they aspire to maintain an export-led development strategy in textiles and clothing. For net importing countries, their suppliers will be exposed to strengthened competitive pressure and retail groups will have greater liberty to source products on a global basis. Hence, net importing countries also have to reassess their competitive strengths and weaknesses with a view to implementing measures that improve the overall economic environment, taking into account both their producing and consuming interests.

Achieving greater policy synergy among distinct policy areas that affect the competitive position of national firms is in essence the purpose of a business facilitation agenda. This chapter highlights the policy and regulatory dimensions that have an impact on the cost competitiveness of national firms and complements discussions of policy areas covered in earlier chapters.

Policy makers generally recognise the need to pursue a business facilitation agenda under which domestic regulations and sectoral programmes are updated to keep pace with technological development and to meet the expectations of dynamic firms in their quest for growth opportunities in both domestic and foreign markets. For the purpose of this chapter, the scope of the business facilitation agenda includes trade-related regulatory and policy issues in: logistical dimensions of the international movement of goods; essential services that are key inputs for industrial activities, *e.g.* electricity, telecommunications and water; customs procedures or trade facilitation; standards harmonisation; and small and medium-sized enterprises (SMEs). Thus, the scope of business facilitation is much broader than that of trade facilitation, which focuses more directly on customs-related issues.[2] Trade facilitation is here considered as a subset of business facilitation.

This chapter first highlights the overarching business environment in which trade in textiles and clothing takes place, underscoring the importance of a sound and dynamic macroeconomic environment to facilitate the process of structural adjustment and the redeployment of resources to other productive areas. It then discusses first the logistical dimensions of the international movement of goods and then customs facilitation. The following section emphasises the value of modern and efficient electricity and telecommunications services for underpinning the competitiveness of domestic textile and clothing firms. Next are examined the trade implications of standards heterogeneity in textiles and clothing and the importance of nurturing a culture of entrepreneurship to support the textile and clothing industries where SMEs predominate. Some concluding remarks close the chapter.

The overarching environment in textiles and clothing

The elimination of quantitative trade restrictions is taking place in an increasingly globalised world economy, where production and marketing activities depend on business decisions that reflect competitive opportunities around the world. Trade policy measures have had a major impact on production and investment decisions in textiles and clothing and on trade flows (see Chapter 2). In particular, MFA restrictions have contributed to the international fragmentation of the supply chain by accelerating the diversification of supply to the benefit of less competitive suppliers when quota-constrained suppliers have sub-contracted clothing assembly into third low-cost countries. The scheduled elimination of quantitative restrictions at the end of December 2004 marks the end of these industries' dependency on a derogative trade regime.

Trade liberalisation heightens the pressure on firms to adapt their production mix to meet changing consumer requirements in terms of design, quality and prices, while implementing efficient production methods that minimise production costs. However, their adjustment may be hampered by various domestic obstacles, such as the lack of backward linkages to national high-quality fabrics, unreliable or obsolete port infrastructure, transport systems, telecommunications and electricity networks, inefficient customs procedures and distorted market structures.

The textile and clothing industries are characterised by multiple suppliers who exert little influence on market prices. In this environment, the cost of inefficiencies resulting from deficient or obsolete regulations or essential services is ultimately borne by the firms that are affected. These pressures squeeze operating margins and may in some cases make it impossible to support an export-led development strategy based on textile and clothing production.

Many studies have recently assessed the trade benefits of facilitation measures that include streamlined regulatory environments, deeper harmonisation of standards, and conformity to international regulations.[3] Wilson *et al.* (2002) have estimated for Asia-Pacific Economic Cooperation (APEC) Forum members the trade impact of reductions in indicators of facilitation efforts encompassing port logistics, customs procedures, the domestic regulatory environment, standards harmonisation, business mobility, e–business activity and administrative transparency. They estimated that bringing the below-average APEC members half-way to the APEC average indicators would increase intra–APEC trade by about USD 280 billion, of which half would come from the improvement of port logistics.[4] A study by Wilson, Bagai and Fink (2003) extended this scenario analysis of improvements in facilitation-related efforts halfway to average performance beyond the APEC region to 75 countries and suggested that improvements in port efficiency, customs environment, regulatory environment and services sector infrastructure would increase trade among these countries by USD 377 billion, or equivalent to an increase of 9.7%. These studies imply that business facilitation measures complement trade liberalisation initiatives and improve the international competitiveness of national suppliers.

A recent report by the International Trade Commission (2004) also underscores the importance of infrastructure and proximity to markets as major competitive determinants for textile and clothing suppliers. In particular, it stresses the following factors: short shipping times and frequency of maritime services; reliability of infrastructure in telecommunications, electricity and water services; and accessibility to high-quality fabrics. Since several exporting countries rely on imported fabrics, accessibility to high–quality fabrics is itself influenced by the reliability and efficiency of transport infrastructure and customs procedures.

The overall macroeconomic environment in which market adjustment initiatives take place is probably the most influential policy area for promoting structural adjustment and cannot be ignored by policy makers. A sound and dynamic macroeconomic environment that aims at sustaining non-inflationary economic growth sets the stage for low inflation and low nominal interest rates and, in turn, facilitates the financing of operating capital by firms and stimulates investment in updated equipment. Obtaining financial credits at reasonable rates is a concern widely shared among SMEs, which are prevalent in the textile and clothing industries, and this underscores the importance for governments to pursue sound macroeconomic policies and to foster competitive conditions among financial institutions.

Moreover, as mentioned in Chapter 3 on labour adjustment policies, a sound and dynamic macroeconomic environment is the most important factor in addressing labour market pressures. Labour adjustment programmes and policies are only effective if they result in workers finding new employment. There is strong evidence that real economic growth and, in turn, net employment creation are stimulated in a low-inflationary environment. The pursuit of sound macroeconomic policies fosters market adjustment to change in the competitive environment and facilitates the redeployment of affected resources to other productive sectors without the need to revert to trade protection measures that are costly for taxpayers and consumers. Against this background, pursuing a business facilitation agenda complements other government actions at the macroeconomic and microeconomic levels, *i.e.* trade, labour adjustment and innovation, and brings benefits that go well beyond the textile and clothing industries.

Logistical dimensions of the international movement of goods

There is little information on the apportionment of world trade by mode of transport. This is partly due to the integrated nature of transport chains, which involve more than one mode to complete door-to-door shipments. A typical door-to-door journey for containerised international shipments involves the interaction of approximately 25 different stakeholders, generates 30–40 documents, uses two to three different transport modes and is handled in 12–15 physical locations (OECD, 2003a). There is also considerable reluctance among shippers to release price and route information that might be used by competitors. To illustrate the integrated nature of transport chains, Chart 5.1 shows a simplified representation of the transport chain for traded goods in containers.

Chart 5.1. Transport chain for traded goods in containers

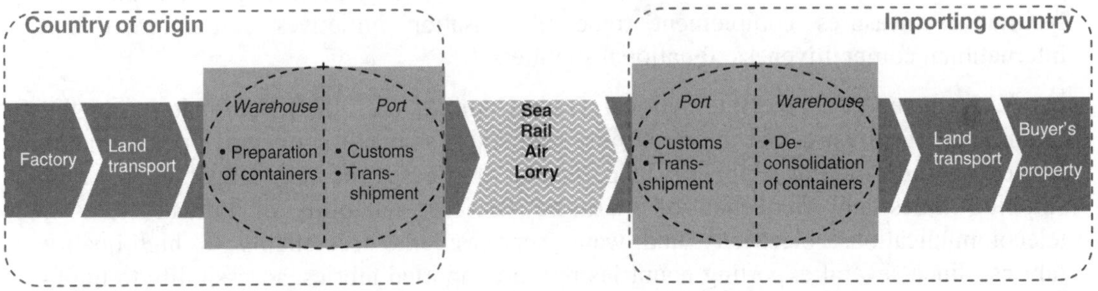

Freight costs and modes of transport for international shipments of textile and clothing products are not generally available even though several countries include international freight costs and insurance charges in the dutiable value of imports. However, based on detailed trade data by mode of transport for US imports of textile and clothing products in 2003 (Table 5.1), seaborne transport is the dominant transport mode, accounting for 83% of total US imports, followed by rail (12.4%), air (3.2%) and lorries (1.4%). Table 5.1 also shows the average shares of freight cost in percentage of the concerned import values for each mode of transport. It reveals that, on average, transport by rail is the least expensive mode, with freight costs accounting for 0.7% of the relevant import values; whereas they represent on average 11.1% by air freight; 4.7% for transport by lorries; and 4.5% by seaborne vessels.

Average freight costs by mode of transport mask considerable differences at country level, which are explained by various factors, including the distance involved, the geography, the regularity of freight services, the competitive conditions on various transport routes, and the composition of the imported goods (standard *versus* fashion articles). Annex Table 5.A1.1 provides detailed freight costs by country of origin and by mode of transport. It shows that freight costs by seaborne vessels vary in a range of 1.7% for shipments originating from the Dominican Republic to 6.4% for shipments originating from Pakistan. The cost range for air shipments is considerably wider, ranging from 3.7% for the Dominican Republic, 14.5% for China, 24.8% for Pakistan and a hefty 41% for Cambodia.

Table 5.1. US imports of textiles and clothing by mode of transport, 2003

	Air	Rail	Seaborne	Lorry	Total
Percentage of imports by mode[1]					
North and Central Americas	0.1%	53.0%	41.0%	5.9%	
Other countries[2]	4.1%		95.9%		
Total	3.2%	12.4%	83.0%	1.4%	
Percentage freight cost/import value					
North and Central Americas	6.9%	0.7%	2.1%	4.7%	1.5%
Other countries	11.1%		4.5%		5.9%

1. The mode of transport is the one by which the imported merchandise entered the US port of arrival from the last foreign country. The North and Central American countries are: Canada, Costa Rica, El Salvador, Guatemala, Honduras, Nicaragua and Mexico.

2. Shipments that were originally attributed to rail and truck for imports from countries other than North and Central America were reallocated on a pro rata basis of 20% for air and 80% for seaborne transport.

Source: OECD, based on data from the US Department of Commerce, Bureau of the Census.

The US data by mode of transport highlight the importance of maritime and rail transport for trade in textile and clothing products, which together accounted for 95.4% of total US imports in 2003. More importantly, the data underscore the importance of efficient transport infrastructure and competitive conditions in transport modes to underpin the competitive position of textile and clothing suppliers. With low-cost railroad access to the US textile and clothing markets, Mexican and Canadian suppliers benefit from a cost advantage over Asian suppliers, whose shipments must be transported by sea or air. Strictly on the basis of freight cost differentials among countries (thus ignoring differences in transit time and customs duty), Mexican shipments transported by rail to the US market have a 5.2% cost advantage over similar imports originating from China and shipped on seaborne vessels (Annex Table 5.A1.1).

The economic literature on the impact of transport on trade of manufactured products illustrates the tyranny of time and distance for countries that aspire to sustain an export-led strategy. Hummels (2000) estimates that each day saved in shipping time is equivalent to a reduction of 0.5% in import tariffs: lengthy shipping times impose inventory-holding and spoilage costs on shippers. Verma (2002) has estimated that Indian firms suffered a 23% cost disadvantage in shipping containers of clothing products from Mumbai or Chennai to the east coast of the United States in 2002 relative to similar container shipments originating from Bangkok, Thailand, owing to delays and inefficiencies at Indian ports. They suffered a 37% cost disadvantage relative to Shanghai, China.

The ITC (2004) quotes shipping data obtained from US retailers that show that the shipping time to the west coast of the United States generally averages: 12 to 18 days from Chinese Taipei, Hong Kong (China) and China; as much as 45 days from some member countries of the Association of South East Asian Nations (ASEAN); and two to seven days (for east coast delivery) for the countries covered under the Caribbean Basin Economic Recovery Act (CBERA). The ITC argues that shipping time and frequency of maritime services can make geographically distant locations competitive from a shipping standpoint. In the country assessment section of the ITC report concerning the competitiveness of the Philippines, it is noted that certain restrictions on domestic cabotage, *e.g.* shipments must be transported on domestic carriers, have the effect of increasing shipping costs and discouraging investors from locating projects on remote islands of the Philippines that have otherwise significant potential for export-led projects. It further noted that the Philippines' high cargo handling fees and its limited containerised cargo handling capacity are contributing to slow ship turnaround time, *i.e.* the total time from entry to departure spent by a vessel at a port.

Radelet and Sachs (1998) compared transport costs for 97 developing countries and estimated that the costs of freight and insurance for landlocked developing countries were on average 50% higher than for coastal economies. The higher shipping costs reflect several factors, including: the higher proportion of transit by land, which tends to be more expensive than maritime transport,[5] the extra cost of transhipment between intermodal transport media; the bureaucratic costs of crossing at least one additional border; and the absence of co-ordinated road infrastructure and customs facilities among the countries concerned.[6] Their work suggests that high shipping costs can essentially eliminate more remote countries from international competition and that policy emphasis should be placed on cutting red tape in port operations to expedite customs clearance.

Limão and Venables (2001) have investigated the dependence of transport costs on geography and infrastructure for over 100 countries, including developed and developing countries, and estimated that a 10 percentage point increase in transport costs typically reduces trade volumes by approximately 20%. They calculated that in 1995 landlocked countries had on average an import share in GDP of 11%, compared with 28% for coastal economies. They also estimated that poor infrastructure accounted for 40% of predicted transport costs for coastal countries and up to 60% for landlocked countries. Their work shows the relative importance of infrastructure in determining transport costs and highlights the priority that should be placed on policies in support of investment in transport infrastructure.

With a view to evaluating the costs involved in the international movement of textile and clothing products, Table 5.2 compares the total logistical and dutiable costs involved in shipping textile and clothing products to the US market from various exporting countries under various trade arrangements. The total cost is the sum of: *i)* the transit cost measured at the rate of 0.5% of import value for each transit day (Hummels, 2000); *ii)* the freight cost incurred on the relevant transport routes (Annex Table 5.A1.1); and *iii)* the applied customs duties which vary on the basis of the prevailing preferential trade arrangements. The last column gives an indication of the total cost advantage or disadvantage of the various countries relative to competing imports from China subject to the regular MFN duty rate.

For example, the total cost for a trade transaction involving one-way shipments of clothing articles originating from Mexico that qualify for duty-free entry under NAFTA amounts to 1.6% of the import value of the shipment, *i.e.* 1% for two days of transit plus 0.6% for rail freight costs. If the same clothing articles were imported directly from China on seaborne vessels, the total cost would be 24.1% (6% for transit time, plus 5.8% for freight cost, plus 12.3% for customs duty). In this case, Mexico enjoys a cost advantage of 22.5% over similar articles originating from China. More than half of this cost advantage is attributed to Mexico's preferential access under NAFTA, about a quarter to freight cost advantage and the other quarter to the time factor due to shorter transit period. The total cost advantage for Mexico over China would be even larger for clothing articles that are subject to higher customs duties: the maximum US duty on clothing products is 32.5% (see Table 5.5).

The transit period by seaborne transport from China is just a few days behind the transit period for countries located near the United States, such as Colombia. This underscores that the reliability of transport infrastructure and efficiency in customs procedures complement each other in minimising total transit time and can make geographically remote countries more competitive from a logistical point of view.

Table 5.2 shows the total cost for trade transactions incurred on the basis of outward processing programmes (OPP) that require two-way shipments: pre-cut fabrics are shipped to offshore centres for final assembly and are re-imported on a duty-free basis to the United States as finished clothing articles. It also shows the net cost advantage or disadvantage of OPP transactions over competing imports from China subject to the regular MFN duty rate. On the basis of these comparisons, OPP transactions provide a net cost advantage of 15.7% for the Dominican Republic and of 11.2% for Colombia and a cost disadvantage of –15.4% for South Africa; and -47.2% for Kenya over competing Chinese imports. With distance and time acting as trade barriers, OPP transactions designed to encourage the final assembly of clothing articles from imported fabrics at low-wage offshore centres remain economically attractive only if the margin of preferential duty exceeds the difference between the OPP-related cost and the logistical cost incurred for competitive suppliers.

For Dominican Republic suppliers, duty-free OPP transactions enable them to take advantage of their geographical proximity to the US market and to compete more effectively with Mexican suppliers. However, for geographically remote suppliers, such as South Africa and Kenya, duty-free OPP transactions offer no net cost advantages. In fact, OPP transactions are the least competitive transactions of all trade possibilities. Even for Kenyan suppliers that can temporarily use third-country fabrics for duty-free OPP transactions, these transactions offer no net cost advantages.[7] These results demonstrate that the cost effectiveness of OPP transactions diminishes as the transit period increases, with obvious negative consequences for suppliers located in geographically remote locations. The trade policy implications of these cost comparisons in the post-ATC period are discussed in Chapter 2.

Total logistical and dutiable costs would vary if other modes of transport were used for comparison purposes. For air shipments, even if air freight is more expensive than seaborne freight (see Annex Table 5.A1.1), the shorter transit period would partially or completely offset the added freight cost involved and, accordingly, modify cost competitiveness among suppliers. However, for countries like Pakistan and Cambodia, air freight costs are very high and air shipment may not improve their competitiveness. In the absence of more detailed data on transit periods for air shipments, it is not possible to make reliable country comparisons. For China, assuming a transit period of two days, air shipments instead of seaborne shipments would increase total cost by only 3.7 percentage points (27.8% instead of 24.1%). Given this small cost differential, Chinese suppliers should be more or less indifferent as to whether they use seaborne or air transport modes for exports to the United States. Hence, it is quite likely that air freight services could capture an increasing share of total trade in textiles and clothing as the air freight industry becomes more competitive.

Table 5.2. Transit, freight and duty cost on US imports of textiles and clothing

Percentage of import values

Country of origin	Transit in days [1]			Time, freight and duty costs				Advantage
	Outbound from USA	Inbound for USA	Transit days	Time factor 0.5%/day	Freight cost	Customs duty [2]	Total cost	Relative to China
Mexico								
Two-way shipments	2	2	4	2.0%	1.2%	0.0%	3.2%	20.9%
One-way shipment		2	2	1.0%	0.6%	0.0%	1.6%	22.5%
Canada								
Two-way shipments	2	2	4	2.0%	1.8%	0.0%	3.8%	20.3%
One-way shipment		2	2	1.0%	0.9%	0.0%	1.9%	22.2%
Dominican Republic (Puerto Plata-Port Everglade)								
Two-way shipments [2]	5	5	10	5.0%	3.4%	0.0%	8.4%	15.7%
MFN shipment		5	5	2.5%	1.7%	12.3%	16.5%	7.6%
Colombia (Cartagena-Miami)								
Two-way shipments [2]	9	10	19	9.5%	3.4%	0.0%	12.9%	11.2%
MFN shipment		10	10	5.0%	1.7%	12.3%	19.0%	5.1%
China								
MFN shipment by sea		12	12	6.0%	5.8%	12.3%	24.1%	-
MFN shipment by air		2	2	1.0%	14.5%	12.3%	27.8%	-
Hong Kong, China (to Long Beach)								
Two-way shipments	18	12	30	15.0%	6.2%	12.3%	33.5%	-9.4%
MFN shipment		12	12	6.0%	3.1%	12.3%	21.4%	2.7%
South Africa (Cape Town-New York)								
Two-way shipments [2]	34	25	59	29.5%	10.0%	0.0%	39.5%	-15.4%
MFN shipment		25	25	12.5%	5.0%	12.3%	29.8%	-5.7%
Kenya (Nairobi-New York)								
Two-way shipments [2]	62	61	123	61.5%	9.8%	0.0%	71.3%	-47.2%
One-way shipment [3]		61	61	30.5%	4.9%	0.0%	35.4%	-11.3%
MFN shipment		61	61	30.5%	4.9%	12.3%	47.7%	-23.6%

1. The outbound and inbound periods are average seaborne shipping and customs clearance periods calculated by ShipGuide.com. For Mexico and Canada, the transit periods are OECD estimates for rail shipments and customs clearance. For China, the transit period for air shipments is an OECD estimate.

2. The average US customs duty on clothing imports was 12.3% MFN in 2002, see Table 5.5. Under various OPP-type programmes, the United States grants duty-free entry on imports of clothing articles assembled abroad from components produced in the United States.

3. Until the end of September 2004, duty-free entry is granted on clothing imports originating from AGOA's LDCs which are assembled from third-country fabrics. In this case, the reported transit period is underestimated since no time period is factored in for the importation of fabrics from third countries.

Source: USAID (2003) for the transit data based on ShipGuide.com; OECD calculation for freight costs based on data from the US Department of Commerce, Bureau of the Census; and Hummels (2000) for the time factor per day.

The data on logistical costs incurred in the international movement of textile and clothing products underscore the importance of efficient port infrastructure, reliable and competitive modes of transport and efficient customs procedures for maintaining a competitive edge in the highly competitive, time-sensitive and fashion-oriented textile and clothing markets. Although the above discussion has focused on US textile and clothing imports owing to the availability of detailed trade data by mode of transport, it is assumed that the related policy and regulatory considerations are equally relevant for other countries. Some of the policy issues in respect of promoting greater efficiency in port infrastructure and competitive conditions in maritime and rail shipping are examined below.[8] Moreover, in the aftermath of the attacks of 11 September 2001 on the World Trade Center, concerns about potential transport disruptions caused by terrorist attacks have become more prominent and are also discussed. Customs-related procedures are discussed in the section dealing with customs facilitation.

Greater efficiency in port infrastructure

Given the importance of seaborne transport for trade in textiles and clothing, efficiency (or lack thereof) in port infrastructure can have a significant effect on the international competitiveness of national firms. Various studies on port infrastructure point to the support roles governments can play in promoting sound investment in port infrastructure.[9] The objectives of government policy may include, for example: *i)* vesting autonomy and financial responsibility to the port authorities themselves;[10] *ii)* encouraging private sector participation; and *iii)* promoting services competition in the delivery of various port services, *e.g.* piloting, towing, loading, handling and other ancillary services, that may operate in monopoly or near monopoly conditions within the confines of port facilities.

Another area of government action relates to the various administrative and inspection tasks carried out directly by customs authorities, and directly or indirectly in the enforcement of national regulations in the fields of environment, sanitary inspection, tax collection and security requirements. Lack of co-ordination among all service providers in ports can result in unnecessary delays in cargo movements, as measured by ship turnaround time. Ship turnaround time is an indicator of port efficiency and should be regularly monitored by stakeholders.[11] Improved co-ordination among service providers should be identified as a priority area for port authorities with a view to minimising unnecessary delays for vessels without compromising on law enforcement requirements. The current energy shortages in China referred to in Box 5.2, which are partly compounded by bottlenecks in transport and port infrastructure, underscore the importance of efficient port infrastructure for the just-in-time manufacturing sectors.

The government policy agenda that nurtures greater efficiency in port infrastructure is rather broad and brings benefits that go well beyond the textile and clothing industries. Ultimately, governments should assess their policy framework and port infrastructure with a view to strengthening the support role of government policies and regulations by: *i)* encouraging sound investment in infrastructure modernisation projects by stakeholders; *ii)* setting up a competition-enhancing environment in various port services; and *iii)* better integrating the enforcement of national laws and regulations, *e.g.* customs procedures, taxation, sanitary and environment protection, with other services providers in ports.

Competition conditions in maritime shipping

The advent of containerised transport in the mid-1960s brought profound changes to the international transport of goods. Transhipment of goods between transport modes was greatly facilitated, ships became larger and more specialised, and there was significant investment in port infrastructure. Together, these developments have brought considerable productivity gains and downward pressures on transport costs. Concurrently, the globalisation of industrial activities, spurred by improved market access and declining telecommunications costs, has multiplied trade opportunities and resulted in added demand for international transport services.

Maritime transport in 40–foot containers is the dominant transport mode for the increasing world trade in textiles and clothing between distant assembly operations and consumption regions. For decades, there were concerns about competition-restraining practices among shipping lines and port terminal operators. The principal organisational feature of the liner sector has been the ability of operators to enter into a variety of co–operation arrangements and agreements which, in most other sectors, would contravene competition laws. These organisational arrangements have traditionally taken the form of liner conferences, *e.g.* co–operation arrangements that limit capacity and set common rates. More recently, new forms of co-operation, such as consortia and strategic alliances, have emerged with the advent of containerisation and new independent operators and have eroded the control of these conferences.

These organisational arrangements have elicited strong and opposing reactions from carriers and shippers. On the one hand, carriers argue that these practices are necessary to prevent destructive competition in maritime services. On the other, shippers remain unconvinced of the benefits of price fixing and consider that these arrangements lead to abuses of power and freight rates above what they would be in a fully competitive market. Despite the perennial disputes, "governments of all major trading nations have continued to provide carriers with exemptions from national antitrust statutes governing price and capacity fixing" (OECD, 2002a, p. 19).

A recent OECD study (2002a) examined the rationale and impacts of the various co-operation arrangements and recommended that "limited antitrust exemptions not be allowed to cover price fixing and rate discussions". It further offered three principles that countries could use to guide future reassessments of the validity of antitrust exemptions for price fixing, rate discussions and capacity agreements between competitors in the liner shipping sector. The three principles are: *i)* shippers and carriers should always have the option of freely negotiating rates, surcharges and other terms of carriage on an individual and confidential basis; *ii)* shippers and carriers should always be able to contractually protect key terms of negotiated service contracts, including information regarding rates, and this confidentiality should be given maximum protection; and *iii)* carriers should be able to pursue operational and/or capacity agreements with other carriers as long as these do not confer undue market power to the parties involved.

Figure 5.1 shows the average freight rates per twenty-foot equivalent unit (TEU) in 2001 for eastbound and westbound maritime shipments over the three main shipping routes, *e.g.* Asia-Europe, Asia-North America, and Europe-North America. It is assumed that they also reflect the freight rates applied to textile and clothing shipments. The striking feature of these shipping costs is that all routes display price imbalances between their eastbound and westbound directions, which lead to an oversupply of capacity in the weak trade direction in order to provide adequate service in the strong direction. These cost differences are explained by: *i)* the rapid industrialisation of the Asia-Pacific region; *ii)* the different composition of the products transported, *e.g.* higher values of traded goods originating from Asia; and *iii)* different competitive conditions prevailing on shipping routes.

The rate imbalance is considerably smaller on the Europe-North America route than on the two Asian routes. This is partly due to the passage of the US Ocean Shipping and Reform Act in 1998 which granted shippers and carriers the right to enter into confidential contracts without prior notice and thus undermined the dominance of conference tariffs. It is estimated that less than 10% of the United States-Europe traffic now takes place directly under conference terms (OECD, 2002a, p. 22).

Figure 5.1. Freight rates per TEU, 2001

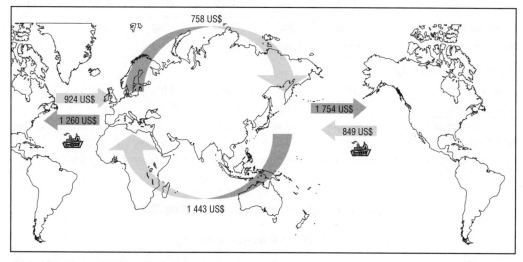

Note: Information sourced from six major liner companies. All rates are all-in, including the inland intermodal portion, if relevant. All rates are average rates of all commodities carried by major carriers. Rates to and from the United States refer to the average for all coasts. Rates to and from Europe refer to the average for North and Mediterranean Europe. Rates to and from Asia refer to the whole of Southeast Asia, East Asia and Japan/Korea.

Source: Containerisation International's Freight Rate Indicators.

Competition conditions in freight shipping by rail

As shown in Table 5.1, in 2003, rail haulage was the second most important mode for transporting imports of textile and clothing products in the United States, exceeding air freight by a considerable margin (12.4% *versus* 3.2%). The re-regulation of US railroad rate setting, under the Staggers Rail Act of 1980, is widely credited for the renewal of the US rail industry and the tangible benefits that it brought to shippers between 1981 and 2002: inflation-adjusted rail rates declined by 60%; productivity increased by almost 200%; train accidents declined by nearly 70%; and railroad firms invested over USD 320 billion in their rail infrastructure (AAR, 2004). The Act removed most barriers to commercial management of railroads but granted the Surface Transportation Board the authority to set maximum rates and to take action if it finds anticompetitive behaviour or market power abuse.

As US rail companies responded to the re–regulation of railroad rate setting, productivity gains per employee between 1983 and 1992 allowed railways to compete with trucks and barges for the first time in decades. Railways have also recaptured the movement of bulk commodities from trucks and have developed long distance trailer-on-flatcar/container–on–flatcar routes (OECD, 1997). Under the new regulatory framework, rail haulage in the United States maintained its market share of total freight at about 41% from 1970 to 2001 (Table 5.3), thereby keeping pace with the expansion of more than 90% of the total freight market. During the same period, the share of total freight carried by rail in the European Union fell from 20% to 7.8%. The breakdown of freight transport by mode is shown in Table 5.4 for five regions and reveals very high shares of total freight carried by rail in Russia and China, *e.g.* two former centrally planned economies, and a low rail share for Japan.

Table 5.3. Rail transport in the EU and the United States, 1970-2001

Billions of tonne-kilometres

	1970	1980	1990	2000	2001	2000/1990
European Union (15)	282	290	255	250	242	-2.0%
United States	1 117	1 342	1 510	2 140		41.7%
Percentage of total freight						
European Union (15)	20.0%	14.6%	11.0%	8.0%	7.8%	
United States	41.5%	39.1%	38.2%	41.3%		

Note: US rail, Class 1 railways (approximately 90% of rail freight traffic). Total freight covers rail, road, inland water, pipeline and sea.

Source: EUROPA, *Energy and Transport: Figures and Main Facts* (annual), based on data from the US Department of Transport and Eurostat.

Table 5.4. Freight transport in five regions, 2000

Billions of tonne-kilometres

	EU15	United States	Japan	China	Russia
Rail	250	2 140	22	1 362	1 373
Road	1 378	1 667	313	597	23
Sea (domestic/intra-EU)	1 270	414	242		165
Inland waterways	125	527	-		65
Oil pipeline	85	843			1 916

Note: US rail, Class 1 railways (approximately 90% of rail freight traffic).

Source: EUROPA, *Energy and Transport: Figures and Main Facts* (annual), based on data from the US Department of Transport; Eurostat; Japan Statistics Bureau; Goskom STAT (Russia); and National Bureau of Statistics of China.

Within the European Union, the implementation of the single European market has required member states to reduce state involvement and to increase the competitive power of railway companies by: introducing commercial financial management; separating infrastructure accounts from the operating business; and providing third parties with access to the infrastructure. Apart from payments for public service and specific funding for infrastructure provision, the railways were required to finance their operational activities without state subsidies. Although some reforms were undertaken in Sweden, Germany and the United Kingdom, these initiatives had not increased competition in international rail services by the mid–1990s (OECD, 1997).

With a view to revitalise the EU railways, the European Commission adopted in 2001 the so–called first railway package of reforms to break down national barriers and to speed up the introduction of market forces in international rail transport.[12] In early 2002, a second railway package was unveiled that aimed at speeding up the implementation of the first package and extended the reform process to national freight services. This package provides for improved safety and greater interoperability and established the European Agency for Rail Safety and Interoperability. In March 2004, the European Council and Parliament reached an agreement that provides for full market opening for international freight services by 1 January 2006 and for all freight services by 1 January 2007.

Campos and Cantos (1999) assessed railway deregulation and privatisation experiences in eight countries and concluded that regulation of the railway sector should remain simple and flexible in order to protect its share of transport markets.[13] The worldwide rail industry has undergone deep restructuring, varying from simple reorganisation measures to more comprehensive restructuring, involving private participation and vertical separation of infrastructure from services when the ownership of facilities is fully separated from other rail functions. They argue that the regulatory framework should be governed by principles that foster competition and market mechanisms, wherever possible. Moreover, they show that important increases in efficiency can be achieved without full privatisation of the industry.

In the large US textile and clothing markets, national suppliers as well as Mexican and Canadian suppliers benefit from meaningful cost advantages over overseas suppliers because they can use rail services as their main mode of transport. This suggests that national suppliers in the large EU textile and clothing market and those located in land-adjacent countries could achieve similar rail-related cost advantages. Furthermore, in countries where railroad re-regulation is less advanced, fostering competition and market mechanisms in the domestic regulatory framework would likely bring tangible cost-competitive advantages to national suppliers of textile and clothing products.

Vulnerability in transport systems

World trade is dependent on efficient and secure transport systems, and great strides have been made in recent years to render these systems as open and frictionless as possible in order to spur even greater economic growth. New security requirements are affecting the cost of transporting goods across borders, through both higher direct costs and longer delivery times. The openness that has allowed transport systems to become more efficient also renders them vulnerable to terrorist attacks that could disrupt or shut them down. Targeted attacks could result in port closures and significant disruptions in the supply of essential materials and would have numerous indirect adverse impacts.

In the aftermath of the 11 September 2001 World Trade Center attacks, the US air transport system was shut down for several days and passage at the US-Canadian land borders was severely affected by the tightening of security measures. The slowdown in customs clearance and border crossings had a major impact on just-in-time manufacturing sectors and led to several factory shutdowns on both sides of the border, especially in the automobile industry (Andrea and Smith, 2002). These dramatic events have led governments to reassess the vulnerability and risks of their transport systems and to strengthen their security dispositions throughout the entire transport system. They have implemented new customs procedures and strengthened border co-operation among customs administrations with the aim of a return to close to normal border crossings.[14]

Under the auspices of the International Maritime Organisation (IMO) – the UN body responsible for developing the common regulatory framework for international maritime transport – new security measures were negotiated that have resulted in the adoption of the International Ship and Port Safety (ISPS) Code which introduced changes in the Convention on the Safety of Life at Sea (SOLAS) that became effective in July 2004. For its part, the United States enacted the American Maritime Transportation Security Act of 2002 which largely adopts the security-related provisions of SOLAS and the ISPS Code. This Act also includes several new measures, such as the requirement for transport security cards for port personnel; new secure seafarer identification papers; and the development of a system of foreign port security assessments.

The implementation of new security-related measures comes with additional costs for carriers in terms of various security assessment procedures, the training of staff and expenditures in security-related equipment. More careful background checks are required from incoming carriers, the transport of hazardous materials is more closely regulated, insurance rates were raised and security surcharges were added. These security-related measures involve additional costs and make transit periods more unpredictable.[15] As suggested by the transit data in Table 5.2, small variations in transit periods of textile and clothing shipments due to delays caused by new customs security measures can modify the relative cost competitiveness of suppliers. In particular, new security measures may have a disproportionate impact on small developing countries which may not be covered under recently signed border co-operation agreements between large trading partners.

An OECD study has estimated the initial burden imposed on ship operators to be at least USD 1.28 billion and then 730 million per year thereafter (OECD, 2003a, page 56). While the study notes the difficulties involved in estimating some port-related security costs, it stresses that these costs are still substantially below those that might result from a major attack. Moreover, many security-related measures bring benefits that go beyond protection against terrorist attacks owing to progress in implementing integrated information technology (IT) systems. These benefits result from "reduced delays, faster processing times, better asset control, decreased payroll, fewer losses due to theft, and decreased insurance costs" (OECD, 2003a, p. 57). Furthermore, it is thought that these improvements have the potential to change long-established practices and lead to shorter vessel turnaround times and accelerated customs clearing measures.

Even though a trade-off between security and efficiency in border crossings is unavoidable in the short term, it is likely to be lessened in the medium term. In implementing new security measures, governments should not lose sight of the beneficiary effects of smoothly functioning transport systems. New security measures might be subjected to risk-management analysis to ensure that they address the most critical risks. The additional costs can be minimised by furthering a co-operative approach among stakeholders in both the design and implementation phases. Efforts could be devoted to enlarging the country coverage of border agreements recently signed between large trading partners with a view to avoiding potentially negative impacts on trade flows from developing and least developed countries.

Customs facilitation dimensions

In the post-ATC period, trade in textile and clothing products will benefit from the elimination of a series of MFA-related controls, but it will remain vulnerable to customs-related inefficiencies given the international fragmentation of the supply chain. In the aftermath of the 11 September 2001 World Trade Center attacks, many exporting countries expressed concern over the compliance cost implications of the enforcement of more stringent security and safety measures. Also, there are considerable disparities among countries in the number of tariff lines used for classifying textile and clothing products for trade purposes under the Harmonised System of classification, with some countries having a more simplified tariff structure than others.

Streamlined border treatment for textiles and clothing

In the post–ATC period, trade in textile and clothing products will benefit from streamlined border treatment. Traders will be spared the bureaucratic arrangements involved in obtaining MFA-related export permits or visas in the exporting country. These bureaucratic arrangements differ among exporting countries. Some have set up highly automated and transparent issuance process, and most traders have learned to deal with them without undue costs. Others, however, have less transparent procedures, *e.g.* discretionary power, and their traders stand to benefit in the post-ATC period from the elimination of these bureaucratic arrangements. The magnitude of the cost saving should be proportional to the level of bureaucratic difficulties currently encountered in obtaining MFA export permits.

On the import side, customs officials in formally constrained importing countries will no longer have to review export permits for accuracy and completeness. The latter typically involves the verification of: *i)* the specific quota category number; *ii)* the quantity; *iii)* the trader's signature; *iv)* the accuracy of the permit number; *v)* the validity period of the permit; and *vi)* the declared merchandise to ensure that they match the shipment concerned and in particular the origin. It is only after these verifications have been completed and charged against the appropriate quota (category and country) that the shipment is released from customs to the importer. Consequently, the elimination of MFA–related controls is expected to translate into: *i)* fewer bureaucratic arrangements for traders; *ii)* faster customs clearance for concerned shipments; and *iii)* fewer customs verification tasks in both the exporting and importing countries.

Inefficient customs procedures undermine export-led strategies

Some countries may have cumbersome and outdated customs procedures, which are unrelated to MFA procedures, and act as non-tariff barriers in their own right. Moreover, in the aftermath of the 11 September attacks, new customs security measures can cause significant delays in customs clearance if these measures are not implemented promptly. Significant cost overruns and production schedule delays are incurred when shipments are held in customs warehouses owing to inefficient customs procedures or lack of co-ordination among border services providers. The internationally fragmented supply chain in textiles and clothing is particularly vulnerable to customs-related inefficiencies, since the crossing of at least two borders is involved: first when imported inputs enter the country where the final assembly takes place, and second, when the final product is imported into the country of final consumption.

In particular, inefficiency in customs procedures and opaque border regulations can seriously undermine export-led strategies that rely on imported inputs for a significant share of production. Similarly, in large net-consuming regions, cumbersome import procedures adversely affect the operations of national producers and retailers that rely on imported products. Even though great strides in modernising customs systems have been made in OECD countries through risk-management principles, industrial partnerships and advanced technology, continuing emphasis on customs modernisation is the right policy direction to underpin the competitiveness of national firms. In many developing countries, the emphasis on customs modernisation may need to be strengthened given the adverse impact of inefficient customs procedures on national textile and clothing firms. Three examples, shown in Box 5.1, illustrate this point.

A recent OECD study (2003b) examined customs reform in various developing countries with a view to deeper understanding of the costs and benefits of trade facilitation measures. While the study does not focus on any particular sector, it usefully reminds textile-dependent developing countries of the need to pursue customs modernisation and reform. The study highlights the importance of correctly identifying problematic customs areas that need to be addressed as a first step; a common cause of failed reform is inadequate or insufficient initial analysis or diagnosis. Moreover, complexities in cross–border trade often owe less to the applicable regulatory framework than to approaches to implementation developed over the years. A fair number of procedural burdens could be addressed by focusing on human resource policies in customs authorities.

Box 5.1. Adverse impacts of customs delays on textile and clothing production

Sri Lanka

In examining the interplay between customs procedures and e-commerce, Mann *et al.* (2000) refer to one Sri Lankan clothing firm which failed to win a long-term contract because input shipments were held up in the local port. The firm obtained a performance-test contract from a major retail chain in Europe which had to be completed within 72 hours. While the firm successfully downloaded the specification order from electronic applications and assembled the shipment in advance of the deadline, the shipment was held up in the local port due to red tape. The missed deadline resulted in the loss of a long-term contract for clothing items of higher value-added content than previous orders filled by Sri Lankan firms.

Madagascar

A diagnostic study undertaken in 2001 under the Integrated Framework for Trade-related Technical Assistance (Integrated Framework 2001) highlights the constraints imposed by the inefficient functioning of customs on low labour cost manufacturing activities, such as clothing. It is reported that customs clearance is the subject of considerable complaints: incoming or outgoing textile and clothing containers took on average four to five days to clear. One major clothing exporter estimated that reducing clearance times to one day would be equivalent to a 3% to 5% cost savings.

Bangladesh customs reform

With more than 75% of total Bangladeshi exports accounted for by clothing in 2001, Bangladesh is pursuing a comprehensive customs reform programme which is carried out with support from the World Bank and the World Customs Organisation. In an interim review, Draper (2001) stresses some of the progress made in modernising customs procedures and identifies risk factors that still challenge Bangladesh reformers. Some of the recommendations include: *i)* setting up a coalition of reformers and potential beneficiaries of reforms to move the reform process forward; *ii)* providing training and appropriate financial incentives for professional work; *iii)* proceeding with additional tariff simplification programmes; and *iv)* pursuing equipment modernisation and automation to further reduce the potential for discretionary interventions.

Operational problems may also have a number of interrelated causes which must be comprehensively addressed to ensure the success and sustainability of reform programmes. Although every reform project is subject to capacity constraints that may not favour exhaustiveness, comprehensiveness and coherence are essential for success. For instance, investments in infrastructure facilities and equipment will not reduce commercial transaction costs unless operations related to foreign trade are free from unnecessary institutional or physical interference. Finally, the OECD study (2003b) acknowledges that the adoption of efficiency-enhancing measures in customs procedures brings tangible benefits for the trading communities in terms of reduction in customs clearance times and in undue transaction costs.

Customs tariff simplification

Another dimension of customs facilitation relates to the classification of textile and clothing products for trade purposes. The Harmonised System (HS) is widely applied by WTO member countries and offers a harmonised structure of product headings that are defined at two-, four- and six-digit levels. The actual tariff lines are defined at eight- and ten-digit levels and each WTO member has some flexibility in specifying the content of its relevant tariff lines. Corresponding tariff rates are set up in accordance with each country's binding commitments. The result is that some countries define fewer tariff lines or set a simpler structure of tariff rates than others, which makes their tariff regime more transparent and relatively easier to administer. Moreover, the multiplicity of tariff lines with different tariff rates makes the system prone to incorrect or fraudulent customs declarations by traders and provides more opportunities for discretionary interpretations by customs officials in countries where integrity concerns prevail.

Figure 5.2. Average applied tariffs and number of tariff lines for clothing products

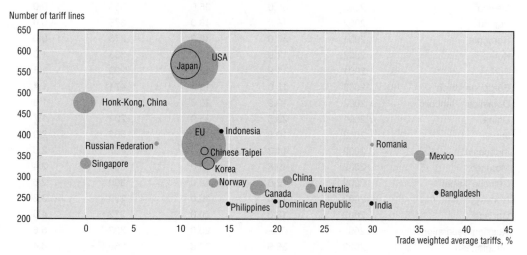

Notes: Trade-weighted average tariffs for the most recent year available. Country circles are proportional to the corresponding country's share of world clothing imports. To present this graph within reasonable proportions, it has not been possible to include the country circles for Turkey and Thailand.

Source: World integrated Trade Solution, WITS.

Tables 5.5 and 5.6 compare the structure of tariff lines and their applied tariff rates for clothing and textile products for the most recent year available for several economies. The economies are ranked in increasing order of their tariff rate dispersion as measured by the standard deviation. For clothing products (Table 5.5 and Figure 5.2), there is considerable disparity in the number of tariff lines, with 990 tariff lines for Turkey and only 233 for the Philippines under the same HS 61 and 62 headings. For textile products (Table 5.6 and Figure 5.3), the number of tariff lines is considerably larger than for clothing products, hovering between 613 for Singapore and 2 834 for Morocco. The standard deviation indicators are generally higher on textiles than on clothing products for most economies, with the exception of the Russian Federation, the United States, Thailand and Australia. This suggests a higher prevalence of tariff peaks on textiles than on clothing products. Chapter 2 discusses the issues of tariff escalation and peaks.

Table 5.5. Structure of customs tariffs on clothing products

	Clothing (HS 61-62)				
	Latest year available	Average tariff (%)	Maximum tariff (%)	Number of tariff lines	Standard deviation
Philippines	2002	15.0	15.0	233	0.0
Singapore	2002	0.0	0.0	235	0.0
Pakistan	2002	25.0	25.0	243	0.0
Mexico	2002	35.0	35.0	353	0.0
Poland	2002	18.0	18.0	375	0.0
Romania	2001	30.0	30.0	375	0.0
Korea	2002	12.9	13.0	333	1.0
Turkey	2001	11.9	12.6	990	1.3
European Union	2002	12.0	12.4	471	1.4
Dominican Republic	2002	19.9	20.0	238	1.6
China	2001	23.5	25.0	292	1.7
Japan	2002	10.8	14.2	563	2.0
Indonesia	2002	14.3	15.0	407	2.3
Morocco	2002	49.8	50.0	561	2.4
Chinese Taipei	2002	12.6	19.0	360	2.6
Norway	2002	13.4	16.0	289	3.3
Canada	2002	18.0	20.0	272	4.6
Russian Federation	2002	7.5	20.0	392	5.6
Bangladesh	2002	36.9	37.5	260	6.4
United States	2002	12.3	32.5	568	7.9
Australia	2002	23.6	25.0	278	8.7
Thailand	2001	38.3	60.0	305	12.0
Switzerland	2002	-	-	329	-

Note: Weighted average applied tariffs for the most recent year available. Since Switzerland applies specific duties as opposed to ad valorem tariffs, there is no average tariffs are mentioned for this country. Since Norway also applies a fair number of specific *ad valorem* tariffs, its average tariffs should be interpreted with caution.

Source: World Integrated Trade Solution, WITS.

There are no direct relationships between the number of tariff lines and the degree of protection afforded. For example, the Philippines has about the same number of tariff lines as Singapore but while the former applied a uniform 15% tariff rate on all clothing tariff lines in 2002, Singapore granted duty-free entry on all lines. Leaving aside the economic aspects of tariff rates, the tariff regime of the Philippines and Singapore are relatively easy to administer from a strict trade-facilitation viewpoint given their flat rate structure and small number of tariff lines.

For several developing countries undertaking customs reforms without the financial resources to invest in paperless customs systems, simplicity in tariff definitions combined with a simplified tariff rate structure often represents a cost-effective approach to protecting government revenue sources and to address fraudulency and integrity concerns. In most advanced countries where IT customs services are effectively enforced, more complex tariff structure can be managed without compromising transparency and high compliance standards. Nevertheless, more complex tariff structures offer a greater possibility for deliberate or accidental misclassification.

Figure 5.3. Average applied tariffs and number of tariff lines for textile products

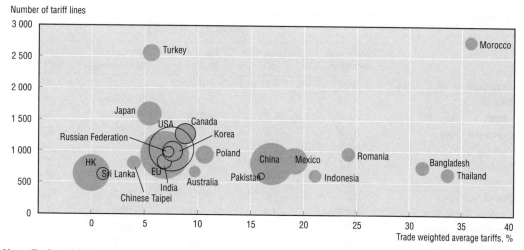

Notes: Trade-weighted average tariffs for the most recent year available. Country circles are proportional to the corresponding country's share of world textile imports.

Source: World Integrated Trade Solution, WITS.

A large number of tariff lines grants more flexibility to calibrate the level of protection with the level of trade sensitivity of the products concerned. A large number of tariff lines may also reflect a statistical objective, *i.e.* to gather detailed trade data on imported products. For example, a given article may be specified under several tariff lines according to the fabric composition of the article, *e.g.* a given article made of cotton, rayon and polyester would be specified under three distinct tariff lines. Japan and the United States acknowledge the use of a multiplicity of tariff lines for statistical purposes. Reconciling customs simplification with either flexibility of calibration or statistical objectives is not necessarily problematic if high transparency and integrity standards are applied by countries throughout their customs procedures. In the context of the Doha Round of multilateral trade negotiations, WTO members have an opportunity to work toward achieving greater tariff simplification and eventual reductions in tariff rates.

Table 5.6. Structure of customs tariffs on textile products

	Textiles (HS 50-60, 63)				
	Latest year available	Average tariff (%)	Maximum tariff (%)	Number of tariff lines	Standard deviation
Singapore	2002	0.0	0.0	613	0.0
Switzerland	2002	-	-	800	-
Japan	2002	5.1	15.8	1 587	2.8
European Union	2002	6.9	12.4	1 251	2.8
Turkey	2001	5.6	12.6	2 557	2.9
Indonesia	2002	6.8	15.0	822	3.9
Korea	2002	7.9	52.9	985	4.0
Philippines	2002	6.0	15.0	607	4.0
Chinese Taipei	2002	4.2	19.0	806	4.6
Russian Federation	2002	7.6	20.0	952	4.9
Poland	2002	10.6	38.0	936	5.0
United States	2002	7.6	27.2	1 026	5.2
Thailand	2001	12.4	30.0	1 496	5.9
Mexico	2002	19.9	35.0	856	6.1
Norway	2002	7.3	16.0	698	6.2
Australia	2002	9.8	25.0	687	6.4
Canada	2002	9.1	19.0	1 155	6.9
China	2001	20.1	90.0	775	7.5
Dominican Republic	2002	5.7	38.0	639	7.8
Sri Lanka	2001	1.1	25.0	624	8.0
Pakistan	2002	13.5	25.0	670	8.1
Romania	2001	22.8	76.0	917	8.3
Morocco	2002	35.9	50.0	2 834	10.2
Bangladesh	2002	28.4	37.5	680	12.8

Note: Weighted average applied tariffs for the most recent year available. Since Switzerland applies specific duties as opposed to ad valorem tariffs, there is no average tariffs are mentioned for this country. As Norway also applies a fair number of specific *ad valorem* tariffs, its average tariffs should be interpreted with caution.

Source: World Integrated Trade Solution, WITS.

Essential business services

After raw materials and labour, electricity, telecommunications and water services are among the important inputs required in the production of textile and clothing products. Modern and reliable electricity services play a crucial role in the increasingly capital–intensive textile fabrication process. Specialised equipment is required for the weaving, knitting, washing, dyeing and finishing of textiles, and each fabrication stage relies on electricity as the main energy source. Since each process uses different energy-intensive equipment, it is difficult to quantify the share of total production costs accounted for by electricity.

In the same vein, modern and reliable telecommunications services play a crucial role in effectively managing internationally fragmented clothing operations on a just-in-time basis. They reduce the occurrence of errors in specifications and also facilitate business-to-business (B2B) contacts. Hence, without reliable telecommunications, the risks of production errors and delays are multiplied and hamper the process of production fragmentation on the basis of comparative advantages. A business survey of major textile and clothing producers in Hong Kong (China) identified the quality of the telecommunications infrastructure as one of the most important investment factors: more important than policies affecting trade and investment, labour costs and education and training of workers (Spinanger, 2001). Fink *et al.* (2002) assessed the impact of communication costs on international trade and found that international variations in communication costs have a significant influence on trade patterns. In particular, their work reveals that the impact of communication costs on trade in differentiated products is larger than in homogenous products, by as much as one-third. They estimated the elasticity of trade flows in clothing products with respect to a bilateral calling price to be -1.112. This means that an increase of 1% in the cost of bilateral communication calls would lead to a drop in trade flows of 1.112%.[16]

ITC (2004) underscores the importance of telecommunications infrastructure for US clothing firms and retailers for communications with suppliers as they seek to reduce lead production time and exercise effective control over all elements of the supply chain. The ITC report also stresses the importance of access to reliable sources of electricity for all the segments of the industry and to reliable supplies of water. In respect of water, certain production segments of the textile supply chain, such as washing, dyeing, finishing of fabrics yarns and denim jeans require reliable supplies of clean water. Economic instruments – the use of water meters, the polluter pays principle, water tariffs set on a cost-recovery basis, and fines and compensation for damage to water bodies – can help countries improve the efficiency of their water management policies. For countries that are poorly endowed with domestic sources of fresh water, such as small islands and countries in hot climates, care should be exercised in respect of water-intensive production processes and water conservation programmes should be actively promoted.

High telecommunications and electricity costs due to outdated regulatory frameworks act as taxes on textile and clothing firms and, more importantly, undermine their capacity to focus production on the higher value-added segments of the supply chain that are critically dependent on reliable equipment to ensure quick market responses. Considerable cost overruns occur when production and shipment deliveries are delayed as a result of inefficiencies in information transmission systems. Moreover, Mann *et al.* (2000) argue that where production, distribution and delivery are not co-ordinated, the private sector loses the incentive to innovate and invest in new technology. They suggest that policy makers must adjust to a more networked global economy and adapt the national regulatory framework to rapidly changing technology to ensure that stakeholders are well positioned to reap the market opportunities offered by innovative telecommunications equipment and services.

Business telephone charges

There are considerable disparities in business telephone charges among OECD countries. Some of the leading textile- and clothing-producing OECD countries are relatively less well off than others, *e.g.* Mexico, the Czech Republic, Poland, Hungary and Turkey. In 2000, these countries' average business phone charges exceeded by at least 50% the OECD average charges (Table 5.7). The regulatory framework of the telecommunications industry changed radically during the past decade in almost all OECD countries. As technological innovation made competition increasingly possible in the long-distance and international telephony markets, policy makers sought to liberalise the access of new entrants.

Table 5.7. Business telephone charges in OECD countries

	Fixed	Usage	Total	% of OECD average
		USD (in PPPs)		
Australia	237.1	1 192.0	1 429.1	102.5%
Austria	228.7	949.5	1 178.2	84.5%
Belgium	178.4	1 298.3	1 476.8	106.0%
Canada	415.7	329.8	745.5	53.5%
Czech Republic	179.7	2 828.6	3 008.3	215.9%
Denmark	139.1	565.6	704.8	50.6%
Finland	128.4	736.3	864.7	62.0%
France	184.5	891.6	1 076.1	77.2%
Germany	135.7	1 041.3	1 177.0	84.5%
Greece	116.3	1 300.5	1 416.8	101.7%
Hungary	357.6	2 100.1	2 457.7	176.4%
Iceland	119.8	349.4	469.2	33.7%
Ireland	190.2	945.6	1 135.8	81.5%
Italy	205.2	1 238.3	1 443.4	103.6%
Japan	399.8	1 166.1	1 565.9	112.4%
Korea	45.7	1 473.5	1 519.3	109.0%
Luxembourg	152.7	639.1	791.8	56.8%
Mexico	449.2	2 728.8	3 178.0	228.0%
Netherlands	172.6	679.3	851.9	61.1%
New Zealand	437.2	894.4	1 331.6	95.6%
Norway	151.7	526.4	678.1	48.7%
Poland	172.0	2 459.0	2 630.9	188.8%
Portugal	206.7	1 355.3	1 562.0	112.1%
Spain	160.6	1 426.9	1 587.4	113.9%
Sweden	151.7	570.2	721.9	51.8%
Switzerland	166.0	835.5	1 001.6	71.9%
Turkey	71.6	2 057.0	2 128.6	152.7%
United Kingdom	247.1	820.0	1 067.1	76.6%
United States	298.8	916.1	1 214.9	87.2%
OECD average	210.3	1 183.3	1 393.6	100.0%

Note: Annual composite charges measured in August 2000, excluding VAT.

Source: OECD and Telïgen.

In developing countries, no reliable data are available to compare the cost advantage (disadvantage) among them and relative to OECD countries. Anecdotal information suggests that international business telephone charges and Internet services are relatively more expensive in developing countries than in developed countries, with few exceptions, such as Hong Kong (China) and Singapore which have modern infrastructure.

Within OECD countries, new independent regulatory agencies were established with a mandate to open markets to competition, prevent incumbents from abusing their position and avoid collusion between operators. As a result, competition has intensified and consumers have benefited from greater choice, lower prices and higher-quality services. However, the intensity of competition has not been the same among all telecommunications services, and some countries have opened up their markets sooner than others. In the new markets of mobile telephony and Internet dial-up (low–speed) access services, the absence of pre-established market positions has facilitated competition (OECD, 2003c).

In the aftermath of the telecommunications bubble, telecommunications firms encountered severe financial difficulties and undertook restructuring programmes to cut costs and strengthen their balance sheets. In this context of consolidation and painful restructuring, governments and regulators should resist the temptation to ease competition requirements. In the post–ATC period, the international competitiveness of textile and clothing firms will be enhanced in countries that maintain a competitive environment, spurring new investment in innovative telecommunications equipment and services and providing lower cost opportunities for consumers.

Industrial electricity prices

There are disparities in industrial electricity prices among OECD countries (Table 5.8), as measured in US dollars (computed on a purchasing power parity exchange rate basis) for kilowatt per hour (kWh). Some of the leading textile and clothing producers have relatively high electricity costs which hamper the competitiveness of their firms. Some of the highest industrial electricity prices are found in Turkey, the Slovak Republic, Hungary, Italy, the Czech Republic, Portugal and Korea, where average electricity prices are more than twice the OECD average. At the other end, the Nordic countries, Canada and the United States enjoy lower than average prices. Table 5.8 also shows nominal electricity prices for some non-OECD countries; they are not computed on a PPP basis, hence are not strictly comparable with the quoted OECD country prices. Within these countries, there are also considerable disparities in industrial electricity prices. For example, Indian electricity prices exceeded by a factor of more than four prevailing prices in South Africa and a factor of two those in Indonesia. Moreover, the electricity prices mentioned for some countries are no longer relevant, particularly for China, which now has recurrent power shortages and blackouts. Box 5.2 illustrates the importance of reliable electricity systems to foster the competitiveness of national textile and clothing suppliers in several developing countries.

Electricity cost is one of many factors that affect production costs and international competitiveness but its relative importance should not be underestimated for certain more energy-intensive production segments. In the post-ATC period, the international competitiveness of textile and clothing firms will be enhanced in countries with reliable systems that maintain a competitive environment in electricity generation and distribution systems.

Table 5.8. Industrial electricity charges in OECD and non-OECD countries

OECD	US Dollars/kWh (using PPPs)				% of OECD average		
	1990	1995	2000	2002	1990	1995	2000
Australia	0.042	0.048	0.044	0.048	67.7%	78.7%	97.8%
Austria	0.053	0.06	0.046		85.5%	98.4%	102.2%
Belgium	0.059	0.061	0.057		95.2%	100.0%	126.7%
Canada	0.032	0.042			51.6%	66.7%	
Czech Republic	0.101	0.149	0.119	0.113	162.9%	244.3%	264.4%
Denmark	0.041	0.046	0.056	0.065	66.1%	75.4%	124.4%
Finland	0.038	0.045	0.042	0.048	61.3%	73.8%	93.3%
France	0.046	0.048	0.041	0.042	74.2%	78.7%	91.1%
Germany	0.071	0.071	0.047	0.051	114.5%	116.4%	104.4%
Greece	0.073	0.071	0.064	0.065	117.7%	116.4%	142.2%
Hungary	0.18	0.093	0.13	0.132	290.3%	152.5%	288.9%
Ireland	0.059	0.064	0.055	0.078	95.2%	104.9%	122.2%
Italy	0.082	0.097	0.12		132.3%	159.0%	266.7%
Japan	0.091	0.103	0.1		146.8%	168.9%	178.6%
Korea	0.088	0.078	0.096	0.101	141.9%	127.9%	213.3%
Mexico	0.074	0.059	0.078	0.078	119.4%	96.7%	173.3%
Netherlands	0.044	0.059	0.067	0.072	71.0%	96.7%	148.9%
New Zealand	0.036	0.04	0.046	0.049	58.1%	65.6%	102.2%
Norway	0.023			0.033	37.1%		
Poland	0.08	0.084	0.086	0.105	129.0%	137.7%	191.1%
Portugal	0.135	0.148	0.108	0.104	217.7%	242.6%	240.0%
Slovak Republic		0.122	0.131	0.138	0.0%	200.0%	291.1%
Spain	0.091	0.077	0.061	0.061	146.8%	126.2%	135.6%
Sweden	0.032	0.029			51.6%	47.5%	
Switzerland	0.056	0.074	0.061	0.059	90.3%	121.3%	135.6%
Turkey	0.144	0.156	0.168	0.215	232.3%	255.7%	373.3%
United Kingdom	0.066	0.066	0.057	0.053	106.5%	108.2%	126.7%
United States	0.048	0.047	0.04	0.049	77.4%	77.0%	88.9%
OECD Europe	0.067	0.07	0.064		108.1%	114.8%	142.2%
OECD Total	0.062	0.061	0.045		100.0%	100.0%	100.0%

Non-OECD	US Dollars/kWh (nominal)			
	1990	1995	2000	2002
Brazil	0.093	0.057		
China	0.025	0.028		
Chinese Taipei	0.077	0.076	0.061	0.053
India		0.068	0.080	
Indonesia	0.049	0.066	0.040	
Kazakhstan		0.021	0.013	0.014
Romania		0.040	0.044	0.053
Russia		0.000	0.000	0.024
South Africa	0.028	0.029	0.017	0.012
Thailand	0.061	0.066	0.057	
Venezuela	0.019	0.054	0.055	

Notes: 1995 data for Canada, 2000 data for Japan and Venezuela, 2002 data for Germany, Korea, Mexico, Netherlands, Norway, Spain and Kazakhstan refer to the previous year. 1995 data for Kazakhstan refer to the next year. Price for Australia and the United States excludes tax.

Source: International Energy Agency (2003), Energy Prices and Taxes, Quarterly Statistics.

Box 5.2. Adverse impacts of high electricity costs and unreliable electricity systems on textile and clothing production in several developing countries

Bangladesh

The limited attractiveness of Bangladesh for foreign investors is partly attributed to its underdeveloped electricity system, *e.g.* the national electrification rate of 30%, and the inadequacy of its port facilities (ITC, 2004).

China

China's stellar economic growth has outpaced the growth of electricity supply and cumulated in power shortages in 2003. Blackout measures were imposed to limit electricity consumption in many regions, especially in east and south China. The State Electricity Regulatory Commission predicts a shortfall of more than 20 million kilowatts in 2004: electricity demand rose by 15% in 2003 and is forecast to rise by 12% to 2 100 billion megawatts in 2004. China's power shortage is not expected to alter fundamentally until new generation capacity is installed and the distribution system is improved (2006). The power shortage is further exacerbated by bottlenecks in transport infrastructure which delay the distribution of imported coal and oil feeds. Power shortages are forcing plants to halve production temporarily in several regions and are putting upward pressures on energy and transport costs. Although it is considered too early to evaluate the risks of inflation on the cost competitiveness of Chinese exporters, the emergence of infrastructure bottlenecks is raising questions about the reliability of Chinese suppliers for meeting tight delivery requirements in the just-in-time manufacturing sectors.

Dominican Republic

The relative scarcity of low-cost electricity and clean water in the Dominican Republic makes this country less attractive as an investment location in the post–ATC period for energy-intensive and water-intensive production processes, such as the spinning of yarns, and the weaving and finishing of fabrics (USAID, 2003).

India

High industrial energy prices in India due to cross-subsidisation between different Indian states and huge transmission and distribution losses are considered a major obstacle to improving the competitiveness of the Indian textile and clothing industries (Verma, 2002).

Philippines

Owing to high electricity costs, energy-intensive textile production, such as woven fabrics used in the production of most shirts and blouses, is too expensive to be manufactured domestically and must be imported (ITC, 2004).

Other dimensions

Standards heterogeneity and labelling

With the advent of new fabrics and public awareness of making sustainable development part of the life cycle of textile and clothing products, producers and consumers face various standards and labelling schemes. There is increased awareness of the need to protect consumer health from potentially allergenic, carcinogenic or poisonous substances in fabrics and to protect the environment against potentially harmful effects in terms of air pollution, the generation of waste and the contamination of water and soil.

The textile production process makes fairly intensive use of chemicals and is subject to various safety regulations. Starting with natural fibres, crops like cotton are very prone to pests and are sprayed with different types of pesticides. The spinning of man–made fibres requires many additives to provide the desirable fibre properties, such as fire retardant, hydrophilic or antistatic. The highest incidence of textile contamination occurs in the dyeing and finishing processes, as traces of heavy metal in certain dyestuffs, chlorinated products and stain removers are likely to be present. In the clothing assembly process, the use of stain removers containing chlorinated products and some sprayed products containing chloro–fluorocarbon and fluorides are subject to various safety regulations.

Compliance with different standards and regulations in different countries for like products can present firms wishing to engage in international trade with significant and sometimes prohibitive costs. For textile manufacturers, differentiated national standards may entail engineering costs and the purchase of specialised equipment or chemicals that are required to satisfy a limited number of foreign customers. Higher manufacturing costs result from the loss of economies of scale when smaller production runs are necessary to meet different national standards. Responses to changing consumer demand can also be delayed. SMEs are usually more vulnerable than larger enterprises to regulatory heterogeneity as they are the least able to afford the investment in costly equipment and chemical treatment.

The extra costs incurred in complying with different regulatory regimes are ultimately borne by consumers. To some extent, consumers are willing to pay for qualitative features and more environmentally friendly products, but they would pay less if production inefficiencies resulting from the absence of regulatory harmonisation are minimised. Consumers also need to be protected from voluntary labelling schemes that do not confer real and verifiable qualitative or ecological advantages.

In the post-ATC period, some countries are concerned that constraining standards-related regulations may be developed as a way to shield domestic production from foreign competition. Eco-labelling schemes and standards-related regulations may be captured by domestic vested interests, *e.g.* retailers and producers, to promote their products, thereby adding to the regulatory heterogeneity and making trade more difficult. The validity of these concerns should be weighed against the multilateral and regional frameworks put in place to help avoid unnecessary obstacles to trade in the preparation, adoption and application of standards-related systems.

The process of preparation, adoption and application of standards-related systems in textiles and clothing are covered by the WTO Agreement on Technical Barriers to Trade (TBT). This Agreement provides for the application of WTO principles, such as transparency and national treatment, and it encourages the use of internationally recognised standards and systems. The WTO Committee on Technical Barriers to Trade oversees its application and regularly prepares a review of the operation and implementation of the Agreement. The third triennial review was completed in November 2003 and highlighted a number of generic trade concerns (not necessarily related to textiles and clothing) concerning the lack of transparency in certain labelling requirements involving procedural problems, *e.g.* failures to notify, short periods for comments and inadequate handling of comments (WTO, 2003, paragraph 19). With regard to the Code of Good Practice for the Preparation, Adoption and Application of Standards (the Code), the Committee also noted that, in some cases concerning voluntary labelling requirements, the related standards were developed by bodies that are not commonly considered as standards bodies and have not accepted the Code (WTO, 2003, paragraph 25). These comments underscore the continuing trade sensitivity of WTO members to standards in respect of voluntary labelling requirements.

Concurrently, harmonisation and/or mutual recognition provisions are pursued within the framework of regional groupings, such as the European Union, the North American

Free Trade Agreement (NAFTA) and the Asia-Pacific Economic Cooperation (APEC) Forum. They also contribute to the process of minimising regulatory heterogeneity and the incidence of standards-related trade conflicts in their respective region.

Hence, heterogeneity of standards in textile and clothing products may contribute to regulatory inefficiencies and trade restrictiveness, while standards adopted in a manner consistent with international obligations may reduce such inefficiencies and restrictions. The issue for policy makers is to promote the widest possible participation of stakeholders in the preparation, adoption and application of standards-related regulations, to ensure the transparency of the whole process and to promote various internationally recognised standards and systems. In the segmented clothing markets in which private labelling schemes are promoted to confer qualitative or ecological advantages, policy makers should be vigilant to ensure that such standards are developed in conformity with the WTO Code and that consumers are protected from unverifiable labelling claims.

The importance of involving developing countries in the preparation of standards was highlighted in the UNCTAD (1996) report dealing with eco–labelling requirements in textiles and clothing. With a growing world share of textile and clothing production taking place in developing countries,[17] co-operation is necessary between standards-setting bodies in developed and developing countries. Technical assistance to developing countries can help to improve awareness of the WTO TBT Agreement in these countries and to build their technical capacity.

SME–related dimensions

In recognition of the economic role of SMEs, most governments implement a range of programmes aimed at alleviating the difficulties experienced by SMEs in diverse areas – financing, technology and innovation, e-commerce, management and export promotion – and seek to identify and implement best practices. In SME-related policies, the OECD has a broad mandate to contribute to the implementation of the Bologna Charter on SME Policies (adopted in June 2000) by further deepening analysis of some of the main issues included in the Charter, *e.g.* globalisation, innovation, clusters and partnerships, e-business, partnerships for development, entrepreneurship, etc. In the framework of the Bologna Process, a second OECD Ministerial Conference on SMEs took place in Istanbul on 4-5 June 2004 under the theme "Promoting Entrepreneurship and Innovative SMEs in a Global Economy".[18] The SME policy agenda is broad and horizontal in nature and applicable across sectors, including the textile and clothing industries. While there are many SME-related dimensions that have a bearing on textiles and clothing, the present discussion focuses on entrepreneurship, which is important for the textile and clothing industries given the predominance of SMEs (Table 5.9).

The commercial viability (failure) of SMEs in the textile and clothing industries depends to a large extent on the entrepreneurial skills of thousands of individuals who strive daily in a highly competitive environment. Particularly in the clothing industry, competition may come closest to the perfect competition of economic theory and most firms have no or little influence on selling prices. A vibrant entrepreneurship culture supported by a dynamic entrepreneurial business environment is thus increasingly considered a crucial factor for economic growth and international competitiveness in a global economy.

Relative to other industrial processes, barriers to entry (and exit) in the clothing industry are low; as a result, the industry is characterised by a large number of producers, typically with a very large number of SMEs that concentrate production on just a few product categories. The industry also includes multidivision enterprises producing a wide range of often high-volume products. Table 5.9 shows that 80% of clothing establishments in the United States and 95% in the European Union employ fewer than 49 employees. Nevertheless, establishments employing more than 250 employees account for 37.5% of total clothing employment in the United States and 19.2% in the European Union. In the textile industry, although industrial processes are more capital-intensive than in the clothing industry, the shares of establishments by employment size broadly replicate the composition of the clothing industry.

While it is commonly agreed that entrepreneurship is a driving force behind SMEs, there is no universally accepted definition of entrepreneurship. It appears that entrepreneurs have some common characteristics, whether they are prompted to become entrepreneurs out of necessity (to escape unemployment) or as a result of an observed opportunity. In the fashion-oriented clothing markets, entrepreneurs must combine many skills: creativity, management and commercial flair. In the growing specialised textile applications, entrepreneurs also need science-based knowledge to succeed.

Although it is important to nurture SME-related entrepreneurship, it is important to avoid the danger of granting excessive fiscal advantages and labour law exemptions that may ultimately discourage entrepreneurs from investing in optimal production scale plants and may create strong vested interests that oppose reform. In India, the textile and clothing industries are based on a system of decentralised production, referred to as "reservation of garment manufacture for small-scale industry (SSI)", which provides a series of economic advantages to small-scale, labour-intensive firms. These domestic measures have fragmented the Indian textile and clothing industries which have neither attained optimal economies of scale, nor produced quality clothing products (Verma, 2002). Similarly, Kathuria and Bhardwaj (1998) have argued that India faces formidable domestic hurdles to meet international standards and competition due to the government SSI policy and other inefficiencies in domestic infrastructure. ITC (2004) also argues that India's SSI policy has prevented Indian firms from achieving economies of scale and investing in new state-of-the art technology.

To cultivate an entrepreneurial culture and to foster entrepreneurship values and spirit with a view to building an entrepreneurial society, most governments have set up SME–related entrepreneurship agendas to facilitate the emergence of a larger pool of entrepreneurs. Education and training have been recognised in this context as the single most effective means of achieving this objective (OECD, 2003d). Education and training for entrepreneurship can have two types of effects. First, they can have considerable impact on the performance of entrepreneurs, especially in helping them increase their firm's chances of survival, and to a lesser extent, in helping make the business more profitable. Second, although extremely difficult to measure, education in entrepreneurship is also supposed to have long-term impacts on the level of entrepreneurial spirit and attitudes which are fundamental for an entrepreneurial population and society.

Table 5.9. Establishments by employment size in the United States and the European Union

	Textiles			Clothing		
	No. of	Share of total		No. of	Share of total	
	establishments	Establishments	Employment	establishments	Establishments	Employment
United States (1997) (Employees)						
1-9	6 917	54.9%		7 896	46.5%	
10-49	3 235	25.7%		5 933	34.9%	
50-249	1 812	14.4%		2 618	15.4%	
250-2 499	629	5.0%	49.7%	542	3.2%	36.3%
2 500 or more	3	0.024%		3	0.018%	1.2%
Total	12 593		627 340	16 989		710 796
European Union (2000) (Employees)						
1-9	48 262	66.5%	13.3%	84 738	78.7%	20.9%
10-49	15 079	20.8%	26.7%	18 765	17.4%	35.4%
50-249	6 103	8.4%	33.1%	2 942	2.7%	24.2%
250 or more	3 082	4.2%	26.9%	1 162	1.1%	19.2%
Total	72 575		1 044 756	107 663		1 022 304

Note: Due to rounding, the percentages do not necessarily sum to 100%.

Source: US data: US Bureau of the Census, 1997 Economic Census, June 2001; and EU data: Eurostat, Euratex calculations.

The benefits of education and training in entrepreneurship are widely recognised, and practically all OECD countries have launched initiatives in this respect. An OECD report (2003d) has compared various national experiences with entrepreneurial education and stressed three means of improving the effectiveness of national programmes: *i)* use hands-on teaching methods in schools to introduce children to entrepreneurship; *ii)* teach personal characteristics of entrepreneurs in schools; and *iii)* focus on integrating entrepreneurship at the university level.

Conclusion

In the post-ATC period, there will be neither quantitative restrictions nor MFA–related guaranteed market access to mask the vulnerable situation of national textile and clothing suppliers whose international competitiveness is hampered by inefficient domestic regulatory regimes, obsolete infrastructure in essential business services, cumbersome customs procedures and other distorted market structures. All these dimensions are influenced by the policy and regulatory framework implemented by governments. From a trade policy perspective, efficiency in transport, telecommunications and electricity infrastructure and in customs services is an important determinant of a country's ability to integrate fully the world economy.

The prime responsibility for adjustment in the textile and clothing industries falls on the firms themselves, which are best placed to evaluate how to organise production methods, procure high-quality fabrics, and invest and shift the product mix on the basis of evolving market signals. The role of governments is to support the entire economy, by ensuring that the domestic policy and regulatory framework supports private initiatives and does not impose unnecessary costs on them. Achieving greater policy synergy among distinct policy and regulatory areas that affect the competitive position of national firms is in essence the purpose of a business facilitation agenda.

Above all, the role of government is to pursue a sound and dynamic macroeconomic environment that aims at sustaining non-inflationary economic growth. There is strong evidence that real economic growth and, in turn, net employment creation are stimulated in a low-inflationary environment. Sound macroeconomic policies facilitate market adjustment to change in the competitive environment and facilitate the redeployment of affected resources to other productive sectors without the need to revert to costly trade protection measures. The pursuit of a business facilitation agenda complements other government actions at the macroeconomic and microeconomic levels, *i.e.* in the areas of trade, labour adjustment and innovation, and offers benefits that go well beyond the textile and clothing industries.

This chapter stresses the importance of efficient port infrastructure, reliable and competitive modes of transport and efficient customs procedures for maintaining a competitive edge in the highly competitive, time-sensitive and fashion-oriented textile and clothing markets. The reliability of transport infrastructure and efficiency in customs procedures complement each other to minimise transit periods for shipments involved in international trade and can make geographically remote locations more internationally competitive. The corollary is that long transit periods can essentially eliminate from international competition offshore centres that are geographically remote or that are nearby but have poor infrastructure. Even if long transit periods can be mitigated to some extent by preferential market access arrangements, outward processing programmes requiring two-way shipments offer no net cost advantage for geographically remote suppliers.

Given that every country has a certain geographical position relative to large consumer regions and different transport options, countries should assess the logistical costs involved in export markets with a view to: *i)* setting up an efficiency-enhancing environment in port infrastructure; *ii)* strengthening competition conditions in and between transport modes; *iii)* setting up a competition-enhancing environment in various port services; *iv)* addressing the terrorist risks in transport without losing sight of the beneficial effects of frictionless systems; and *v)* better integrating the enforcement of national laws and regulations, *e.g.* customs procedures, taxation, sanitary and environment protection, with other service providers in ports.

In matters concerning the facilitation of international trade, textile and clothing traders in formerly constrained exporting and importing countries are poised to benefit from streamlined border requirements with the dismantling of MFA export permits and related controls. However, the internationally fragmented supply chain remains vulnerable to cumbersome and outdated customs procedures in countries that are less advanced in the implementation of modern customs systems. When shipments are held up in customs warehouses owing to inefficiencies in customs procedures, export-led strategies are undermined, especially in countries that rely on imported inputs for a significant share of their production.

In the aftermath of the 11 September 2001 World Trade Center attacks, added emphasis has been placed on security and safety measures, and many exporting countries are concerned about the compliance costs resulting from the enforcement of these measures. While a trade-off between security and efficiency in crossing borders is unavoidable in the short term, governments should not lose sight of the beneficial effects of smoothly functioning transport and customs clearance systems. Cost pressures on traders can be minimised by furthering co-operation among stakeholders. Ultimately, these developments can lead to faster interaction between traders and customs authorities.

There are considerable disparities among countries in terms of the number of tariff lines defined for classifying textile and clothing products as well as considerable differences in the tariff protection afforded. Simplicity in tariff definitions combined with a simplified tariff rate structure represents a cost-effective approach to protect government revenues and to address fraudulency and integrity concerns. In the context of the Doha Round of multilateral trade negotiations, WTO members have an opportunity to work towards greater tariff simplification and to reduce tariff rates.

Reliable and modern telecommunications and electricity infrastructure is an important determinant of competitive textile and clothing suppliers. Trade flows in differentiated products, such as textiles and clothing, are sensitive to international variations in communication costs. Moreover, entrepreneurs in Hong Kong (China) consider the quality of telecommunications infrastructure one of the most important factors in deciding on investment projects. An outdated regulatory framework in electricity and telecommunications services acts as a tax on textile and clothing firms and, more importantly, it undermines the capacity of national suppliers to focus production on the higher value-added segments of the supply chain that are critically dependent on reliable infrastructure to ensure quick market response. In the post-ATC period, the international competitiveness of textile and clothing suppliers will be enhanced in countries that maintain an environment that encourages investment in innovative telecommunication equipment, electricity generation and distribution systems.

Some countries are concerned that constraining standards-related regulations and eco-labelling schemes may be developed as a way to shield domestic production or used by domestic vested interests to promote their products, thereby adding to regulatory heterogeneity and making trade more difficult. Differentiated standards in textile and clothing products may contribute to regulatory inefficiencies or trade restrictiveness. Standards that are consistent with international obligations may reduce such inefficiencies and restrictions. Policy makers should promote the widest possible participation of stakeholders in the preparation, adoption and application of standards-related regulations, in order to ensure the transparency of the process and to promote internationally recognised standards and systems. Moreover, efforts could be made to further develop co-operation between standards-setting bodies in developed and developing countries.

In recognition of the economic role of SMEs, most governments apply a range of programmes aimed at alleviating the difficulties that SMEs experience in various areas, *e.g.* financing, technology and innovation, e-commerce, management and export promotion, and seek to identify and implement best practice policies. While it is important to nurture SME-related entrepreneurship, it is equally important to avoid the danger of distorting incentives to invest in sub-optimal productive capacity by offering excessive fiscal advantages and labour law exemptions to small-scale operations. Recent work by the OECD in the context of the Bologna Charter on SME Policies has found that education and training are recognised as the single most effective means for achieving the objective of fostering entrepreneurship in societies and that this policy focus should continue.

Annex 5.A1. Table

Annex Table 5.A1.1. Freight costs by mode of transport for textile and clothing imports in the United States, 2003

	Air	Rail	Seaborne	Lorry	Total
North and Central Americas (NCAs)					
Mexico	7.0%	0.6%	2.0%	2.8%	0.9%
Canada	5.5%	0.9%	3.3%	6.0%	1.1%
Honduras	13.8%	1.1%	1.9%	7.8%	2.1%
Costa Rica	-	0.2%	2.0%	5.3%	2.2%
El Salvador	4.3%	1.9%	2.0%	6.4%	2.3%
Guatemala	7.0%	11.8%	2.4%	8.8%	3.0%
Nicaragua	10.4%	3.0%	2.7%	5.9%	3.0%
Total for NCAs	**6.9%**	**0.7%**	**2.1%**	**4.7%**	**1.5%**
Other countries					
Dominican Republic	3.7%		1.7%		1.9%
Colombia	5.6%		1.7%		3.2%
Peru	5.5%		2.4%		3.8%
Italy	4.5%		3.1%		4.1%
Israel	7.8%		3.5%		4.1%
Japan	16.9%		3.0%		4.2%
United Kingdom	5.9%		3.3%		4.6%
Hong Kong, China	8.7%		3.1%		4.8%
France	5.9%		3.4%		4.9%
Jordan	9.3%		3.8%		5.1%
Macau (China)	11.6%		3.5%		5.3%
Malaysia	21.2%		4.0%		5.6%
Philippines	9.7%		4.2%		5.6%
Cambodia	41.0%		4.3%		5.8%
Turkey	14.1%		4.4%		5.8%
Egypt	16.6%		4.3%		5.8%
Thailand	9.8%		4.7%		6.1%
Chinese Taipei	12.8%		4.6%		6.2%
Indonesia	16.3%		4.5%		6.2%
Sri Lanka (Ceylon)	13.4%		4.4%		6.3%
Russia	9.0%		5.7%		6.6%
Korea	11.0%		4.8%		6.7%
Bangladesh	14.1%		5.6%		6.8%
China	14.5%		5.8%		6.9%
Brazil	13.9%		5.1%		7.1%
South Africa	13.9%		5.0%		7.2%
Vietnam	10.6%		5.0%		7.3%
India	14.4%		5.0%		7.3%
Pakistan	24.8%		6.4%		8.0%
Rest of the world	9.3%		4.3%		5.7%
Total non–NCAs	**11.1%**		**4.5%**		**5.9%**

1. The mode of transport is the one by which the imported merchandise entered the US port of arrival from the last foreign country.

Source: OECD calculation based on data from the US Department of Commerce, Bureau of the Census.

Notes

1. The WTO Agreement on Textiles and Clothing (ATC) superseded the Multi-Fibre Arrangement (MFA) regime of quantitative trade restrictions when it entered into force in January 1995 and provided the multilateral trade framework applicable for trade in textiles and clothing for all WTO members. The ATC provides for the elimination by 31 December 2004 of all forms of quantitative restrictions applied to trade in textile and clothing products, including those that originated under the MFA regime. The ATC phases itself out of existence at the end of 2004. For the purpose of qualifying the period when there will be no more quantitative restrictions applied to trade in textile and clothing products, the term "the post-ATC period" is used throughout this publication.

2. Trade facilitation is defined in WTO reference materials as the "simplification and harmonisation of international trade procedures, with trade procedures being the activities, practices and formalities involved in collecting, presenting, communicating and processing data required for the movement of goods in international trade".

3. See Batra *et al.* (2002); SWEPRO (2002); Wilson, Mann and Otsuki (2003); Wilson *et al.* (2002); and Woo *et al.* (2000).

4. They estimated that the elasticity of trade with respect to port logistics is 5.2, implying that an increase of 1% in the average APEC indicator of port logistics would increase intra-APEC trade in manufactured goods by 5.2%. In a similar quantitative study for APEC trade, Wilson, Mann and Otsuki (2003) estimated that the trade benefits of specific facilitation efforts would be USD 254 billion for intra-APEC trade, equivalent to an increase in APEC average per capita GDP of 4.3%.

5. The general rule of thumb for total delivery costs involving seaborne movements, *e.g.* from the seller's door to the buyer's door, is that the maritime leg usually accounts for between one-third and one-half of total delivery costs.

6. UNCTAD (2002a) reports that imports from African landlocked countries suffer from high freight costs that ranged between 16.2% and 27.6% of the value of the goods imported in 2000. Moreover, it argues that the situation of landlocked African countries "reflects inefficient transport organisation and facilities; poor utilisation of assets; weak managerial, procedural, regulatory and institutional systems; apart from overall inadequate infrastructure conditions".

7. AGOA's LDCs are temporarily entitled to use non-US fabrics and still enjoy duty-free access, but this special provision expires at the end of September 2004.

8. While achieving more competitive conditions in air shipping should remain a policy objective for trading countries, the relative importance of maritime and rail shipping modes for trade in textile and clothing products explains the focus on maritime and rail shipping conditions in the following discussion.

9.   For comprehensive reviews of policy reforms in the seaport industry, see Trujillo and Nombela (1999), Trujillo and Estache (2001), Hoffman (1998), Juhel (1997) and UNCTAD (2002b).

10.   This is important given the fact that, over the years, port activities have become more capital-intensive, requiring significant investment to accommodate larger and more specialised ships.

11.   Generally, port authorities do not publicly release information on ship turnaround time for fear of losing business to competitors. Another performance indicator to evaluate the efficiency of ports is the container handling charge per TEU (20 foot equivalent unit), which typically represents between 70% and 90% of total port charges. Under normal business circumstances, port authorities pass on to users their operating and infrastructure improvement costs and the container handling charge ultimately reflects these costs. The container handling charge per TEU is another indicator for comparing and benchmarking ports, but it is recognised that local conditions may vary considerably.

12.   Three Directives were adopted requiring implementation by 15 March 2003. Directive 2001/12/EC requires the legal separation (not just accounting separation) between infrastructure managers and railway undertakings. Under Directive 2001/14/EC, infrastructure managers are required to provide a number of mandatory access services on a non-discriminatory basis. Finally, Directive 2001/14 provides for the creation of an organisation to co-ordinate the international allocation of capacity on different networks, in order to allow for the creation of international train paths.

13.   The eight countries reviewed are: the United States, the United Kingdom, Argentina, Sweden, Brazil, Chile, New Zealand and Japan.

14.   For example, the United States and Canada signed the "Smart Border" initiative to facilitate trade through improved co-ordination and information sharing in December 2001, and a similar initiative between the United States and Mexico was unveiled in March 2002. More recently, the United States launched the Customs-Trade Partnership against Terrorism (C-TPAT), which aims at increasing the integrity and security of the supply chain by offering expedited clearance to carriers and importers enrolled in this programme. In Canada, the programme "Partners in Protection" has similar objectives. In the European Union, the Commission has recently proposed a series of measures to address security issues, including amendments to the "Community Customs Code" to harmonise risk assessment systems and to launch a "Container Security Initiative" that provides for enhanced co-operation in transport security.

15.   With an estimated elasticity of trade flows with respect to transaction costs at about -2 (Limão and Venables, 2001), this means that an increase of 1% in the cost of trading internationally would lead to a drop in trade flows of 2%.

16.   Their estimated elasticity of trade flows to bilateral calling price is: -0.764 for textile fibres (SITC 2 code 26); -1.112 for clothing (SITC 2 code 84); and -1.15 for textile yarns, fabrics and made-up articles.

17.   Between 1985 and 2001, the developing countries' share of world textile production increased from 23% to 33%. During the same period, their share of world clothing, leather and footwear increased from 22.7% to 27.8% (see Chapter 2).

18.   The following issues were addressed during the Conference: *i)* fostering entrepreneurship, including women's entrepreneurship; *ii)* fostering SMEs' access to innovation and technology through access to financing and through clusters, networks and partnerships; *iii)* financing innovation SMEs in a global economy; *iv)* clusters, networks and partnerships: opportunities and challenges for innovative SMEs in a Global economy; *v)* promoting ICT use and e-business adoption by SMEs; *vi)* alternative dispute resolution mechanisms online for SMEs; *vii)* promoting SMEs for development; *viii)* cross-cutting themes; *ix)* SME statistics; and *x)* evaluation of SME policies and programmes.

References

Andrea, D. and B. Smith (2002), "The Canada-US Border: an Automotive Case Study", Center for Automation Research, Altarum Institute, Ann Arbor, Michigan, January.

AAR (Association of American Railroads) (2004), "Why the Rail Reregulation Debate is Important", Position Paper, Washington, DC, January.

Batra, G., D. Kaufmann and A.H.W. Stone (2002), *Voices of the Firms 2000: Investment Climate and Governance Findings of the World Business Environment Survey (WBES)*, The World Bank Group, Washington, DC.

Campos J. and P. Cantos (1999), "Regulating Privatised Rail Transport", Working Paper 2064, The World Bank Group, Washington DC, February.

Draper, C. (2001), "Reforming Customs Administration: The Unlikely Case of Bangladesh?", The World Bank, Washington, DC.

Fink C., A. Mattoo and I.C. Neagu (2002), "Assessing the Impacts of Communication Costs on International Trade", World Bank Policy Research Working Paper 2929, November.

Hoffman, J. (1998), "What are the Obstacles, Advantages, and Disadvantages of Port Privatisations? It all Depends!", mimeo, Economic Commission for Latin America and the Caribbean, United Nations, Santiago de Chile.

Hummels, D. (2000), "Time as a Trade Barrier", Purdue University.

Integrated Framework (2001), "Madagascar – Increasing Integration into World markets as a Poverty Reduction Strategy", November, www.integratedframework.org/countries/madagascar.htm.

IEA (International Energy Agency) (2003), *Energy Prices and Taxes, Quarterly Statistics*, Second Quarter 2003, IEA, Paris.

ITC (International Trade Commission) (2004), *Textiles and Apparels: Assessments of the Competitiveness of Certain Foreign Suppliers to the U.S. Market*, Investigation No. 332-448, Washington, DC, February.

Juhel, M. (1997), "Government Regulation of Port Activities: What Balance Between Public and Private Sectors?", International Course on Privatisation and Regulation of Transport Services, The World Bank, Washington, DC.

Kathuria, S. and A. Bhardwaj (1998), "Export Quotas and Policy Constraints in the Indian Textile and Garment Industries", Policy Research Working Paper, No. WPS 2012, The World Bank, New Delhi Office.

Limão, N. and A.J. Venables (2001), "Infrastructure, Geographical Disadvantage, Transport Costs and Trade, *The World Bank Economic Review*, Vol. 15, No. 3, p. 451–479, Washington, DC.

Mann, C.L., S. Eckert and S.C. Knight (2000), *Global Electronic Commerce: A Policy Primer*, Institute for International Economics, Washington, DC.

OECD (1997), "Freight and the Environment: Effects of Trade Liberalisation and Transport Sector Reforms", OCDE/DG(97)213.

OECD (2002a), "Competition Policy in Liner Shipping", DSTI/DOT(2002)2.

OECD (2002b), *Regional Trade Agreements and the Multilateral Trading System*, OECD, Paris.

OECD (2003a), "Security in Maritime Transports: Risk Factors and Economic Impact", DSTI/DOT/MTC(2003)47/FINAL.

OECD (2003b), "Trade Facilitation Reforms in the Service of Development", TD/TC/WP(2003)11/FINAL.

OECD (2003c), *Communications Outlook 2003*, OECD, Paris.

OECD (2003d), "The Bologna Process, The 2nd Session OECD Conference of Ministers Responsible for SMEs, Theme 1: Fostering Entrepreneurship and Firm Creation as a Driver of Growth in a Global Economy", OECD internal working document.

Radelet, S. and J. Sachs (1998), Shipping Costs, Manufactured Exports and Economic Growth, Mimeo, Harvard Institute for International Development, Cambridge.

Spinanger, D. (2001), "Beyond Eternity: What Will happen When the ATC Gives Way to MFN Principles Beyond 2004?", paper presented at the EU-LDC Conference on Trade and Poverty Reduction, Rotterdam, May.

SWEPRO (2002), "Trade Facilitation – Impact and Potential Gains, Swedish Trade Procedures Council", Stockholm.

Trujillo, L. and A. Estache (2001), "Surfing a Wave of Fine Tuning Reform in Argentina's Ports", The World Bank, Washington, DC.

Trujillo, L. and G. Nombela (1999), "Privatisation and Regulation of the Seaport Industry", Policy Research Working Paper, No. 2181, The World Bank, Washington, DC.

UNCTAD (1996), *Eco-labelling and Other Environmental Quality Requirements in Textiles and Clothing: Implications for Developing Countries*, United Nations, New York and Geneva.

UNCTAD (2002a), *Review of Maritime Transport 2002*, United Nations, New York and Geneva.

UNCTAD (2002b), *Global Economic Prospects 2002, Part 4: Transport Services: Reducing Barriers to Trade*, United Nations, New York and Geneva.

USAID (United States Agency for International Development) (2003), "Economic and Employment Impacts on the Dominican Republic of Changing Global Trade Rules for Textiles and Apparel", prepared by Nathan Associates Inc., Washington, DC, June.

Verma, S. (2002), "Export Competitiveness of Indian Textile and Garment Industry", Indian Council for Research on International Economic Relations, Working Paper No. 94, New Delhi.

Wilson, J., C.L. Mann, Y.P. Woo, N. Assanie and I. Choi (2002), *Trade Facilitation: A Development Perspective in the Asia-Pacific Region*, Asia-Pacific Economic Cooperation, Singapore.

Wilson, J., S. Bagai and C. Fink (2003), "Reducing Trading Costs in a New Area of Security", Part 5 in *Global Economic Prospects 2004 – Realizing the Development Promise of the Doha Agenda*, World Bank, Washington, DC.

Wilson, J., C.L. Mann and T. Otsuki, (2003), "Trade Facilitation and Economic Development: Measuring the Impact", World Bank Policy Research Working Paper 2988, Washington, DC.

Woo, Y., J. Wilson and the World Bank (2000), *Cutting through the Red Tape: New Directions for APEC's Trade Facilitation Agenda*, Asia-Pacific Economic Cooperation, Singapore.

World Bank (2003), *Global Economic Prospects 2002, Part 4: Transport Services: Reducing Barriers to Trade*, Washington, DC.

WTO (World Trade Organisation) (2002), *International Trade Statistics 2002*, Geneva.

WTO (2003), "Report of the Committee on Technical Barriers to Trade", Geneva, G/L/657, November.

Annex A

Literature Review of Quantitative Studies

Introduction

A considerable body of analysis by a number of analysts at national and international institutions aims at quantifying the economic and trade effects of the liberalisation of the textile and clothing markets. Different tools and approaches have been used to evaluate the impact of textile trade reforms at the regional or global level. Given the economic importance of the textile and clothing industries in some developed and developing countries and the economy–wide repercussions that changes in the scale and pattern of textile production tend to trigger, most studies have used general equilibrium models, but some have adopted partial equilibrium approaches. Most of this research was published during the 1990s, and this annex summarises and compares the findings of pertinent quantitative studies. References to earlier analyses of the effects of liberalising textile and clothing trade can be found, for example, in Pelzman (1983), Goto (1989) and Spinanger (1991).

The annex is organised under four headings. The first provides background information by discussing some of the major economic effects to be expected from the WTO Agreement on Textiles and Clothing (ATC) reforms, as well as the implications of different modelling approaches and assumptions. It aims to help the reader understand the factors that drive the modelling results. There follows a review of quantitative studies of ATC reforms at the global level. Next, relevant studies with a country or regional focus are discussed. A brief conclusion summarises the main findings.

Quantitative aspects of trade liberalisation in the textile and clothing industries

Under the Multi-Fibre Arrangement (MFA), developed and developing countries negotiated bilateral quotas regulating trade in textiles and clothing.[1] In order to implement these quantitative restrictions, it was agreed that exporting developing countries would voluntarily restrain supplies. Export rights became scarce and turned into valuable assets, generating rents for internationally competitive suppliers. Governments generally distributed the quotas free of charge to domestic firms based on criteria such as past export performance (Hamilton, 1990). In most countries, quotas were not tradable. Such allocation schemes favouring *status quo* exporters, as well as requirements that related annual quota renewal to export performance in unrestricted markets, for example, generated substantial efficiency losses in developing countries over time (Trela and Whalley, 1995). In some cases, developing country exporters had to share part of their quota rents with importing firms that were able to exercise market power at the individual product level (Krishna *et al.*, 1994). Yet, most of the rents generated under the MFA accrued to developing country exporters. Table A1 shows estimates of quota rents for a number of countries, as reported by Harrison *et al.* (1997).

Table A.1. Estimates of MFA quota rents and price premiums for textiles and clothing, 1994

	Textiles				Clothing			
	Value of quota rents (USD millions)	Share of exports constrained (%)	Quota premium (%)		Value of quota rents (USD millions)	Share of exports constrained (%)	Quota premium (%)	
			EU	USA			EU	USA
Korea	119	16	10	10	555	55	19	23
Indonesia	97	24	17	12	512	52	48	47
Malaysia	65	100	12	10	330	100	32	37
Philippines	7	50	10	9	363	81	28	34
Singapore	7	11	10	8	365	100	28	31
Thailand	53	40	13	9	396	42	36	35
China	378	19	27	18	2 223	31	36	40
Hong Kong, China	48	13	8	8	1 249	100	16	18
Chinese Taipei	95	13	12	8	515	81	22	19
Brazil	65	100	14	9	43	77	18	20
Mexico	41	60	14	9	181	99	18	20
Latin America	46	45	14	9	619	86	18	20
Middle East and North Africa	84	78	7	5	390	97	9	10
Eastern Europe and FSU	87	78	9	6	430	97	12	13
South Asia	566	46	27	18	1 375	85	36	40

FSU = Former Soviet Union

Source: Harrison *et al.* (1997).

The system of bilateral quotas has frequently been accompanied by high tariffs applied on imports of textiles and clothing. Countries engaged in tariff reduction commitments during the Uruguay Round, but tariffs on textiles and clothing frequently remain significant even after the cuts, and, as illustrated in Table A.2 for the European Union, are on average considerably higher than in the manufacturing sector overall. Also, textile and clothing tariffs appear to be consistently high across a large number of products and show lower than average variation. Moreover, high tariffs on textile and clothing exports are not confined to OECD countries. Large developing country exporters in the Association of South East Asian Nations (ASEAN), and South Asia have tariffs ranging from 20% to 33% on textiles and 30% to 35% on clothing, which impede the increasingly important trade among developing countries (Lankes, 2002).

Table A.2. Structure of EU pre- and post-Uruguay Round tariffs in the textile and clothing industries

Pre-Uruguay Round (1994)				Tariff rate distribution (%)										
	HS lines	Mean	CoV[1]	0-2	2-4	4-6	6-8	8-10	10-12	12-14	14-16	16-18	18-20	20-22
Textiles	3943	10.1	0.26	0.8	0.3	2.7	11.2	6.6	64.9	6.1	4.6	2.8	0.0	0.0
Clothing	447	12.3	0.26	0.4	1.1	5.6	4.7	5.4	2.7	13.6	66.4	0.0	0.0	0.0
All manuf.	17760	6.5	0.53	6.8	5.2	29.7	22.3	11.3	17.0	3.6	3.2	0.7	0.0	0.2

Post-Uruguay Round (2004)				Tariff rate distribution (%)										
	HS lines	Mean	CoV[1]	0-2	2-4	4-6	6-8	8-10	10-12	12-14	14-16	16-18	18-20	20-22
Textiles	3941	7.3	0.25	0.9	0.4	16.2	2.5	68.0	8.1	2.7	0.5	0.8	0.0	0.0
Clothing	447	10.6	0.29	2.0	6.3	1.1	3.1	5.6	1.8	72.7	7.4	0.0	0.0	0.0
All manuf.	17324	4.0	0.96	14.6	27.4	24.6	11.4	17.7	2.8	3.1	0.6	0.4	0.0	0.0

1. CoV = coefficient of variation.

Source: Spinanger (1999b).

The complexity of the quota system, the interaction between quotas and tariffs, and the simultaneous Uruguay Round changes in other sectors of the economy make the evaluation of ATC reforms difficult. Empirical analysis is necessary to quantify the relative magnitude of different impacts. Some of the welfare effects from tariff reduction and quota phase-out that need to be considered are:

- The removal of quantitative restrictions eliminates the basis for quota rents. The latter are passed from exporters to consumers in previously import-constrained markets in the form of lower prices. There are also efficiency gains from specialisation according to comparative advantage, which, for the United States, the European Union and other quota-constrained countries, is likely to imply increasing domestic consumption and reducing production. As the MFA arrangements were motivated by potential adjustment problems within developed importing countries caused by surges of lower-cost imports, the shift of labour and capital resources out of the textile and clothing industries is likely to entail sizeable adjustment costs. Hence, developed importing countries face advantages and disadvantages from ATC reforms.

- Importers of textiles and clothing that were previously unconstrained, such as Japan, could well experience reductions in welfare from the removal of textile quotas. Exporters will tend to divert sales to previously constrained markets, possibly resulting in import price increases and a terms-of-trade deterioration in previously unconstrained importing countries.

- The lowering of tariffs applied to textile and clothing imports will affect the amount of tariff revenues collected by governments. If the demand for imports is very price elastic, such that a reduction in tariffs (to non-zero levels) triggers a large increase in imports, tariff revenue might increase. Otherwise it will decrease.

- For quota-constrained exporting countries, the welfare effects are mixed (Yang et al., 1997). On the one hand, there is the loss of quota rent in export markets that were previously constrained. On the other hand, exporters might gain in efficiency by shifting resources into textiles and clothing, assuming they have an ex post comparative advantage in these industries, which in many cases will be based on their low labour costs (Figure A.1). In addition, there is the potential improvement in terms of trade on sales of textile and clothing products to previously unconstrained markets, such as Japan. The size of the terms-of-trade effects will depend largely on the share of sales to previously constrained versus unconstrained markets.

- ATC reforms will also influence the country composition of exports, most likely in the direction of a concentration of suppliers. Whenever textile and clothing quotas became binding in one country under the MFA, investment was directed to initially unconstrained exporting countries, which later also became constrained, so that investment then flowed elsewhere. Removal of discriminatory restraints will tend to lead to a reversion to more country-concentrated patterns of exports, with many higher-cost developing countries, where the production of textiles and clothing might have been the first stage in the industrialisation process, possibly losing out (Whalley, 1999).

Figure A.1. Hourly labour costs in the primary textile industry, 1993 (in USD)

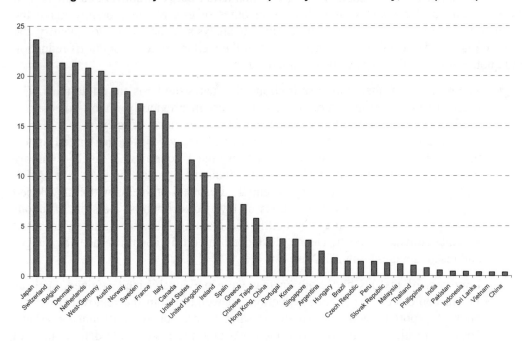

Source: Werner International, reproduced from Brugnoli and Resmini (1996).

One major challenge for applied economic modelling of textile and clothing liberalisation is to represent existing quantitative restrictions appropriately. The restrictiveness of the applied MFA quotas varies from product to product and from supplier to supplier, and aggregate measures have to be interpreted with care. Some researchers have modelled the phase-out of quotas as an increase in exporting efficiency in order to capture the effect of removing the constraint on exports (Diao and Somwaru, 2001), while most liken the effects of the MFA quotas to price wedges and use estimates of export tax equivalents, such as those derived by Francois and Spinanger (2000) and generalised in the GTAP database, in their simulations.

There are a number of other differences among the available empirical studies. Analysts emphasise different economic relationships in the textile and clothing industries and choose their methods and simplifying assumptions accordingly. It is not surprising that different modelling approaches and sets of behavioural and structural hypotheses generate differing results. The following list describes some major aspects of frequently encountered analytical approaches to ATC reforms and provides the background for the subsequent discussion of individual studies.

- *General equilibrium versus partial equilibrium analysis*: Computable general equilibrium (CGE) models make it possible to consider changes simultaneously, in different parts of the economy, linkages between sectors and economy-wide resource constraints at the national and international level (Francois and Reinert, 1998). However, these tools rely on a number of simplifying assumptions, such as full employment of resources, and depend on a large amount of empirical information. If the sector to be analysed is small and not closely linked to other parts of the economy, partial equilibrium analysis focusing on the sector under consideration will tend to yield similar results, while being less data-intensive. However, most ATC reform studies employ CGE models.

- Base year: The base year influences the modelling results in several ways. Prices and quantities change over time, so that models that are calibrated on data for different time periods are not fully comparable. Also, knowledge about policy parameters evolves. For example, available estimates of the export tax equivalents of MFA quota restrictions have undergone major revisions during the 1990s. Moreover, when comparing absolute welfare effects across studies that use different base periods, the effects of inflation should be taken into account.

- Level of aggregation: The sectoral and regional aggregation of a model varies with the study's objective and data availability. Some aggregation seems inevitable, because it is virtually impossible to model the hundreds of product lines that are involved in product-specific MFA quotas. A relatively high level of aggregation has the advantage of reducing computational complexity and the need to estimate unknown model parameters. However, aggregation reduces the dispersion of distortions in the economy, so that welfare estimates of the removal of these distortions will be biased downwards. For example, when using a 12-region model, Harrison et al. (1997) found global welfare gains from the Uruguay Round that are 5% to 10% lower than those obtained from an otherwise identical model that differentiates among 24 regions.

- Homogenous versus heterogeneous imports: One important modelling issue concerns the degree to which domestically produced goods and imports from different countries are substitutes for each other. If imports from different countries are taken to be imperfect substitutes (the so-called Armington assumption), intra-industry trade can be represented. Most studies of ATC reforms differentiate textile and clothing products by place of origin and thus allow for intra-industry trade. This heterogeneity assumption tends to lead to smaller quantity changes in simulations than would be the case for homogenous products, as consumers are taken to express a preference for domestically produced goods over foreign goods.

- *Constant versus increasing returns to scale:* Several ATC studies depart from the standard framework of perfect competition and constant returns to scale by assuming that manufacturing, including textile and clothing production, is characterised by increasing returns to scale. This assumption implies some degree of market power and the representation of firms' behaviour as monopolistic competition. Both domestic and imported products are heterogeneous, so that there is no "home bias" and import price changes are transmitted symmetrically to the domestic market. As a result, simulations of ATC reforms generally show stronger impacts than under constant returns to scale and "Armington preferences".

- Static versus dynamic analysis: Analysis using comparative static models is generally based on a medium-term horizon that allows for some adjustments, such as employment shifts, to take place, while assuming a fixed stock of capital. Longer-run dynamic models incorporate additional linkages over time, such as those between policy reform, savings and investment. Changes in investment, in turn, trigger further changes in production and income. Hence, dynamic models tend to predict more pronounced economic effects from policy reform than static ones.

A number of analysts have aimed to quantify the impacts of the complex set of trade policy changes contained in the Uruguay Round Agreement. The information requirements for such an undertaking are considerable and analysts have had to compromise between comprehensiveness of sector and country coverage and the detail of structural and trade policy representation. For example, Haaland and Tollefsen (1994) and Brown *et al.* (1996) place the emphasis of their CGE analysis on tariff and services trade liberalisation and do not model the phasing out of MFA quotas. Their sectoral results contain estimates of the impact of the Uruguay Round on textiles and clothing, but as the central liberalisation feature in this sector was not represented, the findings should be interpreted with care. The following discussion concentrates on quantitative analysis that explicitly deals with MFA quota elimination. Some structural features and the central results of some of the main studies are summarised in Annex Tables A.4 and A.5.

Studies at the global level

The global effects of trade liberalisation in textile and clothing were considered and quantified before the ATC was conceived. For example, Trela and Whalley (1990) analyse the removal of quotas and tariffs between Canada, the European Union, the United States and 34 supplying developing countries, using a static CGE model under assumptions of perfect competition and constant returns to scale.[2] Traded products are assumed to be homogenous. Their analysis is explicitly geared towards the textile sector by specifying 14 textile and clothing categories and one other composite sector in their model. The researchers expect global welfare gains from quota and tariff elimination to total USD 23 billion a year, with the three developed country/region importers together accounting for about two-thirds of the gains and developing countries for one-third. A number of developing countries are expected to be able to increase their exports by several hundred per cent at the expense of production in developed countries. Nevertheless, a few developing countries are expected to face welfare losses from textile trade liberalisation, as improved access to developed-country markets would in their cases not compensate for the loss in quota rents. These losses would be more widespread and pronounced if the liberalisation of the textile market consisted of eliminating quotas but leaving tariffs unchanged, as assumed by the analysts in a second policy scenario.

In a follow-up study (Trela and Whalley, 1995), the authors expand their CGE model to capture effects related to internal quota-allocation schemes in exporting countries.[3] This is done by distinguishing two types of producers in exporting developing countries: established high-cost producers that supply restricted export markets, and new and more efficient producers that are confined to supplying the domestic market. Removal of MFA restrictions and quota-allocation procedures would allow textile and clothing production to shift to the most efficient producer, both internationally and domestically. The authors estimate that the welfare losses from inefficient quota-allocation schemes exceed those from the country quotas, so that the global benefits of quota and tariff elimination would amount to USD 49.7 billion annually. The benefits of removing the inefficient quota-allocation scheme would mainly accrue to developing country exporters, even though some of the efficiency improvements would be passed on to developed country importers in the form of lower prices.

Like Trela and Whalley, Yang (1994) concludes that the abolition of the MFA would benefit most countries and result in a substantial global welfare gain.[4] However, his study, based on a partial equilibrium model of two sectors (textiles and clothing) across eight country groups, finds aggregate welfare improvements that are substantially lower than those expected by Trela and Whalley. Moreover, the gains do not fall mainly on developed countries but are about equally divided between developed and developing countries, even though internal inefficiencies due to quota-allocation schemes in developing countries are not explicitly considered. The differences in findings seem to be mainly due to the lower tariff equivalents used to represent the quota protection of developed-country markets and to the differentiation between restricted and unrestricted products in the United States, the European Union and other restricted markets in Yang's study.

The first quantitative assessments of the Uruguay Round Agreement have predicted very substantial impacts from the opening of textile and clothing markets. Nguyen *et al.* (1993) evaluate the implications of the Draft Final Act of the Uruguay Round for nine sectors and ten country groups using a static CGE model. They find that the aggregate welfare gains from textile quota expansion would exceed those of the scheduled agriculture and service market liberalisation and account for USD 84.5 billion a year, or almost 40% of the total Uruguay Round gains.[5] The welfare gains would fall roughly equally on developed and developing countries and world trade in textiles would increase by an estimated 6%. Large-scale labour market adjustments are predicted, with the country group comprising Korea, Chinese Taipei, Hong Kong (China) and Singapore expected to see employment in textile and clothing production increase by more than 80%, while the textile labour force in Australia and New Zealand, Canada, the United States and western Europe is foreseen to contract by 22% to 36%.[6]

Large shares in overall Uruguay Round welfare gains from textile trade liberalisation are also found by other analysts. Using a dynamic CGE model under assumptions of perfect competition and constant returns to scale, Francois *et al.* (1994) estimate the global gains from the removal of textile and clothing quotas to amount to USD 47 billion annually, which corresponds to 42% of their estimate of total Uruguay Round welfare increases.[7] In a second scenario, in which the authors assume monopolistic competition and increasing returns to scale, the predicted welfare gains from textiles market liberalisation are, at USD 189 billion, more than four times higher than in their first scenario and account for no less than two-thirds of all Uruguay Round gains. Moreover, in the second scenario, all countries, including developing countries, see welfare improvements from the elimination of textile quotas, while developing countries lose in the case of perfect competition and constant returns to scale. This result is due to the greater price elasticity of import demand under monopolistic competition and increasing returns to scale, so that the benefits from the improved access of developing countries to developed-country markets more easily compensate for the loss of quota rents.[8]

In a subsequent study (Francois *et al.*, 1996), the authors use a similar modelling set-up for a different baseline period and a more detailed sectoral and regional breakdown. In addition, they explore alternative linkages between trade, income and capital accumulation. In particular, different assumptions concerning the capital stock (fixed or endogenous) and the savings rate (fixed or endogenous) are considered in order to study longer-term capital accumulation effects that can magnify income gains or losses. The results indicate that incorporation of "full dynamics" (both capital-stock and savings-rate endogenous) leads to estimates of global welfare gains from the liberalisation of textile and clothing market that are almost twice as high as those under the assumption of a fixed capital stock and a fixed savings rate.

Yang *et al.* (1997) analyse textile and clothing market liberalisation using the Global Trade Analysis Project (GTAP) and a CGE model calibrated on data for the year 1992. They distinguish ten sectors, including two for textiles and clothing, and ten regions. Their results suggest that the ATC would account for aggregate annual benefits of USD 28.6 billion, or 38% of all global welfare gains from the Uruguay Round. The authors also report expected terms-of-trade changes due to the phase-out of MFA quotas, which show improvements in export-to-import price ratios for Australasia, North America and the European Union, while Japan and developing countries are expected to see a worsening in their terms of trade (Figure A.2).

Figure A.2. Expected changes in terms of trade after MFA quota removal

Percentages

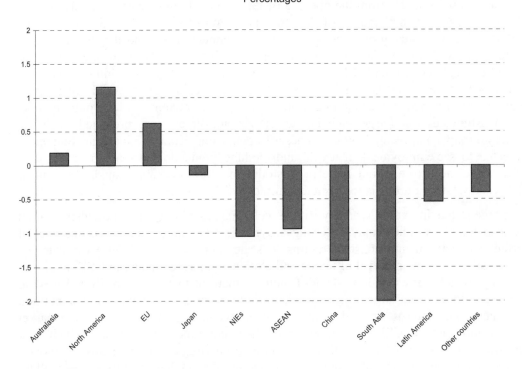

Note: No changes are assumed in pre-Uruguay Round tariffs.

Source: Yang *et al.* (1997).

A version of the GTAP model is also used by Hertel *et al.* (1996) when analysing the liberalisation of manufacturing trade. However, their estimates are based on ATC reforms in a projected economy of 2005. They find that MFA quotas would become more binding over time for virtually all exporters, taking into account projected economic growth, structural changes and ATC quota growth. The increases in restrictiveness are particularly pronounced for exports of clothing from China, Indonesia, Malaysia and the Philippines. Removing textile and clothing quotas under these circumstances would lead to global welfare gains of USD 37.3 billion a year.

Bach *et al.* (2000) explicitly compare liberalisation scenarios with and without projected changes in the economy during the Uruguay Round implementation period. Simulations of MFA removal using the high export tax equivalents for 2005 yield estimates of global welfare gains that are more than 140% higher (in 1992 USD) than those obtained using export taxes for the year 1992. The differences in simulation results for other parts of the Uruguay Round package, such as tariff reform, are much less pronounced, suggesting that economic growth and structural changes in the textile and clothing sector warrant particular attention by analysts.

Yang (1996) also analyses MFA reforms for an economy projected to 2005. He first evaluates the impacts of quota acceleration during the ATC transition period, before proceeding to an assessment of the elimination of MFA quotas. He finds limited production and welfare impacts during the three phases of transition. One reason for the small effects might be that the integration requirements are defined in volume terms so that importing countries can minimise their adjustment needs by first integrating product items that are high in volume but low in value (Bagchi, 1994). The global welfare improvement from full elimination of MFA quotas is projected to amount to USD 52.9 billion annually. In a further scenario, the author evaluates the implications of induced technological change on the outcome of liberalisation and estimates that the benefits of reform would be magnified substantially and would, under his assumptions, lead to welfare gains for all country groups concerned.

The substantial size of the expected welfare gains in some of the early studies of ATC reforms may be partly due to an overestimation of the tariff equivalents of textile and clothing quotas and, hence, the benefits of removing existing protection. Using updated figures for tariff equivalents and a static CGE model under constant returns to scale, Harrison *et al.* (1997) estimate the annual benefits of ATC reforms to amount to USD 16 billion, or 27% of total Uruguay Round gains.[9] An increasing-returns-to-scale version of their model predicted slightly higher global welfare gains from textile and clothing liberalisation of USD 16.4 billion, and the simultaneous consideration of dynamic capital accumulation effects resulted in a benefit estimate of USD 20.3 billion. As in the analysis by Francois *et al.* (1996), the incorporation of dynamic linkages in the model led to more optimistic estimates concerning the impact of ATC reforms on developing countries. Harrison *et al.* (1997) also conducted sensitivity analysis with respect to the elasticities of demand, and found that developing countries would experience higher and more widely spread welfare increases if demand was assumed to be relatively more inelastic, as reductions in import prices would trigger larger demand increases in developed importing countries and higher terms-of-trade gains in unconstrained markets. Moreover, larger elasticities of substitution between different export markets would benefit developing countries in the aggregate, but efficient producers, such as China, South Asia, Indonesia, Thailand and Malaysia would gain from the possibility of breaking more easily into previously constrained markets at the expense of high-cost producers in Latin America, the Middle East, North Africa, Eastern Europe and the former Soviet Union.

Diao and Somwaru (2001) stress the impacts of liberalisation over time in their analysis. They model ATC reforms as a reduction in tariffs by 30- 40% and an annual increase in export efficiency by 0.5% over 20 years. They predict that textile and clothing trade levels after trade policy reform would be 5% to 16% higher than they would have been without trade liberalisation, with trade increasing twice as fast in clothing products as in textiles. Clothing and textile exports from non-OECD countries would increase, but so, to some extent, would textile exports from OECD countries. This finding hints at the international interrelationships in production patterns, with lower prices for clothing stimulating demand in developed countries and exports from developing countries, which then increase their imports of capital-intensive textile products used as inputs for the production of labour-intensive clothing. Asian and Middle Eastern exporters are expected to gain world market share, at the expense of producers in eastern Europe, Latin America and developed countries. As the authors assume that no MFA quota rents exist, the improved resource allocation after trade liberalisation leads to welfare gains in all countries. Global benefits are expected to amount to USD 88 billion a year in the short run (year 5) and USD 203 billion in the long run (year 20). More than two-thirds of all welfare gains accrue to developing countries.

Recent International Monetary Fund (IMF) analysis using the GTAP model covers impacts on labour market and upstream sectors (Lankes, 2002). It is estimated that each job saved in a developed country by tariffs and quotas costs about 35 jobs in developing countries. Eliminating MFA quotas and tariffs on textiles and clothing in developed countries would generate employment for as many as 27 million workers in developing countries. Global welfare gains are estimated to amount to USD 34.7 billion a year, with more than two-thirds of the total accruing to developing countries. Some of these gains would be captured by fibre crop producers. For example, cotton exports from Sub–Saharan Africa are expected to increase by 9%, or USD 132 million, as a result of textile and clothing liberalisation. The study also evaluates the impact of further liberalisation of textile and clothing trade, including tariff reductions in developing countries, and finds that developing countries would be able to capture almost all of the welfare gains from such liberalisation efforts.

Regional trade agreements, like the Europe Agreements and NAFTA, and the establishment of offshore processing legislation, which enabled firms to circumvent MFA quotas, had a major impact on textile and clothing trade flows during the 1990s (Brugnoli and Resmini, 1996; Spinanger, 1999a). Fouquin *et al.* (2002) quantify the impacts of further regional integration in addition to analysing the elimination of MFA quotas. In particular, they simulate the impact of hypothetical free trade areas between the European Union and Mediterranean countries, and between North and Latin American countries. They find that removing the remaining EU tariffs on textile and clothing imports from Mediterranean countries would boost production of textiles and clothing by 20% and more than 50%, respectively. Clothing exports to the European Union would more than double. In terms of welfare effects, the Mediterranean countries would gain USD 3 billion a year compared to a welfare loss under a scenario of elimination of MFA quotas without regional preferences. Owing to trade diversion, Asian exporters, notably China, would lose in exports and economic welfare. Qualitatively similar effects are predicted from the creation of a free trade area of the Americas, even though the quantitative impacts are expected to be less pronounced.

Studies with a regional focus

In addition to studies of the global impacts of ATC reforms, a number of studies focus on the effects of liberalising textile and clothing trade in particular regions. Francois *et al.* (2000) analyse the impacts of ATC reforms for the European Union using a CGE model. In particular, they evaluate the relative effects of MFA quota phase-out and Uruguay Round tariff reductions. They find that the European Union would reap total welfare gains of EUR 25.3 billion a year, of which 97% would derive from MFA elimination and 3% from tariff reform. Moreover, they estimate the distribution of reform benefits across member countries (Table A.3). Germany, France and the United Kingdom are the main beneficiaries of ATC reforms in absolute terms, while Denmark, Germany and Austria gain most if the welfare increases are related to population size. Southern European countries would carry relatively large shares of negative sectoral impacts, but these would be more than compensated through estimated consumer gains. Nevertheless,

Greek families would on average gain only about a fifth as much from ATC reforms as Danish ones. The authors also assess the annual costs of protection per job saved. For textiles, the latter amount to about EUR 28 500 per worker, and for clothing to about EUR 41 100.

Table A.3. Annual welfare gains from ATC reforms in the European Union, 1997

	MFA elimination EUR millions	UR tariff cuts EUR millions	Total ATC reforms	
			EUR millions	EUR per family of four
Austria	639	18	661	327
Belgium/Lux.	789	22	815	307
Denmark	494	14	511	386
Finland	350	10	362	281
France	4 428	124	4 581	312
Germany	6 752	196	6 999	341
Greece	211	5	217	83
Ireland	175	5	181	196
Italy	3 356	83	3 453	240
Netherlands	1 101	32	1 140	291
Portugal	230	5	235	94
Spain	1 580	43	1 633	166
Sweden	517	15	536	242
United Kingdom	3 824	106	3 956	268
Total EU	24 446	677	25 282	270

Source: Francois *et al.* (2000).

The production and labour market effects of ATC reforms on the German textile and clothing industries are investigated and quantified by Schöppenau *et al.* (2002). They first simulate the impact of the European Union's eastward enlargement on textile and clothing markets, as the final stage of ATC reforms is scheduled to take place after ten new members have joined the European Union. In Germany, enlargement is expected to have a moderately positive effect on textile production (+2.9%) and a moderately negative impact on clothing output (–1.5%). The removal of MFA quotas will have more pronounced though still limited effects, with expected reductions of textile output and employment of about 4.4% and a contraction of clothing production and employment by about 6.4%. In a further simulation, the authors assess the impact of a worldwide cut in textile and clothing tariffs by 20% and find that it would only have minimal effects in Germany and the European Union. The general equilibrium analysis is complemented by partial equilibrium assessments of the effects on industries related to textiles and clothing, such as spinning, weaving and machinery. The expected impacts on these industries vary, as they are affected to a differing extent by the removal of MFA quotas and the subsequent adjustments in the textile and clothing industries. The output of the spinning sector in Germany is expected to contract by 3.4%, while production in the weaving and machinery industry is foreseen to fall more than proportionally (10.4% and 9.2%, respectively). The study did not report any estimates of welfare impacts, but Francois *et al.* (2000) indicate that Germany can be expected to be among the main beneficiaries of ATC reforms in the European Union, owing to lower consumer prices and more efficient use of resources.

The United States is also expected to gain considerably from the liberalisation of textile and clothing trade. Using a partial equilibrium approach, Cline (1987) estimates the net welfare gains from complete liberalisation to amount to USD 7.3 billion annually for clothing and USD 0.8 billion for textiles.[10] He also investigates the income distribution effects of textile and clothing protection. When taking employment effects, consumption patterns and enterprise profits into account, he finds that protection tends to benefit primarily the higher-income groups that obtain most of the protection-inflated industry profits.

De Melo and Tarr (1990) use a CGE model of the US economy to examine the effects of quota removal. They estimate that improvements in efficiency would generate annual benefits of USD 5.9 billion and capturing rents from foreigners would result in additional gains of USD 6 billion, resulting in an overall annual welfare improvement of USD 11.9 billion. The authors also assess concerns regarding adjustment costs in the domestic quota-protected industries. When measuring social hardship as the earnings losses of displaced workers over six years, they estimate that the benefits of quota elimination would largely outweigh the adjustment costs, to the extent that for every dollar of worker income saved, the economy would lose USD 65.[11]

Reinert (1993) uses an approach similar to that of De Melo and Tarr, while differentiating between the textile and clothing industries and explicitly considering five upstream supplier sectors: cotton, cellulosic man-made fibres, non-cellulosic organic fibres, textile machinery, and needles, pins and fasteners. He estimates US welfare gains from the elimination of MFA quotas to amount to USD 7.3 billion. About 90% of these gains are due to the removal of clothing quotas and 10% to the liberalisation of textile trade. Employment in the textile and clothing industries is expected to contract by 16 100 and 21 300 full-time equivalent employees, respectively, and by an aggregate 2 560 workers in the five upstream sectors.[12]

In a related study, Hanson and Reinert (1997) investigate the distributional effects of textile and clothing protection in the United States. Using the CGE model of Reinert (1993), they disaggregate households into eleven income groups and assess the effects of the removal of MFA quotas on the different groups. Contrary to Cline (1987), they find textile and clothing protection to be slightly progressive. In particular, the losses in employment opportunities for low–wage workers in textile and clothing production following the elimination of the MFA are not entirely offset by lower consumer prices. Hence, removing quota protection is predicted to affect the US income distribution slightly in the direction of greater inequality.

The impact of ATC reforms on some major developing-country exporters, notably Asian countries, has also been subject to quantitative investigations. For example, Yang and Zhong (1998) use the GTAP-CGE model to compare projected annual changes in output and trade for some major textile and clothing exporters with and without trade liberalisation. One of their findings is that while trade liberalisation would accelerate output growth in China, textile output would continue to grow much less rapidly than GDP. In contrast, growth in clothing production exceeds overall economic growth. The group of newly industrialised economies (NIEs) shows an opposite growth pattern, with fiercer competition from China in clothing production after trade liberalisation, while increased textile demand in China and other efficient clothing producers helps boost textile production in the NIEs. In a related study (Zhong and Yang, 2000), the authors estimate that China would realise welfare gains of as much as USD 8.6 billion a year from the phasing out of the MFA. This would correspond to almost two–thirds of the country's total gains from liberalisation according to Uruguay Round patterns.

Ianchovichina *et al.* (2000) evaluate the impact of China's accession to the WTO, based on the "accession offer" of November 1999. Their GTAP analysis uses economic projections for the period 1995-2005. They find that the most important sectoral impacts of China's accession to the WTO would concern the clothing industry. Production of clothing is expected to rise by 249% over the ten-year period following accession, compared to 54% in a counterfactual scenario of no accession. Exports would increase by 330%, compared to 43% without accession. The expansion of clothing production is predicted to stimulate input demand for imported textiles, to the extent that the latter would increase by 163%.

Walmsley and Hertel (2000) use a dynamic version of the GTAP model to analyse the effects of alternative target dates for the elimination of China's MFA quotas following WTO accession. In particular, they compare a scenario in which quotas levied by North American and European countries are assumed to be eliminated at the beginning of 2005 with one in which safeguards are invoked to delay the removal of quotas on Chinese textiles and clothing until 2010. The results indicate that China, North America and Europe would all experience lower welfare gains from deferred liberalisation. Moreover, the authors find that job losses in the textile and clothing industries of OECD countries are delayed, but not avoided, when quotas are phased out more gradually.

China's and Chinese Taipei's accession to the WTO is also the subject of analysis by Francois and Spinanger (2002). Like other analysts, they see textiles and clothing as sectors with very strong production and export potential, particularly in China. ATC reforms alone are expected to increase China's GDP by 1.1%, which corresponds to about a fifth of the economy-wide impact of WTO accession on growth. According to the authors' GTAP results, WTO accession and ATC reforms increase textile exports significantly both in China (+39%) and Chinese Taipei (+14%). For clothing, exports from China are expected to explode (+168%), while those from Chinese Taipei (-53%) will likely contract. More generally, countries that have profited from preferential market access to industrial countries through the MFA are expected to suffer substantial losses in international market share. The authors also evaluate the prospective impact of China's WTO accession and ATC reforms on Hong Kong (China) and conclude that Hong Kong (China) will remain a major sourcing hub for textile and clothing production, but will face fiercer competition in world markets.

India is another developing country that is expected to experience significant production, export and welfare increases from ATC reforms. In their study of the impact of global trade policy, Chadha *et al.* (2000) expect India to experience welfare improvements of USD 1.9 billion (in 1995 USD) from the phase-out of MFA quotas, which correspond to more than half of the country's total Uruguay Round gain.[13] These gains are likely to have further increased in recent years, as export tax equivalents of Indian MFA quotas for textiles and clothing have risen over time (Kathuria and Bhardwaj, 1998; Kathuria *et al.*, 2001). Moreover, when studying the implications of domestic policy reforms in India in the context of trade liberalisation, Elbehri *et al.* (2003) find that if labour productivity in Indian textile and clothing industries increased by 67% to reach the level enjoyed by China, the benefits from ATC reforms would more than double.

Conclusion

The preceding sections survey various quantitative analyses of ATC reforms. The key characteristics and main results of 29 assessments, drawn from 16 different studies, are summarised in Annex Tables A.4 and A.5. The ATC reform simulations rely on differing modelling approaches, base data and structural assumptions, which, as discussed above, drive the results. It seems *a priori* impossible to judge which assessments are right or wrong. In any case, having several estimates derived under different circumstances can help to increase one's confidence about some consistently obtained simulation outcomes, and at the same time help to identify issues that might warrant further analysis.

For example, the modelling results consistently indicate considerable shifts in textile and clothing production and trade as the ATC is implemented. There is pressure for a large-scale reallocation of resources, with production of textiles and clothing expanding in Asian and other developing countries. In parallel, textile and clothing production in OECD countries is expected to contract significantly, while imports of textiles and clothing from developing countries increase.

All the reviewed studies foresee increases in global welfare as a result of liberalisation of trade in textiles and clothing. However, the estimates of welfare gains vary significantly, with expected annual global benefits ranging from USD 6.5 billion to USD 324 billion. Some studies predict ATC reforms to account for up to two-thirds of all gains from the Uruguay Round, while others put the contribution of textile and clothing liberalisation at a mere 5%. There is a similar discrepancy with respect to the distribution of welfare gains. A number of analysts see developing countries as the main beneficiaries of ATC reforms, while others expect them to lose in the aggregate from the policy changes. There is also variation in the direction and magnitude of expected welfare impacts at the level of many individual developing countries.

In this context of uncertainty regarding the outcome of the reform, it is striking that developing countries have consistently supported the removal of the MFA. As some of the quantitative studies show, this stance is understandable in a dynamic world where capital accumulation effects are taken into account and where inefficient quota-allocation schemes can lead to a dissipation of quota rents over time. Under these circumstances, elimination of the MFA might make it possible for developing countries to seize their comparative advantage in textiles and clothing and increase their export revenues and incomes.

Another significant result from the empirical studies is that Canada, the European Union and the United States are expected to experience substantial increases in welfare from ATC reforms, although these countries were among the initiators of the MFA. The optimistic modelling results seem partly due to the implicit assumption that resources that are released from some activity can switch to another without major disruption. In other words, any potential short– or medium–term adjustment problem is assumed away. This assumption makes it difficult to understand properly the purpose of quotas. Of the reviewed studies, only De Melo and Tarr (1990) try to incorporate adjustment costs into their assessment, and this in a rather *ad hoc* way. While substantial welfare gains seem likely for most OECD countries from lower consumer prices and more efficient resource allocation in the longer run, potential adjustment problems following MFA phase-out are an important policy consideration.

Annex Table A.4. Structural characteristics of ATC reform studies

	Scenario	Author affiliation	Approach	Base year	Dynamics	Competition	Imports	Sectors (T and C)	Regions	Policy reform
Trela and Whalley (1990)	a	Univ.-CAN	CGE	1986	Static	Perfect	Homogeneous	15 (14)	37	Quota and tariff elimination
	b		CGE	1986	Static	Perfect	Homogeneous	15 (14)	37	Quota elimination
Trela and Whalley (1995)	a	Univ.-CAN	CGE	1986	Static	Perfect	Homogeneous	15 (14)	37	Quota and tariff elimination
	b		CGE	1986	Static	Perfect	Homogeneous	15 (14)	37	Quota elimination
Nguyen et al. (1993).		Univ.-CAN	CGE	1986	Static	Perfect	Heterogeneous	9 (1)	10	Exp. of quotas by a factor of 4
Yang (1994)		Univ.-AUS	PE	1986	Static	Perfect	Heterogeneous	2 (2)	8	Quota elimination
Francois et al. (1994)	a	GATT	CGE	1990	Dynamic	Perfect	Heterogeneous	15 (2)	9	Quota elimination and tariff red.
	b		CGE	1990	Dynamic	Monop.	Heterogeneous	15 (2)	9	Quota elimination and tariff red.
	c		CGE	1990 and 2005	Dynamic	Perfect	Heterogeneous	15 (2)	9	Quota elimination and tariff red.
	d		CGE	1990 and 2005	Dynamic	Monop.	Heterogeneous	15 (2)	9	Quota elimination and tariff red.
Francois et al. (1996)	a	GATT	CGE	1992	Static	Perfect	Heterogeneous	19 (2)	13	Quota elimination and tariff red.
	b		CGE	1992	Semi-dyn.	Perfect	Heterogeneous	19 (2)	13	Quota elimination and tariff red.
	c		CGE	1992	Dynamic	Perfect	Heterogeneous	19 (2)	13	Quota elimination and tariff red.
	d		CGE	1992	Static	Monop.	Heterogeneous	19 (2)	13	Quota elimination and tariff red.
	e		CGE	1992	Semi-dyn.	Monop.	Heterogeneous	19 (2)	13	Quota elimination and tariff red.
	f		CGE	1992	Dynamic	Monop.	Heterogeneous	19 (2)	13	Quota elimination and tariff red.
Yang et al. (1997)		Univ.-AUS and WB	CGE	1992	Static	Perfect	Heterogeneous	10 (2)	10	Quota elimination and tariff red.
Hertel et al. (1996)		Univ.-USA and WB	CGE	1992	Static	Perfect	Heterogeneous	10 (2)	15	Quota elimination
Bach et al. (2000)	a	Univ.-DNK/USA and WB	CGE	1992	Static	Perfect	Heterogeneous	8 (2)	13	Quota elimination
	b		CGE	1992 and 2005	Static	Perfect	Heterogeneous	8 (2)	13	Quota elimination
Harrison et al. (1997)	a	Univ.-USA and WB	CGE	1992 and 94	Static	Perfect	Heterogeneous	22 (2)	24	Quota elimination and tariff red.
	b		CGE	1992 and 94	Static	Monop.	Heterogeneous	22 (2)	24	Quota elimination and tariff red.
	c		CGE	1992 and 94	Dynamic	Monop.	Heterogeneous	22 (2)	24	Quota elimination and tariff red.
Yang (1996)		UN	CGE	1992 and 2005	Static	Perfect	Heterogeneous	6 (2)	15	Quota elimination
Chadha et al. (2000)		R-Inst.-IND	CGE	1995	Static	Monop.	Heterogeneous	23 (2)	7	Quota elimination
Diao and Somwaru (2001)		IFPRI and Gov.-USA	CGE	1997	Dynamic	Perfect	Heterogeneous	7 (2)	13	Exp. efficiency incr. and tariff red.
Fouquin et al. (2002)		R-Inst.-FRA	CGE	1997	Static	Perfect	Heterogeneous	7 (2)	13	Quota elimination
Lankes (2002)		IMF	CGE	1997	Static	Perfect	Heterogeneous	7 (3)	17	Quota and tariff elimin. in indust. countries.

Source: OECD.

Annex Table A.5. Estimates of annual welfare gains from ATC reforms

Base year USD billions

	Scenario	Global	Canada	EU	Japan	United States	China	India	All dev. countries (% of tot gains)	Share of UR (% of total gains)	Comment
Trela and Whalley (1990)	a	23.4	0.8	2.2		12.3	1.8	0.1	35%		Capturing effects of inefficient quota allocation
	b	21.9	0.9	3.0		15.0	0.9	-0.1	13%		Capturing effects of inefficient quota allocation
Trela and Whalley (1995)	a	49.7	1.1	3.7		16.4	1.9	0.5	57%		
	b	48.3	1.2	4.7		19.2	1.2	0.3	48%		
Nguyen et al. (1993).		84.5	1.6	17.2	-0.5	21.6			49%	40%	
Yang (1994)		7.3		1.0	-0.1	2.2	0.4		52%		
Francois et al. (1994)	a	47.0	1.7	26.4	-0.3	23.6	-1.0		-16%	42%	Dynamics through endogenous capital stock
	b	189.0	6.3	70.7	1.3	62.9	1.6		19%	65%	Dynamics through endogenous capital stock
	c	71.0	2.7	42.9	-0.4	38.4	-3.5		-24%	39%	Dynamics and 2005 projected economy
	d	324.0	10.2	115.1	2.1	102.3	5.4		23%	64%	Dynamics and 2005 projected economy
Francois et al. (1996)	a	18.4	0.3	5.9	-0.6	7.1	3.3		27%	46%	Endogenous capital stock and fixed savings rate
	b	28.4	0.7	8.6	-0.8	10.8	5.4		28%	44%	Endogenous savings rate and end. capital stock.
	c	35.7	1.0	9.4	-0.6	11.9	5.9		36%	35%	
	d	58.7	-0.2	10.3	2.0	11.7	9.4		61%	59%	Endogenous capital stock and fixed savings rate
	e	118.1	-0.1	17.3	3.3	19.2	19.0		68%	61%	Endogenous savings rate and end. capital stock.
	f	107.7	0.4	18.5	4.2	22.6	11.2		59%	50%	
Yang et al. (1997)		28.6		13.5	-1.7		5.6		-4%	38%	
Hertel et al. (1996)		37.3		24.9	0.8		5.9		-32%	14%	Based on 2005 projected economy
Bach et al. (2000)	a	16.2		8.1	0.2		1.9	1.4	-11%	30%	Based on 2005 projected economy
	b	38.9		23.3	0.7		7.2	1.9	-20%	38%	
Harrison et al. (1997)	a	16.0	0.9	7.6	-0.5	10.1	0.9		-14%	27%	Dynamics through endogenous capital stock
	b	16.4	0.9	7.6	-0.6	10.0	1.0		-9%	17%	
	c	20.3	1.0	7.8	-0.5	9.2	1.7		17%	12%	
Yang (1996)		52.9		30.7	3.7		5.1		-31%	49%	
Chadha et al. (2000)		6.5	0.8		-1.7	4.4	0.6	1.9	37%	5%	
Diao and Somwaru (2001)		203.0		19.4			23.7	10.8	72%		Welfare effects after year 20
Fouquin et al. (2002)		9.8		1.5	-0.8		6.0	4.1	69%		
Lankes (2002)		34.7									

Source: OECD.

Notes

1. Quotas on exports from developing countries were to grow by 6% annually, although the growth rate of bilateral quotas often fell short of this target. The MFA also foresaw some limited flexibility that allowed countries to transfer a portion of an unfilled quota from one category to another ("swing"), to use the unfilled quota from the previous year ("carryover"), or to borrow quota from the next year ("carry forward").

2. An earlier version of the analysis was published as a working paper (Trela and Whalley, 1988).

3. This study was completed before the ATC came into effect, so that it does not assess the ATC as such.

4. The analysis draws on a doctoral dissertation (Yang, 1992a) and a working paper (Yang, 1992b).

5. In the Nguyen *et al.* analysis, textiles and clothing are grouped together with furniture into a "light industries" sector, so that a part of the reported welfare gains from trade liberalisation will be due to improved furniture market access.

6. Yet, employment losses have to be seen in the context of ongoing restructuring in the textile and clothing industries, which in the United States, for example, resulted in the contraction of employment by 725 000 jobs between 1994 and 2002.

7. The estimates apply to the removal of industrial quotas, which in the authors' analysis comprise quotas on Japanese car exports alongside textile and clothing quotas.

8. In the case of increasing returns to scale and imperfect competition, there is no dichotomy between homogenous domestic products and heterogeneous imported products. Both domestic and imported products are heterogeneous, while with perfect competition and constant returns to scale the use of the so-called "Armington assumption", which implies that imports from different regions are imperfect substitutes, leads to an inherent home bias with a relatively low transmission of import price changes to the domestic market.

9. The study was also published as a chapter in Harrison *et al.* (1996).

10. This study was completed before the ATC came into effect and therefore does not directly assess the ATC.

11. Concerning adjustment impacts on capital owners in the textiles industry, the losses can be expected to be relatively modest, as the US textile industry has consistently lagged the sector average in terms of profitability. This study was also completed before the ATC came into effect and therefore does not directly assess the ATC.

12. This study was completed before the ATC came into effect and therefore does not directly assess the ATC. It should also be noted, however, in retrospect, that these

estimates of employment effects far understate the employment losses experienced by the US textile and clothing industries, which exceeded 800 000 between 1994 and 2002.

13.   This study is related to an earlier study by Chadha *et al*. (1999).

References

Bach, C.F., B. Dimaranan, T. Hertel and W. Martin (2000), "Market Growth, Structural Change, and the Gains from the Uruguay Round", *Review of International Economics* 8(2), pp. 295-310.

Bagchi, S. (1994), "The Integration of the Textile Trade in GATT." *Journal of World Trade* 28(6), pp. 31-42.

Brown, D.K., A.V. Deardorff, A.K. Fox and R.M. Stern (1996), "The Liberalization of Services Trade: Potential Impacts in the Aftermath of the Uruguay Round", pp. 183-215 in W. Martin and L.A. Winters (eds.), *The Uruguay Round and the Developing Countries*. Cambridge University Press, Cambridge.

Brugnoli, A. and L. Resmini (1996), "Textiles and Clothing Trade: Trends and Development after the Europe Agreements and the Uruguay Round", paper presented at the third European Community Studies Association Conference on "The European Union in a Changing World", Brussels.

Chadha, R., S. Pohit, R.M. Stern and A.V. Deardorff (1999), "Phasing out the Multi-fibre Arrangement: Implications for India", paper presented at the Second Annual Conference on Global Economic Analysis, Copenhagen.

Chadha, R., D. Pratap, S. Bandyopadhyay, P. Sachdeva and B. Kurien (2000), *The Impact of Changing Global Trade Policies on India*. Sanei Project Report, National Council of Applied Economic Research, New Delhi.

Cline, W.R. (1987), *The Future of World Trade in Textiles and Apparel*. Institute for International Economics, Washington, DC.

De Melo, J. and D. Tarr (1990), "Welfare Costs of U.S. Quotas in Textiles, Steel and Autos", *Review of Economics and Statistics* 72, pp. 489-497.

Diao, X. and A. Somwaru (2001), "Impact of MFA Phase-Out on the World Economy: An Intertemporal, Global General Equilibrium Analysis", TMD Discussion Paper No. 79. International Food Policy Research Institute, Washington, DC.

Elbehri, A., T. Hertel and W. Martin (2003), "Estimating the Impact of WTO and Domestic Reforms on the Indian Cotton and Textile Sectors: A General Equilibrium Approach", *Review of Development Economics* 7.

Fouquin, M., P. Morand, R. Avisse, G. Minvielle and P. Dumont (2002), "Mondialisation et Régionalisation: Le Cas des Industries du Textile et de l'Habillement", Working Paper 2002-08, Centre d'Etudes Prospectives et d'Informations Internationales, Paris.

Francois, J.F., H.H. Glismann and D. Spinanger (2000), "The Cost of EU Trade Protection in Textiles and Clothing", Working Paper No. 997, Kiel Institute of World Economics, Kiel.

Francois, J.F., B. McDonald and H. Nordström (1994), "The Uruguay Round: A Global General Equilibrium Assessment", Discussion Paper No. 1067. Centre for Economic Policy Research, London.

Francois, J.F., B. McDonald and H. Nordström (1996), "The Uruguay Round: A Numerically Based Qualitative Assessment", pp. 183-215, in W. Martin and L.A. Winters (eds.), *The Uruguay Round and the Developing Countries,* Cambridge University Press, Cambridge.

Francois, J.F. and K.A. Reinert (editors) (1998), *Applied Methods for Trade Policy Analysis: A Handbook.*, Cambridge University Press, Cambridge.

Francois, J.F. and D. Spinanger (2000), "Hong Kong's Textile and Clothing Industry: The Impact of Quotas, the UR and China's WTO Accession", Working Paper, Kiel Institute of World Economics, Kiel.

Francois, J.F. and D. Spinanger (2002), "Greater China's Accession to the WTO: Implications for International Trade/Production and for Hong Kong", paper presented at the Fifth Annual Conference on Global Economic Analysis, Chinese Taipei.

Goto, J. (1989), "The Multifibre Arrangement and Its Effects on Developing Countries", *World Bank Research Observer* 4, pp. 203-227.

Haaland, J.I. and T.C. Tollefsen (1994), "The Uruguay Round and Trade in Manufactures and Services: General Equilibrium Simulations of Production, Trade and Welfare Effects of Liberalization", Discussion Paper No. 1008, Centre for Economic Policy Research, London.

Hamilton, C.B. (ed.) (1990), *Textiles and Trade and the Developing Countries: Eliminating the Multi-Fibre Arrangement in the 1990s.* The World Bank, Washington, DC.

Hanson, K.A. and K.A. Reinert (1997), "The Distributional Effects of U.S. Textile and Apparel Protection", *International Economic Journal* 11(3), pp. 1-12.

Harrison, G.W., T.F. Rutherford and D.G. Tarr (1996), "Quantifying the Uruguay Round", pp. 216-252 in W. Martin and L.A. Winters (eds.), *The Uruguay Round and the Developing Countries*, Cambridge University Press, Cambridge.

Harrison, G.W., T.F. Rutherford and D.G. Tarr (1997), "Quantifying the Uruguay Round", *Economic Journal* 107, pp. 1405-1430.

Hertel, T.W., W. Martin, K. Yanagishima and B. Dimaranan (1996), "Liberalising Manufactures Trade in a Changing World Economy", pp. 183-215 in W. Martin and L.A. Winters (eds.), *The Uruguay Round and the Developing Countries,* Cambridge University Press, Cambridge.

Ianchovichina, E., W. Martin and E. Fukase (2000), "Assessing the Implications of Merchandise Trade Liberalization in China's Accession to WTO", paper presented to the Roundtable on China's Accession to the WTO sponsored by the Chinese Economic Society and the World Bank, Pudong/Shanghai.

Kathuria, S. and A. Bhardwaj (1998), "Export Quotas and Policy Constraints in the Indian Textile and Garment Industries", Policy Research Working Paper No. 2012, The World Bank, Washington, DC.

Kathuria, S., W. Martin and A. Bhardwaj (2001), "Implications for South Asian Countries of Abolishing the Multifibre Arrangement", Policy Research Working Paper No. 2721, The World Bank, Washington, DC.

Krishna, K., R. Erzan and L. Tan (1994), "Rent Sharing in the Multi-Fibre Arrangement: Theory and Evidence from US Apparel Imports from Hong Kong", *Review of International Economics* 2(1), pp. 62–73.

Lankes, H.P. (2002), "Market Access for Developing Country Exports", *Finance and Development* (September 2002), pp. 8–13.

Nguyen, T.T., C. Perroni and R.M. Wigle (1993), "An Evaluation of the Draft Final Act of the Uruguay Round", *Economic Journal* 103, pp. 1540–1549.

Pelzman, J. (1983), "Economic Costs of Tariffs and Quotas on Textile and Apparel Products Imported into the United States: A Survey of the Literature and Implications for Policies", *Weltwirtschaftliches Archiv* 119(3), pp. 523–542.

Reinert, K.A., (1993), "Textile and Apparel Protection in the United States: A General Equilibrium Analysis", *World Economy* 16, pp. 359–376.

Schöppenau P.V., J. Egerer, P. Brenton and C. Buelens (2002), *Die Auswirkungen der ATC-Liberalisierung auf die Deutsche Textilwirtschaft*, Project Report, European Public Policy Advisers and Centre for European Policy Studies, Brussels.

Spinanger, D. (1991), "Experiences with Liberalization Policies: The Case of Textiles", *European Economic Review* 35, pp. 543–551.

Spinanger, D. (1999a), "Textiles Beyond the MFA Phase-Out", *World Economy* 22(4), pp. 455–476.

Spinanger, D. (1999b), "Faking Liberalization and Finagling Protectionism: The ATC at Its Best", paper presented at the ERF/IAI/World Bank Workshop on Preparing for the WTO 2000 Negotiations: Mediterranean Interests and Perspectives, Cairo.

Trela, I. and J. Whalley (1988), "Do Developing Countries Lose from the MFA?", Working Paper No. 2618, National Bureau of Economic Research, Cambridge, Massachusetts.

Trela, I. and J. Whalley (1990), "Global Effects of Developed Country Trade Restrictions on Textiles and Apparel", *Economic Journal* 100, pp. 1190–1205.

Trela, I. and J. Whalley (1995), "Internal Quota-Allocation Schemes and the Costs of the MFA", *Review of International Economics* 3(3), pp. 284–306.

Walmsley, T.L. and T.W. Hertel (2000), "China's Accession to the WTO: Timing is Everything", GTAP Working Paper No. 13, Center for Global Trade Analysis, West Lafayette, Indiana.

Whalley, J. (1999), "Notes on Textiles and Apparel in the Next Trade Round", paper presented at the Harvard University Conference on Developing Countries in the Next WTO Trade Round, Cambridge, Massachusetts.

Yang, Y. (1992a), "The Impact of the Multifibre Arrangement on World Clothing and Textile Markets with Special Reference to China", Ph.D. dissertation, Australian National University, Canberra.

Yang, Y. (1992b), "The MFA, World Markets and East Asian Exporters", Economics Division Working Paper 92/3, Australian National University, Canberra.

Yang, Y. (1994), "The Impact of MFA Phasing Out on World Clothing and Textile Markets", *Journal of Development Studies* 30(3), pp. 892–915.

Yang, Y. (1996), *Prospects for the Textile and Clothing Sector of the ESCAP Region in the Post-Uruguay Round Context*, Studies in Trade and Investment No. 17, United Nations Economic and Social Commission for Asia and the Pacific, New York.

Yang, Y., W. Martin and K. Yanagishima (1997), "Evaluating the Benefits of Abolishing the MFA in the Uruguay Round Package," in T. Hertel (ed.), *Global Trade Analysis: Modeling and Applications*, Cambridge University Press, Cambridge, New York and Melbourne.

Yang, Y. and C. Zhong (1998), "China's Textile and Clothing Exports in a Changing World Economy", *Developing Economies* 36(1), pp. 3–23.

Zhong, C. and Y. Yang (2000), "China's Textile and Clothing Exports in the Post Uruguay Round", pp.175–193 in P. Drysdale and L. Song (eds.), *China's Entry to the WTO: Strategic Issues and Quantitative Assessments*, Routledge, London.

OECD PUBLICATIONS, 2, rue André-Pascal, 75775 PARIS CEDEX 16
PRINTED IN FRANCE
(22 2004 05 1 P) ISBN 92-64-01853-0 – No. 53789 2004